Key Topics in Psychiatry

Dedication
To our parents

For Elsevier:

Commissioning Editor: **Mike Parkinson**

Development Editor: **Barbara Simmons**

Project Manager: **Nancy Arnott**

Design Direction: **Stewart Larking**

Key **Topics** in **Psychiatry**

Sheena Jones
MBChB DRCOG MRCPsych

Specialist Registrar in General Adult and Learning Disabilities Psychiatry,
West of Scotland Higher Training Scheme, Glasgow, UK

Kate Roberts
BSc(Med Sci) MBChB MRCPsych

Senior Registrar in Forensic Psychiatry, Victorian Institute of Forensic Mental Health
(Forensicare), Australia; previously West of Scotland Basic Training Scheme, Glasgow, UK

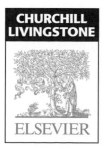

CHURCHILL
LIVINGSTONE

ELSEVIER

EDINBURGH LONDON NEW YORK OXFORD PHILADELPHIA ST LOUIS SYDNEY TORONTO 2007

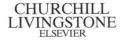

First published 2007

ISBN-13: 9780443101656
ISBN-10: 0 4431 0165 5

British Library Cataloguing in Publication Data
A catalogue record for this book is available from the British Library

Library of Congress Cataloging in Publication Data
A catalog record for this book is available from the Library of Congress

Notice
Knowledge and best practice in this field are constantly changing. As new research and experience broaden our knowledge, changes in practice, treatment and drug therapy may become necessary or appropriate. Readers are advised to check the most current information provided (i) on procedures featured or (ii) by the manufacturer of each product to be administered, to verify the recommended dose or formula, the method and duration of administration, and contraindications. It is the responsibility of the practitioner, relying on their own experience and knowledge of the patient, to make diagnoses, to determine dosages and the best treatment for each individual patient, and to take all appropriate safety precautions. To the fullest extent of the law, neither the Publisher nor the Editors assume any liability for any injury and/or damage to persons or property arising out of or related to any use of the material contained in this book.

The Publisher

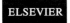
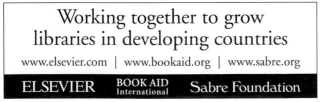
Printed in China

Contents

Acknowledgements

We are grateful to Alison Gordon for her contribution to the chapter on old age psychiatry (Chapter 17), and to Selwyn McIlhinney for his contributions to the chapters on education and training, and policy and legislation (Chapters 8 and 9, respectively).

We would like to thank our friends and colleagues for their support, encouragement, amusement and general disbelief. With particular thanks to Forensicare and to Dan.

Contributors

Alison Gordon
MBChB MRCPsych

Specialist Registrar in Old Age Psychiatry, West of Scotland
Higher Training Scheme, Glasgow, Scotland, UK

Selwyn McIlhinney
MBChB, MRCPsych

Specialist Registrar in General Adult Psychiatry, West of Scotland
Higher Training Scheme, Glasgow, Scotland, UK

Preface

Introduction and aim

The idea for this book came soon after we had taken the membership exams because we had spent many, many hours searching for all the information not covered by clinical textbooks and study guides. Our aim, then, was to identify relevant articles and sources of information on key subjects and present them in one book – in particular, topical clinical issues, legislation, mental health policy and reform. We have summarised the findings as presented by the original authors as opposed to critically appraising each item.

Layout

Each chapter of the book has the same layout. Within each chapter the items are grouped under a set order of subheadings. These are:
- Ethical issues
- General topics
- Policy and legislation
- Treatment – Psychopharmacology
- Treatment – Psychological therapies
- Treatment – Others
- Assessment tools and rating scales
- Guidelines.

Each item is identified by the reference to its original source. Web addresses for related subjects and links are also given. Where an item is placed in one chapter, but is equally relevant to another, the reader is advised of this in the text.

Sources

The focus was topical issues. Articles adequately covered by clinical textbooks and study guides were not included. We have summarised relevant articles from the *British Journal of Psychiatry*, the *Psychiatric Bulletin* and *Advances in Psychiatric Treatment* from the beginning of 2004 until Spring 2006. Additional important articles from other sources were included. The *British Medical Journal*, *Cochrane Reviews* and reports from the Department of Health, Royal College of Psychiatrists, the General Medical Council and the National Health Service Executive were also reviewed.

Excerpts from guidelines produced by the National Institute of Clinical Evidence, the Scottish Intercollegiate Guidelines Network and the Department of Health have been reproduced. Whilst neither NICE nor SIGN guidelines apply throughout the country, both were included as they raise and discuss evidence-based practice. Guidelines are constantly under review. We used the most up-to-date information available to us, but some guidelines may have been updated after we finished writing this book.

We hope that our efforts in producing this book will reduce the significant effort required in exam preparation as well as providing a user-friendly text on topical issues.

Addictions psychiatry

1

Chapter contents

Ethical Issues

Alcohol dependence and driving

Culshaw M, Wootton L, Wylie S 2005 Alcohol dependence and driving. A survey of patients' knowledge of DVLA regulations and possible clinical implications. Psychiatric Bulletin 29: 90–93

The Driver and Vehicle Licensing Agency (DVLA) is responsible for making the decision about whether a person should continue to drive. The doctor is seen only as a source of information and advice. Drivers have a duty to keep the DVLA informed of any condition that may impair their ability to drive. Doctors have a duty to advise their patients to inform the DVLA of any condition likely to make driving dangerous. If the patient fails to take this advice, the doctor may contact the DVLA directly.

With regard to alcohol problems, Group 1 entitlement is affected if a diagnosis of alcohol misuse or alcohol dependency is confirmed by medical enquiry. Alcohol dependency requires a recommended 12-month period of licence revocation or refusal, to attain abstinence or controlled drinking with normal blood parameters if relevant. License restoration requires satisfactory independent medical examination, arranged by the DVLA, with satisfactory blood results and medical reports from the patient's doctor.

Method

- 56 driver patients with alcohol dependence were included.

Results

- A total of 89% of responders had driven in the last year.
- 55% were driving daily.
- It became clear that nearly all of the participants were unaware that there were any restrictions for drivers with significant alcohol problems.
- Many thought the restrictions were purely to do with driving under the influence of alcohol, rather than there being long-term implications for their drinking behaviour.
- 86% stated that no health professional had ever discussed driving with them.
- 45% indicated they would be unlikely to seek medical treatment if they had a duty to inform the DVLA regarding their driving.

See also the 'Ethical issues' section in Chapter 9 (Ethical issues), page 119.

General Topics

Aggression in drug-dependent inpatients

Rajesh GS, Day E 2005 Aggression in drug dependent inpatients. Psychiatric Bulletin 29: 141–143

There is evidence regarding associations between substance misuse and violence. The majority of the research has been conducted in psychiatric hospitals, with little evidence from specialist treatment units for substance misuse.

Aims

- This study aimed to determine the rates of aggression among drug-dependent inpatients during their admission and to describe the nature of violent episodes in terms of target and severity of injury.
- The demographic and diagnostic categories of patients that present a greater risk of aggressive incidents were also investigated.

Method

- The study was based in an English 16-bed inpatient unit that provides a detoxification service for alcohol and other substances.
- A retrospective review of incident reports from an 11-month period was performed.
- Clinical notes were also examined in order to establish any incidents of unreported aggression.
- An 'incident' was defined as any act of physical or verbal aggression with a hostile intent by a patient towards a fellow patient, member of staff or property.
- A severity of assault scale was used.
- Demographic and ICD-10 diagnoses were recorded.

Results

- Physical aggression was rare, occurring in 4% of admissions.
- Staff and fellow patients were the victims in eight incidents and property was damaged in two incidents.
- Aggressive patients were significantly younger than patients in the non-aggressive group.
- Patients with polysubstance dependency were significantly more aggressive than everyone else put together.
- Those dependent on alcohol were significantly less aggressive than the other groups.
- There was no statistical difference between the aggressive and non-aggressive groups in terms of gender, race, employment status and the presence or absence of additional diagnosis.
- Previous forensic history was not associated with aggression although a past history of aggression was.

Discussion

- The lower rates of aggression in this group, when compared with previous studies, may reflect the fact that patients were voluntary admissions and motivated to change.
- The study showed that people using more than one illegal drug were more likely to be aggressive than others.
- The need for clear treatment contracts before admission is suggested.

Blomhoff S, Seim S, Friis S 1990 Can prediction of violence among psychiatric inpatients be improved? Hospital and Community Psychiatry 41: 771–775

- Reported the link between inpatient aggression and psychoactive substance use.

Swanson JW, Holzer CE, Ganju VK et al 1990 Violence and psychiatric disorders in the community: evidence from the Epidemiological Catchment Area Surveys. Hospital and Community Psychiatry 41: 761–770

- Found a link between violence and psycho-active substance misuse in community samples.

Scott H, Johnson S, Menzes P et al 1998 Substance misuse and risk of aggression and offending among the severely mentally ill. British Journal of Psychiatry 172: 345–350

- Dual diagnosis of a severe mental illness and a substance misuse disorder has a highly significant association with aggression.

Miles H, Johnson S, Amponsahafuwape S et al 2003 Characteristics of subgroups of individuals with psychotic illness and a comorbid substance use disorder. Psychiatric Services 54: 554–561

- Stimulant drugs such as cocaine or amphetamine increase the risk of violence.

Alcohol consumption as a risk factor for anxiety and depression

Haynes J, Farrell M, Singleton N et al 2005 Alcohol consumption as a risk factor for anxiety and depression. Results from the longitudinal follow up of the National Psychiatric Morbidity Survey. British Journal of Psychiatry 187: 544–551

To date, the results of existing longitudinal studies examining the relationship between alcohol and depression and anxiety are conflicting.

Hartka E, Johnstone B, Leino V et al 1996 A meta-analysis of depressive symptomatology and alcohol consumption over time. British Journal of Addiction 86: 1283–1298

- Found from eight early meta-analyses that baseline alcohol consumption was associated with depression later in life.

Wang J, Patten SB 2001 Alcohol consumption and major depression: findings from follow up study. Canadian Journal of Psychiatry 46: 632–638

- Found no association between alcohol consumption and depressive illness.

Gilman SE, Abraham HD 2001 A longitudinal study of the order of onset of alcohol dependence and major depression. Drug and Alcohol Dependence 63: 277–286

- Found some evidence that women may be at greater risk of concurrent alcohol dependence and major depression.

Singleton N, Lewis G 2003 Better or worse: a longitudinal study of the mental health of adults living in private households in Great Britain. The Stationery Office, London

- An 18 month follow-up study performed in 2000.
- Data were derived from the Psychiatric Morbidity Among Adults Living in Private Households survey.
- Examined whether alcohol consumption and misuse are risk factors for incident anxiety and depression.
- The reverse relationship was also examined, whether anxiety and depression are risk factors for increased alcohol consumption.
- Alcohol use was recorded at baseline and after 18 months using the Alcohol Use Disorders Identification Test (AUDIT).
- Those who scored 10 or more on the AUDIT were asked to complete the Severity of Alcohol Dependence Questionnaire.
- Alcohol use was classified in four ways:
  - hazardous drinking: AUDIT score ≥ 8
  - above government guidelines (21 units for men and 14 units for women)
  - binge drinking: six or more drinks on one occasion on at least a monthly basis
  - dependence: AUDIT score ≥ 10 and SAD-Q score ≥ 4.

Results

- After weighting, hazardous drinking was at 24% in the general population.
- Only 6% of the population reported drinking above government guidelines.
- The prevalence of binge drinking was 31%.
- 18% reported binge drinking at least once a week.
- Overall alcohol use was more prevalent in men.
- Men were six times more likely to be dependent than women.
- Hazardous drinkers did not have increased odds of developing anxiety and depression compared with non-hazardous drinkers.
- Those who had not consumed alcohol in the preceding 12 months were less likely than non-hazardous drinkers to develop anxiety and depression.
- Binge drinking was associated with incident anxiety and depression but this was not significant.

- Those abstinent from alcohol were less likely to have new-onset anxiety and depression at follow-up.
- There was weak evidence that subthreshold symptoms of anxiety or depression were associated with the development of alcohol dependence. There was no association with hazardous drinking or binge drinking.

See also the 'General topics' section in Chapter 2 (Affective disorders), page 29.

Cannabis-induced psychosis and subsequent schizophrenia-spectrum disorder

Arendt M, Rosenberg R, Foldager L et al 2005 Cannabis-induced psychosis and subsequent schizophrenia-spectrum disorders: follow-up study of 545 incident cases. British Journal of Psychiatry 187: 510–515

Method

- This study describes the outcomes for patients treated for cannabis-induced psychotic disorder who had no prior history of psychotic symptoms.
- The follow-up period was 3 years.
- The aim of the study was to determine the number of people who went on to develop schizophrenia-spectrum disorders.
- Data was extracted from the Danish Psychiatric Central Register.
- Specifically looked at those treated from de novo cannabis-induced psychosis between 1994 and 1999.
- In a separate analysis the group was compared with a cohort who were referred with first episode schizophrenia-spectrum disorders but without the history of cannabis-induced psychosis.

Results

- 535 cases were followed up for 3 years.
- The mean age for people with cannabis-induced psychosis was 27.
- 82.4% of the patients were male.
- 379 patients were admitted to hospital, with 156 receiving outpatient treatment only.
- 44.5% of people with cannabis-induced psychosis went on to develop a schizophrenia-spectrum disorder, the proportion increasing with length of follow-up.
- 9% of people developed persistent delusional disorder, unspecified non-organic psychosis or bipolar affective disorder within the follow-up time.
- 77.2% experienced new psychotic symptoms.
- Only 15.9% remained out of psychiatric care throughout the 3-year follow-up.

- Men had an increased risk of developing schizophrenia-spectrum disorder compared to women.
- Younger age was also related to increased risk.
- Paranoid schizophrenia was the most common diagnosis, followed by acute and transient psychotic disorders, personality disorder and unspecified schizophrenia.
- Most patients were treated numerous times for schizophrenia-spectrum disorders.
- For the majority of patients, cannabis-induced psychosis led to later schizophrenia which is inconsistent with multiple previous studies. Previous studies were of much shorter duration – up to 3 months.
- Patients with cannabis-induced psychosis responded much faster to treatment than patients with psychoses that were not substance dependent.

Conclusions

- This is the first study to show that symptoms of cannabis-induced psychosis can be the initial manifestations of long-term psychotic illness.
- The results do not disprove the existence of 'cannabis psychosis' but must be regarded as an important risk factor for the development of subsequent schizophrenia-spectrum psychosis.
- The findings in this study cannot definitely be defined as causal as the study design does not allow factors such as hereditary predisposition to be controlled for.
- The fact, however, that those with cannabis-induced psychosis go on to develop schizophrenia at a younger age indicates that cannabis use may hasten pathogenesis.
- Half of the patients treated for cannabis-induced psychosis will subsequently develop a schizophrenia-spectrum disorder, with almost a third developing schizophrenia.
- The onset of such psychopathology is substantially delayed in most patients.
- First episode schizophrenia occurs several years earlier in these patients compared with those with no history of cannabis-induced psychosis.

Arseneault L, Cannon M, Witton J et al 2004 Causal association between cannabis and psychosis: examination of the evidence. British Journal of Psychiatry 184: 110–117

- Linked cannabis use and schizophrenia.
- Little is known about the clinical implications and prognostic significance of cannabis-induced psychotic symptoms.
- Has shown that cannabis use increases the risk of developing severe psychotic disorders.

Johns A 2001 Psychiatric effects of cannabis. British Journal of Psychiatry 178: 116–122

- Psychotic symptoms may follow cannabis intake.
- Such symptoms are usually short lived and total remission is achievable.
- This is in agreement with a number of other studies.

Macleod J, Oakes R, Copello A et al 2004 Psychological and social sequelae of cannabis and other illicit drug use by young people: a systematic review of longitudinal, general population studies. Lancet 363: 1579–1588

- The results are inconclusive.

Veen ND, Selten JP, van der Tweed I et al 2004 Cannabis use and age at onset of schizophrenia. American Journal of Psychiatry 161: 501–506

- Also found that people using cannabis had a lower age of onset of schizophrenia, further validating the significant findings.

See also the 'General topics' section in Chapter 26 (Schizophrenia), page 368.

Cannabis use and misuse prevalence among people with psychosis

Green B, Young R, Kavanagh D 2005 Cannabis use and misuse prevalence among people with psychosis. British Journal of Psychiatry 187: 306–313

Cannabis is the most widely used illegal substance in Europe, the US and Australia. There are associations between cannabis use and psychotic illness. Little research has been done to look into factors contributing to the variability in prevalence estimates.

This study aimed to examine factors associated with variability in prevalence estimates and to compare prevalence estimates of individuals with and without psychosis. Most studies did not distinguish between misuse and dependence.

Results

- Systematic reviews found that 12-month misuse prevalence provided a sound indication of lifetime misuse prevalence.
- Prevalence estimates were calculated as:
    - current use (23%)
    - current misuse (11.3%)
    - 12-month use (29.2%)
    - 12-month misuse (18.8%)
    - lifetime use (42.1%)
    - lifetime misuse (22.5%).
- There was a consistently higher prevalence of cannabis use and misuse in people with psychosis.

Degenhardt L, Hall W, Lynskey M 2003 Testing hypotheses about the relationship between cannabis use and psychosis. Drug and Alcohol Dependence 71: 37–48

- Reported that the sharp increase in cannabis use has not been reflected in an increased prevalence of schizophrenia.

Rabinowitz J, Bromet EJ, Lavelle J et al 1998 Prevalence and severity of substance use disorders and onset of psychosis in first-admission psychotic parents. Psychological Medicine 28: 1411–1419

- Found conflicting results regarding the prevalence of substance use and associated outcomes on psychosis.

See also the 'General topics' section in Chapter 26 (Schizophrenia), page 368.

Causal association between cannabis and psychosis

Arsneeault L, Cannon M, Witton A, Murray R 2004 Causal association between cannabis and psychosis: examination of the evidence. British Journal of Psychiatry 184: 110–117

Controversy remains as to whether cannabis acts as a causal risk factor for schizophrenia and related disorders. It is recognised that cannabis can exacerbate psychotic symptoms and lead to their recurrence. Four recent epidemiological studies have provided further evidence of the causal relationship between cannabis and schizophrenia.

D'Souza C, Cho H-S, Perry E et al 2004 A cannabinoid model psychosis, dopamine–cannabinoid interactions and implications for schizophrenia. In: Castle DJ, Murray R (eds) Marijuana and madness. Cambridge University Press, Cambridge

- Cannabis intoxication can lead to acute transient psychotic episodes in some individuals.

Johns A 2001 Psychiatric effects of cannabis. British Journal of Psychiatry 178: 116–122

- Controversy remains as to whether cannabis can actually cause schizophrenia or other functional psychotic illness in the long term.

Andreasson S, Allebeck P, Engstom A et al 1988 Cannabis and schizophrenia: a longitudinal study of Swedish Conscripts. Lancet 1988; 11: 1483–1485

- The first paper that suggested cannabis may have a causal role in the development of later schizophrenia.

- Cohort study which observed a dose–response relationship between cannabis use at conscription (aged 18) and schizophrenia diagnosed 15 years later.
- Cannabis users were six times more likely to develop schizophrenia 15 years later.
- The risk remained significant after correction for confounding.
- Authors concluded 'cannabis should be viewed as an additional clue to the still elusive aetiology of schizophrenia'.

Further evidence for causality

The following cross-sectional studies from the US, Australia and The Netherlands found that the rates of cannabis use are approximately twice as high among people with schizophrenia as among the general population:

Regier D, Farmer ME, Rae DS et al 1990 Comorbidity of mental disorders with alcohol and other drug abuse: results from the epidemiological catchment area (ECA) study. Journal of the American Medical Association 264: 2511–2518

Tien AY, Anthony JC 1990 Epidemiological analysis of alcohol and drug use as risk factors for psychotic experiences. Journal of Nervous and Mental Disease 178: 473–480

Robins LN, Regier DA 1991 Psychiatric disorders in America: The Epidemiological Catchment Area Study. The Free Press, New York

Hall W, Degenhardt L 2000 Cannabis use and psychosis: a review of clinical and epidemiological evidence. Australian and New Zealand Journal of Psychiatry 34: 26–34

van Os J, Bak M, Bijl RV et al 2002 Cannabis use and psychosis: a longitudinal population-based study. American Journal of Epidemiology 156: 319–327

- The Netherlands Mental Health Survey and Incidence Study.
- Compared with non-users, individuals using cannabis were over three times more likely to manifest psychotic symptoms at follow-up (1 and 3 years after baseline).
- The risk remained significant after adjustment.
- Further analysis revealed that a lifetime history of cannabis use at baseline, as opposed to use of cannabis at follow-up, was a stronger predictor of psychosis 3 years on, suggesting that it is not merely the short-term effects which lead to acute psychosis.

- 'Cannabis use is an independent risk factor for the emergence of psychosis in psychosis-free persons and that those with an established vulnerability to psychotic disorders are particularly sensitive to its effects, resulting in poor outcome.'

Duke PJ, Pantelis C, McPhillips MA et al 2001 Comorbid non-alcohol substance misuse among people with schizophrenia. Epidemiological study in central London. British Journal of Psychiatry 179: 509–513

- This London study corroborated previous work and found that between 20 and 40% of patients with psychotic illnesses report lifetime cannabis use.

Wheatly M 1998 The prevalence and relevance of substance use in detained schizophrenic patients. Journal of Forensic Psychiatry 9: 114–129

- Higher rates of cannabis use were found in people detained under the Mental Health Act.

McCreadie RG 2002 Use of drugs, alcohol and tobacco by people with schizophrenia: case-control study. British Journal of Psychiatry 181: 321–325

- Found that rates of cannabis use seem to be about twice as high in those with psychosis than among controls.

Hambrecht M, Hafner H 1996 Substance abuse and the onset of schizophrenia. Biological Psychiatry 40: 1155–1163

- A retrospective study of 232 patients with schizophrenia.
- One-third of the sample had used drugs for over a year before the onset of illness.
- One-third had used drugs in the year prior to developing the illness.
- One-third started using cannabis after the occurrence of symptoms.

Cantwell R, Brewin J, Glazebrook C et al 1999 Prevalence of substance misuse in first episode psychosis. British Journal of Psychiatry 174: 150–153

- Investigated 168 patients with first episode psychosis.
- 37% had used substances and alcohol prior to presentation.

Zammit S, Allebeck P, Andreasson S et al 2002 Self-reported cannabis use as a risk factor for schizophrenia: further analysis of the 1969 Swedish conscript cohort. British Medical Journal 325: 1199–1201

- Examined the Swedish conscript cohort.

- Heavy cannabis use at age 18 was associated with 6.7 times the risk of a diagnosis of schizophrenia 27 years later.
- The risk reduced but did remain when controlled for confounders.

Fergusson DM, Horwood LJ, Swain-Campbell NR 2003 Cannabis dependence and psychotic symptoms in young people. Psychological Medicine 33: 15–21

- Examined the association between cannabis-dependence disorder and the presence of psychotic symptoms at ages 18 and 21.
- They controlled for confounding factors including previous psychotic symptoms.
- Individuals who met the diagnostic criteria for cannabis-dependence disorder at age 18 had a 3.7-fold increased risk of psychotic symptoms than those without cannabis-dependence disorder.
- At 21, the risk was 2.3 times higher for those with cannabis-dependence problems.
- 'The findings are clearly consistent with the view that heavy cannabis use may make a causal contribution to the development of psychotic symptoms since they know that, independently of pre-existing psychotic symptoms and a wide range of social and contextual factors, young people who develop cannabis dependence show an elevated rate of psychotic symptoms.'

Arseneault L, Canon M, Poulton R et al 2002 Cannabis use in adolescence and risk for adult psychosis: longitudinal study of Swedish conscripts. British Medical Journal 325: 1212–1213

- Individuals using cannabis at 15 and 18 had higher rates of psychosis aged 26 compared with non-users.
- The effect was stronger with earlier use.
- 10.3% of cannabis users aged 15 were diagnosed with schizophreniform psychosis at aged 26 compared with 3% of controls.
- A significant exacerbation was found between psychotic symptoms at age 11 and cannabis use at 18.
- 'Using cannabis in adolescence increases the likelihood of experiencing symptoms of schizophrenia in adulthood.'

Summary

All the studies found cannabis use is associated with later schizophrenic outcomes. All the studies supported the argument for a temporal relationship by showing that cannabis use most probably preceded schizophrenia. Overall, cannabis seems to confer a two-fold risk of later schizophrenia and schizophreniform disorder. However, it does not seem either a sufficient or necessary cause for psychosis. It is part of the component leading to the complex number of factors that result in psychosis. Psychosis could be prevented by discouraging cannabis use among vulnerable youths. Further research is required to establish the causal mechanisms.

See also the 'General topics' section in Chapter 26 (Schizophrenia), page 368.

Desperately seeking solutions: the search for appropriate treatment for comorbid substance misuse and psychosis

Tyrer P, Weaver T 2004 Desperately seeking solutions: the search for appropriate treatment for comorbid substance misuse and psychosis. Psychiatric Bulletin 28: 1–2

The authors suggest that dual diagnosis is an incorrectly used term and that comorbidity is the correct term. Treatment of substance misuse and treatment of mental health problems have different aims and purposes. Treatment of substance misuse requires patients to avoid psychoactive substances and generally requires a degree of patient motivation; treatment of mental health problems may rely on medication and at times may require compulsory treatment.

Treatment could be aided if there was a better understanding of the theoretical model for the association between psychosis and substance misuse. The extent of an association in terms of social and biological vulnerabilities is not clear.

The authors suggest that 'sensitive anticipatory action' may be a more helpful treatment approach than assertive outreach. This method focuses on:
- prevention of relapse – via thorough medication review
- avoidance of crises – by arranging accommodation
- advance joint planning.

Weaver T, Madden P, Charles V et al 2003 Comorbidity of substance misuse and mental illness in community mental health and substance misuse services. British Journal of Psychiatry 183: 304–313

- The Comorbidity of Substance Misuse and Mental Illness Collaborative (COSMIC) study.
- 40% of patients managed by community mental health teams reported problem drug use and/or harmful alcohol use in the past year.
- This is much greater than could be expected by random association.
- Found that even modest drug use can reduce the benefits of treatments with proven efficacy.

Hunt GE, Bergen J, Bashir M 2002 Medication compliance and comorbid substance abuse in schizophrenia: impact

on community survival 4 years after relapse. Schizophrenia Research 54: 253–264

- Public opinion suggests that comorbidity has a greater impact on services than single components, with increased psychiatric admission and more negative treatment outcomes.

Scott H, Johnson S, Manezes P et al 1998 Substance misuse and risk of aggression and offending among the severely mentally ill. British Journal of Psychiatry 172: 345–350

- Comorbidity is associated with increased levels of violence.

Cantwell R 2003 Substance use and schizophrenia: effects on symptoms, social functioning and service use. British Journal of Psychiatry 182: 324–329

- There was no increase in service use and minimal influence on other clinical variables in patients with comorbidity.

Ley A, Jeffery JP, McLaren S et al 2001 Treatment programmes for people with both severe mental illness and substance misuse **(Cochrane Review)**. In: The Cochrane Library, Issue 1. Update Software, Oxford

- There was no definite evidence that any type of substance misuse programme for those with severe mental illness had an advantage over treatment as normal.

Reis R 1993 Clinical treatment matching models for dually diagnosed patients. Psychiatric Clinics of North America 16: 167–175

- There was no evidence to support an 'integrated programme'.
- Integrated programmes treat both conditions together with care provided by a dedicated team, in comparison to serial treatment or parallel programmes.

Barrawclough C, Haddock G, Tarrier N et al 2001 Randomised controlled trial of motivational interviewing, cognitive behaviour therapy and family intervention for patients with comorbid schizophrenia and substance use disorders. American Journal of Psychiatry 158: 1706–1713

- Has shown some promising results in patients living with family members.
- The study showed success with a combination of cognitive therapy, motivational interviewing and family intervention.
- The combination of treatments led to increased abstinence and better functioning in both the short and longer term.

- The Medical Research Council are now supporting a larger trial using the same intervention.

Chambers RA, Krystal JH, Self DW 2001 A neurobiological basis for substance abuse comorbidity in schizophrenia. Biological Psychiatry 50: 71–83

- Suggested that the cortical and hippocampal dysfunctions in schizophrenia could also be responsible for the greater reinforcing properties of drugs of misuse.

See also the 'General topics' section in Chapter 26 (Schizophrenia), page 368.

Dual diagnosis: management within a psychosocial context

Abou-Saleh MT 2004 Dual diagnosis: management within a psychosocial context. Advances in Psychiatric Treatment 10: 352–360

This paper discusses treatment models for the care of individuals with comorbid substance misuse and psychiatric disorders. Current policies are discussed and the evidence examined.

Drake RE, Mercer-McFadden C, Mueser KT 1998 Review of integrated mental health and substance abuse treatment for patients with dual disorders. Schizophrenia Bulletin 24: 589–608

- Review of 36 studies of integrated treatment for dual diagnosis patients.
- Included 10 studies of comprehensive integrated outpatient treatment programmes.
- These programmes were effective in engaging patients in services, reducing substance use and sustaining remission.
- Outcomes relating to hospital use, psychiatric symptoms and other domains were less consistent.
- The use of assertive outreach, case management and a longitudinal, stage-wise, motivational approach to the treatment of substance misuse were associated with effectiveness.

Features of the integrated approach include:
- focus on anxiety reduction versus overcoming denial
- trust and education versus confrontation and criticism
- harm reduction versus abstinence
- long-term focus versus rapid withdrawal, short-term treatment
- motivational techniques versus confrontation
- 12-step groups available versus mandatory.

Drake RE, Bartels SJ, Teague GB et al 1993 Treatment of substance abuse in severely mentally ill patients. Journal of Nervous and Mental Disease 181: 606–611

- Identified nine principles for the treatment of substance misuse in severely mentally ill patients.
- An evidence-based approach was used.
- Principles included:
  - assertive outreach to facilitate engagement
  - close monitoring to provide structure and social reinforcement
  - integrated service
  - comprehensive, wide range of interventions
  - stable living situation
  - flexibility and specialisation
  - staged treatment
  - a longitudinal perspective
  - instilling optimism in both patients and carers.
- The stages of treatment included:
  - engagement: regular contact and development of a therapeutic alliance and meeting basic needs
  - persuasion: motivational techniques
  - active treatment: harm reduction to abstinence-orientated approaches
  - relapse prevention: identification of high-risk situations for relapse and management of future relapses.

Drake RE, Mueser KT 2000 Psychosocial approaches to dual diagnosis. Schizophrenia Bulletin 26: 105–117

Identified the common components of integrated care:
- Case management: multidisciplinary case management with assertive outreach to engage and retain patients in community services.
- Close monitoring: medication supervision, urine drug screening and coercive approaches.
- Substance misuse treatment: motivational approaches; harm reduction and CBT in individual, group and family settings; self-help (12-step programme) and social skills training.
- Rehabilitation: provision of long-term support in the community, whether day care or residential care, to enable restoration of social and occupational function (supported education and employment).
- Housing: both supported and independent.
- Pharmacotherapy: provision of antipsychotic medication (particularly clozapine) in those with schizophrenia, and improvement of compliance by providing education and medication supervision.

Drake RE, McHugo GJ, Clark RE et al 1998 Assertive community treatment for patients with co-occurring severe mental illness and substance use disorder: a clinical trial. American Journal of Orthopsychiatry 68: 201–215

- RCT of assertive community treatment (ACT) versus standard care in patients with dual diagnosis.
- ACT was more effective with regard to substance misuse and quality of life.

Weiss RD, Grifin ML, Greenfield SF et al 2000 Group therapy for patient with bipolar disorder and substance dependence: results of a pilot study. Journal of Clinical Psychiatry 61: 361–367

- A trial of integrated group therapy with a focus on rapid intervention in patients with bipolar disorder and substance misuse.
- Those who received group therapy had greater improvements in terms of drug use, manic symptoms and medication compliance.

Barrowclough C, Haddock G, Tarrier N et al 2001 Randomized controlled trial of motivational interviewing, cognitive behaviour therapy, and family intervention for patients with comorbid schizophrenia and substance use disorders. American Journal of Psychiatry 158: 1706–1713

- A RCT of family intervention in comorbid psychosis and substance misuse.
- Therapy comprised five weekly sessions of motivational interviewing, six sessions of cognitive therapy held fortnightly and 10–16 sessions of family intervention.
- The treatment was found to be better than standard care in terms of general function, psychopathology and days of abstinence from substance misuse over 12 months.

Definition

Dual diagnosis – the co-occurrence of substance misuse with other psychiatric disorders which may include:

- – severe psychiatric disorder with problematic substance misuse, with or without an underlying personality disorder
- – substance-induced psychiatric disorder
- – substance dependence with personality disorder, without comorbid psychiatric disorder.

See also the 'Treatment – Psychological therapies' section in Chapter 26 (Schizophrenia), page 395.

Inpatient treatment of opiate dependence

Smyth BP, Barry J, Lane A et al 2005 In-patient treatment of opiate dependence: medium-term follow-up outcomes. British Journal of Psychiatry 187: 360–265

The hypothesis for this study was that a substantial minority of patients would have attained abstinence when followed-up after inpatient treatment. Studies have shown that treatment for opioid dependence is associated with early relapse and high levels of attrition.

Method

- 149 patients were included.
- Abstinence was the aim.
- 67% were male and the median age was 23 years.
- 79% had reported injecting at some point in the past.
- The Maudsley Addiction Profile, a structured interview, was used to establish drug use in the previous month.

Results

- 81% of patients achieved detoxification with methadone.
- Five patients died prior to follow-up.
- 76% were interviewed at follow-up.
- 41% reported heroin misuse and 18% reported methadone misuse at follow-up.
- 50% reported misuse of at least one opiate.
- 15% were using heroin daily.
- Of the 86 who completed methadone maintenance, 53% reported no recent opiate misuse and 57% were on methadone treatment at follow-up.
- Over half the cohort were on methadone maintenance treatment at follow-up, meaning that many patients relapsed following discharge and subsequently re-accessed treatment.
- 89% of patients were admitted with a primary problem of heroin dependence.
- Only 41% reported recent heroin misuse at follow-up.
- 15% reported daily heroin use.
- This supports the view that inpatient treatment is effective in reducing heroin misuse. However, the inpatient treatment cannot be presumed to be the sole reason for the reduction in heroin use as many were on methadone maintenance at follow-up which will have contributed to the reduced rates of use.
- Abstinence was associated positively with completion of the 6-week inpatient programme and attendance at aftercare.
- It was negatively linked to a family history of substance misuse.
- Treatment adherence was the principal influence on prolonged abstinence, suggesting that treatment units should focus on adherence to the programme.

Gossop M, Marsden J, Stewart D et al 1999 Treatment retention and 1 year outcomes for residential programmes in England. Drug and Alcohol Dependence 57: 89–98

- The UK National Treatment Outcome Research Study (NTORS) showed that inpatient treatment reduces mean levels of opiate use.
- Similar findings have been shown in America.

Ghodse AH, London M, Bewley TH et al 2002 Treating an opiate-dependent inpatient population: a one-year follow-up study of treatment completers and non-completers. Addictive Behaviours 27: 765–778

- Pre-treatment patient characteristics are poor predictors of treatment outcome.
- Patients who spend a longer time in treatment have better outcomes.

See also the 'General topics' section in Chapter 30 (Treatment settings), page 435.

National survey of methadone prescribing for maintenance treatment

Joseph R, Moselhy H 2005 National survey of methadone prescribing for maintenance treatment: 'opioidphobia' among substance misuse services? Psychiatric Bulletin 29: 459–461

Methadone maintenance treatment is the most widely known, well-researched, cost-effective treatment for opioid dependence. Its use varies widely across the UK, although the common goal is to enable patients to refrain from heroin use. There are concerns that the doses of methadone prescribed are not sufficient.

Aims

To describe the characteristics of methadone maintenance treatment services across England and to determine the average doses. The views of the prescribing teams were also examined.

Method

- The DrugScope database of methadone services was used.
- Questionnaires were sent to all of the specialist treatment centres.

Results

- 298 substance misuse treatment centres were identified; 157 prescribed methadone.
- Service types were:
  - community drug teams (71%)
  - addiction treatment units (27%)
  - general practices (2%).
- 79.6% had doctors attached to the services.
- 20.4% of the scripts were written by GPs.
- 15,931 patients received methadone from 157 centres.
- On average, 101 patients attended each centre.

Prescribing

- The most common formulation was oral methadone mixture.
- The maximum mean dose of methadone prescribed for maintenance was 116 mg, with a maximum dose of 325 mg.
- The minimum dose ranged from 1 to 70 mg.
- The mean dose was 47 mg.
- 4% used serum levels to find optimum dose.

Views on methadone prescribing

- 49% of centres expressed the view that there should be a maximum and a minimum dose of methadone.
- 40% of centres felt that methadone maintenance treatment should be restricted to specialised services.
- 24% of centres thought that methadone treatment should be time-limited but the majority disagreed with this.
- 13% thought that people should purely receive methadone with no counselling or social interventions.
- It was speculated that there may be a fear of prescribing higher doses.
- It was suggested that monitoring serum levels of methadone is a better way of predicting appropriate dose compared to arbitrary clinical judgement.

Department of Health 1996 The task force to review services for drug misusers. The Stationery Office, London

- Found that those on doses of methadone greater than 50 mg have higher rates of abstinence.

Farrell M, Ware J, Mattick R et al 1994 Methadone maintenance treatment in opiate dependence: a review. British Medical Journal 309: 997–1001

- Also found that patients on higher doses have better outcomes.

Strang J, Sheridan J 2001 Methadone prescribing to opiate addicts by private doctors: comparison with NHS practice in South East England. Addiction 95: 567–576

- Investigated community pharmacies and found that 50% of patients are on less than 50 mg of methadone.

Dunn J 2003 A survey of methadone prescribing at an inner-city drug service and comparison with national data. Psychiatric Bulletin 27: 167–170

- Inner-city study finding that a significant minority of patients were on subtherapeutic doses.

Home Office 2000 Reducing drug related deaths. The Stationery Office, London, p 72

- Advised against the use of controlled drugs in drug users because of the risk of injecting.
- Stated that deaths would be reduced if the prescription of controlled drugs in tablet form or in ampoules was stopped.

Ward J, Hall W, Mattick RP 1999 Role of maintenance treatment in opioid dependence. Lancet 353: 221–226

- International research showing outcomes were better on higher doses of methadone.

Weblink DrugScope – www.drugscope.org.uk.

Stimulant psychosis

Curran C, Byrappa N, McBride A 2004 Stimulant psychosis: systematic review. British Journal of Psychiatry 184: 196–204

It is increasingly recognised that stimulant misuse is associated with psychotic illness.

Aims

- The purpose of this study was to critically examine the evidence for sensitisation.
- It is hypothesised that stimulant psychosis can be divided into two different types:
  - the toxic type
  - the chronic persisting response, resulting from longer-term use.

Method

- A systematic review of studies that had investigated stimulant use and psychosis in humans.
- The main outcome measures were:
  - increases in psychosis with stimulant use
  - differences between stimulant use and non-users.

Results

- 43 studies met the criteria and were included in the review.
- A single dose of stimulant drug can produce a brief increase in psychosis ratings (a 'response') in 50–70% of participants with schizophrenia and pre-existing acute psychotic symptoms.
- The presence of antipsychotic medication does not appear to block the action of the stimulants.
- Only 30% of patients with schizophrenia in remission show increases in psychotic ratings.

Discussion

- There is evidence that, irrespective of mental state, stimulants cause a brief psychotic reaction, usually

lasting only hours and, in the majority of cases, being self-limiting.
- Antipsychotic medication in a patient with schizophrenia will not prevent relapse or worsening of psychotic symptoms if stimulants are used.
- Low dose antipsychotics may be beneficial in stimulant users, to prevent sensitisation.

Koyama T, Muraki A, Nakayame M et al 1991 CNS stimulant abuse; long lasting symptoms of amphetamine psychosis. Biological Psychiatry 2: 63–65

- Reported an epidemic of stimulant psychosis with a prolonged and chronic course.

Ellingwood EH, Kilbey MM 1980 Fundamental mechanisms underlying altered behaviour following chronic administration of psychomotor stimulants. Biological Psychiatry 15: 749–757

- Wrote about the 'kindling' effect.
- This is described as producing a psychotic illness similar to schizophrenia by way of repeated low doses of stimulant leading to changes in the central nervous system.

Brabbins C, Poole R 1996 Psychiatrists' knowledge of drug induced psychosis. Psychiatric Bulletin 20: 410–412

- Dispute the theory of sensitisation.

Srisurapanont N, Kittiratanapaiboon P, Jarusuraisin N 2004 Treatment for amphetamine psychosis **(Cochrane Review)**. In: The Cochrane Library, Issue 2. Update Software, Oxford

- A recent Cochrane Review found no relevant studies.

Supervised injecting centres

Wright NMJ, Tompkins CNE 2004 Supervised injecting centres. British Medical Journal 328: 100–102

In 2001, the first medically supervised injecting centre was opened in Sydney, Australia. Since then, over 40 others have opened in Germany, the Netherlands, Switzerland and Spain.

Government Reply to the Third Report from the Home Affairs Committee 2002 The Government's drugs policy: is it working? Session 2001–2002, HC 318. The Stationery Office, London

- The UK Home Affairs Select Committee recommended that 'an evaluated pilot programme of safe injecting houses for heroin users is established without delay and that if this is successful, the programme is extended across the country'.

- This applied only to those undergoing a heroin prescribing programme.

Medically Supervised Injecting Centre Evaluation Committee 2003 Final report on the evaluation report of the Sydney medically supervised centre. MSIC Evaluation Committee, Sydney

- 18-month trial of the Sydney Centre.
- Staff intervened in 329 overdoses in 12 months with an estimated four lives saved per year.
- There was a rise in hepatitis B and C infections occurring elsewhere in Sydney during that time, but not in the area served by the medically supervised injecting centre.
- There was a decrease in injecting-related problems in those using the centre and subjective reports of lower-risk injecting practices.
- Those attending the centre were more likely to seek treatment for their drug misuse (referral rate of 11%).
- Economic evaluation showed costs were comparable for the supervised injecting centre and alternative public health measures.
- Local sightings of public injection decreased, as did syringe counts in the local vicinity.
- Rates of theft and robbery did not increase in the local area.
- Acceptance by local businesses and residents increased over the time of the study.

Yamey G 2000 UN condemns Australian plans for 'safe injecting rooms'. British Medical Journal 320: 667

- The United Nations International Narcotics Control Board has stated that the supervised injecting centres violate international drugs conventions.
- The authors argue that the pilot of safe injecting houses should not be limited to those undergoing a heroin prescribing programme.
- Social exclusion and homelessness would exclude target patients from the services they need and the continuation of unsafe injection practices.
- There is little evidence from other countries regarding supervised injecting centres, but there have been no deaths reported from any centre.
- The centres are beneficial in that they openly address unsafe injecting practice in a safe, structured clinical environment and integrate it with other harm reduction methods, such as needle exchange programmes.

Definitions

Medically supervised **injecting centres** are 'legally sanctioned facilities designed to reduce the health and public order problems associated with illegal injection drug use'. Alternative names are health rooms, supervised injecting centres, drug consumption rooms and safer injecting rooms or facilities. (*Source*: as weblink below.)

'Shooting galleries' differ, as users pay to inject on site. (*Source*: Carlson RG 2000 Shooting galleries, dope houses and injection doctors: examining the social ecology of HIV risk behaviours amid drug injectors in Dayton, Ohio. Human Organization 59: 325.)

Weblink Consumption rooms as a professional service in addictions health 1999 International Conference for the Development of Guidelines. Guidelines for the operation and use of consumption rooms – www.adf.org.au.

Policy and Legislation

Alcohol harm reduction strategy for England

Prime Minister's Strategy Unit 2004 Alcohol harm reduction strategy for England. Cabinet Office, London

This report outlines plans to tackle excessive drinking.

Four key groups of alcohol-related harms are to be addressed:
- Health harms
  - The annual cost of alcohol misuse is estimated at £1.7bn per annum
  - £95m is spent per annum on specialist alcohol treatment
  - There are over 30,000 hospital admissions for alcohol dependence per annum
  - There are approximately 22,000 premature deaths per year
  - Up to 70% of all admissions to A&E at peak times are alcohol related
  - There are increasing numbers of deaths from chronic liver disease.
- Crime and antisocial behaviour harms
  - An annual cost of £7.3bn is estimated (alcohol misuse related only)
  - 1.2m violent incidents (approximately half of all violent crimes) and 360,000 incidents of domestic violence (approximately a third) are alcohol related.
- Loss of productivity and profitability
  - An estimated cost of £6.4bn per year
  - Up to 17m working days are lost each year.
- Harms to family and society
  - Approximately 1m children are affected by parental alcohol problems
  - Marriages are twice as likely to end in divorce where there are alcohol problems

- There is an estimated cost of £4.7bn per annum in terms of human and emotional impact suffered by victims of alcohol-related crime.

There are four key ways that government can act to reduce alcohol-related harms:

- through improved and better targeted education and communication
- through better identification and treatment of alcohol problems
- through better coordination and enforcement of the current framework to tackle crime and antisocial behaviour
- through encouraging the alcoholic drinks industry to promote more responsible drinking and take a role in reducing alcohol-related harms.

Specific examples are education regarding 'safe drinking', alcohol education in schools, health warnings on alcohol bottles, and the responsible portrayal of alcohol use in the media and advertising.

The government's recommended sensible drinking guidelines

Government-recommended 'sensible drinking' guidelines were developed on the basis of careful consideration of the harmful, and some beneficial, effects of drinking at different levels.

The 'sensible drinking' message was first referred to in the government's 1992 *Health of the Nation* White Paper. This recommended that men should consume no more than 21 units and women no more than 14 units per week.

In 1995, in recognition of the dangers of excessive drinking in a single session, the sensible drinking message was changed to focus on daily guidelines. It suggests:

- a maximum intake of 2–3 units per day for women and 3–4 for men, with two alcohol-free days after heavy drinking; continued alcohol consumption at the upper level is not advised
- that intake of up to 2 units a day can have a moderate effect against heart disease for men over 40 and postmenopausal women
- that some groups, such as pregnant women and those engaging in potentially dangerous activities (such as operating heavy machinery), should drink less or nothing at all.

Weblink Prime Minister's Strategy Unit – www.strategy.gov.uk.

Plant M 2004 The alcohol harm reduction strategy for England [editorial]. British Medical Journal 328: 905–906

Reports on the government's *Alcohol Harm Reduction Strategy for England*. There are increasing levels of adverse effects from alcohol in the UK in both males and females and across all ages. The harm minimisation strategy states that binge drinking and chronic drinking are the main

targets of proposed action to reduce the 'further increase in alcohol related harm in England'.

The author stresses that binge drinking is not new and drinking patterns are not fixed. It is felt that the cultural aspects of drinking are not sufficiently acknowledged in the report. The editorial suggests that much more focus should be directed on family and friends, where most drinking habits are learned. There is also a limited comment on treatment – despite the good evidence base.

McBride N, Farrington F, Midford R et al 2003 Harm minimisation in school drug education: final results of the school health and alcohol harm reduction programme (SHAHRP). Addiction 99: 278–291

- The Australian School Health and Alcohol Harm Reduction Programme (SHAHRP) is a harm minimisation programme which produced positive outcomes.
- The document focuses on crime and disorder.
- While useful initiatives are cited, it is felt that mandatory and evaluated local action programmes would be much better – for example, toughened glasses have been examined in Queensland, Australia and in the UK.

See also Project MATCH (p. 19).

The dual diagnosis good practice guide

Department of Health 2002 Mental health policy implementation guide: the dual diagnosis good practice guide. DH, London[†]

The National Service Framework (NSF) for Mental Health emphasised the importance of addressing dual diagnosis but did not set standards and service models to address the issues for patients with either dual diagnosis or substance use disorders.

Background

Historically, substance misuse and mental health services have evolved separately. Few services currently exist which explicitly deal with clients with both substance misuse and mental health problems. These clients have tended either to be treated within one service alone, which has meant that some aspects of their cluster of problems have not been dealt with as they might, or have been shuttled between services, with a corresponding loss of continuity of care. Some potential clients or patients have almost certainly been excluded from all the available services.

This guide is focused on people with severe mental health problems and problematic substance misuse. Services will often have developed their own local definitions of severe

---

[†] Crown copyright. Reproduced with permission.

mental health problems. Many of these will be based on the five 'SIDDS' dimensions of severity, informal and formal care, diagnosis, disability and duration. Risks of harm to self or others, or of severe self-neglect, are also relevant.

This guide covers the problematic use of all types of substances, whether licit or illicit. Crucially it includes alcohol. Tobacco, however, is not included. The guide also covers non-dependent but nonetheless problematic substance misuse.

Prevalence

Increased rates of substance misuse are found in individuals with mental health problems, affecting around a third to a half of people with severe mental health problems. Alcohol is the most common form of substance misuse. Where drug misuse occurs, it often coexists with alcohol misuse. Homelessness is frequently associated with substance misuse problems.

Community mental health teams report that 8–15% of their clients have dual diagnosis problems although higher rates may be found in inner cities.

Prisons have a high prevalence of drug dependency and dual diagnosis.

Clinical implications

Substance misuse among individuals with psychiatric disorders has been associated with significantly poorer outcomes, including:
- worsening psychiatric symptoms
- increased use of institutional services
- poor medication adherence
- homelessness
- increased risk of HIV infection
- poor social outcomes, including impact on carers and family
- contact with the criminal justice system.

Implementation

Substance misuse is usual rather than exceptional amongst people with severe mental health problems and the relationship between the two is complex. Individuals with these dual problems deserve high-quality, patient-focused, integrated care. This should be delivered within mental health services. This policy is referred to as 'mainstreaming'.

'Mainstreaming' will only work if the following policy requirements are delivered:
- Local services must develop focused definitions of dual diagnosis which reflect patterns of need and clarify the target group for services.
- These definitions must be agreed between relevant agencies.
- Where they exist, specialist teams of dual diagnosis workers should provide support to mainstream mental health services.

- All staff in assertive outreach teams must be trained and equipped to work with dual diagnosis.
- Adequate numbers of staff in crisis resolution, early intervention, community mental health teams and inpatient services must also be suitably trained.
- All services, including drug and alcohol services, must ensure that clients with severe mental health problems and substance misuse are subject to the care programme approach and have a full risk assessment.

Integrated care – delivered by one team – appears to produce better outcomes than serial care or parallel care. However, more UK-based research is required and well-organised parallel care can be used as a stepping stone to integration. Integrated care in this country can be delivered by existing mental health services following training and with support from substance misuse services.

Specific groups

Certain groups of individuals are emphasised in the literature as warranting specific attention, as follows:
1. Young people: substance misuse is a major contributory factor in the development of mental health problems in the young. For example, early onset of substance misuse is linked with higher rates of major depressive disorders and it is estimated that a third of young people committing suicide are intoxicated with alcohol at the time of death.
2. Homeless people: studies have identified high levels of concurrent substance misuse and mental health problems among groups of homeless people and rough sleepers. Homelessness almost trebles a young person's chance of developing a mental health problem. Assertive outreach to these groups and inreach to hostels are necessary.
3. Offenders including prisoners: both mental health problems and substance misuse play a major role in youth offending, and their combination (together with low adherence to medication) may lead to a higher risk of violence among adults with severe mental health problems.
4. Women: significant differences between men and women have been found in their patterns of substance misuse and psychiatric comorbidity:
   - Women who misuse substances are significantly more likely than other women or men to have experienced sexual, physical and/or emotional abuse as children
   - Substance misuse lifestyles can impact on women's sexual health and establish a pattern of re-victimisation
   - Women are more likely to present at mental health or primary care services for psychological difficulties rather than for any associated substance misuse problem

- Women therefore tend to access alcohol and drug services later than men, and this may explain their more severe presentation
- Women may have children, or want children, and this can deter them from contact with statutory services for fear of their children being removed.

5. People from ethnic minorities: although definitive studies on the influence of culture and ethnicity upon individuals with a dual diagnosis have yet to be conducted, it is known that severe mental illness and substance misuse present differently across cultures and ethnic groups.

Treatment – key points

Assessment of substance misuse forms an integral part of standard assessment procedures for mental health problems:

- Services need to develop routine screening procedures and, where substance misuse is identified, the nature and severity of that misuse and its associated risks should be assessed.
- An awareness of specific groups for whom these dual conditions generate specific needs must inform the assessment process.
- Treatments should be staged according to an individual's readiness for change and engagement with services.
- Staff should avoid prematurely pushing clients towards abstinence but adopt a harm reduction approach.
- An optimistic and longitudinal perspective regarding the substance misuse problem and its treatment are necessary.
- A flexible and adaptive therapeutic response is important for the integrated management of these dual conditions.
- Attention must be paid to social networks of clients, to meaningful daytime activity and to sound pharmacological management.

Definitions

Serial care – sequential referrals to different services.

Parallel care – more than one service engaging the client at the same time.

Models of care for the treatment of drug misusers

NHS National Treatment Agency for Substance Misuse 2002 Models of care for the treatment of drug misusers. Promoting quality, efficiency and effectiveness in drug misuse treatment services in England. DH, London

This National Service Framework for the treatment of adults who misuse substances in England is in two parts, where part one is aimed at the commissioning of services for drug treatment commissioners and part two is directed at drug treatment providers. The framework aims to provide 'equity, parity and consistency' in substance misuse treatment in England. There is specific guidance for coordinating drug misuse services, general health care and social services. The framework suggests a systems approach with explicit links to the criminal justice system. It is an evidence-based plan which is in line with key national documents including *The NHS Plan* (2000).

It does not cover alcohol, under 18s, prisoners or misuse of prescribed medication specifically.

Aims

- Reductions in the waiting times for treatment
- Development of integrated care pathways
- Tiered system of care
- Development of various drug misuse treatment modalities, including:
  - needle exchange facilities
  - care-planned counselling
  - structured day programmes
  - community prescribing
  - inpatient substance misuse treatment
  - residential rehabilitation.

A tiered model of care is suggested where all patients will have access to all tiers of care.

- Tier 1: Non-substance misuse specific services requiring interface with drug and alcohol treatment – consists of services offered by a wide range of professionals (e.g. primary care or general medical services, social workers, teachers, community pharmacists, probation officers, homeless persons units).
- Tier 2: Open access drug and alcohol treatment services – these include needle exchange, drug (and alcohol) advice and information services, and ad hoc support.
- Tier 3: Structured community-based drug treatment services – which include psychotherapeutic interventions and structured counselling, motivational interventions, methadone maintenance programmes, community detoxification and day care.
- Tier 4: Residential services for drug and alcohol misusers.
- Tier 4a: Residential drug and alcohol misuse specific services – these may include inpatient drug and alcohol detoxification or stabilisation services, drug and alcohol residential rehabilitation units and residential drug crisis intervention services.
- Tier 4b: Highly specialist non-substance misuse specific services – these may include specialist liver units and forensic services for mentally ill offenders.

The framework requires the development of evidence-based standards, recommendations and justification for each treatment modality outlined. It also details the provision of treatment to pregnant women and to special groups. The latter includes stimulant users, women drug users, black and ethnic minority populations, young people, parents, and those with combined alcohol and drug use.

Cross-cutting issues include:

- overdose
- blood-borne diseases
- psychiatric comorbidity (dual diagnosis)
- outreach work
- criminal justice
- users, carers and self-help groups
- complementary therapies.

Weblink   National Treatment Agency for Substance Misuse – www.nta.nhs.uk/publications/MOCPART2/mocpart2_feb03-old.pdf.

See also the 'Policy and legislation' section in Chapter 27 (Service provision), page 405.

Treatment – Psychopharmacology

Buprenorphine in substance misuse

Taikato M, Kidd B, Baldacchino A 2005 What every psychiatrist should know about buprenorphine in substance misuse. Psychiatric Bulletin 29: 225–227

Buprenorphine was introduced in 1996 in Europe and is now the main treatment modality in some countries. Its use in Britain was affected by its potential for abuse in the 1980s; this was particularly true in Scotland.

Ward J, Mattick RP, Hall W 1997 Methadone maintenance treatment and other opioid replacement therapies. Harwood Academic, Sydney

- Methadone substitute prescribing is the primary maintenance treatment in the UK for opioid dependence.

Walsh SL, Preston K, Stitzer ML et al 1994 Clinical pharmacology of buprenorphine: ceiling effects at high doses. Clinical Pharmacology and Therapeutics 55: 569–580

Detailed adverse effects relating to treatment with buprenorphine as:

- death following overdose
- the need for daily dosing
- the risk of the drug being abused by others
- stigma.

Sakol MS, Stark C, Sykes R 1989 Buprenorphine and temazepam abuse by drug takers in Glasgow – an increase. Clinical Pharmacology and Therapeutics 55: 569–580

- Discussed buprenorphine abuse in the 1980s in Glasgow.

Kintz P 2001 Deaths involving buprenorphine: a compendium of French cases. Forensic Science International 121: 65–69

- Combination of benzodiazepines and buprenorphine, with or without alcohol, can be fatal.
- Tricyclic antidepressants and MAOIs can compound the central depressant effect.
- Antipsychotics can also interact because they are metabolised by similar enzymes.

Kakko J, Svanborg K, Kreek M et al 2003 1 year retention and social function after buprenorphine-assisted relapse prevention treatment for heroin dependence in Sweden: a randomised, placebo-controlled trial. Lancet 361: 662–668

- Suggested that psychosocial treatments should be included in treatment programmes for heroin dependence.

See also Cochrane Review of buprenorphine and methadone (p. 17).

Buprenorphine for the management of opioid withdrawal

Gowing L, Ali R, White J 2006 Buprenorphine for the management of opioid withdrawal **(Cochrane Review)**. In: The Cochrane Library, Issue 1. Update Software, Oxford

- 14 studies were included ($n = 784$).
- Buprenorphine was compared with clonidine (seven studies), methadone (three studies) and oxazepam (one study).
- Four of the studies compared different buprenorphine dosing regimens.
- Compared with treatment with clonidine, treatment with buprenorphine is associated with:
  - less severe withdrawal symptoms
  - reduced numbers of adverse effects
  - reduced rates of dropout.
- Treatment with buprenorphine causes withdrawal symptoms as severe as with treatment with methadone, but of shorter duration.
- There were no differences between the two treatments with regard to dropout rates.
- Rapid reduction in buprenorphine dose after a period of maintenance therapy leads to more severe symptoms of withdrawal.

Weblink The Cochrane Collaboration – www.cochrane.org.

Buprenorphine maintenance versus placebo or methadone maintenance for opioid dependence

Mattick RP, Kimber J, Breen C et al 2006 Buprenorphine maintenance versus placebo or methadone maintenance for opioid dependence **(Cochrane Review)**. In: The Cochrane Library, Issue 1. Update Software, Oxford

- 13 randomised studies were included.
- Treatment of opioid dependence with a flexible buprenorphine regimen resulted in lower numbers of patients remaining in treatment compared with a methadone treatment programme.
- There were no differences in outcomes for buprenorphine or methadone when compared at low dose.
- High doses of buprenorphine, in comparison with low dose methadone treatment, may reduce concurrent heroin use but with no beneficial effects on dropout rates.
- Buprenorphine at high dose was no better than high dose methadone in terms of dropout rates and was less effective with regard to concurrent heroin use.
- High and very high doses of buprenorphine were required before benefits were seen over placebo in terms of dropout rates.

Weblink The Cochrane Collaboration – www.cochrane.org.

Medical prescription of heroin

van den Brink W, Hendricks VM, Blanken P, Koeter MWJ, van Zwieten BJ, van Ree JM 2003 Medical prescription of heroin to treatment resistant heroin addicts: two randomised controlled trials. British Medical Journal 327: 310

- Two open-label randomised controlled trials were included (n = 549) set in methadone maintenance programmes in six Dutch cities.
- Injectable and inhalable heroin were prescribed over 1 year.
- Up to 1 gram of heroin was prescribed per day (with up to 150 mg of methadone) and was compared with methadone prescribed alone (up to 150 mg).
- Control group patients were offered 6 months of combination therapy at the end of the year.
- Medically prescribed heroin was withdrawn for at least 2 months at the end of the treatment period, in all cases.
- Outcome measures included validated indicators of physical health, mental status and social function.

These included the Maudsley Addiction Profile and the Symptom Checklist.
- Improvement was taken as a greater than 40% improvement in one of the three domains (physical, mental and social).
- Intention to treat analysis was used, although adherence was good, with 1-year outcome data available in 94% of cases.

Results

- Heroin and methadone in combination were significantly more effective than methadone alone for both injectable and inhalable heroin.
- Between 45 and 88% of the participants did not respond to co-prescription of heroin (depending on response criterion used).
- Completion rates were highest in the control groups.
- On average, those who completed treatment visited the heroin dispensing units 2.1 times a day, used 260 mg heroin a visit and 548 mg a day.
- Discontinuation of heroin prescription was associated with a rapid deterioration.
- The numbers of serious adverse events was similar in all groups.

Rehm J, Geschwend P, Steffen T, Gutzwiller F, Dobler-Mikola A, Uchtenhagen A 2001 Feasibility, safety and efficacy of injectable heroin for refractory opioid addicts: a follow up study. Lancet 358: 1417–1420

- A large Swiss cohort study (n = 1969) of medical prescription of injectable heroin.
- 237 patients completed the 18-month programme.
- Found benefits for physical and mental health, in social integration and for illegal drug use.
- No controls were available.
- There was mandatory psychosocial counselling and care.

Pharmacotherapy in dual diagnosis

Crome IB, Myton T 2004 Pharmacotherapy in dual diagnosis. Advances in Psychiatric Treatment 10: 413–424

- Dual diagnosis, in its use here, covers a complex and heterogeneous group of patients.
- Drug problems may not present alone.
- Concurrent smoking and alcohol use mean that there can be dual or triple dependencies.
- Comorbid substance misuse and psychiatric disorders result in multiple social, physical and psychological complications.

- Large numbers of RCTs have investigated substance misuse; however, those with mental disorder are often excluded.

Regier DA, Farmer ME, Rae DS et al 1990 Comorbidity of mental disorders with alcohol and other drug misuse: results from The Epidemiologic Catchment Area Study. Journal of the American Medical Association 264: 2511–2518

- Men with opioid dependence had lifetime anxiety rates of 6.1% compared with 10.7% in women.
- 47% of people with schizophrenia had comorbid substance misuse (alcohol 37%, cannabis 23%, stimulants/hallucinogenics 13%).
- 32% of people with affective disorder had comorbid substance misuse.
- The lifetime prevalence of alcohol misuse and dependence in people with social anxiety was 22%.

Coutlhard M, Farrell M, Singleton N et al 2002 Tobacco, alcohol and drug use and mental health. The Stationery Office, London

- National comorbidity study.
- The prevalence of drug taking by 16–64 year olds had increased from 5 to 12% since 1993.
- 4% of those who had ever used drugs (estimated 27% of total population surveyed) had experienced an accidental overdose.

Fricher M, Collins J, Millson D et al 2004 Prevalence of comorbid psychiatric illness and substance abuse in primary care in England and Wales. Journal of Epidemiology and Community Health 58: 1036–1041

- The only study of comorbidity in the primary care population in the UK.
- Data were collected between 1993 and 1998.
- During the study the annual prevalence of dual diagnosis (determined by the co-occurrence of a substance misuse diagnosis and psychiatric diagnosis in the same month) in England and Wales increased by 62%.
- Comorbid psychosis increased by 147%.
- Schizophrenia increased by 128%.
- Paranoia increased by 144%.

Granholm E, Anthenelli R, Monteiro R et al 2003 Brief integrated outpatient dual-diagnosis treatment reduces psychiatric hospitalisations. American Journal on Addictions 12: 306–313

- Comorbidity leads to more frequent recurrence of psychiatric disorder, increased time spent in hospital, increased violence, homelessness and alienation from families and carers.
- The dual diagnosis group may do better than those without substance misuse once they are abstinent.

Buckley P, Thompson PA, Way L et al 1994 Substance abuse and clozapine treatment. Journal of Clinical Psychiatry 55 (Suppl B): 114–116; Zimmet SV, Strous RD, Burgess ES 2000 Effects of clozapine on substance use in patients with schizophrenia and schizoaffective disorder. Journal of Clinical Psychopharmacology 20: 94–98

- There is good evidence to suggest that clozapine reduces substance misuse (nicotine and alcohol) in patients with schizophrenia.
- The findings were less consistent for cannabis.
- In patients with treatment-resistant illness and substance misuse there are also improvements in psychopathology and psychosocial function comparable to those with treatment-resistant illness who do not misuse substances.

Littrell KH, Petty RG, Hilligross NM et al 2001 Olanzapine treatment for patients with schizophrenia and substance abuse. Journal of Substance Abuse Treatment 21: 217–221

- Olanzapine led to improvements in patients with psychosis and substance misuse.

Levin FR, Evans SM, Coomaraswammy S et al 1998 Flupenthixol treatment for cocaine abusers with schizophrenia: a pilot study. American Journal of Drug and Alcohol Abuse 24: 343–360

- A small pilot of flupenthixol treatment in comorbid schizophrenia and cocaine use.
- Flupenthixol was associated with improvements in psychopathology (positive and negative symptoms).
- It also led to a reduction in cocaine use.

McGrath PJ, Nunes EV, Stewart JW et al 1996 Imipramine treatment of alcoholics with primary depression. Archives of General Psychiatry 53: 232–240

- 12-week RCT of imipramine in patients with harmful use of alcohol.
- Depression improved in the imipramine-treated group.
- There was no significant decrease in numbers of drinking days or in alcohol consumed per day.

Cornelius JR, Salloum IM, Haskett RF et al 2000 Fluoxetine versus placebo in depressed alcoholics: a one year follow-up study. Addictive Behaviour 25: 307–310

- 12-month, double-blind, placebo-controlled trial of fluoxetine in depression and alcohol dependence.
- Fluoxetine had significant effects on reducing the number of days drinking to intoxication.
- The reduction in total drinking days was not significant.

Kranzler HR, Burleson JA, Korner P et al 1995 Placebo-controlled trial of fluoxetine as an adjunction to relapse prevention in alcoholics. American Journal of Psychiatry 152: 391–397

- This study showed that fluoxetine (up to 60 mg) was not effective in reducing drinking when used for relapse prevention.

Hertzman M 2000 Divalproex sodium used to treat concomitant substance abuse and mood disorders. Journal of Substance Abuse Treatment 18: 371–372

- Retrospective study of valproate in patients with bipolar disorder and substance misuse.
- Half of the patients reduced their substance misuse.

Nunes EV, Quitkin FM, Donovan SJ et al 1998 Imipramine treatment of opiate-dependent patients with depressive disorders. A placebo-controlled trial. Archives of General Psychiatry 55:153–160

- Imipramine was effective in reducing depressive symptoms compared to placebo in a group of opioid-dependent patients receiving methadone maintenance.
- Abstinence was achieved in 14% of the imipramine group and 2% of the placebo group.
- Although the reductions in depressive symptoms and substance misuse were associated, a causal relationship was not established.

Petrakis I, Carroll K, Gordon L et al 1994 Fluoxetine treatment for dually diagnosed methadone maintained opioid addicts: a pilot study. Journal of Addictive Diseases 13: 25–32

- This small pilot study showed a significant reduction in self-reported drug use in methadone-maintained, opioid-dependent patients prescribed fluoxetine.
- The patients had either comorbid depression or concurrent cocaine use.
- The reduction in depressive symptoms was not significant.

Cheeta S, Schifano F, Oyesfeso A et al 2004 Antidepressant-related deaths and antidepressant prescriptions in England and Wales, 1998–2000. British Journal of Psychiatry 184: 41–47

- Deaths involving antidepressants in combination with other drugs are significantly more likely to occur in those who misuse drugs.
- Caution is therefore required.

Malec TS, Malec EA, Dongier M 1996 Efficacy of buspirone in alcohol dependence: a review. Alcoholism: Clinical and Experimental Research 20: 853–858

- This review of five studies of buspirone in comorbid alcohol dependence and anxiety showed the

effectiveness of buspirone on anxiety symptoms and length of treatment.
- There was no consistent reduction in alcohol use.

Definition

Dual diagnosis in this article refers to people with coexisting mental disorder and substance misuse (including alcohol, nicotine and illicit drugs).

See also the 'Treatment – Psychopharmacology' section in Chapter 26 (Schizophrenia), page 379.

Treatment – Psychological Therapies

Project MATCH

Project MATCH Research Group 1993 Project MATCH: rationale and methods for a multisite clinical trial matching patients to alcoholism treatment. Alcoholism: Clinical and Experimental Research 17: 1130–1145

Project MATCH (a multisite clinical trial of alcohol treatment) was designed to test two a priori hypotheses on how patient–treatment interactions relate to outcome.

Method

- Two parallel matching studies were conducted.
- One study recruited from outpatient settings and the other from patients receiving follow-up after discharge from an inpatient unit.
- Patients were randomly assigned to:
  - 12-step facilitation
  - cognitive behavioural coping skills
  - motivational enhancement therapy.
- There was a 12-week treatment period with follow-up every 3 months for a year.
- Changes in drinking patterns, functional status, quality of life and the utilisation of treatment services were evaluated.

Results

- There was a significant association between low psychiatric severity and the 12-step facilitation therapy.
- The 12-step facilitation therapy led to more abstinent days than those treated with cognitive behavioural therapy.

See also the 'Treatment – Psychological therapies' section in Chapter 25 (Psychological therapies), page 360.

Assessment Tools and Rating Scales

AUDIT

> Saunders J, Aasland O, Babor T et al 1993 Development of the alcohol use disorders identification test (AUDIT): WHO collaborative project on early detection of persons with harmful alcohol consumption. Addiction 88: 791–804; Babor T, Higgins-Biddle J, Saunders J et al 2001 The alcohol use disorders identification test: guidelines for use in primary care, 2nd edn. World Health Organization, Geneva

- 10-item self-report questionnaire which acts as a screening instrument for alcohol use disorders.
- Items are scored 0–4, giving a total between 0 (no problems) and 40 (severe problems.)
- Covers three domains:
  - excessive alcohol intake
  - dependence
  - problems related to drinking.
- A score of more than 8 out of 40 has been deemed to indicate hazardous use.
- A score of over 10 has been used in some studies to indicate dependence.

Severity of Alcohol Dependence Questionnaire (SAD-Q)

> Stockwell T, Murphy D, Hodgson R 1983 The severity of alcohol dependence questionnaire: its use, reliability and validity. British Journal of Addiction 78: 145–155

- 20 questions covering a range of topics regarding dependence (marked from 0 to 3), inquiring about the past 6 months.
- Score:
  - No dependence   <3
  - Mild dependence   4–19
  - Moderate dependence   20–34
  - Severe dependence   35–60

The value of the CAGE in screening for alcohol abuse and alcohol dependence in general clinical populations

> Aertgeerts B, Buntinx F, Kester A 2004 The value of the CAGE in screening for alcohol abuse and alcohol dependence in general clinical populations: a diagnostic meta-analysis. Journal of Clinical Epidemiology 57: 30–39

- Meta-analysis to assess the diagnostic characteristics of the CAGE in screening for alcohol abuse or dependence in a general population.
- The CAGE is of limited diagnostic value using this test for screening purposes at the recommended cut-off of ≥ 2.

Guidelines

Guidance on the use of nicotine replacement therapy (NRT) and bupropion for smoking cessation. NICE Technology Appraisal No. 39*

Guidance

Nicotine replacement therapy (NRT) and bupropion are recommended for smokers who have expressed a desire to quit smoking. NRT or bupropion should normally only be prescribed as part of an abstinent-contingent treatment (ACT), in which the smoker makes a commitment to stop smoking on or before a particular date (target stop date). Smokers should be offered advice and encouragement to aid their attempt to quit. Ideally, initial prescription of NRT or bupropion should be sufficient to last only until 2 weeks after the target stop date. Normally, this will be after 2 weeks of NRT therapy, and 3–4 weeks of bupropion, to allow for the different methods of administration and mode of action. Second prescriptions should be given only to people who have demonstrated that their quit attempt is continuing on reassessment. It is recommended that smokers who are under the age of 18 years, who are pregnant or breastfeeding, or who have unstable cardiovascular disorders should discuss the use of NRT with a relevant healthcare professional before it is prescribed.

Bupropion is not recommended for smokers under the age of 18 years, as its safety and efficacy have not been evaluated for this group. Women who are pregnant or breastfeeding should not use bupropion. If a smoker's attempt to quit is unsuccessful using either NRT or bupropion, the NHS should normally fund no further attempts within 6 months. However, if external factors interfere with an individual's initial attempt to stop smoking, it may be reasonable to try again sooner. There is currently insufficient evidence to recommend the use of NRT and bupropion in combination.

In deciding which of the available therapies to use, and in which order they should be prescribed, practitioners should take into account:
- intention and motivation to quit, and likelihood of compliance
- the availability of counselling or support
- previous usage of smoking cessation aids
- contraindications and potential for adverse effects

* personal preferences of the smoker.

* Reproduced with permission from the National Institute for Health and Clinical Excellence, London.

Management of harmful drinking and alcohol dependence in primary care. SIGN Guideline 74**

Detection and assessment

D   Primary care workers should be alerted by certain presentations and physical signs, to the possibility that alcohol is a contributing factor and should ask about alcohol consumption.

B   Abbreviated forms of AUDIT[†] (*e.g. FAST[†]*) or CAGE[†] plus two consumption questions should be used in primary care when alcohol is a possible contributory factor.

C   In A&E, FAST[†] or PAT[†] should be used for people with an alcohol-related injury.

B   TWEAK[†] and T-ACE[†] (*or shortened versions of AUDIT*) should be used in antenatal and preconception consultations.

Brief interventions

A   General Practitioners (*GPs*) and other primary care health professionals should opportunistically identify hazardous and harmful drinkers and deliver a brief (*10 minute*) intervention.

B   Motivational interviewing techniques should be considered when delivering brief interventions for harmful drinking in primary care.

☑   Staff who deliver motivational interviewing should be appropriately trained.

B   Training for GPs, practice nurses, community nurses and health visitors in the identification of hazardous drinkers and delivery of a brief intervention should be available.

☑   Patients who screen positive for harmful drinking or alcohol dependence in A&E should be encouraged to seek advice from their GP or given information on how to contact another relevant agency.

[†] Details of these screening tests are available in the full guideline or from the SIGN website www.sign.ac.uk

Detoxification

Hospital detoxification is advised if the patient:
* is confused or has hallucinations
* has a history of previous complicated withdrawal
* has epilepsy or a history of fits

* is undernourished
* has severe vomiting or diarrhoea
* is at risk of suicide
* has severe dependence and is unwilling to be seen daily
* has a previously failed home-assisted withdrawal
* has uncontrollable withdrawal symptoms
* has an acute physical or psychiatric illness
* has multiple substance misuse
* has a home environment unsupportive of abstinence.

Community detoxification
Community detoxification is an effective and safe treatment for patients with mild to moderate withdrawal symptoms.

☑   Where community detoxification is offered, it should be delivered using protocols specifying daily monitoring of breath alcohol level and withdrawal symptoms, and dosage adjustment.

☑   Intoxicated patients presenting in GP practice, out-of-hours services and A&E, requesting detoxification should be advised to make a primary care appointment and be given written information about available community agencies.

Pharmacological detoxification
Medication may not be necessary if:
* the patient reports consumption is less than 15 units/day in men or 10 units/day in women and reports neither recent withdrawal symptoms nor recent drinking to prevent withdrawal symptoms
* the patient has no alcohol on breath test, and no withdrawal signs or symptoms.

D   When medication to manage withdrawal is not needed, patients should be informed that at the start of detoxification they may feel nervous or anxious for several days, with difficulty in going to sleep for several nights.

A   Benzodiazepines should be used in primary care to manage withdrawal symptoms in alcohol detoxification, but for a maximum period of 7 days.

D   For patients managed in the community, chlordiazepoxide is the preferred benzodiazepine.

Vitamin supplements

D   Patients with any sign of Wernicke-Korsakov syndrome should receive Pabrinex in a setting with adequate resuscitation facilities. The treatment should be according to British National Formulary (*BNF*) recommendations and should continue over several days, ideally in an inpatient setting.

☑   Patients detoxifying in the community should be given intramuscular Pabrinex (one pair of ampoules daily for 3 days) if they present with features which put them at risk of Wernicke–Korsakov syndrome.

☑   Patients who have a chronic alcohol problem and whose diet may be deficient should be given oral thiamine indefinitely.

Delirium tremens

D   Local protocols for admitting patients with delirium tremens should be in place.

Referral and follow up

A   Access to relapse prevention treatments of established efficacy should be facilitated for alcohol dependent patients.

B   When the patient has an alcohol-related physical disorder, the alcohol treatment agency should have close links with the medical and primary care team.

B   Primary care teams should maintain contact over the long term with patients previously treated by specialist services for alcohol dependence.

Lay services

C   Alcohol-dependent patients should be encouraged to attend Alcoholics Anonymous.

D   If patients are referred to a lay service, agencies where lay counsellors use motivational interviewing and coping skills training should be utilised.

Alcohol dependence and psychiatric illness

B   Patients with an alcohol problem and anxiety or depression should be treated for the alcohol problem first.

☑   Patients with psychoses should be referred for psychiatric advice.

Alternative therapies

There is insufficient evidence to make any recommendations about the use of acupuncture, transcendental meditation or other alternative therapies in treating patients with an alcohol problem.

Patients and families

C   The primary care team should help family members to use behavioural methods which will reinforce reduction of drinking and increase the likelihood that the drinker will seek help.

There is widespread acceptance that the GP is the most appropriate first point of contact once a patient has decided to seek help. However, there are considerable fears or reservations associated with seeking such help even where a good relationship exists with the GP.

Patients often progress from mild misuse of alcohol to more extreme stages so it is important to try to address any problem at an early stage, seeking medical assistance necessary.

Having a family member with an alcohol problem can seriously affect a family, where family members and friends can become anxious, depressed or alienated. Financial problems caused by the purchase of alcohol, coupled with reduced earnings potential also impact on the family.

☑   It should be stressed to patients that stopping or cutting down their drinking can only result from their own decision to do so. Any treatment, from whatever source, can only be an aid to taking this decision and following it through.

Websites

Alcoholics Anonymous
www.alcoholics-anonymous.co.uk
Down Your Drink
Online program for reducing drinking
www.downyourdrink.org.uk

A, B, C and **D** indicate grades of recommendation; ☑ indicates a good practice point (see Appendix II for full details). ** Reproduced with permission from the Scottish Intercollegiate Guidelines Network, Edinburgh.

Annex 3 to SIGN Guideline 74**: The fast alcohol screening test (FAST) for the detection of probable hazardous drinking

For the following questions please circle the answer which best applies. 1 drink = 1 unit = 1/2 pint of beer or 1 glass of wine or 1 single spirits

1. MEN: How often do you have EIGHT or more drinks on one occasion?

    WOMEN: How often do you have SIX or more drinks on one occasion?

    Never
    Less than monthly
    Monthly
    Weekly
    Daily
    or almost daily

    Only ask Questions 2, 3 and 4 if the response to Question 1 is 'Less than monthly' or 'Monthly'

2. How often during the last year have you been unable to remember what happened the night before because you had been drinking?

    Never
    Less than monthly
    Monthly
    Weekly
    Daily
    or almost daily

3. How often during the last year have you failed to do what was normally expected of you because of drink?
   Never
   Less than monthly
   Monthly
   Weekly
   Daily
   or almost daily
4. In the last year has a relative or friend, or a doctor or other health worker been concerned about your drinking or suggested you cut down?
   No
   Yes, on one occasion
   Yes, on more than one occasion

Scoring is quick and can be completed with just a glance at the pattern of responses as follow:

Stage 1

The first stage only involves Question 1.
If the response to Question 1 is Never, then the patient is not misusing alcohol. If the response to Question 1 is Weekly/Daily or Almost Daily, then the patient is a hazardous, harmful or dependent drinker. Over 50% of people will be classified using just this one question. Only consider Questions 2,3 and 4 if the response to Question 1 is Less than monthly or Monthly.

Stage 2

If the response to Question 1 is Less than monthly or Monthly, then each of the four questions is scored 0 to 4. These are then added, resulting in a total score between 0 and 16. The person is misusing alcohol in the total score for all four questions is 3 or more.
Score Questions 1,2 and 3 as follows:
Never = 0
Less than monthly = 1
Monthly = 2
Weekly = 3
Daily or almost daily = 4
Score Question 4 as follows:
No = 0
Yes, on one occasion = 2
Yes, on more than one accasion = 4
In summary, score Questions 1,2 and 3: 0, 1, 2, 3, 4. Score Question 4: 0, 2, 4
The minimum score is 0
The maximum score is 16
The score for hazardous drinking is 3 or more.

** Reproduced with permission from the Scottish Intercollegiate Guidelines Network, Edinburgh.

Annex 4 to SIGN Guideline 74**: The one minute Paddington Alcohol Test (PAT)

Please complete for ALL A&E PATIENTS where there is any INDICATION OF ALCOHOL MISUSE:
e.g. assault, head (especially facial injury), fall, non-specific gastrointestinal problem, 'unwell', fit, blackout, collapse, insomnia, sweating, hypo/hyperglycaemia, palpitations, chest pain, gout, rashes, depression, overdose; note **REPEAT** attendance (perhaps with unexplained symptoms) and **DELAYED** attendance >4 hours (perhaps intoxicated at the time of 'incident').
Remember the elderly presenting with: falls. confusion, incontinence and self-neglect.
1. Quite a number of people have times when they drink more than usual; what is the most you will drink in any one day?
   N.B. Please note if home or pub measures. Units (1 unit = 8 grams alcohol) relating to pub measures, are shown in brackets
2. If this is more than 8 units/day for a man, or 6 units/day for a woman, does this happen:
   Once a week or more? YES: PAT +ve
   or
   Between once a month and once a week? YES: PAT +ve
   or
   Neither (i.e. once a month or less)? YES: PAT -ve (go to Question 3)
3. Do you feel your current attendance in A&E is related to alcohol?
   YES: PAT +ve
   NO: PAT -ve
   i.e. PAT +ve if > 8 units male or 6 units female more than once a month, and/or YES to Question 3.

** Reproduced with permission from the Scottish Intercollegiate Guidelines Network, Edinburgh.

Annex 5 to SIGN Guideline 74**: Important elements of motivational interviewing

Portraying empathy

* Use of open-ended questions and avoiding premature closure
* Respect for individual differences
* Reflective listening so that patients sense you are trying to 'get on their wavelength'
* Expressing interest/concern
* Acceptance that ambivalence is normal.

Type of drink	Amount
Beer/Larger/Cider	Pints (2) or Cans (1.5) = Units/day
Strong Beer/Larger/ Cider	Pints (5) or Cans (4)
Wine	Glasses (1.5) or Bottles (9)
Fortified Wine (Sherry, Martini)	Glasses (1) or Bottles (12)
Spirits (Gin, Whisky, Vodka)	Singles (1) or Doubles (2) or Bottles (30)

Developing discrepancy

- Patients are helped to see the gap between the drinking and its consequences and their own goals/values – the gap between *'where I see myself, and where I want to be'*
- Enhancing their awareness of consequences, perhaps adding feedback about medical symptoms and test results: *'How does this fit in?' 'Would you like the medical research information on this?'*
- Weighting up the pros and cons of change and of not changing
- Progressing the interview so that patients present their own reasons for change.

Avoiding argument (*'in rolling with resistance'*)

- Resistance, if it occurs (such as arguing, denial, interrupting, ignoring) is not dealt with head-on, but accepted as understandable, or sidestepped by shifting focus
- Labelling, such as *'I think you have an alcohol problem'* is unnecessary, and can lead to counterproductive arguing.

Supporting self-efficacy

- Encouraging the belief that change is possible
- Encouraging a collaborative approach (patients are the experts on how they think and feel, and can choose from a menu of possibilities)
- The patient is responsible for choosing and carrying out actions towards change.

Facilitating and reinforcing 'self-motivating statements'

- Recognising that alcohol has caused adverse consequences
- Expressing concern about the effects of drinking
- Expressing the intention to change
- Being optimistic about change.

A tenet of motivational interviewing is *'People believe what they hear themselves say'*.

** Reproduced with permission from the Scottish Intercollegiate Guidelines Network, Edinburgh.

Affective disorders

2

Chapter contents

General topics

Antidepressant-related deaths and antidepressant prescriptions

Cheeta S, Schifaio F, Oyefeso A et al 2004 Antidepressant-related deaths and antidepressant prescriptions in England and Wales, 1998–2000. British Journal of Psychiatry 184: 41–47

It is recognised that newer SSRIs are safer in overdose than the TCAs. However, several questions remain regarding the toxicity of various antidepressants.
- Previous studies have failed to differentiate between accidental deaths and those with suicidal intent.
- Studies have not previously looked at whether certain antidepressants are more likely to be used in multiple overdoses.
- Studies have not examined whether some antidepressants are more likely to be taken in combination with other antidepressants or other psychoactive substances.

Aims

- This study examines the relative toxicity of the major classes of antidepressant drugs, with the specific objective of assessing if the cause of death was accidental or intentional.
- It also analysed deaths where other drugs were present in combination with antidepressants.

Method

- Data were collected from the National Programme of Substance Abuse Deaths (NP-SAD) database.
- Demographics and information regarding the drugs implicated were supplied by the coroner.

Results

- 11.2% of all drug-related deaths involved antidepressant drugs.
- There was substantial variation in the risk of death from different antidepressants.
- TCAs and MAOIs were more often involved than SSRIs.
- The mentions per million prescriptions were:
  - TCAs   12
  - MAOIs   14
  - SSRIs   2
- Dothiepin, amitriptyline and lofepramine were the most frequently prescribed tricyclics.
- Dothiepin and amitriptyline were associated with significantly more deaths, and lofepramine with significantly less.
- The SSRIs were associated with significantly fewer mentions when standardised for the number of prescriptions.
- For the other class of antidepressants, venlafaxine was associated with 88% of fatalities.
- Venlafaxine had mortality rates similar to that of the tricyclics – 13 mentions per million prescriptions of this drug.
- There were 468 deaths in total.

- 60% of deaths had antidepressants solely implicated in death.
- SSRI antidepressants in combinations with other drugs (including alcohol and substances) were three times more likely to cause death than TCAs.
- 20% of deaths were accidental.
- Most deaths related to antidepressants are due to suicide.
- Tricylics were associated with a higher number of accidental and intentional deaths than would be expected, and SSRIs less than would be expected for both.

Limitations

- Non-compliance, undertreatment and non-response to antidepressant therapy contributing to the fatal outcome were not examined.
- Quantity of drugs at postmortem was not available.
- The number of deaths from antidepressants is likely to be underestimated as not all coroners report to NP-SAD.

Witchel HJ, Hancox JC, Nutt DJ 2003 Psychotropic drugs, cardiac arrhythmia, and sudden death. Journal Clinical of Psychopharmacology 23: 58–77

- Toxicity in overdose may be due to modulation of the ion channel function within the myocardium.
- Amitriptyline in particular is associated with inhibition of both the cardiac sodium and potassium channels, which is associated with an increased risk of cardiac arrhythmia and sudden death.

Darcy P, Kelly JP, Leonard BE et al 2002 The effect of lofepramine and other related agents on the motility of Tatrahymena pyriformis. Toxicology Letters 128: 207–214

- The mechanism of lower toxicity of lofepramine is yet to be clarified.
- Lofepramine has membrane-stabilising activities much lower than amitriptyline or desipramine.
- Membrane stabilisation can be associated with cardiac arrhythmias.

Ables AZ, Baughman OL 2003 Antidepressants: update on new agents and indications. American Family Physician 67: 547–554

- SSRIs are more likely than other classes of antidepressant to be prescribed for disorders other than depression, which in turn carry a lower risk of suicide.
- This could therefore account for the lower toxicity of these drugs in overdose.

Fava M 2001 Augmentation and combination strategies in treatment-resistant depression. Journal of Clinical Psychiatry 62 (Suppl 18): 4–11

- Augmentation therapy involving prescribing one antidepressant alongside another is used in treatment-resistant depression or in patients who have only partially responded.
- This may explain the increased number of combination deaths with SSRIs.
- Individuals suffering from treatment-resistant depression may have TCAs and SSRIs prescribed, resulting in more fatal outcomes.
- Augmentation therapy in resistant patients should be monitored carefully given the risk of suicide.

Richelson E 1997 Pharmokinetic drug interactions of new antidepressants: a review of the effects on the metabolism of other drugs. Mayo Clinic Proceedings 72: 835–847

- SSRIs have been shown to differ in their extent of cytochrome p450 enzymes of the liver, which are crucial in the metabolism of numerous drugs.
- This raises the possibility of drug–drug interactions.
- SSRIs inhibit CYP2D6 which can increase the plasma levels of TCAs and increase the toxic effects.

Birth weight and later risk of depression

Gale C, Martyn CN 2004 Birth weight and later risk of depression in a national birth cohort. British Journal of Psychiatry 184: 28–33

There are well-recognised links between childhood circumstances, environment and the risk of affective disorders in adolescence and adulthood. Whether the environment in fetal life is as important is less clear.

Method

- The 1970 British Cohort Study – a longitudinal study of individuals born between 5th and 11th April in England, Wales and Scotland – was used.
- It examined the relationship between birth weight and the risk of psychological distress at the age of 16 years and depression at age 26.
- At age 16 the subjects completed the General Household Questionnaire and the Malaise Inventory.

Results

- Women whose birth weight was ≤ 3 kg had an increased risk of depression at 26 years.
- There was no association found between psychological distress at age 16 in women.
- Men who weighed ≤ 2.5 kg were more likely to be psychologically distressed at age 16 and to report depression at 26.
- Neurodevelopment during fetal life may increase susceptibility to depression.

Kelly TL, Nazaroo JY, McMunn A et al 2001 Birthweight and behavioural problems in children: a modifiable effect. International Journal of Epidemiology 30: 88–94

- Low birth weight leads to behavioural problems in childhood.
- The vulnerability to depression in adolescence or adult life is lacking in direct evidence.

Depression in young adults

Smith DJ, Blackwood DHR 2004 Depression in young adults. Advances in Psychiatric Treatment 10: 4–12

- Earlier age at onset in depression is associated with higher genetic loading and poorer long-term outcome.
- Adolescents and young adults with depression are also at high risk of developing a bipolar illness.

Agerbo E, Nordentoft M, Mortensen PB 2002 Familial, psychiatric and socioeconomic risk factors for suicide in young people: nested case control study. British Medical Journal 325: 74–77

- The commonest cause of death in young men between age 25 and 34 is suicide.
- The strongest risk factors are a history of mental illness and a family history of suicide and mental illness.
- Poor schooling, poverty and unemployment are also important.

Houston K, Hawton K, Shepperd R 2001 Suicide in young people aged 15–24: a psychological autopsy study. Journal of Affective Disorders 63: 159–170

- 70% suffered from mental illness.
- Depression was the most common diagnosis, with 56% affected.
- 30% had a personality disorder.
- 33% had a comorbid psychiatric disorder.
- Few were receiving psychiatric care when they died.

Aalto-Setala T, Marttunen M, Tuulio-Henriksson A et al 2002 Depressive symptoms in adolescence as predictors of early adulthood depressive disorders and maladjustment. American Journal of Psychiatry 159: 1235–1237

- Adolescents with subdiagnostic levels of depressive symptoms show higher rates of early-adulthood depression, substance misuse and adverse psychological and social functioning.

Fombonne E, Wostear G, Cooper V et al 2001 The Maudsley long term follow up of child and adolescent depression.

1: Psychiatric outcomes in adulthood. British Journal of Psychiatry 179: 210–217

- The study followed 149 participants over 20 years.
- 62% experienced a recurrence of major depression.

Fombonne E, Wostear G, Cooper V et al 2001 The Maudsley long term follow up of child and adolescent depression. 2: Suicidality, criminality and social dysfunction in adulthood. British Journal of Psychiatry 179: 218–223

- Suicidal behaviour was high.
- 44% attempted suicide at least once.

Cryanowski J, Ellen F, Young E et al 2000 Adolescent onset of the gender difference in lifetime rates of major depression: a theoretical model. Archives of General Psychiatry 57: 21–27

- Women are twice as likely as men to have depression.
- Before puberty boys are slightly more likely than girls to be depressed.
- Between the ages of 11 and 13 the trend reverses and girls are twice as likely as boys to be depressed.
- The female predominance persists for the next 35–40 years.

Geller B, Zimerman B, Williams M et al 2001 Bipolar disorder at prospective follow up of adults who had pre-pubertal major depressive disorder. American Journal of Psychiatry 158: 125–127

- Prepubertal onset of depression is a strong marker for bipolar disorder.
- Some studies find that at least one-third of depressed children will develop bipolar disorder in adult life.

Rao UM, Ryan ND, Birmaher B et al 1995 Unipolar depression in adolescents: clinical outcome in adulthood. Journal of the American Academy of Child and Adolescent Psychiatry 34: 566–578

- A 7-year prospective study of 28 outpatient adolescents with depression.
- The rate of bipolar disorder in adulthood was almost 20%.

Goldberg JF, Harrow M, Whiteside JE 2001 Risk for bipolar illness in patients initially hospitalized for unipolar depression. American Journal of Psychiatry 158: 1265–1270

- 15-year follow-up of 74 young adults hospitalised for unipolar depression.
- 27% developed subsequent hypomania.
- An additional 19% experienced at least one episode of mania.

- The presence of psychotic symptoms during the index depressive episode was strongly predictive of bipolar disorder.
- Psychotic depression led to bipolar disorder in eight out of 10 patients.
- Bipolar disorder was also associated with a positive family history of mania.

Sullivan P, Neale MC, Kendler KS 2000 Genetic epidemiology of major depression: review and meta-analysis. American Journal of Psychiatry 157: 1552–1562

- Depression runs in families.
- Most of the familiality occurs as a result of genetic rather than environmental influences.

Zubenko G, Zubenko WN, Spiker DG et al 2001 Malignancy of recurrent, early onset depression: a family study. American Journal of Medical Genetics 105: 690–699

- Recurrent, early onset depression (defined as two or more episodes before the age of 25) is associated with a strong family history of affective disorder.
- It appears to run a particularly malignant course, with frequent recurrence, poor response to treatment and high psychiatric and physical comorbidity.
- The heritability estimate of major depression across the lifespan is between 31 and 42%.
- Recurrent early onset depression carries an estimated heritability of 70%.
- Over one-third of first-degree relatives and one-fifth of extended relatives had a history of depression.

Maher B, Marazita ML, Zubenko WN et al 2002 Genetic segregation analysis of recurrent, early onset depression: evidence for single major locus transmission. American Journal of Medical Genetics 114: 214–221

- Segregation analysis of these families was consistent with a single major locus being responsible for the expression of the disorder.

Tambs K, Sundet JM, Eaves L et al 1991 Pedigree analysis of Eysenck Personality Questionnaire scores in monozygotic twin families. Behaviour Genetics 21: 369–382

- Neuroticism (general vulnerability to neurotic breakdown under stress) is a heritable personality trait.

Krueger RF, Caspi A, Moffitt TE et al 1996 Personality traits are differentially linked to mental disorders: a multi-trait–multi-diagnosis study of an adolescent birth cohort. Journal of Abnormal Psychology 105: 299–312

- There is a strong association between high premorbid neuroticism and the subsequent development of a depressive illness.

Kendler KS, Neale MC, Kessler RC et al 1993 A longitudinal twin study of personality and major depression in women. Archives of General Psychiatry 50: 853–862

- Genes that predispose to mood disorders overlap with those implicated in neuroticism.

Farmer A, Redman K, Harris T et al 2002 Neuroticism, extraversion, life events and depression. British Journal of Psychiatry 181: 118–122

- Individuals with high levels of neuroticism are more likely to experience depression after stressful life events than those with low levels.

van Os J, Park SBG, Jones PB 2001 Neuroticism, life events and mental health: evidence for person–environment correlation. British Journal of Psychiatry 178 (Suppl 40): S72–S77

- Evidence is emerging for a significant person–environment interaction whereby individuals with high neuroticism scores select themselves into high-risk environments and as a result become more likely to experience stressful life events.

Ghaziuddin M, Ghaziuddin N, Stein GS 1990 Life events and the recurrence of depression. Canadian Journal of Psychiatry 35: 239–242

- In recurrent depressive disorder, the association between life events and depression is strongest for early episodes and becomes weaker as the number of episodes increases.

Post R 1992 Transduction of psychosocial stress into the neurobiology of recurrent affective disorder. American Journal of Psychiatry 149: 191–201

- Recurrent depressive episodes tend to become more autonomous and are progressively less linked to environmental adversity.
- This process is called kindling.

Kendler K, Thornton L, Gardner C 2001 Genetic risk, number of previous depressive episodes and stressful life events in predicting onset of major depression. American Journal of Psychiatry 158: 582–586

- Kindling tends to be most marked in individuals at low genetic risk of depression.
- Those at high genetic risk of depression tend to exhibit 'prekindling'.
- 'Prekindled' individuals appear to become depressed after only minimal environmental provocation.
- This would suggest that young people with a strong family history of affective disorder are constitutionally

vulnerable to the effects of even minor psychosocial stressors.

Rao U, Daley SE, Hammen C 2000 Relationship between depression and substance use disorders in adolescent women during the transition to adulthood. Journal of the American Academy of Child and Adolescent Psychiatry 39: 215–222

- 5-year longitudinal study of 155 adolescent females.
- 19% developed a substance use disorder.
- Substance use was a marker for the eventual occurrence of depression.

Lewinsohn PM, Rhode P, Seeley JR et al 2000 Natural course of adolescent major depressive disorder in a community sample: predictors of recurrence in young adults. American Journal of Psychiatry 157: 1584–1591

- Prospective follow-up of 274 formerly depressed adolescents to age 24.
- Two-thirds experienced another depressive episode.
- 77% of the third who did not have a further depressive episode were found to have a substance misuse disorder.

Paton GC, Coffey C, Carlin JB et al 2002 Cannabis use and mental health in young people: a cohort study. British Medical Journal 325: 1195–1198

- It may be that those who are premorbidly depressed are more likely to use cannabis as a form of self-medication.
- Daily use of cannabis in adolescence is associated with a significant risk of anxiety and depression by early adulthood.
- This was particularly true for teenage girls – those who used cannabis on a daily basis were five times more likely to have depression than non-users.

Kandel DB, Davies M, Karis D et al 1986 The consequences in young adulthood of adolescent drug involvement. An overview. Archives of General Psychiatry 43: 746–754

- Higher use of cannabis in depressed groups may be related to confounding factors such as social deprivation, early adjustment problems and poor academic achievement.

Brook DW, Brook JS, Zhang C et al 2002 Drug use and the risk of major depressive disorder, alcohol dependence, and substance use disorders. Archives of General Psychiatry 59: 1039–1044

- New York State Children in the Community Study.

- 736 children were followed between the ages of 14 and 27.
- Regular cannabis use was strongly predictive of depression in young adulthood.
- Those who began to use cannabis in their early teens were at much higher risk than those who began in their early twenties.
- Alcohol use at a young age leads to a higher risk of depression in young adulthood.
- Earlier alcohol use predicted not only depression but also any substance use disorder and alcohol dependence by age 27.

Angst J 1998 The emerging epidemiology of hypomania and bipolar II disorder. Journal of Affective disorders 50: 143–151

- When less restrictive diagnostic criteria for bipolar affective disorder are used, the true prevalence of bipolar disorders in the community is at least 5%.
- The diagnostic criterion used was duration of mania less than 7 days.
- Modal duration of manic episodes in bipolar disorder is between 1 and 3 days.

Ghaemi SN, Ko JY, Goodwin FK 2002 Cade's disease and beyond: misdiagnosis, antidepressant use and a proposed definition for bipolar spectrum disorder. Canadian Journal of Psychiatry 47: 125–134

Proposed diagnostic criteria for bipolar spectrum disorder for patients who do not meet the strict DSM-IV criteria for bipolar disorder but who have significant symptoms, i.e.:

A. A major depressive disorder

B. No spontaneous DSM-IV hypomanic or manic episodes

C. Either of the following plus two from D, or both plus one from D:
   a) first-degree relative with bipolar disorder
   b) antidepressant-induced mania or hypomania

D. If none from C, at least six of the following:
   a) hyperthermic personality
   b) more than three depressive episodes
   c) brief major depressive episodes (less than 3 months)
   d) atypical depressive symptoms
   e) psychotic major depressive episodes
   f) early age of onset (under 25 years)
   g) postpartum depression
   h) antidepressant 'wear-off' (acute but not prophylactic response)
   i) lack of response to more than two antidepressant trials.

Ghaemi et al 2002 (as above) and Pies R 2002 The 'softer' end of the bipolar spectrum. Journal of Psychiatric Practice 8: 189–195

Proposed indicators to bipolarity, including:
* early age of onset (under 25)
* multiple episodes of depression, each usually of short duration (under 3 months)
* racing thoughts during depressive episodes
* hyperphagia and weight gain
* lethargy or psychomotor slowing
* poor or short-lived response to antidepressants
* history of bipolar disorder in a first-degree relative, or multiple family members affected by unipolar depression
* psychotic features
* postpartum onset
* manic symptoms induced by electroconvulsive therapy or antidepressants
* hyperthermic personality traits at baseline.

See also the 'General topics' section in Chapter 5 (Child and adolescent psychiatry), pages 72 and 75.

Life events, difficulties and recovery from chronic depression

Brown GW, Adler Z, Bifulco A 1988 Life events, difficulties and recovery from chronic depression. British Journal of Psychiatry 152: 487–498

* In this general population survey for women with chronic depression, 395 women were originally interviewed. Of these, 353 were interviewed again 12 months later. Of 34 women with a diagnosis of clinical depression, 29 were interviewed on a third occasion.
* The Present State Examination (PSE) and the Life Events and Difficulties Schedule (LEDS) were completed. Chronic depression was defined as having episodes lasting 12 months or more. Anxiety disorders were not included.
* It was found that recovery and/or improvement were often preceded by a decrease in ongoing difficulties and by the occurrence of an event which suggested a better time ahead (a 'fresh start' event).
* Examples of difficulty reducing events (or neutralising events) included husband being sent to prison, mother surviving major surgery and husband getting a job.
* Fresh start events included husband being sent to prison, reversal of sterilisation and rehousing.

Brown GW, Harris TO 1978 Social origins of depression: a study of psychiatric disorder in women. Tavistock, London

* This was the first study of depression to use the investigator-based LEDS.
* It linked ongoing major difficulties and perpetuation of depression in a group of women from Camberwell.

Quality of life and function after ECT

McCall WV, Dunn A, Rosenquist PB 2004 Quality of life and function after electroconvulsive therapy. British Journal of Psychiatry 185: 405–409

Aims

This study examines the effects that antidepressant medication and cognitive side effects make in terms of changes in function and quality of life in patients given ECT.

The hypotheses under examination were:
* whether antidepressant efficacy would be associated with improvement in function and quality of life
* whether cognitive side effects would be associated with a dampening of function and quality of life in patients treated with ECT.

Method

* Patients were examined within the month following therapy.
* Patients had a diagnosis of major depressive disorder, were over 18 years and scored over 18 on MMSE.
* Patients were not included if they has received ECT in the preceding 4 months.
* Depression was rated using the BDI and the HRSD at baseline, at the end of treatment and after 4 weeks.
* Cognitive function was assessed with the MMSE.
* Retrograde autobiographical memory was assessed with the Personal Memory Questionnaire.
* Anterograde amnesia was assessed with the Rey Auditory Verbal Learning Test (RAVLT) and the Rey Complex Figure Test.
* Function and quality of life were measured with the Instrumental Activities of Daily Living scale (IADL) and the Personal Self Maintenance Scale (PSMS).
* Quality of life was assessed with the Daily Living and Role Functioning (DLRF) subscale and the Relationship to Self and Others (RSO) subscale of the BASIS-32.

Results

* Prior to ECT the participants had:
  – severe depression
  – minimal cognitive dysfunction
  – significant deficits in quality of life and functional status.
* The immediate post-ECT responder rate was 66%.
* 37% of responders relapsed within the first month of ECT.
* The sample showed improvement in every measure at the 2-week and 4-week time points.

- No improvements were noted on the autobiographical memory test – it records only decline.
- All measures were statistically significant bar the RAVLT.
- Most patients experienced improved quality of life, although some patients had a deterioration on their scores.
- A key finding is that patients experience improvement of quality of life as early as 2 weeks after completion of ECT.

See also Electroconvulsive therapy, Step 5 of NICE Clinical Guideline 23, page 45.

See also the 'Treatment –Others' section in Chapter 17 (Old age psychiatry), page 269.

Treatment – Psychopharmacology

Active placebo versus antidepressants for depression

Moncrieff J, Wessely S, Hardy R A 2004 Active placebo versus antidepressants for depression **(Cochrane Review)**. In: The Cochrane Library, Issue 1. CD003012. Update Software, Oxford

- Nine studies ($n = 751$) were included.
- Two studies produced effect sizes which showed a consistent and statistically significant difference in favour of the active drug.
- The combined results of all the studies favoured the antidepressant in efficacy measured by improvement in mood.
- It may be that in trials using inactive (inert) placebos unblinding effects may increase the benefits of antidepressants. Further examination of this is warranted.

Amitriptyline versus other types of pharmacotherapy for depression

Guaiana G, Barbui C, Hotopf M 2003 Amitriptyline versus other types of pharmacotherapy for depression **(Cochrane Review)**. In: The Cochrane Library, Issue 2. CD004186. Update Software, Oxford

- Treatment with amitriptyline was associated with a greater response than treatment with placebo.
- The number needed to treat (NNT) is 50.
- When compared on continuous outcomes, amitriptyline showed better results than the control agents.

- After stratification by drug class, the efficacy analysis showed no differences in outcome between amitriptyline and either TCAs or SSRIs.
- Dropout rates were similar between groups, although those taking amitriptyline had more side effects.
- Amitriptyline was less well tolerated than SSRIs (NNH 40).
- For treatment setting, amitriptyline was more effective than control antidepressants in inpatients (NNT 24) but not in outpatients (NNT 200).

Antidepressants and benzodiazepines for major depression

Furukawa TA, Streiner DL, Young LT et al 2001 Antidepressants and benzodiazepines for major depression **(Cochrane Review)**. In: The Cochrane Library, Issue 3. CD001026. Update Software, Oxford

- 10 studies ($n = 731$) were identified.
- Those treated with antidepressants and benzodiazepines were less likely to drop out than those receiving antidepressants alone.
- At 4 weeks those receiving antidepressants and benzodiazepines were more likely to improve in terms of their depression (as shown by 50% or greater reduction in the depression scale from baseline).
- At 6–12 weeks the difference was no longer significant.
- Those who received combination treatment were less likely to drop out due to side effects than those receiving antidepressant alone.
- Equal numbers from the two groups reported at least one side effect.

Antidepressant use in clinical practice: efficacy versus effectiveness

Donoghue J, Hylan TR 2001 Antidepressant use in clinical practice: efficacy v. effectiveness. British Journal of Psychiatry 179: S9–S17

How effective an antidepressant is in clinical practice may not be the same as how effective it is in a clinical trial. An antidepressant taken at sufficient dose over an adequate period of time reduces morbidity, improves function and reduces later relapse or recurrence.

Method

- A review of studies of antidepressant prescribing comparing different drugs and different classes.

Results

- Patients treated with TCAs often receive subtherapeutic doses for an insufficient length of time.
- Patients treated with SSRIs are more likely to receive therapy at a sufficient dose for a sufficient length of time.

Balance trials

These ongoing trials of treatment of bipolar depression are outlined in Box 2.1.

Clinical importance of long-term antidepressant treatment

Hirschfeld RMA 2001 Clinical importance of long-term antidepressant treatment. British Journal of Psychiatry 179: S4–S8

Box 2.1

BALANCE trials

BALANCE

- A randomised clinical trial of maintenance treatment for bipolar disorder comparing:
  - lithium and valproate semisodium (Depakote) combination therapy
  - lithium monotherapy
  - valproate semisodium monotherapy.

BALANCE 2

- A two-phase trial comparing treatments for bipolar depression.
- The start-up phase will compare SSRIs with lamotrigine.
- The main trial will compare:
  - SSRIs
  - lamotrigine
  - quetiapine.
- Outcome measures include:
  - number of depressive symptoms at 4 and 12 weeks
  - quality of life
  - time spent in hospital
  - the need for additional treatment for depressive or manic symptoms
  - deliberate self-harm.

Weblink: www.psychiatry.ox.ac.uk/balance.

Depression is increasingly recognised to be a recurrent and, in some, chronic illness.

Method

- A literature review.
- Examined the relationship between the length of antidepressant treatment and the efficacy of treatment.

Results

- One in three patients who responded to initial treatment with an antidepressant will relapse if continuation treatment is not given.
- If medication is continued after an initial response, the relapse rate drops to between 10 and 15%.
- If maintenance treatment is given, between 10 and 30% of patients will relapse.
- Without maintenance treatment up to 60% of patients will have a relapse within 12 months.

Definitions

Initial treatment – stabilisation of acute symptoms, relating to the first 3 months of treatment.

Continuation treatment – the period between the end of the stabilisation phase and the point at which the depression would have spontaneously resolved. This may be a further 6–12 months. Return of symptoms during the continuation phase is termed a relapse of the illness.

Maintenance treatment – prevents further new episodes of illness as well as recurrences, and can extend from the end of continuation treatment for many years.

Drugs versus placebo for dysthymia

Lima MS, Moncrieff J, Soares BGO 2006 Drugs versus placebo for dysthymia **(Cochrane Review)**. In: The Cochrane Library, Issue 2. CD001130. Update Software, Oxford

- 29 trials were included, with 17 providing results on the main outcome measures.
- Drug classes included TCAs, SSRIs, MAOIs and others (sulpiride, amineptine and ritanserin).
- The main measure of outcome used was absence of treatment response.
- For TCAs the RR was 0.68 (NNT 4.3).
- For SSRIs the RR was 0.68 (NNT 5).
- For MAOIs the RR was 0.59 (NNT 2.9).
- The other drugs showed similar results.
- The results were unchanged when full remission was used as the main outcome measure.

- TCAs were more likely than placebo to cause adverse effects and dropouts.

Low dosage tricyclic antidepressants for depression

Furukawa T, McGuire H, Barbui C 2003 Low dosage tricyclic antidepressants for depression (**Cochrane Review**). In: The Cochrane Library, Issue 3. CD003197. Update Software, Oxford

- 35 studies ($n = 2013$) compared low dosage tricyclics with placebo, and six studies ($n = 551$) compared low dosage tricyclics with standard dosage tricyclics.
- At 4 weeks, low dosage tricyclics were 1.65 times more likely to bring about a response than placebo.
- At 6–8 weeks, low dosage tricyclics were 1.47 times more likely to bring about a response than placebo.
- Standard dosage tricyclics were no more effective than low dosage tricyclics.
- Low dosage tricyclics (75–100 mg/day) had fewer dropouts due to side effects than standard dosage tricyclics.

New drugs, old problems: pharmacological management of treatment-resistant depression

Cowen PJ 2005 New drugs, old problems. Revisiting… pharmacological management of treatment resistant depression. Advances in Psychiatric Treatment 11: 19–27

The need for large scale randomised trials of pharmacological treatment in resistant depression is increasingly recognised. A flexible stepped approach is suggested, with earlier use of augmentation strategies for those who have gained limited but definite benefit from an initial treatment, where this will almost certainly be lost when the first preparation is withdrawn.
- It is well recognised that TCAs can be more effective in higher dose, provided tolerance is satisfactory and there are no cardiac issues.
- There is some support for the use of non-selective, irreversible MAOIs in patients resistant to TCAs and other antidepressants.
- There is good evidence from randomised trials that lithium added to ineffective antidepressant treatment can produce useful clinical improvement in partial/non-responders. Lithium appears to be effective in improving antidepressant response when added to different types of treatment including TCAs and SSRIs. The plasma level of lithium required to produce an antidepressant

effect in treatment-resistant depression has not been clearly identified.
- Atypical antipsychotic drugs are increasingly used in depressive psychosis and there have been suggestions that they may be effective as monotherapy. There is preliminary evidence that some atypical antipsychotics may have antidepressant effects when used in combination with SSRIs.
- There is evidence from controlled trials that the addition of L-tryptophan can improve the therapeutic effect of MAOI treatment in patients not selected for treatment resistance. There are no controlled trials to indicate that L-tryptophan produces beneficial effect in patients who have failed to respond to MAOIs or TCAs.
- There is conflicting evidence regarding the augmentation of TCA therapy with thyroid hormone.
- ECT is indicated for treatment-resistant depression, but a history of this may lower the response to ECT.

Nelson JC 2003 Managing treatment resistant major depression. Journal of Clinical Psychiatry 64 (Suppl 1): 5–12

- Switching to a second antidepressant produces benefit in about 50% of patients unresponsive to an initial medication trial.
- Open studies have shown equally good response rates when patients who failed to respond to one SSRI were switched to another (as compared with switching to a different class).
- The results from two controlled trials have not been supportive for the augmentation of SSRI treatment with buspirone.

Fava M 2000 New approaches to the treatment of refractory depression. Journal of Clinical Psychiatry 61 (Suppl 1): 26–32

- 20–30% of patients with major depression fail to respond to treatment with a single antidepressant drug given in adequate dosage for an appropriate period.
- Approximately half of these patients will respond when switched to another antidepressant medication.

Fava M, Rosenbaum JF, McGrath PJ 1994 Lithium and tricyclic augmentation of fluoxetine treatment for major depression: a double blind controlled study. American Journal of Psychiatry 151: 1372–1374

- SSRIs are said to have relatively flat dose–response curves.
- If tolerance permits, increasing the dose of an SSRI can produce symptomatic improvement, particularly in patients who have shown a partial response.

Quitkin FM, McGrath PJ, Stewart JW 1989 Phenelzine and imipramine in mood reactive depressives. Further delineation of the syndrome of atypical depression. Archives of General Psychiatry 46: 787–793

- There is evidence that patients with certain clinical features may have a preferential response to MAOIs.
- The features of atypical depression are mood reactivity, overeating, oversleeping, overwhelming fatigue and rejection sensitivity.
- Patients with atypical depression have significantly higher rates of response to phenelzine than imipramine.

Carpenter LL, Yasmin S, Price LH 2002 A double blind placebo controlled study of antidepressant augmentation with mirtazapine. Biological Psychiatry 51: 183–188

- Best evidence for combination treatment with antidepressants is for the addition of mirtazapine to ineffective SSRI treatment.

Licht RW, Qvitzau S 2002 Treatment strategies in patients with major depression not responding to first-line sertraline treatment. A randomized study of extended duration of treatment, dose increase or mianserin augmentation. Pharmacology 161: 143–151

- A large randomised trial in resistant depression failed to find a benefit of combined sertraline and mianserin (predecessor of mirtazapine) over mianserin alone.

Kennedy N, Paykel ES 2004 Treatment and response in refractory depression: results from a specialist affective disorders service. Journal of Affective Disorders 81: 49–53

- The combination of moclobemide and TCA (combined in some cases with lithium) produced benefit in a significant number of severely depressed, treatment-resistant patients.
- The combination of lithium with MAOIs may be particularly helpful in patients with severe refractory depression.

Bauer M, Dopfmer S 1999 Lithium augmentation in treatment resistant depression: meta-analysis of placebo controlled studies. Archives of General Psychiatry 47: 435–455

- The addition of lithium to antidepressant treatment increased the chance of responding three-fold relative to placebo (OR = 3.3; 95% CI 1.5–7.5).
- The NNT is 3.7.

Shelton RC, Tollefson GD, Tohen M 2001 A novel augmentation strategy for treating resistant major depression. American Journal of Psychiatry 158: 131–134

- A randomised controlled trial of patients resistant to fluoxetine treatment.
- The addition of olanzapine produced a significantly greater response than the addition of placebo or olanzapine monotherapy.

Nemets B, Stahl Z, Belmaker RH 2002 Addition of omega-3 fatty acid to maintenance medication treatment for recurrent unipolar depressive disorder. American Journal of Psychiatry 159: 477–479

- A small double-blind randomised trial.
- 2 g daily of eicosapentanoic acid (EPA) produced a significantly greater response in antidepressant-resistant patients (60%) than did placebo (10%).

Prudic J, Sackheim HA, Devenand DP 1990 Medication resistance and clinical response to ECT. Psychiatric Research 31: 287–296

- In patients whose previous antidepressant therapy had been adequate, the response rate to bilateral ECT was 50%.
- Patients who had not received adequate drug treatment had a response rate of 86%.

Sackheim HA, Prudic J, Devenand DP 1990 The impact of medication resistance and continuation of pharmacotherapy on relapse following response to ECT in major depression. Journal of Clinical Psychopharmacology 10: 96–104

- 50% of patients who responded to ECT relapsed after 1 year.
- The relapse rate in patients who had received adequate antidepressant treatment prior to ECT (64%) was significantly higher than in those who had not (32%).
- Relapse rate after ECT was only weakly influenced by whether or not patients had received adequate antidepressant treatment after the ECT.

Definition

Treatment-resistant depression is one where the depressive syndrome has not responded to a trial of at least one antidepressant medication.

Weblink Texas Medication Algorithm Project – www.dshs.state.tx.us/mhprograms.

Newer versus older antidepressants in long-term pharmacotherapy

Edwards JG 2005 Newer versus older antidepressants in long-term pharmacotherapy. Revisiting... Prevention of relapse and recurrence of depression. Advances in Psychiatric Treatment 11: 184–194

Studies have confirmed the recurrent nature of depression. There are no studies that suggest the choice of one particular antidepressant over another in the treatment of depression, either short or long term. Antidepressant choice may be led by the consideration of unwanted effects. These are discussed in this article, as are effects in overdose and effects in pregnancy.

Lee AS, Murray RM 1988 The long term outcome of Maudsley depressives. British Journal of Psychiatry 153: 741–751

- A 17–19 year follow-up study.
- Found that patients, whose admission to hospital with depression was their first psychiatric contact, had a 50% chance of readmission within their lifetime.
- Patients with previous admissions had a 50% chance of readmission in the subsequent 3 years.
- Fewer than one in five patients remained well.
- More than one in three patients had severe and chronic morbidity or died unnaturally.

Edwards JG 1997 Prevention of relapse and recurrence of depression: newer versus older antidepressants. Advances in Psychiatric Treatment 3: 52–57

- A review of 12 placebo-controlled studies.
- Approximately 59% of patients who respond to an antidepressant treatment will remain in remission, for up to 2 years, when treatment is changed to a placebo.
- This figure is higher in patients who remain on the treatment to which they initially responded.

Geddes JR, Carney SM, Davies C et al 2003 Relapse prevention with antidepressant drug treatment in depressive disorders: a systematic review. Lancet 361: 653–661

- Found a 41% relapse rate on placebo compared with an 18% relapse rate on active treatment.
- Continuing treatment reduced the risk of relapse by 50%.
- Most trials were of 12 months' duration, but the effects of continuing treatment appear to last for 3 years.
- The absolute treatment benefit is greater in patients at higher risk of relapse.

Kessing LV, Hansen MG, Anderson PK 2004 Course of illness in depressive and bipolar disorders. Naturalistic study, 1994–1999. British Journal of Psychiatry 185: 372–377

- This study found that outcomes in severe depression have not changed with the introduction of new antidepressants.

Definitions

Relapse – a worsening of an ongoing or recently treated episode.

Recurrence – a new episode of illness.

Pharmacotherapy for dysthymia

Lima MS, Hotopf M 2003 Pharmacotherapy for dysthymia **(Cochrane Review)**. In: The Cochrane Library, Issue 3. CD004047. Update Software, Oxford

- 14 trials were identified.
- There was no difference between individual antidepressants in terms of clinical response.
- Differences in side effect profiles were noted and should lead clinical management.
- The evidence for TCAs and SSRIs was the strongest in terms of the number of trials and of participants.

Predictors of therapeutic benefit from amitriptyline in mild depression

Paykel ES, Hollyman JA, Freeling P, Sedgwick P 1988 Predictors of therapeutic benefit from amitriptyline in mild depression: a general practice placebo-controlled trial. Journal of Affective Disorders 14: 83–95

General practice patients with depressive disorder as a whole have milder, shorter illnesses than psychiatric patients. It was in the latter group that studies of tricyclic antidepressants had mainly been performed.

Method

- General practice patients with depression ($n = 141$), regarded by the general practitioner to require an antidepressant, were treated for 6 weeks with amitriptyline or placebo in a controlled trial.
- Research Diagnostic Criteria for probable or definite major, minor or intermittent depression were used.
- Exclusion criteria included patients with comorbid psychiatric illness, learning disability, addiction disorder or at high risk of suicide.
- Rating scales included the Present State Examination (PSE), the Research Diagnostic Criteria, the Hamilton Rating Scale for Depression, the Clinical Interview for Depression and the Raskin Three Area Depression Scale.
- Predictor variables were limited to four groups: demographic, illness history, severity of illness and classification of depression (endogenous or not).

Results

- The mean dose of amitriptyline was 119 mg in weeks 4 and 6.
- Amitriptyline was superior to placebo overall in reducing scores on the rating assessments.
- Interactions were examined between drug effects and a number of variables, principally reflecting demographic characteristics, history of illness, severity of illness, and endogenous depression separately in symptoms and stress.
- Only in the area of severity were significant interactions found.
- Amitriptyline was superior to placebo in probable or definite major depression on the Research Diagnostic Criteria, but not in minor depression.
- Amitriptyline was also superior to placebo in subjects with initial scores on the HRSD of 13–15, and 16 or more, but not with lower scores.
- Findings indicate that TCAs are of considerable benefit in relatively mild depression, except in the mildest range.

Selective serotonin reuptake inhibitors versus other antidepressants

Geddes JR, Freemantle N, Mason J, Eccles MP, Boynton J 1999 Selective serotonin reuptake inhibitors (SSRIs) versus other antidepressants for depression **(Cochrane Review)**. In: The Cochrane Library, Issue 4. CD001851. Update Software, Oxford

- 98 trials were included.
- 5044 patients receiving an SSRI or related drug were compared with 4510 patients treated with an alternative antidepressant.
- The standardised effect size for SSRIs and related drugs together versus alternative antidepressants was 0.035 using a fixed effects model.
- No clinically significant differences were found when SSRIs and TCAs were compared in terms of effectiveness.

Treatment discontinuation with selective serotonin reuptake inhibitors versus tricyclic antidepressants

Barbui C, Hotopf M, Freemantle N et al 2000 Treatment discontinuation with selective serotonin reuptake inhibitors (SSRIs) versus tricyclic antidepressants (TCAs) **(Cochrane Review)**. In: The Cochrane Library, Issue 4. CD002791. Update Software, Oxford

- 136 trials were included.
- Patients taking SSRIs were less likely to drop out than those taking TCAs/heterocyclic antidepressants.
- This difference was significant when SSRIs were compared with the older TCAs and the newer TCAs, but not when compared with the heterocyclics alone.
- Differences between SSRIs and TCAs are modest.
- Dropouts for the older TCAs are explained by differences in side effects, not in efficacy.

Tryptophan and 5-hydroxytryptophan for depression

Shaw K, Turner J, Del Mar C 2002 Tryptophan and 5-hydroxytryptophan for depression **(Cochrane Review)**. In: The Cochrane Library, Issue 1. CD003198. Update Software, Oxford

- Of 111 trials, only two ($n = 64$) were of sufficient quality to be included.
- The evidence suggested that these substances were better than placebo (NNT 2.78).
- The data were not of sufficient quality to be conclusive.

Two week delay in onset of action of antidepressants

Mitchell AJ 2006 Two week delay in onset of action of antidepressants: new evidence [editorial]. British Journal of Psychiatry 188: 105–106

- The delay, of several weeks, in the onset of action of antidepressant medication is widely believed.
- Recent evidence has not replicated early trial data regarding the delayed onset hypothesis.
- Very early measurable improvement includes placebo response and additional time is required to distinguish placebo and treatment response.

Posternak MA, Zimmerman M 2005 Is there a delay in the antidepressant effect? A meta-analysis. Journal of Clinical Psychiatry 66: 148–158

- Meta-analysis of 47 double-blind, placebo-controlled antidepressant trials included 5100 patients receiving antidepressants and 3400 receiving placebo.
- Depression outcome was measured with the HRSD.
- Just under a quarter of all differences between the treatment and control groups were apparent by the end of week 1 and 57% by week 2.
- 60% of all improvement occurring in the trials occurred in the first 2 weeks.

- In the majority of the trials the response to treatment was greater in the first 2 weeks than in either the second or the third 2-week period.

Stassen HH, Angst J, Delini-Stula A 1996 Delayed onset of action of antidepressant drugs? Survey of results of Zurich meta-analyses. Pharmacopsychiatry 29: 87–96; Stassen HH, Angst J, Delini-Stula A 1997 Delayed onset of antidepressant drugs? Survey of recent results. European Psychiatry 12: 166–176

- Two large scale studies of 429 and 1277 patients, respectively.
- The effects of medication could be recorded on day 1 regardless of the antidepressant taken.
- By the third day, one in five patients had measurable improvement.
- By the seventh day, one in two patients had measurable improvement.
- 90% of those showing any measurable improvement in the first 3 weeks went on to show full response to treatment.

Parker G, Roy K, Menkes DB et al 2000 How long does it take for antidepressant therapies to act? Australian and New Zealand Journal of Psychiatry 34: 65–70

- This study compared groups who did and did not show response to treatment with antipsychotic medication.
- In all patients there were measurable effects on depression and anxiety symptoms in the first 3 days.
- Non-responders showed little additional improvement in the subsequent 3 days.

Box 2.2

Factors that necessitated admission in clinical trials of outpatient alternatives

All patients

- Severe psychosis
- Violence
- Delusions about the family
- Pathologi amily dynamics
- Assessment of the patient in police custody
- Refusal to take prescribed drugs
- Recurrent overdosing
- Concurrent physical problems

Patients with depression

- Psychosis

Posternak MA, Miller I 2001 Untreated short-term course of major depression: a meta-analysis of outcomes from studies using waiting list control groups. Journal of Affective Disorders 66: 139–146

- This study concluded that spontaneous remission of major depression (derived from waiting list control groups) is around 1 in 10 per month.
- The mean duration of an episode of major depression is 6 months.

Treatment – Psychological Therapies

Treatment of severe depression – non-pharmacological aspects

Porter R, Linsley K, Ferrier N 2001 Treatment of severe depression – non-pharmacological aspects. Advances in Psychiatric Treatment 7: 117–124

A large body of literature exists on the alternatives to inpatient treatment in severe mental illness. It does not establish if relatively rare outcomes, such as suicide, increase if alternatives to hospitalisation are used. Such studies have not generally looked separately at outcomes in patients with affective disorder.

- Inpatient assessment may occur to ensure safety while pharmacological treatment becomes effective (Box 2.2).
- Other aims would include practical and psychological help, education and rehabilitation.
- There is little direct evidence regarding the therapeutic effects of simple supportive nursing or occupational therapy strategies in severe depression.
- Formal nursing observation is usually concentrated on patients who are considered to be at high risk of suicide and may be viewed as negative or punitive.
- Formal nursing observation can ensure that those with severe depressive illness or who are at risk of suicide get one-to-one therapeutic involvement.
- Both cognitive behavioural therapy (CBT) and interpersonal therapy (IPT) have usually been found to be as effective as pharmacotherapy in outpatient depression.
- The studies examining response in severe depression have yielded conflicting results.
- No studies were identified which compare inpatient CBT with standard pharmacotherapy.
- Assessment and investigation of physical health is important in patients with severe depression and

should emphasise adequate hydration, nutrition and mobilisation.

The Sainsbury Centre for Mental Health 1998 Acute problems: a survey of the quality of care in acute psychiatric wards. Sainsbury Centre for Mental Health, London

- 40% of inpatients did not take part in any social or recreational activity during their inpatient stay.
- 30% did not take part in any therapeutic activity.
- Only 5% received psychological therapies.
- Nearly 50% said they had not received enough information about their illness.

Perry A, Tarrier N, Morriss R et al 1999 Randomised controlled trial of efficacy of teaching patients with bipolar disorder to identify early symptoms of relapse and obtain treatment. British Medical Journal 318: 149–153

- Psychological therapies are helpful in bipolar affective disorder and help compliance with medication.

Appleby L 2000 Safer services: conclusions from the report of the National Confidential Inquiry. Advances in Psychiatric Treatment 6: 5–15

- Suicide whilst under intermediate levels of observation (e.g. observation every 10–15 minutes) is relatively common.

Harris EC, Barraclough B 1997 Suicide as an outcome for mental disorders. A meta-analysis. British Journal of Psychiatry 170: 205–228

- Looked at the suicide risk in patients subject to involuntary admission.
- Patients subject to involuntary admission had a standardised mortality ratio (SMR) of 3852 (95% CI 3328–4436).
- The SMR for all patients is 582.
- This probably reflects the greater morbidity and disturbance in the group of patients who require involuntary admission.
- It is important to note that the use of the Mental Health Act does not guarantee the safety of the patient.

DeRubeis RJ, Gelfand LA, Tang TZ et al 1999 Medications versus cognitive behaviour therapy for severely depressed outpatients: meta-analysis of four randomised comparisons. American Journal of Psychiatry 156: 1007–1013

- In the outpatient treatment of severe depression, CBT used twice weekly for the first 4–8 weeks was compared with standard antidepressant medication.

- No statistically significant difference between the treatments, both of which were associated with improvement, was shown.

Elkin I, Shea MT, Watkins JT et al 1989 National Institute of Mental Health Treatment of Depression Collaborative Research Program. General effectiveness of treatments. Archives of General Psychiatry 46: 971–982; discussion 983

- Interpersonal therapy and pharmacotherapy were equally effective in outpatients with severe depression.

Thase ME, Friedman ES 1997 Is psychotherapy an effective treatment for melancholia and other severe depressive states? Journal of Affective Disorders 54: 1–19

- Compared IPT, CBT and IPT in combination with pharmacotherapy.
- Combined therapy was not significantly more effective than psychotherapy alone in milder depression.
- A significant advantage was found for combined therapy in more severe and recurrent depression.

Stuart S, Wright JH, Thase ME et al 1997 Cognitive therapy with inpatients. General Hospital Psychiatry 19: 42–50

- In inpatient depression CBT can be adapted with an increased frequency of sessions.
- It can be used to reduce hopelessness as quickly as possible.
- The programme can be tailored to varied levels of functioning and include significant others as collaborators.

Miller IW, Norman WH, Keitner GI 1989 Cognitive– behavioural treatment of depressed inpatients: six- and twelve-month follow up. American Journal of Psychiatry 146: 1274–1279

- Studied 45 inpatients with depression.
- Patients were assigned to cognitive therapy or social skills training.
- The control group received treatment as usual.
- All treatments began in hospital and continued for 4 months after discharge.
- Significantly higher proportions of the patients who received additional psychotherapy of either kind had responded by the end of the formal treatment period.
- Those who responded did not relapse for the remainder of the 1-year follow-up period.

Inskip HM, Harris EC, Barraclough B 1998 Lifetime risk of suicide for affective disorder, alcoholism and schizophrenia. British Journal of Psychiatry 172: 35–37

- Conclude that about 6% of patients with primary affective disorder will ultimately commit suicide.

Goldstein RB, Black DW, Nasrallah A et al 1991 The prediction of suicide. Sensitivity, specificity and predictive value of a multivariate model applied to suicide among 1906 patients with affective disorders. Archives of General Psychiatry 48: 418–422

- Prospectively followed 1906 patients with affective disorders for up to 13 years.
- 46 suicides occurred during the study period.
- A multiple logistical regression model was created.
- Identified risk factors were male gender, previous suicide attempts (increasing with more attempts), suicidal ideas on admission, less favourable outcome at discharge and unipolar depression with a family history of mania.
- At a threshold of a 50% likelihood of suicide, the multiple regression model did not predict any of the suicides.

Modestin J, Kopp W 1988 Study on suicide in depressed inpatients. Journal of Affective Disorders 15: 157–162

- Examined factors to discriminate between a group of 75 inpatients with depression who committed suicide and 50 non-suicide controls.
- Discriminating factors were male gender, suicidal behaviour at index admission and during hospitalisation, number of previous psychiatric hospitalisations, broken homes and disruption of close interpersonal relationships in the previous year.

Fawcett J, Scheftner WA, Fogg L et al 1990 Time-related predictors of suicide in major affective disorder. American Journal of Psychiatry 147: 1189–1194

- Reported a prospective study of 954 patients with affective disorder, of whom 569 had unipolar depression.
- 32 committed suicide within 10 years.
- Risk factors for suicide within 1 year were anxiety, panic, insomnia, anhedonia, loss of concentration and alcohol misuse.
- Risk factors for later depression were severe hopelessness, suicidal ideation and history of previous suicide attempts.
- In the follow-up study, patients' charts for the week prior to suicide showed that 64% denied suicidal ideation in their last communication.
- 87% were judged to have severe anxiety/agitation in the preceding week.

Dinan TG 1999 The physical consequences of depressive illness [editorial]. British Medical Journal 318: 826

- The acute effects of depressive illness can include dehydration, infection, decubitus ulcer and deep vein thrombosis.
- The long-term effects of depressive illness may include both cardiovascular disease and osteoporosis.

Treatment – Others

Acupuncture for depression

Smith CA, Hay PPJ 2004 Acupuncture for depression **(Cochrane Review)**. In: The Cochrane Library, Issue 3. CD004046. Update Software, Oxford

- Seven trials were included ($n = 517$).
- Five compared acupuncture with medication and two compared acupuncture with sham acupuncture or waiting list control.
- There was no evidence that medication was better than acupuncture in reducing the severity of depression.
- There was no evidence that medication was better than acupuncture in improving depression, where improvement was defined as remission versus no remission.
- Study design was poor, numbers were small and there was insufficient evidence regarding the efficacy of acupuncture in the management of depression.

Distinctive neurocognitive effects of repetitive transcranial magnetic stimulation and ECT in major depression

Schulze-Rauschenbach SC, Harms U, Schlaepfer TE et al 2005 Distinctive neurocognitive effects of repetitive transcranial magnetic stimulation and ECT in major depression. British Journal of Psychiatry 186: 410–416

Looks at the differential impact on cognition between unilateral ECT and left prefrontal rTMS.

Method

- 30 patients with non-psychotic major depression which had not responded to at least two antidepressants for a period of 2 weeks were recruited.
- They had not had previous ECT or rTMS.
- Patients were assessed objectively and subjectively prior to treatment and 1 week post-treatment using HRSD and BDI.
- Psychological battery assessed cognitive effects and the psychologist was masked to treatment assignments.

Results

- Efficacy was comparable.
- 46% of the ECT group and 44% of the rTMS group showed a reduction of 50% or more in HRSD.
- Cognitive performance was unchanged or improved in the rTMS group.
- Subjective memory problems improved in the rTMS group.
- Patients in the ECT group developed memory recall deficits.
- There was no change in their subjective memory problems.

Conclusion

- rTMS has no adverse memory effects in contrast to ECT.
- Self-reported memory impairments after ECT can be related to objective memory deficits and must not be dismissed as being depressive complaints only.
- While the pattern of cognitive findings is in line with previous research, it should be noted that no sham-treated patient control group existed and patients were not randomly assigned.

See also the 'Treatment – Others' section in Chapter 17 (Old age psychiatry), page 269.

Electroconvulsive therapy and newer modalities for the treatment of medication-refractory mental illness

Rasmussen KG, Sampson SM, Rummans TA 2002 Electroconvulsive therapy and newer modalities for the treatment of medication refractory mental illness. Mayo Clinic Proceedings 77(6): 552–556

- Retrograde amnesia related to treatment with ECT can affect recall of events of several months before treatment.
- There can also be sporadic memory loss.
- Memory loss can be permanent.

Abrahams R 1997 Electroconvulsive therapy, 3rd edn. Oxford University Press, New York

- ECT is the most effective treatment for major depression.
- The average response rate is 70–90% which compares with 60–70% for antidepressant medications.

Sackheim HA, Prudic J, Devanand DP 1993 Effects of stimulus intensity and electrode placement on the efficacy and cognitive effects of electroconvulsive therapy. New England Journal of Medicine 328: 839–846

- The anterograde amnesia related to treatment with ECT is temporary.

Definitions

Retrograde amnesia – the inability to recall information learned before the commencement of treatment.

Anterograde amnesia – the inability to recall information learned after the commencement of treatment.

See also the 'Treatment – Others' section in Chapter 17 (Old age psychiatry), page 269.

Light therapy and the management of winter depression

Eagles JM 2004 Light therapy and the management of winter depression. Advances in Psychiatric Treatment 10: 233–240

In winter depression, symptoms typically commence in autumn or winter, peak between December and February and remit during spring and summer. During spring and summer up to a third of patients become hypomanic, usually to a mild degree. Around 3% of adults in the UK are affected to a clinically significant degree. Onset is typically between age 20 and 30. It can occur in children.

Characteristic symptoms include a significant increase in sleep in about three-quarters of patients, with poor quality sleep and associated daytime somnolence which often peaks in the late afternoon. Similar numbers experience increase in weight and in appetite, with prominent cravings for chocolate and carbohydrate.

Increasing appetite, increasing somnolence and decreased activity levels can lead to increasing weight. This in turn can contribute to irritability, deteriorating interpersonal relationships and social withdrawal. Social withdrawal in turn leads to reduced exposure to natural daylight.

Difficulties exist in the methodology of controlled trials of light therapy in terms of selection bias and difficulty with blinding. The evidence to support the use of light visors (baseball caps with light sources in the brim) is not compelling.

Eagles JM, Howie FL, Cameron IM et al 2002 Use of health care services in seasonal affective disorder. British Journal of Psychiatry 180: 449–454

- A primary care study of patients with winter depression.
- These patients undergo more investigations (particularly for anaemia and hypothyroidism) than controls.

- They also receive more prescriptions for a wide range of physical ailments than controls.

Thompson C, Isaacs G 1988 Seasonal affective disorder in a British sample: symptomatology in relation to mode of referral and diagnostic sub-type. Journal of Affective Disorder 14: 1–11

- Anxiety symptoms are common concomitants of winter depression.
- 5–20% of patients experience panic disorder.

Blouin AG, Blouin JH, Aubin P et al 1992 Seasonal patterns of bulimia nervosa. American Journal of Psychiatry 149: 73–81

- Patients with eating disorders, particularly bulimia nervosa, frequently experience a winter exacerbation of their symptoms.

Reichborn-Kjennerud T, Lingjaerde O, Dahl AA 1997 DSM-III personality disorders in seasonal affective disorders: change associated with depression. Comprehensive Psychiatry 38: 43–48

- There are high rates of comorbid personality disorders.
- These lower as patients become euthymic.

Kasper S, Rogers SLB, Yancey A et al 1989 Phototherapy in individuals with and without sub-syndromal seasonal affective disorder. Archives of General Psychiatry 46: 837–844

- Introduced the term 'sub-syndromal seasonal affective disorder' or winter blues to describe a milder form of the condition.
- Symptoms responded to light therapy in a small trial.

Eagles JM, Wileman SM, Cameron IM et al 1999 Seasonal affective disorder among primary care attenders and a community sample in Aberdeen. British Journal of Psychiatry 175: 472–475

- Patients were screened with SPAQ criteria, interviews and DSM-IV criteria.
- The estimated adult community prevalence rates of seasonal affective disorder in Aberdeen were 3.5%.

Michalak EE, Wilkinson C, Dowrick G et al 2001 Seasonal affective disorder: prevalence, detection and current treatment in North Wales. British Journal of Psychiatry 179: 31–34

- Patients were screened with SPAQ criteria, interviews and DSM-IV criteria.
- The estimated adult community prevalence rates of seasonal affective disorder in North Wales were 2.4%.

Swedo SE, Pleeter JD, Richter DM et al 1995 Rates of seasonal affective disorder in children and adolescents. American Journal of Psychiatry 152: 1016–1019

- A large study of seasonal affective disorder among North American children.
- Seasonal affective disorder has low prevalence in young children (male and female).
- After puberty there is a marked rise in the prevalence of seasonal affective disorder in females only.

Mersch PPA, Middendorp HM, Bouhays AL et al 1999 Seasonal affective disorder and latitude: a review of the literature. Journal of Affective Disorders 53: 35–48

- A European study.
- Did not replicate earlier North American studies that showed a clear relationship between prevalence of seasonal affective disorder and increasing latitude of residence.

Magnusson A, Stefansson JG 1993 Prevalence of seasonal affective disorder in Iceland. Archives of General Psychiatry 50: 941–946

- An Icelandic study.
- Found that people who are born and continue to reside at quite northern latitudes experience relatively low rates of seasonal affective disorder.
- It is likely that winter depression would confer a reproductive disadvantage and an increased likelihood of moving south.

Rohan KJ, Sigmon ST, Dorhofer DM 2003 Cognitive–behavioural factors in seasonal affective disorder. Journal of Consulting and Clinical Psychology 71: 22–30

- Trial participants with winter depression tended to have more negative automatic thoughts than controls year round.
- A ruminative thinking style in autumn correlated with the severity of winter symptoms.

Lewy AJ, Bauer BK, Cutler NL et al 1998 Morning vs. evening light treatment of patients with winter depression. Archives of General Psychiatry 55: 890–896

- The best evidence of efficacy for light therapy in seasonal affective disorder is that bright light in the mornings is more helpful than bright light in the evenings.

Thompson C 2001 Evidence-based treatment. In: Partonen T, Magnusson A (eds) Seasonal affective disorder: practice and research. Oxford University Press, Oxford, pp 151–158

- A meta-analysis.
- Treatment with a lightbox in seasonal affective disorder was effective (NNT 5).
- Features associated with a good response to light therapy include hypersomnia, increased appetite, winter weight gain and complete remission of symptoms in summer.
- Less predictable factors include feeling worse in the morning, young age and eating a lot of sweet stuff late in the day.
- Response often commences within days and is usually apparent by the end of week one.
- If treatment adherence is adequate and there has been no response in the first 3 weeks, then subsequent response is unlikely.

Avery DH, Elder DN, Bolte MA et al 2001 Dawn simulation and bright light in the treatment of SAD: a controlled study. Biological Psychiatry 50: 205–216

- Dawn-simulating alarm clocks come on at dim illumination and gradually increase in brightness over a period of 30–90 minutes, leading up to a person's normal waking time.
- They were found to be more efficacious in patients with winter depression and hypersomnia than lightboxes or placebo (dim red) dawn-simulating alarm clocks. This may relate to better compliance with treatment.

Weblink SAD Association – www.sada.org.uk.

Light therapy for non-seasonal depression

Tuunainen A, Kripke DF, Endo T 2004 Light therapy for non-seasonal depression **(Cochrane Review)**. In: The Cochrane Library, Issue 2. CD004050. Update Software, Oxford

- 49 reports from 20 studies were included.
- They combined bright light with drug treatment and/or sleep deprivation.
- Data were limited and the studies were heterogeneous.
- There was no statistical significance between the group receiving bright light and the control treatment group.
- Most studies were short (less than 8 days' duration).
- Statistical significance was reached between the bright light group in the high quality studies, in those using morning light treatment and in sleep deprivation responders.
- Hypomania was more common in the bright light group (NNH 8) compared to the control treatment group.

St John's wort for depression

Linde K, Berner M, Egger M, Mulrow C 2005 St John's wort for depression. Meta analysis of randomised controlled trials. British Journal of Psychiatry 186: 99–107

St John's wort (*Hypericum perforatum*) is widely used for depressive illness.

Method

- A systematic review and meta-analysis.
- This review focuses on factors that may clarify the conflicting results of previous trials – for example, the type and severity of depression and the size of the trials.
- Specific questions examined:
  - Are extracts of St John's wort more effective than placebo and as effective as standard antidepressants in improving symptoms in adults with depression?
  - Are hypericum extracts less effective in patients who meet criteria for major depression than in patients with depressive symptoms who may not meet criteria for major depression?
  - Do trials show that hypericum extracts have less adverse effects than standard antidepressants?

Results

- 37 double-blind randomised controlled trials were included.
- These compared the clinical effects of hypericum (monopreparation) with either placebo or a standard antidepressant in adults with depressive disorder.
- 26 studies compared hypericum with placebo.
- 14 studies compared hypericum with a standard antidepressant.
- *Hypericum perforatum* extracts:
  - improved symptoms more than placebo
  - had a similar effect to standard antidepressants in adults with mild to moderate depression.
- In the larger of the trials there was little difference shown between hypericum extract and placebo in those with major depression.
- The evidence available suggests minor benefits of hypericum in those with major depression and no benefit in patients with prolonged duration of depression.
- There is no evidence of effectiveness for severe depression.
- Hypericum extracts caused fewer adverse effects than older antidepressants.

Gaster B, Holroyd J 2000 St John's wort for depression. A systematic review. Archives of Internal Medicine 160: 152–156

- Systematic reviews conclude that St John's wort is more effective that placebo and is comparable with older antidepressants in the treatment of mild to moderate depression.

Hammerness P, Basch E, Ulbricht C et al 2003 St John's wort: a systematic review of adverse effects and drug interactions for the consultation psychiatrist. Psychosomatics 44: 271–282

- Noted potentially serious interactions with a number of frequently used drugs.

Wurglics M, Schulte-Lobbert S, Dingermann T et al 2003 Rationale and traditionelle Johanniskrautprapaate. Deutsche Apotheker Zeitung 143: 1454–1457

- Found that the preparations can vary greatly, with a number of products containing only a minor amount of the bioactive constituents.

Linde K, Mulrow CD, Berner M, Egger M 2005 St John's wort for depression (Cochrane Review). In: The Cochrane Library, Issue 3. CD000448. Update Software, Oxford

- 37 trials were included.
- 26 compared St John's wort with placebo and 14 with standard antidepressants.
- The placebo-controlled trials showed marked heterogeneity.
- Evidence was inconsistent and confusing.
- For mild to moderate depressive symptoms, St John's wort appeared more efficacious than placebo and as efficacious as standard antidepressants.
- In placebo-controlled studies of patients with major depression, the tested hypericum extracts had minimal beneficial effects.
- Other trials showed hypericum extracts and standard antidepressants to be of similar efficacy.
- Preparations of St John's wort vary widely and these data apply only to those preparations that were tested.

Transcranial magnetic stimulation

Martin JLR, Barbanoj MJ, Schlaepfer TE et al 2001 Transcranial magnetic stimulation for treating depression (Cochrane Review). In: The Cochrane Library, Issue 4. CD003493. Update Software, Oxford

- 16 trials were included, with 14 providing data suitable for quantitative analysis.
- Sample sizes were small.
- There were no differences between rTMS and sham TMS when compared with the BDI or the HRDS.

- There were two exceptions:
  - the first was during the period 2 weeks after treatment for high frequency and left dorsolateral prefrontal cortex stimulation
  - the second was for right dorsolateral prefrontal cortex stimulation of low frequency.
- In both cases the HRDS was used and in both rTMS performed better.
- In patients with psychotic symptoms it was shown using the HRDS that, at 2 weeks after treatment, ECT was more effective than rTMS.

Assessment Tools and Rating Scales

Beck Depression Inventory (BDI)

Beck AT, Ward CH, Mock J, Erbaugh J 1961 An inventory for measuring depression. Archives of General Psychiatry 4: 561–571

- Symptom scale.
- Administered by a health professional or self-rated.
- Designed to measure attitude and symptoms characteristic of depression.
- Covers the 2 weeks prior to evaluation.
- 21 items, each categorised into severity.
- Each item scored from 0 to 3.
- Total is the sum of items.
- <9 indicates no or minimal depression.
- >30 indicates severe depression.
- Reading age of approximately 10 years is required.

Hamilton Depression Rating Scale (HAM-D)

Hamilton M 1960 A rating scale for depression. Journal of Neurology, Neurosurgery and Psychiatry 23: 56–62

- Clinician rated semi-structured interview.
- Designed to measure the severity of depressive symptoms in patients with primary depressive illness. Has been used for depression in other groups.
- Performed by a trained clinician (observation) at a fixed time to avoid influence of diurnal variation.
- 17-item scale.
- Monitors change as well as severity of symptoms during treatment and compares efficacy of various interventions.

- Not diagnostic.
- Validity can be a problem if patients also have somatic symptoms.
- Scores from 0 (no depression) to over 23 (severe depression).

Major Depression Inventory (MDI)

Bech P, Rasmussen N, Olsen R et al 2001 The sensitivity and specificity of the MDI using the Present State Examination as the index of diagnostic validity. Journal of Affective Disorders 66: 159–164

- Self-rated questionnaire used to diagnose depression.
- Measures previous 2 weeks.
- Takes 5–10 minutes to complete.
- Well-researched with good sensitivity and specificity for identifying major depression.
- 10 questions examining how much of the time the patient has experienced the feeling described.
- Answer of 'more than half of the time' in at least half of the questions is indicative of major depression.
- Scored according to DSM-IV and ICD-10 algorithms.

Montgomery–Asberg Depression Rating Scale (MADRS)

Montgomery SA, Asberg M 1979 A new depression scale designed to be sensitive to change. British Journal of Psychiatry 134: 382–389

- Clinician-rated scale for patients with major depressive disorder.
- Measures degree of severity of depressive symptoms and is a particularly sensitive measure of change in symptom severity during treatment.
- Measures current state.
- 10-item checklist.
- Widely used in trials, particularly sensitive to treatment effects.
- Useful for patients with concurrent physical illness as there is a comparative lack of emphasis on somatic symptoms.
- Scores are correlated with global sensitivity measures.

Zung Self-Rated Depression Scale

Zung WW, Durham NC 1965 A self-rating depression scale. Archives of General Psychiatry 12: 63–70

- Self-rated scale to assist in the diagnosis of depression.
- Takes 5–10 minutes to complete.
- 20-item scale, each item scored as how much of the time the feeling has been experienced.

Guidelines

College guidelines on electroconvulsive therapy

Scott AIF 2005 College guidelines on electroconvulsive therapy: an update for prescribers. Advances in Psychiatric Treatment 11: 150–156

The publication of the *ECT Handbook* (Royal College of Psychiatrists 2005) was delayed so that the results of two systematic reviews and the NICE Health Technology Appraisal of ECT in the treatment of depressive illness, mania, schizophrenia and catatonia could be taken into consideration. Changes in mental health legislation were also taken into account – in particular, that mentally competent patients can now refuse ECT. The guidelines are not limited to evidence statements and include the role of other treatments.

The recommendations for ECT in depressive illness differ from NICE guidance in that they allow for the use of ECT as a first-line treatment in other circumstances – for example, continuation or maintenance ECT. It is suggested that in those circumstances the preferences of patients and any previous treatment with ECT are taken into account. True and valid informed consent would be important and there may be a role for a second opinion.

UK ECT Review Group 2003 Efficacy and safety of electro-convulsive therapy in depressive disorders: a systematic review and meta-analysis. Lancet 361: 799–808

- ECT is effective in the short-term treatment of depressive illness.
- ECT is superior to antidepressant medication (the evidence does not include comparison with newer dual-action antidepressants).
- Bilateral ECT is superior to unilateral ECT.
- There is no evidence that ECT given three times a week is more effective than that given twice a week.

Rose D, Wykes T, Leese M et al 2003 Patients' perspectives on electro-convulsive therapy: systematic review. British Medical Journal 326: 1363–1365

- Found that at least one in three patients reported significant memory loss after treatment.

National Institute for Clinical Excellence 2003 Guidance on the use of electroconvulsive therapy. Technology Appraisal 59, April 2003. NICE, London. Online. Available: www.nice. org.uk/pdf/59ectfullguidance.pdf

- The NICE Appraisal Committee recommended that ECT should be restricted to situations where all other options have been tried.
- Life-threatening situations need specific consideration.
- Users reported that the cognitive impairment associated with ECT outweighed any benefit. This requires special consideration.

Van der Broek WW, de Lely A, Mulder PGH et al 2004 Effect of antidepressant medication resistance on short-term response to electroconvulsive therapy. Journal of Clinical Psychopharmacology 24: 400–403

- A prospective study.
- Patients who had failed to respond to antidepressant drug treatment were less likely to respond to subsequent ECT.
- This conflicts with other evidence.

Sackheim HA, Prudic J, Devenand DP et al 2000 A prospective, randomized double-blind comparison of bilateral and right unilateral electroconvulsive therapy at different stimulus intensities. Archives of General Psychiatry 57: 425–434

- Patients who receive bilateral ECT take significantly longer to become reorientated and are more likely to have prolonged disorientation.
- Unilateral ECT was found to be effective for some patients with depressive disorder. Stimulus dosing is important.
- Some patients who did not respond to high dose unilateral ECT will respond to bilateral ECT.

Lisanby SH, Maddox JH, Prudic J et al 2000 The effects of electroconvulsive therapy on memory of autobiographical and public events. Archives of General Psychiatry 57: 581–590

- The loss of autobiographical memory for the months or years preceding a course of ECT is more likely to last longer than 2 months when patients receive bilateral ECT.

Depression: management of depression in primary and secondary care. NICE Clinical Guideline 23*

Step 1: Recognition of depression in primary care and general hospital settings

- In primary care and general hospital settings, screen patients with: [C]
  - a past history of depression
  - significant physical illnesses causing disability
  - other mental health problems, such as dementia.
- Bear in mind the potential physical causes of depression and the possibility that depression can be caused by medication. [C]
- Use two screening questions, such as: [B]
  - 'During the last month, have you often been bothered by feeling down, depressed or hopeless?' *and*
  - 'During the last month, have you often been bothered by having little interest or pleasure in doing things?'

Step 2: Treatment of mild depression in primary care

Watchful waiting
- In mild depression, if the patient does not want treatment or may recover with no intervention, arrange further assessment–normally within 2 weeks. [C]

Sleep and anxiety management
- Consider advice on sleep hygiene and anxiety management. [C]

Exercise
- Advise patients of all ages with mild depression of the benefits of following a structured and supervised exercise programme. Effective duration of such programmes is up to three sessions per week of moderate duration (45 minutes to 1 hour) for between 10 and 12 weeks. [C]

Guided self-help
- For patients with mild depression, consider a guided self-help programme that consists of the provision of appropriate written materials and limited support over 6–9 weeks, including follow-up, from a professional who typically introduces the self-help programme and reviews progress and outcome. [C]

Psychological interventions
- In mild and moderate depression, consider psychological treatment specifically focused on depression (problem-solving therapy, brief CBT and counselling) of 6–8 sessions over 10–12 weeks. [B]

- Offer the same range of treatments to older people as to younger people. [C]
- In psychological interventions, therapist competence and therapeutic alliance have significant bearing on the outcome of intervention. [C]
- Where significant comorbidity exists, consider extending treatment duration or focusing specifically on comorbid problems. [C]

Antidepressants

- Antidepressants are not recommended for the initial treatment of mild depression, because the risk–benefit ratio is poor. [C]
- Where mild depression persists after other interventions, or is associated with psychosocial and medical problems, consider use of an antidepressant. [C]
- If a patient with a history of moderate or severe depression presents with mild depression, consider use of an antidepressant (see Step 3). [C]

Review in mild depression

- Consider contacting all patients with mild depression who do not attend follow-up appointments. [C]

Step 3: Treatment of moderate to severe depression in primary care

Starting treatment

- In moderate depression, offer antidepressant medication to all patients routinely, before psychological interventions. [B]
- Discuss the patient's fears of addiction or other concerns about medication. For example, explain that craving and tolerance do not occur. [GPP]
- When starting treatment, tell patients about: [C]
  – the risk of discontinuation/withdrawal symptoms
  – potential side effects.
- Inform patients about the delay in onset of effect, the time course of treatment and the need to take medication as prescibed. Make available written information appropriate to the patient's needs. [GPP]

Monitoring risk

- See patients who are considered to be at increased risk of suicide or who are younger than 30 years old 1 week after starting treatment. Monitor frequently until the risk is no longer significant. [C]
- If there is a high risk of suicide, prescribe a limited quantity of antidepressants. [C]
- If there is a high risk of suicide consider additional support such as more frequent contacts with primary care staff, or telephone contacts. [C]
- Monitor for signs of akathisia, suicidal ideas, and increased anxiety and agitation, particularly in the early stages of treatment with an SSRI. [C]

- Advise patients of the risk of these symptoms, and that they should seek help promptly if these are at all distressing. [C]
- If a patient develops marked and/or prolonged akathisia or agitation while taking an antidepressant, review the use of the drug. [C]

Continuing treatment

- See patients who are not considered to be at increased risk of suicide 2 weeks after starting treatment and regularly thereafter – for example, every 2–4 weeks in the first 3 months – reducing the frequency if response is good. [C]
- For patients with a moderate or severe depressive episode, continue antidepressants for at least 6 months after remission. [A]
- Once a patient has taken antidepressants for 6 months after remission, review the need for continued antidepressant treatment. This review may include consideration of the number of previous episodes, presence of residual symptoms, and concurrent psychosocial difficulties. [C]

Choice of antidepressants

- For routine care, use an SSRI because they are as effective as tricyclic antidepressants and less likely to be discontinued because of side effects. [A]
- Consider using a generic form of SSRI. Fluoxetine or citalopram, for example, would be reasonable choices because they are generally associated with fewer discontinuation/withdrawal symptoms. Note the higher propensity of fluoxetine for drug interactions. [C]
- Treatments such as dosulepin, phenelzine, combined antidepressants, and lithium augmentation of antidepressants should be routinely initiated only by specialist mental healthcare professionals (including general practitioners with a special interest in mental health). [C]
- Venlafaxine should be initiated only by specialist mental health medical practitioners, including general practitioners with a special interest in mental health. [C]
- Venlafaxine should be managed only under the supervision of specialist mental health medical practitioners, including general practitioners with a special interest in mental health. [C]
- Consider toxicity in overdose; note that tricyclics (with the exception of lofepramine) are more dangerous in overdose. [C]
- If increased agitation develops early in treatment with an SSRI, provide appropriate information and, if the patient prefers, either change to a different antidepressant or consider a brief period of concomitant treatment with a benzodiazepine followed by a clinical review within 2 weeks. [C]
- St. John's wort may be of benefit in mild or moderate depression, but its use should not be prescribed or

advised because of uncertainty about appropriate doses, variation in the nature of preparations, and potential serious interactions with other drugs. [C]

- Tell patients taking St John's wort about the different potencies of the preparations available and the uncertainty that arises from this, and about the interactions of St John's wort with other drugs (including oral contraceptives, anticoagulants and anticonvulsants). [C]

Pharmacological treatment of atypical depression

- Treat patients with features of atypical depression with an SSRI. [C]
- If there is no response to an SSRI and there is significant functional impairment, consider referral to a mental health specialist. [GPP]

Stopping or reducing antidepressants

- Inform patients about the possibility of discontinuation/ withdrawal symptoms on stopping or missing doses or reducing the dose. These symptoms are usually mild and self-limiting but can occasionally be severe, particularly if the drug is stopped abruptly. [C]
- Advise patients to take their drugs as prescribed, particularly drugs with a shorter half-life (such as paroxetine). [C]
- Reduce doses gradually over a 4-week period; some people may require longer periods, and fluoxetine can usually be stopped over a shorter period. [C]
- For mild discontinuation/withdrawal symptoms, reassure the patient and monitor symptoms. [C]
- For severe symptoms, consider reintroducing the original antidepressant at the effective dose (or another antidepressant with a longer half-life from the same class) and reduce gradually while monitoring symptoms. [C]
- Ask patients to seek advice from their medical practitioner if they experience significant discontinuation/withdrawal symptoms. [GPP]

Special patient characteristics

Gender

- Note that women have a poorer toleration of imipramine. [B]

Age

- For older adults with depression, give antidepressant treatment at an age-appropriate dose for a minimum of 6 weeks before considering that it is ineffective. If there is a partial response within this period, treatment should be continued for a further 6 weeks. [C]
- When prescribing antidepressants for older adults, consider:
  - the increased risk of drug interactions [GPP]
  - careful monitoring of side effects, particularly with tricyclic antidepressants. [C]

Patients with dementia

- Treat depression in people with dementia in the same way as depression in other older adults. [C]

Patients with cardiovascular disease

- When initiating antidepressant treatment in patients with ischaemic heart disease, note that sertraline has the best evidence base. [B]
- Consider the increased risks associated with tricyclic antidepressants in patients with cardiovascular disease. [GPP]
- Perform an ECG before prescibing a tricyclic antidepressant for a depressed patient at significant risk of cardiovascular disease. [GPP]
- Venlafaxine should not be prescribed for patients with pre-existing heart disease. [C]

Limited response to initial treatment in moderate and severe depression

Pharmacological approaches

- When a patient fails to respond to the first antidepressant prescribed, check that the drug has been taken regularly and at the prescribed dose. [GPP]
- If response to a standard dose of an antidepressant is inadequate, and there are no significant side effects, consider a gradual increase in dose in line with the schedule suggested by the Summary of Product Characteristics. [C]
- Consider switching to another antidepressant if there has been no response after a month. If there has been a partial response, a decision to switch can be postponed until 6 weeks. [C]
- If an antidepressant has not been effective or is poorly tolerated and, after considering a range of other treatment options, the decision is made to offer a further course of antidepressants, then switch to another single antidepressant. [C]
- Choices for a second antidepressant include a different SSRI or mirtazapine; alternatives include moclobemide, reboxetine and tricyclic antidepressants (except dosulepin) (but see below). [B]
- When switching from one antidepressant to another, be aware of the need for gradual and modest incremental increases of dose, of interactions between antidepressants, and the risk of serotonin syndrome when combinations of serotonergic antidepressants are prescribed. Features include confusion, delirium, shivering, sweating, changes in blood pressure, and myoclonus. [C]

Special considerations when switching to a new antidepressant other than a tricyclic

- If switching to mirtazapine, be aware that it can cause sedation and weight gain. [A]

- If switching to moclobemide, be aware of the need to wash out previously prescribed antidepressants. [**A**]
- If switching to reboxetine, be aware of its relative lack of data on side effects, and monitor carefully. [**B**]

Special considerations when switching to a new tricyclic antidepressant

- Consider their poorer tolerability compared with other equally effective antidepressants, and the increased risk of cardiotoxicity and toxicity in overdose. [**B**]
- Start on a low dose and, if there is a clear clinical response, maintain on that dose with careful monitoring. [**C**]
- Gradually increase dose if there is lack of efficacy and no major side effects. [**GPP**]
- Lofepramine is a reasonable choice because of its relative lack of cardiotoxicity. [**C**]

Psychological treatments

- CBT is the psychological treatment of choice. Consider interpersonal psychotherapy (IPT) if the patient expresses a preference for it or if you think the patient may benefit from it. [**B**]
- CBT and IPT should be delivered by a healthcare professional competent in their use–treatment typically consists of 16–20 sessions over 6–9 months. [**B**]
- Consider CBT (or IPT) for patients with moderate or severe depression who do not take or refuse antidepressant treatment. [**B**]
- For patients who have not made an adequate response to other treatments for depression (e.g. antidepressants and brief psychological interventions), consider giving a course of CBT of 16–20 sessions over 6–9 months. [**C**]
- Consider CBT for patients with severe depression for whom avoiding the side effects often associated with antidepressants is a clinical priority or personal preference. [**B**]
- For patients with severe depression, consider providing two sessions of CBT per week for the first month of treatment. [**C**]
- Where patients have responded to a course of individual CBT or IPT, consider offering follow-up sessions– typically two to four sessions over 12 months. [**C**]

Initial presentation of severe depression

- When patients present initially with severe depression, a combination of antidepressants and individual CBT should be considered as it is more cost effective than either treatment on its own. [**B**]

Couple-focused therapy

- Consider couple-focused therapy for people with depression who have a regular partner and who have not benefited from a brief individual intervention. An adequate course is 15–20 sessions over 5–6 months. [**B**]

Chronic depression

- In chronic depression, offer a combination of individual CBT and antidepressant medication. [**A**]

- For men with chronic depression who have not responded to an SSRI, consider a tricyclic antidepressant, as men tolerate the side effects of tricyclic antidepressants reasonably well. [**C**]
- Consider offering befriending (by trained volunteers offering weekly meetings for 2–6 months) as an adjunct to pharmacological or psychological treatments to people with chronic depression. [**C**]
- Consider a rehabilitation programme for patients who are unemployed, or have been disengaged from social activities over a longer term. [**C**]

Enhanced care in primary care

- For all patients, consider telephone support from the primary care team, informed by clear treatment protocols, particularly for monitoring antidepressant medication regimens. [**B**]
- Primary care organisations should consider establishing multifaceted care programmes, which integrate through clearly specified protocols the delivery and monitoring of appropriate psychological and pharmacological interventions for the care of people with depression. [**C**]

Step 4: Treatment of depression by mental health specialists including crisis teams

- Assess patients with depression referred to specialist care, including their symptom profile and suicide risk and, where appropriate, previous treatment history. Where the depression is chronic or recurrent, assess psychosocial stressors, personality factors and significant relationship difficulties as well. [**GPP**]
- Consider re-introducing any previous treatments that were inadequately delivered or adhered to. [**GPP**]
- Crisis resolution teams should be used as a means of managing crises for patients who have severe depression and are assessed as presenting significant risk. [**C**]
- Medication in specialist services should be initiated under the supervision of a consultant psychiatrist. [**GPP**]

Treatment-resistant depression

- For all people whose depression is treatment resistant, consider the combination of antidepressant medication with individual CBT of 16–20 sessions over 6–9 months. [**B**]
- For patients with treatment-resistant moderate depression who have relapsed while taking, or after finishing, a course of antidepressants, consider the combination of antidepressant medication with CBT. [**B**]

- Consider a trial of lithium augmentation for patients whose depression has failed to respond to several antidepressants and who are prepared to tolerate the burdens associated with its use. [**B**]
- Before initiating lithium augmentation, carry out an ECG. [**C**]
- Venlafaxine may be considered for patients who have failed two adequate trials of alternative antidepressants. The dose can be increased up to *BNF* limits if required, provided patients can tolerate the side effects. [**C**]
- When prescribing venlafaxine, be aware of:
  - the increased likelihood of patients stopping treatment because of side effects, compared with equally effective SSRIs [**A**]
  - its higher cost [**C**]
  - its high propensity for discontinuation/withdrawal symptoms if stopped abruptly [**C**]
  - its toxicity in overdose. [**C**]
- Before prescribing venlafaxine, carry out an ECG and measure blood pressure. [**C**]
- For patients prescribed venlafaxine, consider monitoring cardiac function. Undertake regular monitoring of blood pressure, particularly for patients on higher doses. [**C**]
- Consider augmenting an antidepressant with another antidepressant (there is evidence for benefits of adding mianserin or mirtazapine to SSRIs). [**C**]
- When augmenting one antidepressant with another, monitor carefully (particularly for the symptoms of serotonin syndrome), and explain the importance of this to the patient. [**GPP**]
- When augmenting an antidepressant with mianserin, be aware of the risk of agranulocytosis, particularly in older adults. [**C**]
- Re-evaluate the adequacy or previous treatments and consider seeking a second opinion if considering using combinations of antidepressants other than mianserin or mirtazapine with SSRIs. Document the content of any discussion in the notes. [**C**]
- Consider phenelzine for patients who have failed to respond to alternative antidepressants and who are prepared to tolerate the side effects and dietary restrictions associated with its use. Consider its toxicity in overdose when prescribing for patients at high risk of suicide. [**C**]
- Augmentation of an antidepressant with carbamazepine, lamotrigine, buspirone, pindolol, valproate or thyroid supplementation is not recommended in the routine management of treatment-resistant depression. [**B**]
- Consider referring patients who have failed to respond to various strategies for augmentation and combination treatments to a clinician with a specialist interest in treating depression. [**GPP**]
- Dosulepin should not be used routinely because the evidence supporting its tolerability relative to other

antidepressants is outweighed by the increased cardiac risk and its toxicity in overdose. [**C**]
- There is insufficient evidence to recommend augmentation of antidepressants with benzodiazepines. [**C**]

Recurrent depression and relapse prevention

Pharmacological treatments
- Continue antidepressants for 2 years for people who have had two or more depressive episodes in the recent past and who have experienced significant functional impairment during the episodes. [**B**]
- Re-evaluate patients on maintenance treatment, taking into account age, comorbid conditions and other risk factors in the decision to continue the treatment beyond 2 years. [**GPP**]
- Maintain the antidepressant dose used for relapse prevention at the level at which acute treatment was effective. [**C**]
- Patients who have had multiple episodes of depression, and who have had a good response to treatment with an antidepressant and lithium augmentation, should remain on the combination for at least 6 months. [**B**]
- When patients are taking an antidepressant with lithium augmentation, if one drug is to be discontinued, this should be lithium in preference to the antidepressant. [**C**]

Psychological treatments
- CBT should be considered for:
  - patients with recurrent depression, who have relapsed despite antidepressant treatment, or who express a preference for psychological interventions [**C**]
  - patients with a history of relapse and poor or limited response to other interventions [**B**]
  - patients who have responded to another intervention but are unable or unwilling to continue with that intervention, and are assessed as being at significant risk of relapse. [**B**]
- Mindfulness-based CBT should be considered for patients with recurrent depression. [**B**]

Special considerations

Psychotic depression
- For patients with psychotic depression, consider augmentation of the current treatment plan with antipsychotic medication. [**C**]

Atypical depression
- Consider prescribing phenelzine for women whose depression has atypical features, and who have not responded to, or who cannot tolerate, an SSRI. Consider its toxicity in overdose when prescribing for patients at high risk of suicide. [**C**]
- All patients receiving phenelzine require careful monitoring (including taking blood pressure) and

advice on interactions with other medicines and foodstuffs, and should have their attention drawn to the product information leaflet. [**C**]

Step 5: Inpatient treatment for depression

Inpatient care

* Inpatient treatment should be considered for people with depression where the patient is at significant risk of suicide or self-harm. [**C**]
* Crisis resolution teams should be considered for patients with depression who might benefit from an early discharge from hospital after a period of inpatient care. [**C**]

Electroconvulsive therapy

* Electroconvulsive therapy (ECT) should only be used to achieve rapid and short-term improvement of severe symptoms after an adequate trial of other treatments has proven ineffective, and/or when the condition is considered to be potentially life threatening, in a severe depressive illness. [**N**]
* When considering ECT, review risks and potential benefits to the individual, including: the risks associated with the anaesthetic; current comorbidities; anticipated adverse events, particularly cognitive impairment; and the risks of not having treatment. [**N**]
* Particular care is needed when considering ECT treatment during pregnancy, in older people, and in children and young people, because the risks may be increased. [**N**]
* Valid consent should be obtained in all cases where the individual has the ability to grant or refuse consent. The decision to use ECT should be made jointly by the individual and the clinician(s) responsible for treatment, on the basis of an informed discussion. This discussion should be enabled by the provision of full and appropriate information about the general risks associated with ECT and about the risks and potential benefits specific to that individual. [**N**]
* Advance directives should be taken fully into account and the individual's advocate and/or carer should be consulted. [**N**]
* Clinical status should be assessed after each ECT session and treatment should be stopped when a response has been achieved, or sooner if there is evidence of adverse effects. Cognitive function should be monitored on an ongoing basis, and at a minimum at the end of each course of treatment. [**N**]
* A repeat course of ECT should be considered under the circumstances indicated above only for individuals who have depressive illness, and who have previously responded well to ECT. [**N**]

* In patients who are experiencing an acute episode but have not previously responded, a repeat trial of ECT should be undertaken only after all other options have been considered and following discussion of the risks and benefits with the individual and/or where appropriate their carer/advocate. [**N**]
* As the longer-term benefits and risks of ECT have not been clearly established, it is not recommended as a maintenance therapy in depressive illness. [**N**]

A, B, C and **D** indicate grades of recommendation; **GPP** indicates a good practice point; **N** indicates evidence from NICE technology appraisal guidance (see Appendix II for full details). * Reproduced with permission from the National Institute for Health and Clinical Excellence, London.

NICE, but will they help people with depression?

Whitty P, Gilbody S 2005 NICE, but will they help people with depression? The new National Institute for Clinical Excellence depression guidelines [editorial]. British Journal of Psychiatry 186: 177–178

Background

NICE guidelines on managing depression in primary and secondary care have been in development since 2001 and were delivered in 2004. The guidelines are clear, concise and cover all the key aspects of diagnosis and management:
* screening – for high-risk groups
* distinguishing between mild, moderate and severe depression
* assessing the risk of self-harm and suicide
* benefits of 'watchful waiting' with mild depression
* when to offer CBT
* the use of SSRIs – first line in most circumstances
* early use of combined treatment in severe depression
* guidance on maintenance therapy
* guidance on discontinuing treatment.

They will be most useful in primary care as this is where most depression is treated.

The NICE guidelines do not give any recommendations on the organisational interventions that have been shown to be effective.

Method

* A systematic review.
* Articles on educational and organisational interventions improving the management of depression in primary care were examined.
* Collaborative care includes patient and clinician education, along with shared care between various healthcare professionals (this is a vast enhancement of the working relationship between primary and secondary care).

Results

- Case management seemed to have a positive effect in delivering the care.
- Investment in case management and related organisational interventions in primary care is needed as well as considerably improving the relationship between primary and secondary care.
- Graduate primary care workers should be involved in this process.

Singleton N, Bumpstead R, O'Brian M et al 2001 Office for National Statistics: psychiatric morbidity among adults living in private households, 2000. The Stationery Office, London

- Depression affects 5–10% of individuals in the UK.
- Depression is the third most common reason for consulting a general practitioner.
- Given the different ways it can present, it may well go unrecognised.

Dowrick C, Buchan I 1995 Twelve months outcome of depression in general practice: does detection or disclosure make a difference? British Medical Journal 311: 1274–1276

- Reported that depressive symptoms are not recognised in around half of those attending their GP.

Rost K, Zhang M, Fortney J et al 1998 Persistently poor outcomes of undetected major depression in primary care. General Hospital Psychiatry 20: 12–20

- Found that unrecognised depression is associated with poor treatment outcomes.

Gilbody S, Whitty P, Grimshaw JG et al 2002 Improving the recognition and management of depression in primary care. University of York, York

- Guidelines will not improve the treatment of depression in primary care unless the working relationship between primary and secondary care improves.

Anxiety disorders

3

Chapter contents

Treatment – Psychopharmacology

Antidepressants for generalised anxiety disorder

Kapczinski F, Lima MS, Souza JS et al 2003 Antidepressants for generalized anxiety disorder (**Cochrane Review**). In: The Cochrane Library, Issue 2. CD003592. Update Software, Oxford

- Imipramine, venlafaxine and paroxetine were found to be better than placebo in treating GAD (NNT = 5.15).
- There were no differences in dropout rates.
- Only one study included children and adolescents and it suggested encouraging results in the use of sertraline in this group.
- Further study is warranted.

Pharmacotherapy for social anxiety disorder

Stein DJ, Ipser JC, van Balkom AJ 2006 Pharmacotherapy for social anxiety disorder (**Cochrane Review**). In: The Cochrane Library, Issue 2. Update Software, Oxford

- 37 RCTs were included ($n = 5264$) of a number of different medications.
- 23 trials were of less than 14 weeks' duration.
- Publication bias was evident on funnel plot analysis.

- Short-term superiority was shown for all medications over placebo.
- SSRIs were significantly more effective than moclobemide.
- There were statistically significant differences between medication and placebo for symptom severity and this was most marked for the SSRIs.
- Those in the treatment groups had reduced symptoms of social phobia, fewer comorbid depressive symptoms and less associated disability.
- Eight trials (four maintenance and four relapse prevention) showed the value of longer-term medication in treatment responders.

Assessment Tools and Rating Scales

Hospital Anxiety Depression Scale (HAD)

Zigmind AS, Snaith RP 1983 The hospital anxiety and depression scale. Acta Psychiatrica Scandinavica 67: 361–370

- Self-administered scale which assesses the presence and severity of depression and anxiety in patients in non-psychiatric hospital settings or in primary care or community settings.

- Measures symptoms and functioning for the past few days.
- Very quick to complete.
- Anxiety and depression are assessed as separate components, each with seven items scored from 0 to 3.

See also the 'Assessment tools and rating scales' section in Chapter 2 (Affective disorders), page 43.

Hamilton Anxiety Rating Scale (HAM-A)

Hamilton M 1959 The assessment of anxiety states by rating. British Journal of Medical Psychology 32: 50–55

- Clinician-rated scale which quantifies severity of anxiety symptoms.
- Can also assess the response to therapeutic interventions.

- Assesses symptoms over the past week.
- 14 items scored 0 to 4:
  - anxious mood
  - tension
  - fear
  - insomnia
  - intellectual impairment
  - depressed mood
  - somatic muscular complaints
  - somatic sensory complaints
  - cardiovascular symptoms
  - respiratory symptoms
  - GI symptoms
  - GU symptoms
  - autonomic symptoms
  - patient's behaviour at interview.

Guidelines

Anxiety: management of anxiety (panic disorder, with or without agoraphobia, and generalised anxiety disorder) in adults in primary, secondary and community care. NICE Clinical Guideline 22*: Steps 2–4

see pages 56–59

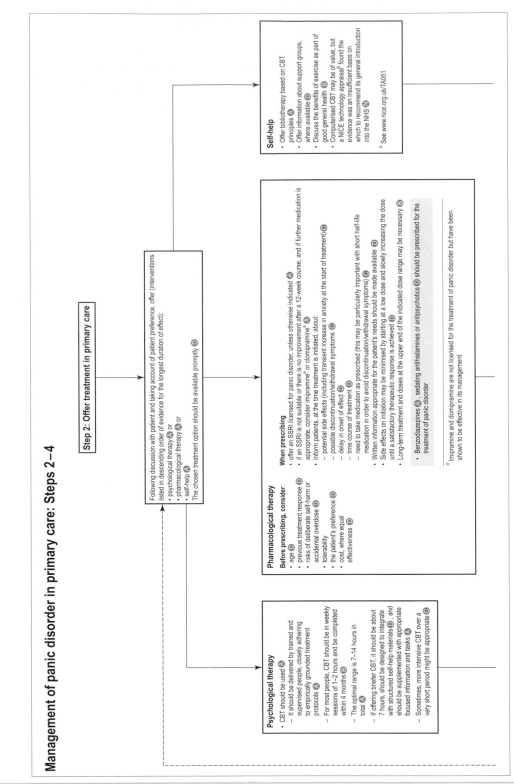

Management of panic disorder in primary care: Steps 2–4

A, B, C and D indicate grades of recommendation (see Appendix II for full details). * Reproduced with permission from the National Institute for Health and Clinical Excellence, London.

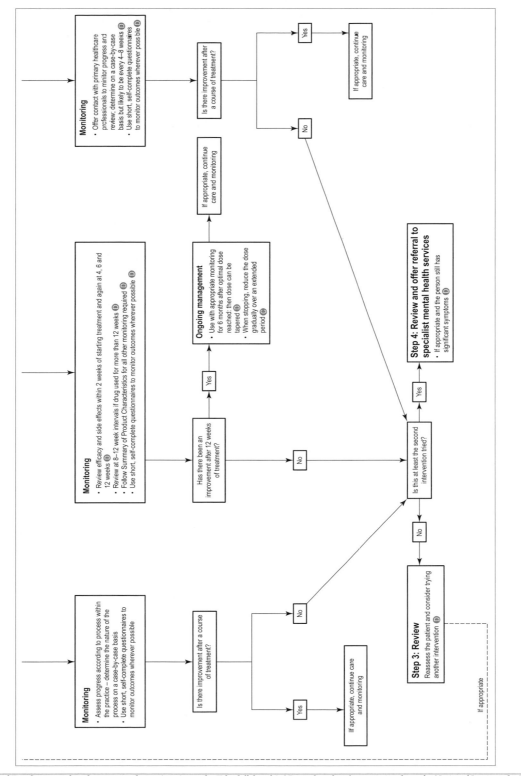

Monitoring
- Offer contact with primary healthcare professionals to monitor progress and review; determine on a case-by-case basis but likely to be every 4–8 weeks to monitor outcomes wherever possible

Is there improvement after a course of treatment?

Yes → If appropriate, continue care and monitoring

No

Monitoring
- Review efficacy and side effects within 2 weeks of starting treatment and again at 4, 6 and 12 weeks
- Review at 8–12 week intervals if drug used for more than 12 weeks
- Follow Summary of Product Characteristics for all other monitoring required
- Use short, self-complete questionnaires to monitor outcomes wherever possible

Has there been an improvement after 12 weeks of treatment?

Yes → **Ongoing management**
- Use with appropriate monitoring for 6 months after optimal dose reached; then dose can be tapered
- When stopping, reduce the dose gradually over an extended period

→ If appropriate, continue care and monitoring

No

Is this at least the second intervention tried?

Yes → **Step 4: Review and offer referral to specialist mental health services**
- If appropriate and the person still has significant symptoms

No → **Step 3: Review**
Reassess the patient and consider trying another intervention

Monitoring
- Assess progress according to process within the practice – determine the nature of the process on a case-by-case basis
- Use short, self-complete questionnaires to monitor outcomes wherever possible

Is there improvement after a course of treatment?

No

Yes → If appropriate, continue care and monitoring

If appropriate

A, B, C and **D** indicate grades of recommendation (see Appendix II for full details). * Reproduced with permission from the National Institute for Health and Clinical Excellence, London.

Management of generalised anxiety disorder disorder in primary care: Steps 2–4

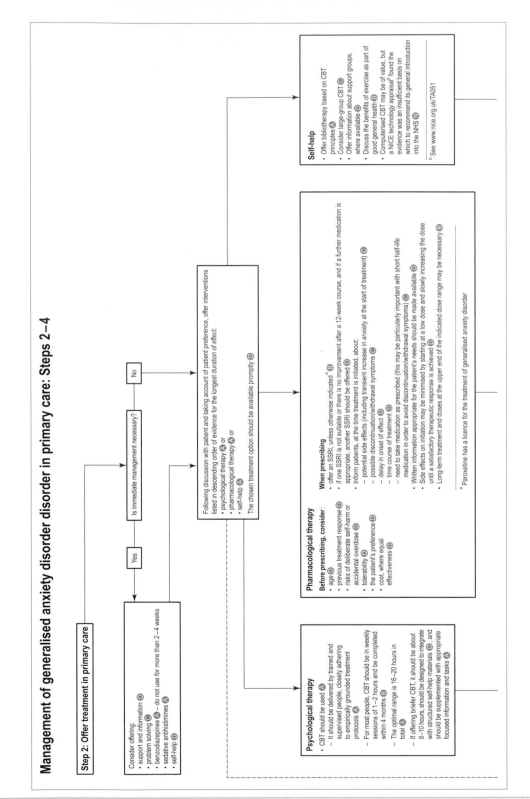

Step 2: Offer treatment in primary care

Consider offering:
- support and information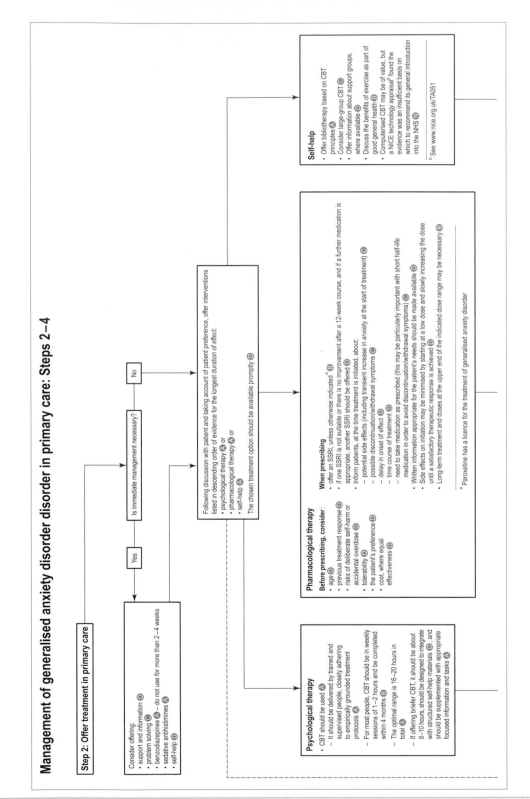
- problem solving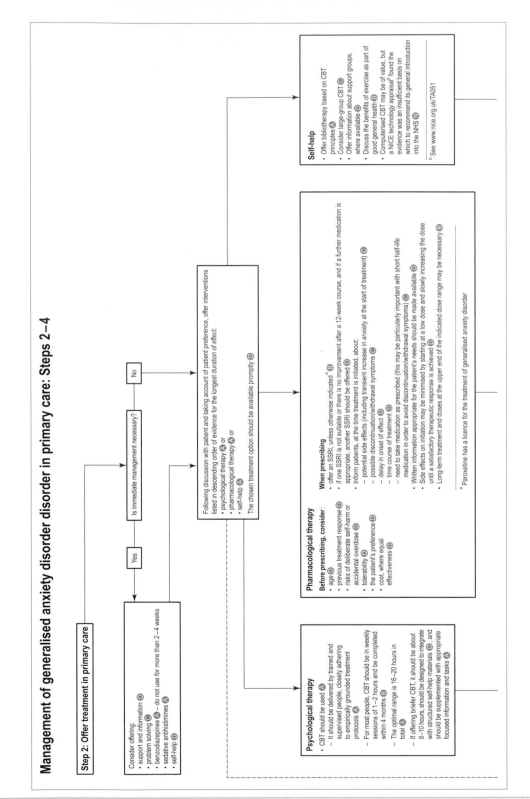
- benzodiazepines 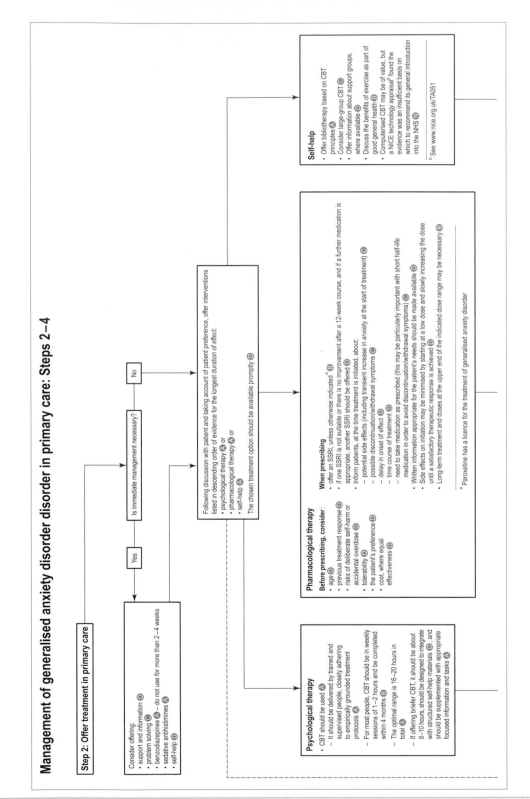 – do not use for more than 2–4 weeks
- sedative antihistimines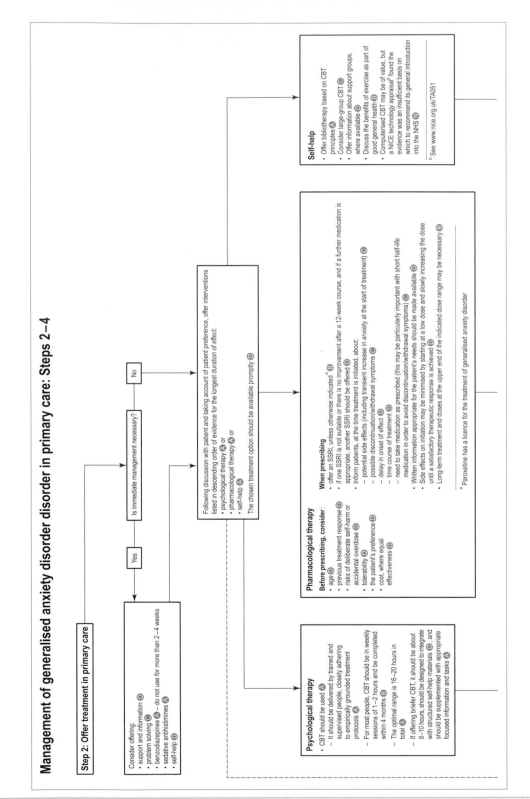
- self-help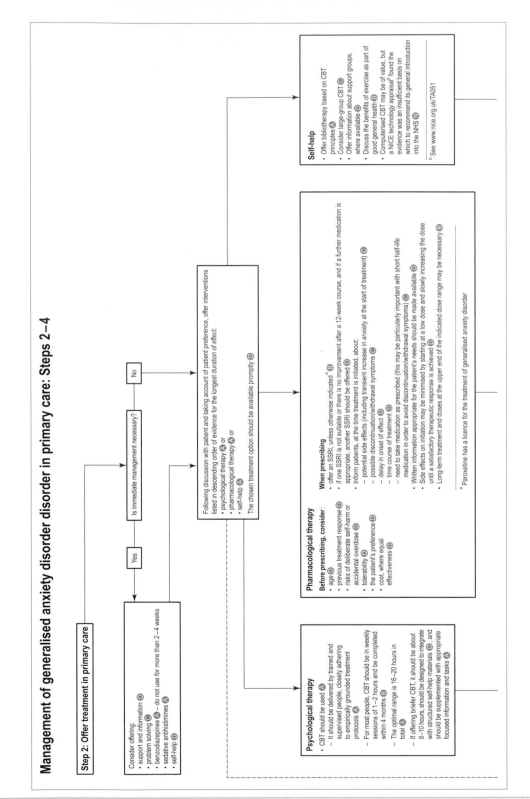

Is immediate management necessary?

Yes

No

Following discussion with patient and taking account of patient preference, offer interventions listed in descending order of evidence for the longest duration of effect:
- psychological therapy 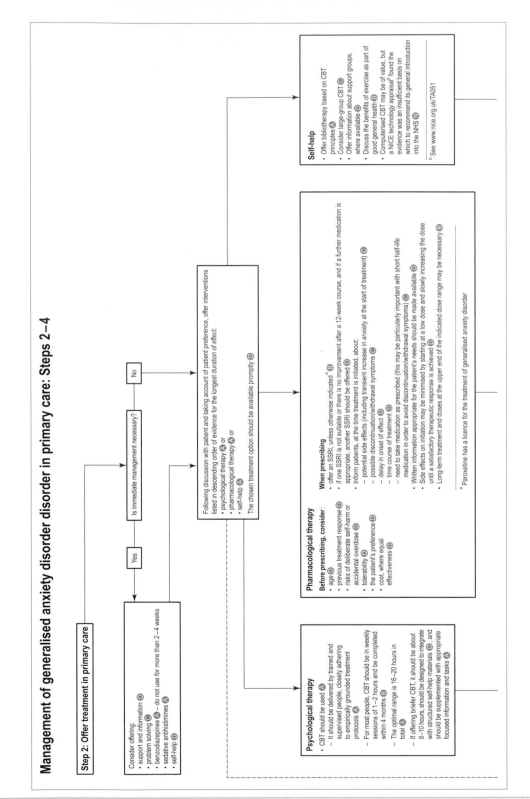 or
- pharmacological therapy 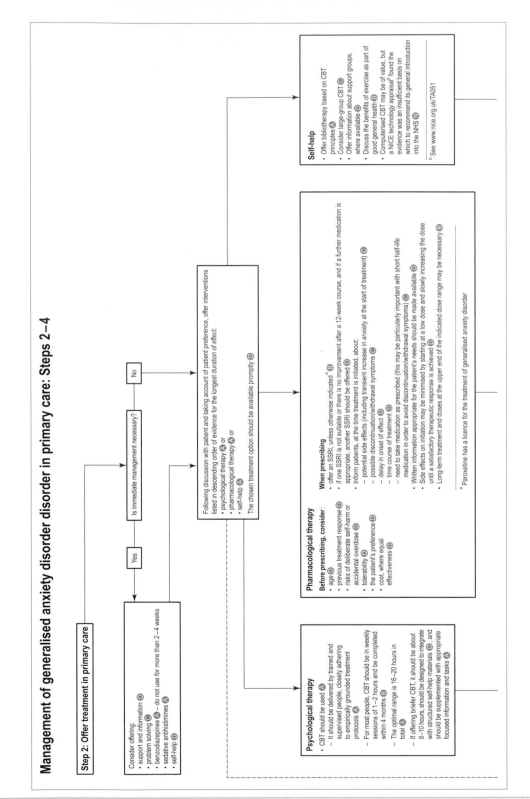 or
- self-help

The chosen treatment option should be available promptly

Psychological therapy

- CBT should be used
  - It should be delivered by trained and supervised people, closely adhering to empirically grounded treatment protocols
  - For most people, CBT should be in weekly sessions of 1–2 hours and be completed within 4 months
  - The optimal range is 16–20 hours in total
  - If offering briefer CBT, it should be about 8–10 hours, should be designed to integrate with structured self-help materials , and should be supplemented with appropriate focused information and tasks

Pharmacological therapy

Before prescribing, consider:
- age
- previous treatment response
- risks of deliberate self-harm or accidental overdose
- tolerability
- the patient's preference
- cost, where equal effectiveness

When prescribing
- offer an SSRI, unless otherwise indicated [a]
- if one SSRI is not suitable or there is no improvement after a 12-week course, and if a further medication is appropriate, another SSRI should be offered
- Inform patients, at the time treatment is initiated, about:
  – potential side effects (including transient increase in anxiety at the start of treatment)
  – possible discontinuation/withdrawal symptoms
  – delay in onset of effect
  – time course of treatment
  – need to take medication as prescribed (this may be particularly important with short half-life medication in order to avoid discontinuation/withdrawal symptoms)
- Written information appropriate for the patient's needs should be made available
- Side effects on initiation may be minimised by starting at a low dose and slowly increasing the dose until a satisfactory therapeutic response is achieved
- Long-term treatment and doses at the upper end of the indicated dose range may be necessary

[a] Paroxetine has a licence for the treatment of generalised anxiety disorder

Self-help

- Offer bibliotherapy based on CBT principles
- Consider large-group CBT
- Offer information about support groups, where available
- Discuss the benefits of exercise as part of good general health
- Computerised CBT may be of value, but a NICE technology appraisal [b] found the evidence was an insufficient basis on which to recommend its general introduction into the NHS

[b] See www.nice.org.uk/TA051

A, B, C and **D** indicate grades of recommendation (see Appendix II for full details). * Reproduced with permission from the National Institute for Health and Clinical Excellence, London.

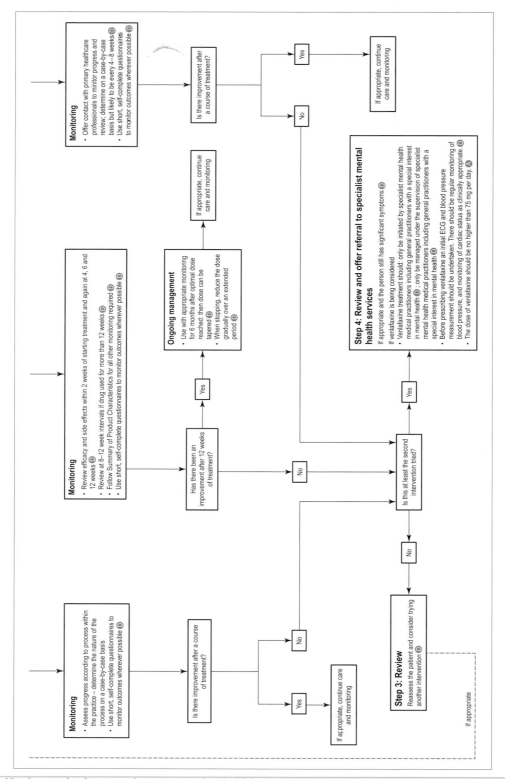

Monitoring
- Offer contact with primary healthcare professionals to monitor progress and review; determine on a case-by-case basis but likely to be every 4–8 weeks ⓓ
- Use short, self-complete questionnaires to monitor outcomes wherever possible ⓓ

Is there improvement after a course of treatment?

Yes → If appropriate, continue care and monitoring

No

Monitoring
- Review efficacy and side effects within 2 weeks of starting treatment and again at 4, 6 and 12 weeks ⓓ
- Review at 8–12 week intervals if drug used for more than 12 weeks ⓓ
- Follow Summary of Product Characteristics for all other monitoring required ⓓ
- Use short, self-complete questionnaires to monitor outcomes wherever possible ⓓ

Has there been an improvement after 12 weeks of treatment?

Yes

Ongoing management
- Use with appropriate monitoring for 6 months after optimal dose reached; then dose can be tapered ⓓ
- When stopping, reduce the dose gradually over an extended period ⓓ

If appropriate, continue care and monitoring

No

Step 4: Review and offer referral to specialist mental health services

If appropriate and the person still has significant symptoms ⓓ

If venlafaxine is being considered
- Venlafaxine treatment should: only be initiated by specialist mental health medical practitioners including general practitioners with a special interest in mental health ⓓ; only be managed under the supervision of specialist mental health medical practitioners including general practitioners with a special interest in mental health ⓓ
- Before prescribing venlafaxine an initial ECG and blood pressure measurement should be undertaken. There should be regular monitoring of blood pressure, and monitoring of cardiac status as clinically appropriate ⓓ
- The dose of venlafaxine should be no higher than 75 mg per day. Ⓐ

Is this at least the second intervention tried?

Yes

No

Monitoring
- Assess progress according to process within the practice – determine the nature of the process on a case-by-case basis
- Use short, self-complete questionnaires to monitor outcomes wherever possible ⓓ

Is there improvement after a course of treatment?

No

Yes → If appropriate, continue care and monitoring

Step 3: Review
Reassess the patient and consider trying another intervention ⓓ

If appropriate

A, B, C and **D** indicate grades of recommendation (see Appendix II for full details). * Reproduced with permission from the National Institute for Health and Clinical Excellence, London.

Anxiety: management of people with generalised anxiety disorder: care in specialist mental health services. NICE Clinical Guideline 22*: Step 5

Care in specialist mental health services

- Specialist mental health services should conduct a thorough, holistic reassessment of the individual, their environment and social circumstances. This reassessment should include evaluation of:
    - previous treatments, including effectiveness and concordance
    - any substance use, including nicotine, alcohol, caffeine and recreational drugs
    - comorbidities
    - day-to-day functioning
    - social networks
    - continuing chronic stressors
    - the role of agoraphobic and other avoidant symptoms.
- A comprehensive risk assessment should be undertaken and an appropriate risk management plan developed. [**D**]
- To undertake these evaluations, and to develop and share a full formulation, more than one session may be required and should be available. [**D**]

- Care and management will be based on the individual's circumstances and shared decisions arrived at. Options include [**D**]:
    - treatment of comorbid conditions
    - CBT with an experienced therapist if not offered already, including home-based CBT if attendance at clinic is problematic
    - structured problem solving
    - full exploration of pharmacotherapy
    - day support to relieve carers and family members
    - referral for advice, assessment or management to tertiary centres.
- There should be accurate and effective communication between all healthcare professionals involved in the care of any person with generalised anxiety disorder and particularly between primary care clinicians (GP and teams) and secondary care clinicians (community mental health teams) if there are existing physical health conditions that also require active management. [**D**]

D indicates grade of recommendation (see Appendix II for full details).
* Reproduced with permission from the National Institute for Health and Clinical Excellence, London.

Bipolar affective disorder

4

Treatment – Psychopharmacology

Does lithium reduce the mortality of recurrent mood disorders?

Coppen A, Standish-Berry H, Bailey J, Houston G, Silcocks P, Hermon C 1991 Does lithium reduce the mortality of recurrent mood disorders? Journal of Affective Disorders 23: 1–7

Method

- An 11-year follow-up study of all 103 patient attendees at a lithium clinic in 1977. Patients had bipolar affective disorder ($n = 30$), recurrent depressive disorder ($n = 67$) and schizoaffective disorder ($n = 6$).
- Actual mortality rates were compared with expected mortality rates estimated on the basis of age/sex/year-specific rates for England and Wales.

Results

- 10 years later, 65% were still attending.
- Only one patient could not be traced and was excluded.
- 70% of the patients traced were continuing to receive medication in 1990.
- There were 10 deaths during the study.

- No deaths were caused by suicide.
- The expected number of deaths was 18.31 ($P = 0.052$, two-tailed).
- After correcting for the prevalence of mood disorder in the general population, the relative risk was 0.60 (95% CI $0.29–1.12$).
- This suggests that lithium reverses the excess mortality associated with recurrent mood disorders, including that from suicide.

Guze SB, Robins E 1970 Suicide and primary affective disorders. British Journal of Psychiatry 117: 437–438

- An extensive review of 17 investigations of mortality in depression.
- Many modern medications were not then available.
- Found that some 15% of these patients could be expected to commit suicide.

Lee AS, Murray RM 1988 The long term outcome of Maudsley depressives. British Journal of Psychiatry 153: 741–751

- In this 18-year study of the above patient group there was increased all-causes mortality in addition to a very high ongoing morbidity.
- The standardised mortality rate was 1.9 ($P < 0.01$).
- At least 45% of the deaths were due to suicide.
- Other studies from the same time showed a range of mortality from 17 to 55%.

Black DW, Winokur G, Nasrallah A 1987 Is death from natural causes still excessive in psychiatric patients? Journal of Nervous and Mental Disease 175: 674–680

- Most of the excess mortality in depression has been due to suicide.

Olanzapine alone or in combination for acute mania

Rendell JM, Gijsman HJ, Keck P, Goodwin GM, Geddes JR 2003 Olanzapine alone or in combination for acute mania **(Cochrane Review)**. In: The Cochrane Library, Issue 1. CD004040. Update Software, Oxford

- Six trials ($n = 1422$) were included.
- Dropout rates were high.
- Olanzapine was better than placebo in reducing manic symptoms when used alone and in combination with lithium/valproate.
- Olanzapine alone was better at reducing psychotic symptoms.
- Olanzapine was better than divalproex in reducing manic symptoms.
- Olanzapine was no more effective than haloperidol.
- More patients dropped out of treatment in the placebo group than the olanzapine group, although olanzapine caused more weight gain and somnolence.
- Olanzapine did not cause more depressive symptoms or movement disorders.
- Olanzapine was associated with greater increases in prolactin elevation than placebo.
- Compared with divalproex, olanzapine caused more weight gain, somnolence and movement disorders but less nausea.
- Olanzapine caused more weight gain than haloperidol but less movement disorder.

Relapse prevention in bipolar I disorder: olanzapine and/or mood stabiliser

Tohen M, Chengappa KNR, Suppes T et al 2004 Relapse prevention in bipolar I disorder: 18 month comparison of olanzapine plus mood stabiliser v. mood stabiliser alone. British Journal of Psychiatry 184: 337–345

The long-term efficacy of medications for bipolar affective disorder has not been well demonstrated. Pharmacological treatments routinely include a mood stabiliser in conjunction with an antipsychotic. Side effects and episodes of depression have implications for treatment.

Atypical antipsychotics may offer some benefits over the older neuroleptics. There have been few controlled trials of atypical antipsychotics in the prophylactic treatment of bipolar disorder.

Method

- An 18-month, double-masked, relapse prevention study of patients with bipolar affective disorder in 29 sites in the US and Canada.
- In an earlier phase of the trial patients were treated with olanzapine in combination with lithium or sodium valproate.
- Patients who had achieved remission were compared in terms of continuation therapy with olanzapine alone or in combination with lithium or sodium valproate.
- Patients had bipolar I disorder, manic or mixed disorder without psychotic features (DSM-IV).
- Patients had to have had persistent manic symptoms using the Young Mania Rating Scale for 2 weeks prior to enrolment and have a therapeutic blood level of lithium or valproate.
- Those who achieved remission with combination therapy were then assigned to either continued combination therapy or monotherapy with either lithium or sodium valproate.
- Relapse was assessed as:
  - syndromic, meeting DSM-IV criteria for manic, mixed or depressive episode
  - symptomatic, using the total score on the YRMS and the 21-item HRSD.

Results

- 99 people were randomised: 48 to monotherapy, 51 to combination therapy.
- The percentage of people completing the 18-month follow-up period was almost three times higher in the combination group.
- Time to relapse into syndromic affective episode, whether depressive or manic, was not significantly different between the groups.
- Time to symptomatic relapse into either mania or depression was significantly longer for the combination treatment group compared with the monotherapy group.
- Women (and Caucasians) showed better results than men with the combination treatment.
- The study found that both the lithium and valproate monotherapies and the combined treatment with olanzapine were generally well tolerated.
- Patients on combination therapy gained on average 2 kg (thought to be due to olanzapine), whereas the monotherapy group lost an average of 1.8 kg.
- Extrapyramidal side effects were similar in both groups.

- There was no abnormal increase in non-fasting blood glucose or cholesterol levels at any time in the study group at 18-month follow-up.

Bowden CL, Calabrese JR, Sachs G et al 2003 A placebo-controlled 18-month trial of lamotrigine and lithium maintenance treatment in recently manic or hypomanic patients with bipolar I disorders. Archives of General Psychiatry 60: 392–400

- Reported similar weight gains with long-term monotherapy with olanzapine, in bipolar disorder.

Sodium valproate or valproate semisodium

Fisher C, Broderick W 2003 Sodium valproate or valproate semisodium. Psychiatric Bulletin: Drug Information Quarterly 27: 446–448

Valproate semisodium is the only form of valproate to be licensed for use in bipolar disorder. The UK Medicines Control Agency favours the use of licensed drugs over unlicensed alternatives. The license is for acute treatment, not for maintenance of bipolar disorder.

There was no evidence that valproate semisodium has different pharmacokinetic properties from those of enteric-coated sodium valproate. Differences in maximum plasma concentration were thought to be related to differences in dose between preparations. Evidence from American studies showing valproate semisodium has better tolerability than valproate (non-enteric coated) does not generalise to the UK where all except the crushable forms of valproate are enteric coated.

Bowden C, Calabrese J, McElroy S 2000 A randomized placebo controlled trial of divalproex and lithium in treatment of outpatients with bipolar disorder. Archives of General Psychiatry 57: 481–489

- The only randomised controlled trial of maintenance treatment of mania.
- Valproate, valproate semisodium and lithium were compared.
- The study failed to show that valproate semisodium or lithium was more efficacious than placebo.

Demoulin L, Landry P 2000 Plasma concentration of valproate following substitution of divalproex sodium by valproic acid. Canadian Journal of Psychiatry 45: 761

- Case report evidence to suggest increased bioavailability of valproate from valproate semisodium compared with the same dose of valproic acid.

- This was demonstrated by higher trough plasma valproate levels.

Valproate for acute mood episodes

Macritchie K, Geddes JR, Scott J, Haslam D, de Lima M, Goodwin G 2003 Valproate for acute mood episodes in bipolar disorder (Cochrane Review). In: The Cochrane Library, Issue 1. CD004052. Update Software, Oxford

- 10 trials were included comparing valproate with placebo (3), lithium (3), olanzapine (2), haloperidol (1), and carbamazepine (2).
- Depression and mixed affective episodes were not examined.
- The studied outcome was failure to respond by the end of the study, measured as a less than 50% reduction in YMRS or SADS-S mania scale.
- Valproate had greater efficacy than placebo in the treatment of mania (RRR 38%).
- There was no significant difference between valproate and lithium or valproate and carbamazepine.
- Olanzapine had greater efficacy than valproate.
- There were no great differences in the number of dropouts.

Valproic acid, valproate and divalproex in the maintenance treatment of bipolar disorder

Macritchie KA, Geddes JR, Scott J, Haslam DR, Goodwin GM 2001 Valproic acid, valproate and divalproex in the maintenance treatment of bipolar disorder (Cochrane Review). In: The Cochrane Library, Issue 3. CD003196. Update Software, Oxford

- The only RCT to meet the inclusion criteria was of 12 months' duration and compared lithium, divalproex and placebo in 372 participants.
- For time to first mood episode there were no significant differences between the treatments.
- Fewer patients receiving divalproex left the study due to a mood episode compared with the placebo group.
- There was no difference in numbers leaving the study due to a mood episode when divalproex was compared with lithium.
- It was not possible to extract any information regarding rapid cycling mood disorder.
- Those receiving divalproex had more tremor, weight gain and alopecia than the placebo group.

- Those receiving divalproex had more frequent sedation and infection than those receiving lithium, but less polyuria and less thirst.
- More patients left the study due to side effects than those on placebo, but fewer than on lithium.

Treatment – Psychological Therapies

Cost-effectiveness of relapse-prevention cognitive therapy for bipolar disorder

> Lam DH, McCrone P, Wright K, Kerr N 2005 Cost-effectiveness of relapse-prevention cognitive therapy for bipolar disorder: 30 month study. British Journal of Psychiatry 186: 500–506

CBT may be cost-effective due to reductions in the use of other NHS services.

Method

- 103 individuals with bipolar I disorder were allocated to either standard treatment (mood stabilisers and psychiatric follow-up) or cognitive therapy plus standard treatment.
- Service use and costs were assessed at 3-month intervals and cost-effectiveness was assessed using a net-benefit approach.

Results

- Patients treated with cognitive therapy had 62.3 fewer days of illness than controls.
- The actuarial cumulative relapse rates were 64% for the cognitive therapy group and 84% for the standard treatment group.
- 38% of the group receiving cognitive therapy, compared to 47% of the comparison group, were admitted to hospital for bipolar episodes – this is not significant.
- There was also a non-significant finding for patients receiving cognitive therapy to spend fewer days in hospital over the 30-month trial period.
- There was wide variation in the resource use throughout the study.
- There was a non-significant reduction in cost for the treatment group at 12 months and at 30 months.
- The majority of costs were for inpatient care.
- Cost-effectiveness analysis shows that cognitive therapy is probably more cost-effective than standard care for a range of different values.

> Lam DH, Hayward P, Watkins E et al 2005 Outcomes of a two year follow-up of a cognitive therapy of relapse prevention in bipolar disorder. American Journal of Psychiatry 162: 324–329

- Found that cognitive therapy is significantly better than standard care with regard to clinical outcomes for relapse prevention.
- There was a trend for a decrease in effectiveness over time.

The early warning symptom intervention

> Morriss R 2004 The early warning symptom intervention for patients with bipolar affective disorder. Advances in Psychiatric Treatment 10: 18–26

There are good RCT data to show the efficacy of interventions that involve the identification and management of early warning symptoms of mania and depressive episodes. Interventions can be provided in a variety of settings, either by members of the multidisciplinary team (nursing staff, psychologists, medical staff, etc.) or by an expert patient. Interventions are likely to be maximally effective if they are a core feature of the care plan and have involved all the relevant team members in their creation. Annual review and review after each relapse are required to ensure relevance and motivation.

The service will need to trust the patients' accounts of their early warning symptoms and must be able to respond within an appropriate time period. The presence of false-positive symptoms must be recognised. The intervention is not suitable if it causes patients with depression to simply focus on their depressive symptoms. There is usually a 2–4 week period between the patient's first detection of early warning symptoms and the moment insight is lost (and the patient becomes unwilling or unable to seek treatment). The 'relapse signature' is individual to each patient and to each relapse pole (mania or depression).

Prodromal symptoms include:
- those characteristic of a full manic or depressive relapse
- those commonly seen in full relapse but not diagnostic in themselves (vivid colours etc.)
- those idiosyncratic to the patient's prodromes (becoming boastful etc.)
- those obvious to other people (but not to the patient) and reported to the patient (playing a certain piece of music etc.)
- situations known to precede the manic or depressive prodrome (e.g. the end of the tax year or air travel).

Box 4.1

Early warning symptom intervention sessions in the management of bipolar affective disorder

Session 1
- Exploration of the patient's illness from their history
- Completion of a mood diary to evaluate interepisode symptoms
- Carers can be involved in both of the above

Session 2
- Symptom history and mood diary are reviewed
- A card-sorting test is used to determine the order of presentation of symptoms and the point of loss of insight, performed for both poles of the illness
- Between four and six symptoms, signs or life situations are used to define the manic relapse signature, two or three of which will prompt more intensive monitoring of mental state
- Patients are asked to identify two people they could contact if prodromal symptoms were identified

- Patients are also asked to identify coping strategies that they previously employed at times of relapse, whether helpful or not

Session 3
- Creation of an action plan, with six components:
  - warning level and danger level early warning symptoms, signs and situations
  - a series of motivational statements
  - a list of good coping strategies (see MDF website, below), including the avoidance of poor coping strategies
  - the names and contact details of three health professionals the patient can contact at the time of relapse
  - an action plan to guide patient management at the time of the danger stage of relapse
  - signing of the created action plan by the patient, RMO and any other relevant professionals who have aided in compiling it.

The timetable for intervention sessions is described in Box 4.1.

Lam D, Wong G 1997 Prodromes, coping strategies, insight and social functioning in bipolar affective disorders. Psychological Medicine 27: 1091–1100

The ideal patient for this intervention has euthymic bipolar I disorder without marked psychiatric comorbidity, who is recognised by the patient themselves and by the clinician as being at high risk of recurrent mania. The intervention (Box 4.2) can provide patients with a sense of control; however, some find the constant vigilance wearing as it only highlights the presence of illness.

Perry A, Tarrier N, Morriss R et al 1999 Randomised controlled trial of efficacy of teaching patients with bipolar disorder to identify early symptoms of relapse and obtain treatment. British Medical Journal 318: 149–153

- Showed the efficacy of using a health professional to teach patients with bipolar affective disorder to recognise the early warning symptoms of manic relapse and to seek conventional psychiatric treatment.
- In this trial of 69 patients the time to the next manic episode was increased four-fold in the intervention group.
- There was a 40% reduction in the number of manic relapses over 18 months in the intervention group.

Box 4.2

Good coping strategies for manic and progressive prodromes

Manic prodromes
- Restrain myself
- Do calming exercises
- Take extra medication as agreed with the doctor
- Prioritise and reduce the number of tasks
- Delay impulsive actions
- Talk to someone to bring reality to thoughts
- Take time off work
- Do not stop prescribed medication
- Do not drink or take street drugs

Depressive prodromes
- Keep busy
- Get myself organised
- Get the support of family/friends
- Meet people
- Distract myself from negative thoughts by doing things
- Recognise unrealistic thoughts and evaluate if they are worth worrying about
- Do not stop medication or take extra medication
- Do not drink alcohol or take street drugs

- The intervention group also showed clinically important improvements in function, particularly in employment.

See also the 'Treatment – Psychological Therapies' section in Chapter 25 (Psychological therapies), page 358.

Cognitive therapy for bipolar illness: relapse prevention

> Lam DH, Bright J, Jones S et al 2000 Cognitive therapy for bipolar illness: a pilot study of relapse prevention. Cognitive Therapy and Research 24: 503–520

- Improved outcomes were found with more experienced therapists.
- The provision of lifestyle advice, including teaching patients additional coping mechanisms for dealing with the first symptoms of depressive relapse, was also beneficial.

> Colom F, Vieta E, Reinares M et al 2003 Psychoeducation efficacy in bipolar disorders beyond compliance enhancement. Journal of Clinical Psychiatry 64(9): 1101–1105

- Improved outcomes associated with psychoeducation do not appear to be related to improved adherence to drug regimens or additional time spent with therapists.

> Miklowitz DJ, Simoneau TL, George EL et al 2000 Family focused treatment of bipolar disorder: 1 year effects of a psychoeducation program in conjunction with pharmacotherapy. Biological Psychiatry 48: 582–592

- A RCT of the use of family therapy sessions in identification and management of early warning symptoms.
- Demonstrated efficacy against depressive relapses but not mania.

> Jolley AG, Hirsch SR, Morrison E et al 1990 Trial of brief intermittent neuroleptic prophylaxis for selected schizophrenic outpatients: clinical and social outcome at two years. British Medical Journal 301: 837–842; Gaebel W, Frick U, Köpcke W et al 1993 Early neuroleptic intervention in schizophrenia: are prodromal symptoms valid predictors of relapse? British Journal of Psychiatry 163 (Suppl): 8–12

- In schizophrenia it has been shown that recognition of early warning symptoms and intermittent use of medication is generally less effective than continuous medication.

Definition

Early warning symptoms and signs – the symptoms and observed behaviour (signs) that constitute the patient's relapse signature in the prodrome.

Interepisode symptom – any mood-related symptom that occurs between manic, hypomanic, mixed affective or depressive episodes.

Prodrome – the build-up in quantity, frequency and severity of interepisode symptoms immediately before each manic, hypomanic, mixed affective or depressive episode. The term is not restricted to the period before the first episode of illness.

Relapse signature – a selection of early warning symptoms that are used in the early warning symptom intervention to indicate that action needs to be taken by the patient and/or clinical team to prevent a manic, hypomanic, mixed affective or depressive episode.

Weblink Manic Depression Fellowship self-management training programme – www.mdf.org.uk.

See also the 'Treatment – Psychological Therapies' section in Chapter 25 (Psychological therapies), page 358.

Assessment tools and rating scales

Bech–Rafaelsen Mania Scale

> Bech P, Bolwig TG, Kramp P, Rafaelsen OJ 1979 The Bech–Rafaelsen Mania Scale and the Hamilton Depression Scale. Acta Psychiatrica Scandinavica 59: 420–430

- Clinician-rated scale designed to assess the presence and severity of clinical features of mania and hypomania and the effectiveness of therapeutic interventions for BPAD.
- Assesses 11 items:
  - elevated mood
  - pressured speech
  - inc. social contact
  - inc. motor activity
  - sleep disturbance
  - social activities and distractibility
  - inc. sexual activity
  - inc. self-esteem
  - flight of ideas
  - noise level of speech
  - other vocal activity.
- Each item is scored from 0 to 4.

- Total score is standardised:
  - mania < 15
  - moderate mania 20+
  - severe mania 28.

Guidelines

Olanzapine and valproate semisodium in the treatment of acute mania associated with bipolar I disorder. NICE Technology Appraisal 66*

Guidance

Olanzapine and valproate semisodium, within their licensed indications, are recommended as options for control of the acute symptoms associated with the manic phase of bipolar I disorder.

Of the drugs available for the treatment of acute mania, the choice of which to prescribe should be made jointly by the individual and the clinician(s) responsible for treatment. The choice should be based on an informed discussion of the relative benefits and side-effect profiles of each drug, and should take into account the needs of the individual and the particular clinical situation.

In all situations where informed discussion is not possible, advance directives should be fully taken into account and the individual's advocate and/or carer should be consulted when appropriate.

---

* Reproduced with permission from the National Institute for Health and Clinical Excellence, London.

Bipolar affective disorder. SIGN Guideline 82**

Diagnosis

☑ Early and accurate diagnosis should be attempted to allow treatment as soon as possible after a first episode.

D A diagnosis of bipolar affective disorder should be made after clinical assessment according to DSM or ICD criteria.

☑ Clinicians should be aware of the instability of diagnosis during clinical review of patients with affective disorder.

Acute treatment for mania

A • Acute manic episodes should be treated with oral administration of an antipsychotic drug or valproate semisodium.

- Lithium can be used if immediate control or overactive or dangerous behaviour is not needed or otherwise should be used in combination with an antipsychotic.

☑ Intramuscular injection of antipsychotics and/or benzodiazepines (lorazepam) should be used in emergency situations, in accordance with local protocols.

☑ Benzodiazepines may be used as adjunctive treatment in acute mania where sedation is a priority.

☑ Patients who suffer an acute manic episode whilst on maintenance treatment with an antimanic drug should have their dose of antimanic drug optimised. Treatment with an antipsychotic or valproic acid should be initiated as appropriate.

☑ Severe, treatment-resistant mania may require electroconvulsive treatment.

☑ Combination therapy with several antimanic agents from different classes may be required in treatment-resistant cases.

☑ Duration of treatment will be determined by the reduction of symptoms, the emergence of side effects and the need to provide treatment for residual symptoms and prevent relapse.

☑ Antidepressant drug treatment should be reduced and discontinued during an acute manic episode.

☑ A clear terminology should be implemented to avoid confusion in the prescription of sodium valproate and valproate semisodium, as well as the different lithium salts and preparation.

Acute treatment for depression

B An antidepressant in combination with an antimanic drug (lithium, valproate semisodium or an antipsychotic drug), or lamotrigine is recommended for the treatment of acute bipolar depression in patients with a history of mania.

☑ • Patients maintained on mood stabilisers who suffer a depressive episode should be started on an antidepressant after optimising their mood stabiliser.

- Interactions between serotonergic antidepressants, antipsychotic drugs and lithium and the risk of triggering mania or rapid cycling should be considered when selecting an antidepressant.

☑ ECT may be considered for patients with bipolar depression at high risk of suicide or self-harm.

Pharmacological relapse prevention

A Lithium is the treatment of choice for relapse prevention in bipolar affective illness.

A Lithium should be prescribed at an appropriate dose with a daily dosing regimen.

A   The withdrawal of lithium should be gradual to minimise the risk of relapse.

☑   In general practice, lithium should be prescribed in the context of a shared care protocol to minimise side effects and toxicity.

☑   Before embarking on maintenance treatment with lithium, patient and doctor should consider the severity of the last episode, number, frequency and severity of previous episodes, personal factors, such as a wish to become pregnant or the wish to avoid sick leave from work or education.

A   Carbamazepine can be used as an alternative to lithium, particularly in patients with bipolar II, or when lithium is ineffective or unacceptable.

A   Lamotrigine can be used as a prophylactic in patients who have initially stabilised with lamotrigine, particularly if depressive relapse is the greater problem.

Psychosocial interventions

B   Evidence-based psychosocial interventions should be available to patients in addition to pharmacological maintenance treatment, especially if complete or continued remission cannot be achieved.

Reproductive health issues

D   • The dose of the combined oral contraceptive should be adjusted accordingly when given with an enzyme-inducing drug.
     • Women should be warned that the efficacy of the COC is reduced.
     • Barrier methods of contraception should also be used for maximal contraceptive effect.

Further information and recommendations on reproductive health issues are available in the full guideline: www.sign. ac.uk.

Suicide prevention

B   Acute and maintenance lithium treatment of patients with bipolar affective disorders should be optimised to make every effort to minimise the risk of suicide.

A, B and **D** indicate grades of recommendation; ☑ indicates a good practice point (see Appendix II for full details). ** Reproduced with permission from the Scottish Intercollegiate Guidelines Network, Edinburgh.

Child and adolescent psychiatry

5

Chapter contents

Ethical issues

Child psychiatry, mental disorder and the law

Potter R, Evans N 2004 Child psychiatry, mental disorder and the law: is a more specific statutory framework necessary? British Journal of Psychiatry 184: 1–2

There has been a recent shift away from parental control to the rights of the young person and parental responsibility. The rights of children with mental health problems may not be sufficiently protected.

According to UK law, children of 10 years are fully responsible and accountable for their criminal activities. A 17-year-old may not be able to refuse medical treatment. Children can be treated for mental disorder without their consent, irrespective of whether or not the child is competent. This is drawn from a combination of statutory and case law.

In the treatment of children with mental disorder it is often appropriate for the parent to make decisions on behalf of the child. The presence of mental illness can have a negative impact on intrafamilial relationships, making decisions difficult. The addition of a doctor to this process further impacts on the decision-making process. Risk, dangerousness and inability to self-care can make it difficult for parents to challenge medical staff. Psychiatrists may be reluctant to use the Mental Health Act.

Bridge C 1997 Adolescents and mental disorder: who consents to treatment? Medical Law International 3: 51–74

- There is a dilemma in acknowledging and respecting a child's autonomy, whilst taking care of and responsibility for the child.

Neilsen v. Denmark [1989] II ECHR 175

- A parent's power to confine and treat a child in a psychiatric hospital against the individual's wishes is seen as an extension of the responsibility to care for the child.

Fennell P 1996 Treatment without consent: law, psychiatry and the treatment of mentally disordered people since 1845. Routledge, London

- Children who refuse treatment and are treated with parental authority have none of the statutory safeguards for the protection of their rights.

The Human Rights Act 1998 and the European Convention on Human Rights do not protect the rights of the child against the wishes of a parent. The framework for treatment has been drawn from adult legislation and does not fully recognise the needs of the children. A specific statutory framework is required.

See ethical decision making (below).
See also the 'Ethical issues' section in Chapter 9 (Ethical issues), page 130.

Decision making about children's mental health care

Paul M 2004 Decision making about children's mental health care: ethical challenges. Determining to whom a duty of care is owed. Advances in Psychiatric Treatment 10: 301–311

Child and adolescent mental health services receive referrals about children, often as a result of the concern of parents or of health, education or social care professionals rather than of the child. The possessor of the primary problem may in fact not be the child. The relationship is complicated by the fact that minors, their guardians and professionals all need to be considered. Parental support and involvement are preferable. The wishes of the child may not be heeded – for example, in child protection issues or when a child is not capable of balancing present and future needs. It may be unclear at times as to whom the duty of care is owed.

The doctor owes the patient a duty of care. It could be that parents and siblings are also owed a duty of care. Parents may act solely as the child's advocate/representative. When the court determines any question with respect to the upbringing of a child, the child's welfare should be the court's principal concern.

Parents may act as proxy decision makers, but they act for the best interests of their family rather than the child in isolation. They have a responsibility to obtain health care for their child. Parental rights may last as long as the legal duration of parenthood but their rights as individuals may be indefinite. Parental responsibility is not automatic. Some non-parents have parental responsibility.

Section 1 of the Children Act 1989 states that when a court is asked to determine on any question concerning a child's upbringing, then welfare should be the most important aspect. The Act should be employed with regard to:
- the ascertainable wishes and feelings of the child
- the needs of the child – physical, emotional and educational
- the effect that any change in circumstances may have on the child
- any relevant background information the court considers relevant
- any harm or risk of harm to the child
- capabilities of the parents in meeting the child's needs.

Eekalaar J 1986 The emergence of children's rights. Oxford Journal of Legal Studies 6: 161–182

Categorised children's interests as:
- basic interests
- developmental interests
- autonomy interests.

The United Nations Convention on the Rights of the Child 1989 and the Children Act confer upon the child participatory decision-making rights.

Lansdown G 2000 Implementing children's rights and health. Archives of Disease in Childhood 83: 286–288

- Healthcare providers are obliged to give minors all the information required to enable them to make a fully informed decision.
- That does not mean that children must then be the final decision makers.

The Human Rights Act 1998. The Stationery Office, London

- Requires the consent of children to be viewed from a rights perspective by acknowledging them as a third party in the relationship where the decision is between adult individuals (the child's parent) and the state.

Bedingfield D 1998 The child in need, the state and the law. Family Law, Bristol

- Discusses the Gillick competence case.
- If it is interpreted narrowly, then physicians only have the authority to provide contraceptive advice and treatment to girls under 16 without parental consent under certain circumstances without fear of criminal or civil liability.
- Interpreted broadly, it means that parents' rights to decide whether or not their child under 16 has treatment ends when the child has achieved a certain level of intelligence and understanding to make the decision for herself.

Tan JOA, Jones DPH 2001 Children's consent. Current Opinion in Psychiatry 14: 303–307

- Separated:
  - capacity – the legal ability of the person to consent to treatment, *from*
  - competence – the clinical ability of the person to consent to treatment.

Alderson P, Montgomery J 1996 Health care choices: making decisions with children. Institute for Public Policy Research, London

Ideally children and parents should come to a decision together about whether to accept treatment or not and should be consulted in relation to four different levels of decision making:
- Being informed
- Expressing a view
- Influencing decision making
- Being the main decision maker.

See also the 'Ethical issues' section in Chapter 9 (Ethical issues), page 127.

Reference Guide to Consent for Examination or Treatment

Department of Health 2001 Reference guide to consent for examination or treatment: children and young people. DH, London[†]

Young people aged 16–17

People aged 16 or 17 are entitled, by virtue of section 8 of the Family Law Reform Act 1969, to consent to their own medical treatment and to any ancillary procedures involved in that treatment, such as an anaesthetic. As for adults, consent will be valid only if it is given voluntarily by an appropriately informed patient capable of consenting to the particular intervention. However, unlike adults, the refusal of a competent person aged 16–17 may, in certain circumstances, be overridden by either a person with parental responsibility or a court.

Section 8 applies only to the young person's own treatment. It does not apply to an intervention which is not potentially of direct health benefit to the young person, such as blood donation or non-therapeutic research on the causes of a disorder. However, a young person may be able to consent to such an intervention under the standard of Gillick competence.

In order to establish whether a young person aged 16 or 17 has the requisite capacity to consent to the proposed intervention, the same criteria as for adults should be used.

If the requirements for valid consent are met, it is not legally necessary to obtain consent from a person with parental responsibility for the young person in addition to that of the young person. It is, however, good practice to involve the young person's family in the decision-making process, unless the young person specifically wishes to exclude them.

Children under 16 – the concept of 'Gillick competence'

Following the case of Gillick, the courts have held that children who have sufficient understanding and intelligence to enable them to understand fully what is involved in a proposed intervention will also have the capacity to consent to that intervention. This is sometimes described as being 'Gillick competent' and may apply to consent to treatment, research or tissue donation. As the understanding required for different interventions will vary considerably, a child under 16 may therefore have the capacity to consent to some interventions but not to others. As with adults, assumptions that a child with learning disability may not

be able to understand the issues should never be made automatically.

The concept of Gillick competence is said to reflect the child's increasing development to maturity. In some cases (e.g. because of a mental disorder) a child's mental state may fluctuate significantly so that on some occasions the child appears Gillick competent in respect of a particular decision and on other occasions does not. In such cases, careful consideration should be given to whether the child is truly Gillick competent at any time to take this decision.

If the child is Gillick competent and is able to give voluntary consent after receiving appropriate information, that consent will be valid, and additional consent by a person with parental responsibility will not be required. However, where the decision will have ongoing implications, such as long-term use of contraception, it is good practice to encourage the child to inform the parents unless it would clearly not be in the child's best interests to do so.

Child or young person with capacity refusing treatment

Where a young person of 16 or 17 who could consent to treatment in accordance with section 8 of the Family Law Reform Act, or a child under 16 who is Gillick competent, refuses treatment, such a refusal can be overruled either by a person with parental responsibility for the child or by the court. If more than one person has parental responsibility for the young person, consent by any one such person is sufficient, irrespective of the refusal of any other individual.

This power to overrule must be exercised on the basis that the welfare of the child/young person is paramount. As with the concept of best interests, 'welfare' does not just mean physical health. The psychological effect of having the decision overruled must be considered. While no definitive guidance has been given as to when it is appropriate to overrule a competent young person's refusal, it has been suggested that it should be restricted to occasions where the child is at risk of suffering 'grave and irreversible mental or physical harm'.

The outcome of such decisions may have a serious impact on the individual concerned. Examples might include a young person with capacity refusing an abortion or further chemotherapy for cancer in the knowledge of a poor prognosis. When a person with parental responsibility wishes to overrule such decisions, consideration should be given to applying to the court for a ruling prior to undertaking the intervention. Such applications can be made at short notice if necessary.

For parents to be in a position to overrule a competent child's refusal, they must inevitably be provided with sufficient information about their child's condition, which the child may not be willing for them to receive. While this will constitute a breach of confidence on the part of the clinician treating the child, this may be justifiable where it is in the child's best interests. Such a justification may only

---

[†] Crown copyright. Reproduced with permission.

apply where the child is at serious risk as a result of their refusal of treatment.

Refusal by a competent child and all persons with parental responsibility for the child can be overruled by the court if the welfare of the child so requires.

A life-threatening emergency may arise when consultation with either a person with parental responsibility or the court is impossible, or the persons with parental responsibility refuse consent despite such emergency treatment appearing to be in the best interests of the child. In such cases the courts have stated that doubt should be resolved in favour of the preservation of life and it is acceptable to undertake treatment to preserve life or prevent serious damage to health.

Child or young person without capacity

Where a child lacks capacity to consent, consent can be given on their behalf by any one person with parental responsibility or by the court. As is the case where patients are giving consent for themselves, those giving consent on behalf of child patients must have the capacity to consent to the intervention in question, be acting voluntarily and be appropriately informed. The power to consent must be exercised according to the 'welfare principle': that the child's 'welfare' or 'best interests' must be paramount. Even where a child lacks capacity to consent on their own behalf, it is good practice to involve the child as much as possible in the decision-making process.

Where necessary, the courts can, as with competent children, overrule a refusal by a person with parental responsibility. It is recommended that certain important decisions, such as sterilization for contraceptive purposes, should be referred to the courts for guidance, even if those with parental responsibility consent to the operation going ahead.

The Children Act 1989 sets out persons who may have parental responsibility. These include:

- the child's parents if married to each other at the time of conception or birth
- the child's mother, but not father, if they were not so married unless the father has acquired parental responsibility via a court order or the couple subsequently marry
- the child's legally appointed guardian
- a person in whose favour the court has made a residence order concerning the child
- a local authority designated in a care order in respect of the child
- a local authority or other authorised person who holds an emergency protection order in respect of the child.

In order to consent on behalf of a child, the person with parental responsibility must themselves have capacity. Where the mother of a child is under 16, she will only be able to give valid consent for her child's treatment if she herself is Gillick competent. Whether or not she has capacity may vary, depending on the seriousness of the decision to be taken.

See also the 'Ethical issues' section in Chapter 9 (Ethical issues), page 127.

General topics

Childhood predictors of future psychiatric morbidity

Niemi L, Suvisaari JM, Haukka JK et al 2005 Childhood predictors of future psychiatric morbidity in offspring of mothers with psychotic illness. Results from the Helsinki high-risk study disorder. British Journal of Psychiatry 186: 108–114

The Helsinki high-risk study, initiated in 1974, is one of the largest ever high-risk investigations. The study includes all eligible mothers and their offspring. The study aimed to compare the development of high-risk and control group children and investigate which factors predicted future psychiatric disorders.

Method

- A follow-up study.
- The childhood and school health cards for 159 offspring of 143 high-risk mothers and 99 controls were examined.
- The health cards examined such features as whether:
  - the child was walking at 12 months and talking words at 2 years
  - the child had a speech problem in childhood or at school
  - there were emotional problems in childhood or at school
  - there were problems in social adjustment in childhood
  - there were problems in neurological development – either 'severe' or 'soft signs'
  - there was failure to reach age-appropriate mental development assessed yearly between 1 and 6
  - there was a need for extra follow-up in the school health system for any reason (assessed at school age)
  - there was a rating of being socially inhibited or having conduct problems or academic impairment.
- Logistic regression examined developmental abnormalities and the prediction of later mental disorders.

Results

- Children in the high-risk group had:
  - more emotional problems before school age

- more attentional problems and social inhibition at school age
- more neurological 'soft signs'.
- Problems in social adjustment at age 5–6 predicted later development of schizophrenia-spectrum disorder (after adjusting for gender and social class).
- Problems in social adjustment at age 5–6 and emotional symptoms at school age tended to predict later development of psychotic disorder.
- Emotional symptoms, conduct problems and social inhibition at school age predicted later development of mood disorder. Attentional problems were most significant.
- Emotional symptoms, conduct problems and attentional problems at school age all predicted later development of substance misuse disorder.
- Delayed mental development, problems in social adjustment at age 5–6, and emotional symptoms, conduct problems and social inhibition at school age predicted later development of personality disorder.
- Delayed mental development, emotional symptoms, conduct problems and social inhibition at school age predicted later development of mental disorder.
- Problems in social adjustment at age 5–6 tended to predict later development of mental disorder.
- Separate analysis of the offspring from mothers with schizophrenia-spectrum disorders changed the results only slightly.
- Neurological soft signs tended to predict later development of schizophrenia-spectrum disorder.
- Problems in preschool social adjustment no longer predicted later development of any psychotic, personality or mental disorder.
- Social inhibition no longer predicted later development of mood disorder.

Summary

- Severe neurological problems and preschool difficulties in social adjustment predicted development of schizophrenia-spectrum disorders.
- In contrast, school age emotional problems and problems in social adjustment were strong predictors of mood, substance-related and personality disorders.
- Only those who developed personality disorders had multiple problems both at preschool and school-age assessments.

Caspi A, Moffitt TE, Newman DL et al 1996 Behavioural observations at age 3 years predict adult psychiatric disorders. Longitudinal evidence from a birth cohort. Archives of General Psychiatry 53: 1033–1039

- Agreed with the finding of the Isle of Wight study (Rutter et al 1970).

- Adults who go on to develop mental illness often have a history of developmental problems in childhood and adolescence.

Niemi LT, Suvisaari JM, Tuulio-Henriksson A et al 2003 Childhood developmental abnormalities in schizophrenia: evidence from the high-risk studies. A review. Schizophrenia Research 60: 239–258

- High-risk research refers to the study of early antecedents of a disorder by investigating those at a higher risk of developing the condition, usually if they have a family history.

Niemi LT, Suvisaari JM, Haukka JK et al 2004 Cumulative incidence of mental disorder among offspring of mothers with psychotic disorder: results from the Helsinki High-Risk Study. British Journal of Psychiatry 185: 11–17

- The original study.
- Children born between 1960 and 1964 in Helsinki to all women born between 1916 and 1948 who had been treated in a psychiatric hospital before 1975 and had a diagnosis of schizophrenia-spectrum disorder were identified.
- A control group was included.
- The final high-risk group consisted of 179 offspring from 161 mothers.
- The control group consisted of 176 offspring from 176 mothers.
- The high-risk mothers were divided into those with schizophrenia, other schizophrenia-spectrum disorders, affective psychosis or schizoaffective psychosis.

See also the 'General topics' section in Chapter 26 (Schizophrenia), page 367.

Impact of child sexual abuse on mental health

Spataro J, Mullen PE, Burgess PM et al 2004 Impact of child sexual abuse on mental health. A prospective study in males and females. British Journal of Psychiatry 184: 416–421

There is a lack of prospective studies and data on male victims, leaving major questions regarding associations between child sexual abuse and subsequent psychopathology unresolved. Most of the evidence to date comes from retrospective ascertainment of child sexual abuse. There is limited evidence regarding subsequent psychological disturbances in adult mental health.

Method

- This study examines males and females who were examined by forensic physicians following allegations of sexual abuse.

- The patients who went on to receive treatment by public mental health were assessed.
- 1612 (1327 female) children were recruited.
- Patients were born between 1950 and 1991.
- The records of the Victorian Institute of Forensic Medicine were scrutinised to identify all the examinations made by police and welfare services following alleged child sexual abuse.
- The cohort positive for abuse were then linked to cases registered on the Victorian Psychiatric Case Register, which records different types of mental disorder.
- Complete psychiatric records were then extracted for the matched cases.
- Although dual diagnosis was common, one primary diagnosis was selected for the purposes of the study.
- The cohort was matched with a population control sample.

Results

- Mean age at examination following suspected sexual abuse was 9.4 years.
- 78.3% were thought to have experienced penetrative sexual abuse.
- The rates of abuse involving penetration were significantly less for males than for females.
- Record of contact with public mental health services was found in 12.4% of cases over the period of a year (3.6% of the control group registered contact).
- Rates of contact were significantly higher for both males and females.
- Major affective disorders were more frequently found amongst cases, with anxiety and acute stress disorders being even more strongly associated with child sexual abuse.
- Personality disorders had the highest relative risk.
- In childhood, conduct disorder was associated with child sexual abuse.
- Rates of schizophrenic disorders, substance dependence and other affective and somatoform diagnoses were not significantly higher than that of the general population.
- When males were compared, anxiety disorders, personality disorders, organic disorders, childhood mental disorders and conduct disorders remained significantly higher in those who had been abused.
- Major affective disorders were not significant in males.
- Females who had been abused were more likely to be recorded on the register for major affective disorders, anxiety disorders, personality disorders, childhood mental disorders and conduct disorders but not for other affective and somatoform disorders.
- Males were significantly more likely than females to have had contact with public mental health services.
- Males were overrepresented for conduct disorder and other childhood mental disorders.

- There were no significant differences between males and females in specific diagnostic categories.
- The study is unique in that it demonstrates prospectively a clear association between child sexual abuse and mental health problems in childhood and adult life.
- The results do not show a relationship between child sexual abuse and schizophrenia, which has previously been hypothesised.

Discussion

- There are methodological biases in that only the more severe cases of CSA are likely to come to the attention of services, and symptoms from the psychiatric register will not reflect all the psychopathology.
- The results do not agree with previous research which found increased rates of drug and alcohol-related disorders and of schizophrenia in people who have experienced CSA.

Darvez-Bornoz JM, Choquet M, Ledoux S et al 1998 Gender differences in symptoms of adolescents reporting sexual assault. Social Psychiatry and Psychiatric Epidemiology 33: 111–117

- There are higher levels of behavioural problems in sexually abused males as opposed to females.
- Conduct disorders are significantly more likely to occur in females who have been sexually abused as children than those who have not.

Pervasive refusal syndrome

Lask B 2004 Pervasive refusal syndrome. Advances in Psychiatric Treatment 10: 153–159

Predominantly affects girls between the ages of 8 and 16. The incidence is unknown. There are no reports of cases in adults. There have been reported cases in boys. Acute onset is usual, although in some there is a more gradual onset. The latter may happen on a background of emotional difficulties such as anxiety or somatisation. There is no social class bias. Other factors may include a normal premorbid personality or high achievement with high self-expectation and difficulty coping with perceived failure. Common precipitants are viral infections and injury. There may be no response to appropriate treatment and subsequent deterioration. Aetiology is unclear, but Seligman's model of learned helplessness offers a psychological explanation.

Associated symptoms include fatigue, lethargy, abdominal pain and nausea. Depressed mood may be present but with insufficient associated features to make the diagnosis of depressive disorder. Distress at separation from parents on admission is common, often later replaced by angry refusal to see the parents. Speech when it occurs is abnormal, barely audible and high pitched. Patients often assume the fetal position, with a tendency to be covered by bedclothes.

Investigations are unremarkable.

Differential diagnosis includes depression, anxiety, eating disorders, selective mutism, catatonic disorders, stupor, somatoform disorder, school refusal, chronic fatigue syndrome and factitious illness.

- Compared with depressive disorder, psychomotor slowing and sleep disturbance are uncommon, although comorbid depression can occur.
- There can be similarities with the eating disorders, but the core features are not present (relentless pursuit of thinness and morbid preoccupation with shape and height).
- Features of generalised psychomotor retardation and increased motor tone do not occur in PRS. Movement still occurs in sleep and when physical contact is attempted. There are no psychotic features.
- While akinesis and negativism occur in both, the diagnosis of stupor is excluded by the wilful negativism of PRS as well as the gradual return of function.
- Compared with somatoform disorders, there are no help-seeking behaviours; indeed, there is treatment resistance. This is also true for chronic fatigue syndrome and factitious illness.
- While there is an inability to go to school, there is also a refusal to take part in any other activity, thus differentiating this from school refusal or phobia.

Treatment

- Hospitalisation is almost always required.
- Patience, time and sympathy are required in treating these patients.
- Initial therapeutic optimism can be counterproductive.
- Recovery generally takes 12 months from the introduction of appropriate treatment. Nursing care is central to the programme, in terms of a detailed daily timetable, nasogastric feeding, skin care and the provision of the ward milieu as a safe, structured and consistent environment.
- Physiotherapy should be introduced in the early stages to release and prevent stiffness, to prevent contractures and to maintain as full a range of movement as possible. Individual therapy, in later stages, can be helpful.
- The use of 'musing' (thinking aloud) seems to be helpful.
- Therapy best focuses on whatever material the child offers, rather than using a specific agenda or therapeutic technique. Letter writing, email and text messaging can all be used to communicate in the period before the return of speech.
- Parents and families should be involved in counselling and therapy to help address anxiety and distress, and to promote consistency in management.

- Medication has a limited role – for example, antidepressants for comorbid depression.
- Short-term use of sedation may be required for periods of distress, such as insertion of feeding tubes or passive physiotherapy.
- Once recovery begins, the focus of treatment moves to a very gradual rehabilitation, the pace determined by the child's progress.
- In general, the symptoms that appear last are the first to recover.

Thompson S, Nunn K 1997 The pervasive refusal syndrome. The Royal Alexandria Hospital for Children experience. Clinical Child Psychology and Psychiatry 2: 145–165

Described diagnostic criteria for pervasive refusal syndrome of:

- clear food refusal and weight loss
- social withdrawal and school refusal
- partial or complete refusal in two or more of the following domains: mobilisation, speaking, attention to self-care
- active and angry resistance to help or encouragement
- no organic condition to account for the severity or degree of symptoms
- no other psychiatric illness that could better account for the symptoms.

Definition

Pervasive refusal syndrome – a disorder characterised by a profound and pervasive refusal to eat, drink, talk, walk and engage in any form of self-care. The varying degrees of refusal are accompanied by dramatic social withdrawal and a determined resistance to treatment, leading to a seriously disabling and potentially life-threatening condition.

Should we prescribe antidepressants to children?

Dubicka B, Goodyer I 2005 Should we prescribe antidepressants to children? Psychiatric Bulletin 29: 164–167

In June 2004, the Committee on Safety of Medicines (CSM) advised that paroxetine should not be prescribed to depressed children and adolescents. This was subsequently followed by similar warnings about other SSRIs with the exception of fluoxetine. The report was based on a detailed review of both published and unpublished data. Negative outcomes had not been reported. It was established that, with the exception of fluoxetine, the risks outweigh the benefits. There is evidence of increased suicidality with most SSRIs compared with placebo.

Another consideration is whether childhood and adolescent depressive disorders share the same aetiology and respond to treatment in the same way. There is some argument that these may be separate disorders.

Whittington CJ, Kendall T, Fonaghy P et al 2004 Selective serotonin reuptake inhibitors in childhood depression: systematic review of published versus unpublished data. Lancet 363: 1341–1345

- Completed a recent meta-analysis which supported the recommendations of the CSM.

Jureidini JN, Doecke CJ, Mansfield PR et al 2004 Efficacy and safety of antidepressants for children and adolescents. British Medical Journal 328: 879–883

- Has criticised the quality of reporting in published trials in a review looking at the safety and efficacy of antidepressants in children and adolescents.
- It concluded that the benefits of all SSRIs have been exaggerated and the adverse effects downplayed.
- They suggest psychological treatments are safer and more effective.

Khan A, Khan S, Kolts R et al 2003 Suicide rates in clinical trials of SSRIs, other antidepressants, and placebo: analysis of FDA reports. American Journal of Psychiatry 160: 790–792

- Found there was no increased risk of suicide in adults taking SSRIs.

Olfson M, Shaffer D, Marcus SC et al 2003 Relationship between antidepressant medication treatment and suicide in adolescents. Archives of General Psychiatry 60: 978–982

- Found that a 1% increase in the use of antidepressants resulted in 0.23 suicides per 100,000 adolescents a year.
- This does not indicate causality but demonstrates we must exercise caution regarding negative associations.

Rice F, Harold GT, Thapar A et al 2002 Assessing the effects of age, sex and shared environment on the genetic aetiology of depression in childhood and adolescence. Journal of Child Psychology and Psychiatry 43: 1039–1051

- Stated that environmental factors are important in depression in childhood and in adolescence but genetic factors are important only in adolescence.

Shaffer D, Gould MS, Fisher P et al 1996 Psychiatric diagnosis in child and adolescent suicide. Archives of General Psychiatry 53: 339–348

- The course of adolescent depression is similar to that in the adult.

- Adolescent depression is the most common adolescent psychiatric disorder associated with suicidal behaviour and completed suicide.

Hazell P, O'Connell D, Heathcote D et al 2003 Tricyclic drugs for depression in children and adolescents **(Cochrane Review)**. In: The Cochrane Library, Issue 4. Update Software, Oxford

- Found no benefit of TCAs in children and only a very modest effect in adolescents.
- Given their side-effect profile in overdose, the risks would outweigh the benefits in suicidal children and adolescents.

Harrington R, Whittaker J, Shoebridge P 1998 Psychological treatment of depression in children and adolescents. A review of treatment research. British Journal of Psychiatry 173: 291–298

- Psychological treatment is effective in mild to moderate depression.

Clarke GN, Hornbrook M, Lynch F et al 2002 Group cognitive–behavioural treatment for depressed adolescent parents in a health maintenance organisation. Journal of the American Academy of Child and Adolescent Psychiatry 41: 305–313

- Studied depressed children of depressed parents.
- Group CBT was no more effective than treatment as usual.

Weblink Committee on Safety of Medicines – www.mhra.gov.uk.

Policy and Legislation

Children Act 2004[†]

Legislates on the strategies for improving children's lives. It includes general services for all children and specific services for children with additional needs.

It aims to encourage the integrated planning, commissioning and delivery of services as well as to improve multidisciplinary working. Local authorities have to provide flexible, coordinated services.

The previous Children Act 1989 legislated to:
- reform the law relating to children
- make provision for local authority services for children in need and others
- amend the law with respect to children's homes, community homes, voluntary homes and voluntary organisations

[†] Crown copyright. Reproduced with permission

- make provision with respect to fostering, child minding and day care for young children and adoption, and for connected purposes.

The Children Act Report 2003

- Collaboration between government and children's services.
- To improve outcomes for all children and young people.
- To narrow the gap in outcomes between the most vulnerable children and their peers.

Every Child Matters (Green Paper, 2003)

- Called for radical improvement in opportunities and outcomes for children.
- Improved outcomes for children and young people.
- Aimed to ensure that all children are healthy, stay safe, enjoy and achieve, make a positive contribution and achieve economic well-being.
- A focus on opportunities for all and narrowing gaps.
- Support for parents, carers and families
- A shift to prevention, early identification and intervention.
- Integrated and personalised services.

The Green Paper set out a number of legislative commitments that have now been taken forward through the Children Act 2004.

Weblinks

The Children Act 1989 – www.hmso.gov.uk

The Children Act 2004 – www.dfes.gov.uk/publications/childrenactreport

Children Act Report – www.dfes.gov.uk

Every Child Matters – information on the implementation of the Act: www.everychildmatters.gov.uk

See also the 'Policy and legislation' section in Chapter 22 (Policy and legislation), page 333.

Treatment – Psychopharmacology

Clozapine prescribing in adolescent psychiatry

Cirulli G 2005 Clozapine prescribing in adolescent psychiatry: survey of prescribing practice in in-patient units. Psychiatric Bulletin 29: 377–380

A number of studies have shown that neuroleptic medication is the mainstay of treatment for schizophrenia in children and adolescents, despite the fact that side effects and treatment resistance occur more often in this group. Some studies have shown that the duration of untreated psychosis is important, with poorer outcomes following delay in treatment. Early treatment may improve later function and reduce morbidity and mortality.

Clozapine is the only drug licensed for treatment-resistant or intolerant psychosis. It can be used in adolescents as young as 16. However, in children under the age of 18 years the manufacturers recommend that patients have EEG assessment prior to and during treatment with clozapine due to the risk of seizures and absences.

The NICE guidelines recommend that in patients resistant to treatment with antipsychotic medication clozapine should be commenced at the earliest opportunity. However, the Clozapine Patient Monitoring Service calculated in April 2004 that only 88 patients under 18 years received treatment with clozapine (total patient number: 21,000).

This paper looks at the prescribing practices and attitudes pertaining to treatment with clozapine in adolescent psychiatry.

Method

Questionnaires were sent to consultants in adolescent psychiatry.

Results

- 12% reported they did not use clozapine because of lack of suitable cases.
- 29% of consultants stated that they just did not use clozapine.
- Unfamiliarity with clozapine and the need for frequent monitoring of side effects appear to influence use.
- Many do not seem to routinely request an EEG before treatment.
- Weight gain seemed to prevent some doctors prescribing the drug to young people.
- 21% reportedly stopped clozapine because of side effects or serious complications.

See also the 'Treatment – Psychopharmacology' section in Chapter 26 (Schizophrenia), page 383.

Efficacy and safety of antidepressants for children and adolescents

Jureidini JN, Doecke CJ, Mansfield PR et al 2004 Efficacy and safety of antidepressants for children and adolescents. British Medical Journal 328: 879–883

The safety of the prescribing of antidepressants to children and adolescents has been of increasing concern in the community and medical circles. SSRIs have been increasingly used to treat depression in children and adolescents since they were introduced in the 1990s. There have been recommendations made against their use from the government and the drug industry.

This paper reviewed the efficacy and safety of newer antidepressants in children.

Results

- Investigators' conclusions on the efficacy of newer antidepressants in childhood depression may have exaggerated the benefits.
- Improvement in the control group is marked with additional benefits from drugs being of doubtful clinical significance.
- Adverse effects have been downplayed.
- Antidepressant drugs cannot confidently be recommended as a treatment option for childhood depression.
- A more critical approach to ensuring the validity of published data is needed.

Tricyclic drugs for depression in children and adolescents

Hazell P, O' Connell D, Heathcote D, Henry D 2002 Tricyclic drugs for depression in children and adolescents **(Cochrane Review)**. In: The Cochrane Library, Issue 2. Update Software, Oxford

- 13 trials ($n = 506$) were included.
- There were no differences between the treatment and placebo groups in terms of overall improvement for children and adolescents.
- A small statistically significant benefit was shown for treatment over placebo in reducing symptoms.
- There is a greater benefit among adolescents.
- There was no benefit among children in subgroup analysis.
- TCAs were associated with more vertigo, orthostatic hypotension, tremor and dry mouth compared with placebo.

See also the 'Treatment – Psychopharmacology' section in Chapter 2 (Affective disorders), page 31.

Treatment – Psychological Therapies

Cognitive–behavioural training interventions for assisting foster carers in the management of difficult behaviour

Turner W, Macdonald GM, Dennis JA 2005 Cognitive–behavioural training interventions for assisting foster carers in the management of difficult behaviour **(Cochrane Review)**. In: The Cochrane Library, Issue 2. Update Software, Oxford

- The evidence was inconclusive.
- There was minimal effect on outcomes relating to looked-after children with regard to psychosocial functioning, extent of behavioural problems and interpersonal functioning.
- There were some positive effects on foster carer outcomes in terms of behavioural management skills, attitudes and psychological functioning.

Psychological and/or educational interventions for the prevention of depression in children and adolescents

Merry S, McDowell H, Hetrick S, Bir J, Muller N 2004 Psychological and/or educational interventions for the prevention of depression in children and adolescents **(Cochrane Review)**. In: The Cochrane Library, Issue 2. CD003380. Update Software, Oxford

- Two studies compared the intervention with an active comparison or placebo. Although neither showed effectiveness, one trial was underpowered and the other used a placebo with active therapeutic elements.
- The remaining studies compared the intervention with waiting list or no-intervention controls.
- In these studies targeted psychological interventions were effective immediately after the intervention was delivered, bringing about a significant reduction on depression rating scale scores.
- The small effect sizes reported translated to a significant reduction in depressive episodes (NNT 10).
- The quality of the studies was generally poor.
- Only two had explicit allocation concealment.
- Boys and girls responded differently to different programmes, but the findings were not consistent.

See also the 'Treatment – Psychological therapies' section in Chapter 25 (Psychological therapies), pages 350, 358, 360-362.

Scared Straight and other juvenile awareness programmes for preventing juvenile delinquency

Petrosino A, Turpin-Petrosino C, Buehler J 2002 Scared Straight and other juvenile awareness programs for preventing juvenile delinquency **(Cochrane Review)**. In: The Cochrane Library, Issue 2. CD002796. Update Software, Oxford

- Nine trials reported narrative results.
- The intervention was found to be more harmful than doing nothing and was associated with an increase in offending behaviour.
- Agencies that use such programmes should rigorously evaluate them to show that they prevent crime and at the very least do not cause more harm than good.

See also the 'Treatment – Psychological therapies' section in Chapter 10 (Forensic psychiatry), pages 350, 358, 360-362.

Guidelines

Depression in children and young people: identification and management in primary, community and secondary care. NICE Clinical Guideline 28*

The guidance follows the following five steps:
1. Detection and recognition of depression and risk profiling in primary care and community settings.
2. Recognition of depression in children and young people referred to CAMHS.
3. Managing recognised depression in primary care and community settings – mild depression.
4. Managing recognised depression in tier 2 or 3 CAMHS – moderate to severe depression.
5. Managing recognised depression in tier 3 or 4 CAMHS – unresponsive, recurrent and psychotic depression, including depression needing inpatient care.

Each step introduces additional interventions; the higher steps assume interventions in the previous step.
See also the 'Guidelines' section in Chapter 2 (Affective disorders), page 45.

Table 5.1 Management of depression in children and young people

Focus	Action	Responsibility
Detection	Risk profiling	Tier 1
Recognition	Identification in presenting children or young people	Tiers 2–4
Mild depression (including dysthymia)	Watchful waiting Non-directive supportive therapy/group, cognitive behavioural therapy/guided self-help	Tier 1
Moderate to severe depression	Brief psychological therapy ± fluoxetine	Tier 1 or 2
Depression unresponsive to treatment/recurrent depression/psychotic depression	Intensive psychological therapy ± fluoxetine, sertraline, citalopram, augmentation with an antipsychotic	Tier 3 or 4

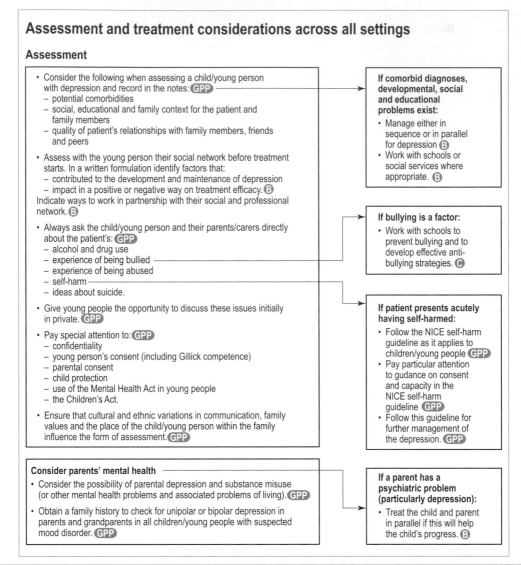

Assessment and treatment considerations across all settings

Assessment

- Consider the following when assessing a child/young person with depression and record in the notes: **GPP**
  - potential comorbidities
  - social, educational and family context for the patient and family members
  - quality of patient's relationships with family members, friends and peers

- Assess with the young person their social network before treatment starts. In a written formulation identify factors that:
  - contributed to the development and maintenance of depression
  - impact in a positive or negative way on treatment efficacy. **B**
  Indicate ways to work in partnership with their social and professional network. **B**

- Always ask the child/young person and their parents/carers directly about the patient's: **GPP**
  - alcohol and drug use
  - experience of being bullied
  - experience of being abused
  - self-harm
  - ideas about suicide.

- Give young people the opportunity to discuss these issues initially in private. **GPP**

- Pay special attention to: **GPP**
  - confidentiality
  - young person's consent (including Gillick competence)
  - parental consent
  - child protection
  - use of the Mental Health Act in young people
  - the Children's Act.

- Ensure that cultural and ethnic variations in communication, family values and the place of the child/young person within the family influence the form of assessment. **GPP**

If comorbid diagnoses, developmental, social and educational problems exist:

- Manage either in sequence or in parallel for depression **B**
- Work with schools or social services where appropriate. **B**

If bullying is a factor:

- Work with schools to prevent bullying and to develop effective anti-bullying strategies. **C**

If patient presents acutely having self-harmed:

- Follow the NICE self-harm guideline as it applies to children/young people **GPP**
- Pay particular attention to gudance on consent and capacity in the NICE self-harm guideline **GPP**
- Follow this guideline for further management of the depression. **GPP**

Consider parents' mental health

- Consider the possibility of parental depression and substance misuse (or other mental health problems and associated problems of living). **GPP**

- Obtain a family history to check for unipolar or bipolar depression in parents and grandparents in all children/young people with suspected mood disorder. **GPP**

If a parent has a psychiatric problem (particularly depression):

- Treat the child and parent in parallel if this will help the child's progress. **B**

A, B, C and D indicate grades of recommendation; **GPP** indicates a good practice point (see Appendix II for full details). * Reproduced with permission from the National Institute for Health and Clinical Excellence, London.

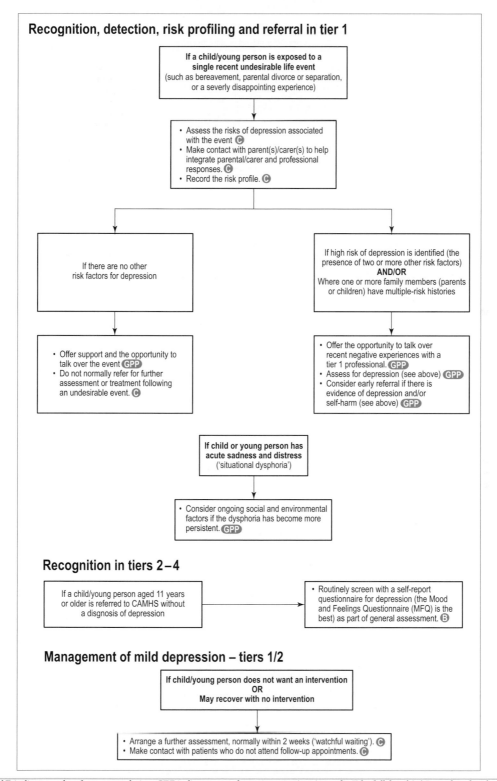

Recognition, detection, risk profiling and referral in tier 1

If a child/young person is exposed to a single recent undesirable life event
(such as bereavement, parental divorce or separation, or a severly disappointing experience)

- Assess the risks of depression associated with the event **C**
- Make contact with parent(s)/carer(s) to help integrate parental/carer and professional responses. **C**
- Record the risk profile. **C**

If there are no other risk factors for depression

If high risk of depression is identified (the presence of two or more other risk factors)
AND/OR
Where one or more family members (parents or children) have multiple-risk histories

- Offer support and the opportunity to talk over the event **GPP**
- Do not normally refer for further assessment or treatment following an undesirable event. **C**

- Offer the opportunity to talk over recent negative experiences with a tier 1 professional. **GPP**
- Assess for depression (see above) **GPP**
- Consider early referral if there is evidence of depression and/or self-harm (see above) **GPP**

If child or young person has acute sadness and distress ('situational dysphoria')

- Consider ongoing social and environmental factors if the dysphoria has become more persistent. **GPP**

Recognition in tiers 2–4

If a child/young person aged 11 years or older is referred to CAMHS without a disgnosis of depression

- Routinely screen with a self-report questionnaire for depression (the Mood and Feelings Questionnaire (MFQ) is the best) as part of general assessment. **B**

Management of mild depression – tiers 1/2

If child/young person does not want an intervention OR May recover with no intervention

- Arrange a further assessment, normally within 2 weeks ('watchful waiting'). **C**
- Make contact with patients who do not attend follow-up appointments. **C**

A, B, C and **D** indicate grades of recommendation; **GPP** indicates a good practice point (see Appendix II for full details). * Reproduced with permission from the National Institute for Health and Clinical Excellence, London.

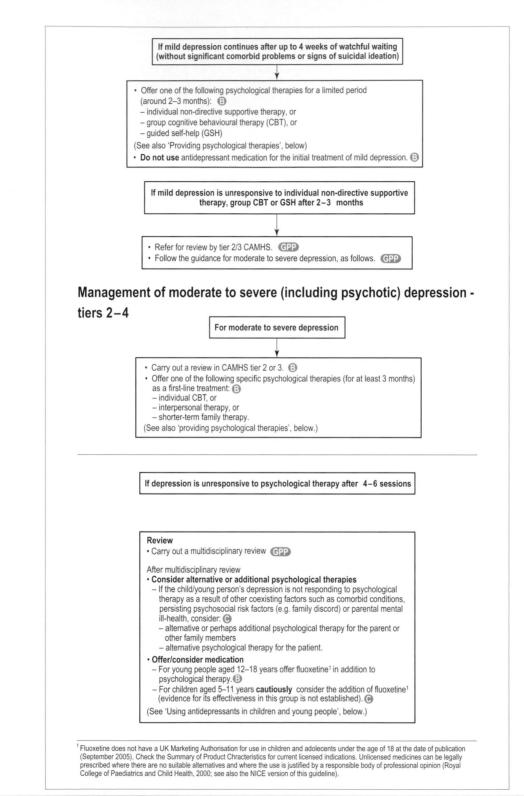

If mild depression continues after up to 4 weeks of watchful waiting (without significant comorbid problems or signs of suicidal ideation)

- Offer one of the following psychological therapies for a limited period (around 2–3 months): Ⓑ
  – individual non-directive supportive therapy, or
  – group cognitive behavioural therapy (CBT), or
  – guided self-help (GSH)
(See also 'Providing psychological therapies', below)
- **Do not use** antidepressant medication for the initial treatment of mild depression. Ⓑ

If mild depression is unresponsive to individual non-directive supportive therapy, group CBT or GSH after 2–3 months

- Refer for review by tier 2/3 CAMHS. GPP
- Follow the guidance for moderate to severe depression, as follows. GPP

Management of moderate to severe (including psychotic) depression - tiers 2–4

For moderate to severe depression

- Carry out a review in CAMHS tier 2 or 3. Ⓑ
- Offer one of the following specific psychological therapies (for at least 3 months) as a first-line treatment: Ⓑ
  – individual CBT, or
  – interpersonal therapy, or
  – shorter-term family therapy.
(See also 'providing psychological therapies', below.)

If depression is unresponsive to psychological therapy after 4–6 sessions

Review
- Carry out a multidisciplinary review GPP

After multidisciplinary review
- **Consider alternative or additional psychological therapies**
  – If the child/young person's depression is not responding to psychological therapy as a result of other coexisting factors such as comorbid conditions, persisting psychosocial risk factors (e.g. family discord) or parental mental ill-health, consider: Ⓒ
    – alternative or perhaps additional psychological therapy for the parent or other family members
    – alternative psychological therapy for the patient.
- **Offer/consider medication**
  – For young people aged 12–18 years offer fluoxetine[1] in addition to psychological therapy. Ⓑ
  – For children aged 5–11 years **cautiously** consider the addition of fluoxetine[1] (evidence for its effectiveness in this group is not established). Ⓒ
(See 'Using antidepressants in children and young people', below.)

[1] Fluoxetine does not have a UK Marketing Authorisation for use in children and adolecents under the age of 18 at the date of publication (September 2005). Check the Summary of Product Chracteristics for current licensed indications. Unlicensed medicines can be legally prescribed where there are no suitable alternatives and where the use is justified by a responsible body of professional opinion (Royal College of Paediatrics and Child Health, 2000; see also the NICE version of this guideline).

A, B, C and **D** indicate grades of recommendation; **GPP** indicates a good practice point (see Appendix II for full details). * Reproduced with permission from the National Institute for Health and Clinical Excellence, London.

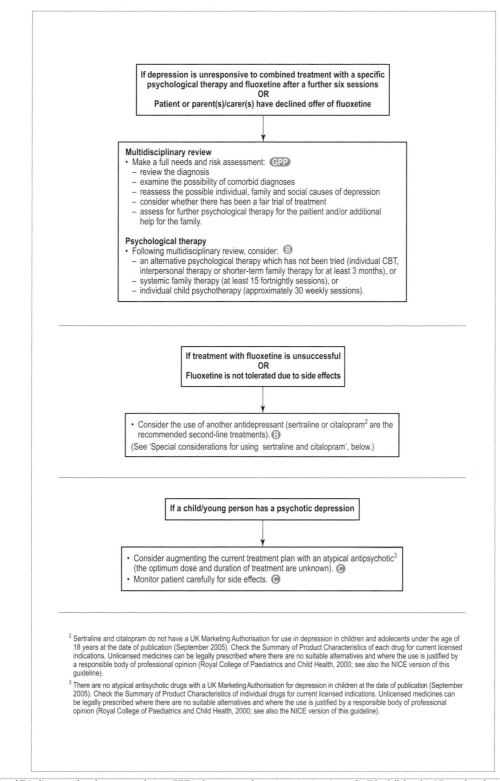

If depression is unresponsive to combined treatment with a specific psychological therapy and fluoxetine after a further six sessions
OR
Patient or parent(s)/carer(s) have declined offer of fluoxetine

Multidisciplinary review
- Make a full needs and risk assessment: **GPP**
  - review the diagnosis
  - examine the possibility of comorbid diagnoses
  - reassess the possible individual, family and social causes of depression
  - consider whether there has been a fair trial of treatment
  - assess for further psychological therapy for the paitient and/or additional help for the family.

Psychological therapy
- Following multidisciplinary review, consider: **B**
  - an alternative psychological therapy which has not been tried (individual CBT, interpersonal therapy or shorter-term family therapy for at least 3 months), or
  - systemic family therapy (at least 15 fortnightly sessions), or
  - individual child psychotherapy (approximately 30 weekly sessions).

If treatment with fluoxetine is unsuccessful
OR
Fluoxetine is not tolerated due to side effects

- Consider the use of another antidepressant (sertraline or citalopram[2] are the recommended second-line treatments). **B**
(See 'Special considerations for using sertraline and citalopram', below.)

If a child/young person has a psychotic depression

- Consider augmenting the current treatment plan with an atypical antipsychotic[3] (the optimum dose and duration of treatment are unknown). **C**
- Monitor patient carefully for side effects. **C**

[2] Sertraline and citalopram do not have a UK Marketing Authorisation for use in depression in children and adolescents under the age of 18 years at the date of publication (September 2005). Check the Summary of Product Characteristics of each drug for current licensed indications. Unlicensed medicines can be legally prescribed where there are no suitable alternatives and where the use is justified by a responsible body of professional opinion (Royal College of Paediatrics and Child Health, 2000; see also the NICE version of this guideline).

[3] There are no atypical antisychotic drugs with a UK Marketing Authorisation for depression in children at the date of publication (September 2005). Check the Summary of Product Characteristics of individual drugs for current licensed indications. Unlicensed medicines can be legally prescribed where there are no suitable alternatives and where the use is justified by a responsible body of professional opinion (Royal College of Paediatrics and Child Health, 2000; see also the NICE version of this guideline).

A, B, C and **D** indicate grades of recommendation; **GPP** indicates a good practice point (see Appendix II for full details). * Reproduced with permission from the National Institute for Health and Clinical Excellence, London.

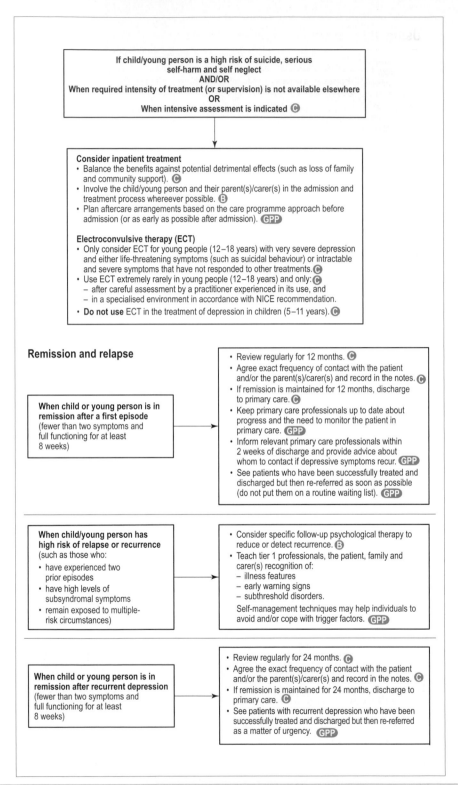

If child/young person is a high risk of suicide, serious
self-harm and self neglect
AND/OR
When required intensity of treatment (or supervision) is not available elsewhere
OR
When intensive assessment is indicated Ⓒ

Consider inpatient treatment
- Balance the benefits against potential detrimental effects (such as loss of family and community support). Ⓒ
- Involve the child/young person and their parent(s)/carer(s) in the admission and treatment process whereever possible. Ⓑ
- Plan aftercare arrangements based on the care programme approach before admission (or as early as possible after admission). **GPP**

Electroconvulsive therapy (ECT)
- Only consider ECT for young people (12–18 years) with very severe depression and either life-threatening symptoms (such as suicidal behaviour) or intractable and severe symptoms that have not responded to other treatments. Ⓒ
- Use ECT extremely rarely in young people (12–18 years) and only: Ⓒ
   – after careful assessment by a practitioner experienced in its use, and
   – in a specialised environment in accordance with NICE recommendation.
- **Do not use** ECT in the treatment of depression in children (5–11 years). Ⓒ

Remission and relapse

When child or young person is in remission after a first episode
(fewer than two symptoms and full functioning for at least 8 weeks)

- Review regularly for 12 months. Ⓒ
- Agree exact frequency of contact with the patient and/or the parent(s)/carer(s) and record in the notes. Ⓒ
- If remission is maintained for 12 months, discharge to primary care. Ⓒ
- Keep primary care professionals up to date about progress and the need to monitor the patient in primary care. **GPP**
- Inform relevant primary care professionals within 2 weeks of discharge and provide advice about whom to contact if depressive symptoms recur. **GPP**
- See patients who have been successfully treated and discharged but then re-referred as soon as possible (do not put them on a routine waiting list). **GPP**

When child/young person has high risk of relapse or recurrence
(such as those who:
- have experienced two prior episodes
- have high levels of subsyndromal symptoms
- remain exposed to multiple-risk circumstances)

- Consider specific follow-up psychological therapy to reduce or detect recurrence. Ⓑ
- Teach tier 1 professionals, the patient, family and carer(s) recognition of:
   – illness features
   – early warning signs
   – subthreshold disorders.
   Self-management techniques may help individuals to avoid and/or cope with trigger factors. **GPP**

When child or young person is in remission after recurrent depression
(fewer than two symptoms and full functioning for at least 8 weeks)

- Review regularly for 24 months. Ⓒ
- Agree the exact frequency of contact with the patient and/or the parent(s)/carer(s) and record in the notes. Ⓒ
- If remission is maintained for 24 months, discharge to primary care. Ⓒ
- See patients with recurrent depression who have been successfully treated and discharged but then re-referred as a matter of urgency. **GPP**

A, B, C and **D** indicate grades of recommendation; **GPP** indicates a good practice point (see Appendix II for full details). * Reproduced with permission from the National Institute for Health and Clinical Excellence, London.

Using antidepressants in children and young people

- Do not offer antidepressant medication except in combeination with a concurrent psychological therapy. **B**
- If psychological therapies are declined, medication may still be given, but monitor regularly and focus on adverse drug reactions. **B**
- Only prescribe following assessment and diagnosis by a child and adolescent psychiatrist. **C**
- Fluoxetine should be prescribed as this is the only antidepressant for which trials show that benefits outweigh the risk. **A**
- Consider the use of another antidepressant (sertraline or citalopram are the recommended second-line treatments). **B** (See 'Special considerations' for using sertraline and citalopram', below.)

Do not use:
- paroxetine and venlafaxine **A**
- tricyclic antidepressants **C**
- St John's-wort **C**

If patient is taking St John's-wort (over the counter)
- Inform of the risks:
  - there are no trials in children and young people upon which to make a clinical decision
  - unknown side effect profile
  - known drug interactions, including contraceptives.
- Advise discontinuation of St John's-wort:
  - monitor for recurrence of depression
  - assess for alternative treatments in accordance with this guideline.

Special considerations for using sertraline and citalopram

Only use when the following criteria have been met: C
- the patient and parent(s)/carer(s) have been fully involved in discussions about the benefits and risks.
- the patient and parent(s)/carer(s) have been provided with appropriate written information covering:
  - rationale for drug treatment
  - delay in onset of ef fect
  - time course of treatment
  - possible side effects
  - need to take medication as prescribed
  - the latest patient information advice from the relevant regulatory authority.
- The depression is sufficiently severe and/or causing sufficiently serious symptoms (e.g. weight loss or suicidal behaviour) to justify trial of another antidepressant.
- There is clear evidence of a fair trial of fluoxetine with a psychological therapy (i.e. all efforts have been made to ensure adherence to the recommended treatment regimen).
- There has been a reassessment of the likely causes of the depression and of treatment resistance (e.g. other diagnoses such as bipolar disorder or substance abuse).
- There has been advice from a senior child and adolescent psychiatrist (usually a consultant).
- The child/young person and/or someone with parental responsibility (or the younger person alone, if over 16 or deemed competent) has signed an appropriate and valid consent form.

Length of treatment
- After remission (no symptoms and full functioning for at least 8 weeks) continue medication for at least 6 months (after the 8-week period). **C**

Providing psychological therapies

- Ensure psychological therapies are provided by:
  - therapists who are also trained child and adolescent mental healthcare professionals **B**
  - healthcare professionals who have been trained to an appropriate level of competence in the therepy being offered. **C**
- Develop a joint treatment alliance with the family. If this proves difficult, consider providing the family with an alternative therapist. **C**

A, B, C and D indicate grades of recommendation; GPP indicates a good practice point (see Appendix II for full details). * Reproduced with permission from the National Institute for Health and Clinical Excellence, London.

Diagnosis and management of epilepsies in children and young people. SIGN Guideline 81**

Diagnosis

Differential diagnosis

There is wide differential diagnosis of paroxysmal episodes in childhood. Misdiagnosis of epilepsy appears to be a significant problem and may have major longer-term implications. A service for children with epilepsy should have specialists with skills and interest in the management of epilepsy and other paroxysmal disorders.

D   The diagnosis of epilepsy should be made by a paediatric neurologist or paediatrician with expertise in childhood epilepsy.

D   An EEG should only be requested after careful clinical evaluation by someone with expertise in childhood epilepsy.

Investigative procedures

ECG and EEG

☑   All children presenting with convulsive seizures should have an ECG with a calculation of the QTc interval.

☑   Home video camera recordings should be used in order to capture recurrent events where the diagnosis is in doubt.

C   All children with recurrent epileptic seizures should have an EEG. An early recording may avoid the need for repeated EEG investigations.

D   For children with recurrent epileptic seizures and a normal standard EEG, a second EEG recording including sleep should be used to aid identification of a specific epilepsy syndrome.

D   Where the clinical diagnosis of epilepsy is uncertain and if events are sufficiently frequent, an ictal EEG should be used to make a diagnosis of an epileptic or non-epileptic seizure.

☑   • An EEG is not indicated for children with recurrent or complex febrile seizures.
      • Antiepileptic drug medication should not usually be started before an EEG recording since it may mask a syndromic diagnosis.

Brain imaging

D   Most children with epilepsy should have an elective MRI brain scan. Children with the following epilepsy syndromes (which are following a typical course) do not need brain imaging:
     • idiopathic (primary) generalised epilepsies (*e.g. childhood absence epilepsy, juvenile myoclonic epilepsy or juvenile absence epilepsy*)

• benign childhood epilepsy with centrotemporal spikes (*benign rolandic epilepsy*)

Management

Information and planning

D   Children with epilepsy should be encouraged to participate in normal activities with their peers. Supervision requirements should be individualised taking into account the type of activity and the seizure history.

☑   A checklist should be used to help healthcare professionals deliver appropriate information to children, families and carers.

D   Families should be advised if the child has an increased risk of SUDEP. They can be reassured if the risk is considered to be low.

Information for schools

☑   Children should be enabled to participate in the full range of school activities.

☑   Children who have epilepsy should have a written care plan for their epilepsy, drawn up in agreement with the school and family.

☑   Epilepsy awareness training and written information should be offered to schools.

Antiepileptic drug treatment

When to start antiepileptic drug treatment

B   Children with febrile seizures, even if recurrent, should not be treated prophylactically with antiepileptic drugs.

A   Long-term prophylactic antiepileptic drug treatment for children with head injuries is not indicated.

A   Antiepileptic drug treatment should not be commenced routinely after a first, unprovoked tonic–clonic seizure.

Which drug to give?

C   The choice of first AED should be determined where possible by syndromic diagnosis and potential adverse effects.

A   When appropriate monotherapy fails to reduce seizure frequency, combination therapy should be considered.

☑   The choice of combination therapy should be guided by the epilepsy syndrome and the adverse effect profile of the AED.

☑   Where there is no response to an appropriate AED, the diagnosis and treatment of epilepsy should be reviewed.

☑   Referral to tertiary specialist care should be considered if a child fails to respond to two AEDs appropriate to the epilepsy in adequate dosages over a period of 6 months.

Antiepileptic drugs which may **WORSEN** specific syndromes or seizures

Antiepileptic drug	Epileptic syndrome/seizure type
Carbamazepine, vigabatrin, tiagabine, phenytoin	Childhood absence epilepsy, juvenile absence epilepsy, juvenile myoclonic epilepsy
Vigabatrin	Absences and absence status
Clonazepam	Generalised tonic status in Lennox–Gastaut syndrome
Lamotrigine	Dravet's syndrome, juvenile myoclonic epilepsy

Management of prolonged or serial seizures and convulsive status epilepticus

B   Prolonged or serial seizures should be treated with either nasal or buccal midazolam or rectal diazepam.

☑   All units admitting children should have a protocol for the management of convulsive status epilepticus.

Adverse effects

☑   Clear advice on the management of the potential adverse effects of AEDs should be discussed with children and parents or carers.

B   Routine AED level monitoring is not indicated in children.

☑   Adolescent girls taking AEDs and their parents should be advised of the risks of fetal malformations and developmental delay.

Withdrawal of antiepileptic drugs

A   Withdrawal of AED treatment should be considered in children who have been seizure free for 2 or more years.
The prescription of any medication requires an assessment of risk and of benefit. In this guideline the efficacy and safety of AEDs have been reviewed using the best available evidence. Where recommendations are graded for individual AEDs, this is done irrespective of the licensing status of that medication.

Behaviour and learning

Although many children with epilepsy have intellectual functioning in the normal range, learning and behavioural problems are more prevalent in this group than in the general childhood population.

☑   All children with epilepsy should have their behavioural and academic progress reviewed on a regular basis by the epilepsy team. Children with academic or behavioural difficulties should have appropriate educational and/or psychological assessment and intervention.

Epilepsy and the use of other medications

D   Neurostimulant treatment should not be withheld, when indicated, from children with epilepsy and ADHD.

D   Epilepsy, or a history of seizures, are not contraindications to the use of melatonin for the treatment of sleep disorders in children and young people.

☑   Selective serotonin reuptake inhibitors and atypical neuroleptics such as risperidone should not be withheld, when indicated, in children and young people with epilepsy and associated behavioural and psychiatric disorders.

Calculation of corrected QT interval

Models of care

☑   • Children with epilepsy should have access to specialist epilepsy services, including dedicated young people and transition clinics.
    • Each child should have an individual management plan agreed with the family and primary care team.
    • Annual review is suggested as a minimum, even for children with well-controlled epilepsy, to identify potential problems, ensure discussion on issues such as withdrawal of treatment, and minimise the possibility of becoming lost to follow-up.

D   Each epilepsy team should include paediatric epilepsy nurse specialist.

☑   Children and families should be advised of the range of services provided by the voluntary sector.

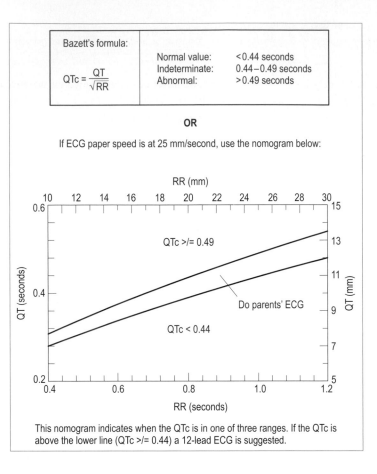

Bazett's formula:

$$QTc = \frac{QT}{\sqrt{RR}}$$

Normal value:	< 0.44 seconds
Indeterminate:	0.44–0.49 seconds
Abnormal:	> 0.49 seconds

OR

If ECG paper speed is at 25 mm/second, use the nomogram below:

RR (mm)

QTc >/= 0.49

Do parents' ECG

QTc < 0.44

QT (seconds)

QT (mm)

RR (seconds)

This nomogram indicates when the QTc is in one of three ranges. If the QTc is above the lower line (QTc >/= 0.44) a 12-lead ECG is suggested.

Websites

Enlighten–Action for Epilepsy
Website: www.enlighten.org.uk
Epilepsy Action
Website: www.epilepy.org.uk
Epilepsy Connections
Website: www.epilepsyconnections.org.uk
Epilepsy Scotland
Website: www.epilepsyscotland.org.uk

A, B, C and **D** indicate grades of recommendation; ☑ indicates a good practice point (see Appendix II for full details). ** Reproduced with permission from the Scottish Intercollegiate Guidelines Network, Edinburgh.

See also the 'Guidelines' section in Chapter 21 (Physical health), page 315.

Cross-cultural psychiatry

6

Ethical Issues

Independent Inquiry into the death of David Bennett

> Norfolk, Suffolk and Cambridgeshire Strategic Health Authority 2003 Independent Inquiry into the death of David Bennett. Online. Available: www.nscha.nhs. uk/4856/11516/David%20Bennett%20Inquiry.pdf

David 'Rocky' Bennett died aged 28 during restraint in a Norwich medium-secure psychiatric unit in 1998. He was an Afro-Caribbean man who had been treated for schizophrenia for 18 years.

Recommendations made by the Inquiry included the following:
- The provision of regularly updated training for all mental health staff in cultural issues and tackling racism.
- Government to acknowledge the presence of institutional racism in mental health services and commit to combating the same.
- Written policies on racist abuse.
- Encourage an ethnically diverse workforce.
- No patients to be restrained prone for more than 3 minutes.
- Strict adherence to upper limits on medication doses.
- CPR and control and restraint training to be improved.
- All patients to be empowered to request an independent second opinion from a doctor of their choice and also to be able to request transfer to another hospital if they have valid reasons for doing so.
- CPA plans to include appropriate details of ethnic and cultural needs.

General topics

Caring for dispersed asylum seekers

> Department of Health 2003 Caring for dispersed asylum seekers: a resource pack. DH, London

Whilst asylum seekers/refugees are a diverse group they will share some common experiences. They may suffer the same mental health problems as the host population, but they may express these in different ways.

The refugee experience

- Pre-flight experience: This may include oppression, persecution, harassment, conflict, witnessing combat, imprisonment, violence, torture, rape, fear, famine, death of family and friends.
- Flight: This may involve escape, paying traffickers to cross borders, hazardous conditions, the fear of being discovered and imprisoned, uncertainty, physical and sexual abuse, deprivation and loss of family members.
- Exile: The most common feelings are anxiety about the outcome of the asylum claim, fear of deportation,

detention, poverty, homelessness, cultural shock, language barrier, racism, isolation, unemployment, boredom, homesickness, separation and loss of family, friends and community, status, occupation, income and home, and guilt and anxiety about those left behind. Feelings of insecurity and powerlessness, and an inability to settle.

Accessing mental health services

Factors inhibiting access to mental health services include:
- More urgent priorities such as immigration, housing, support arrangements, etc.
- Unfamiliarity with UK systems, lack of knowledge of mental health services and rights.
- Fear of institutions and fear of institutionalisation.
- Fear of betrayal of confidence, mistrust of health professionals due to fears of diagnosis being passed on to immigration authorities and others.
- Fear and stigma of being labelled as 'mentally ill'.
- Cultural and linguistic barriers.
- 'Counselling' as understood in a western culture may be an alien concept to many asylum seekers/refugees.
- Reluctance to talk about feelings with people seen as 'outsiders'; also talking about past trauma may not always be a culturally appropriate way of dealing with unhappy memories.
- Some female asylum seekers/refugees actively search for a female counsellor and may not attend if this is not offered.

Mental health in a multicultural context

Cultural factors can have a profound significance – for example:
- The understanding of mental health varies greatly from one culture to another.
- Emotional states may be described by asylum seekers/refugees in ways that are unfamiliar to health professionals.
- There may not be equivalent words for stress, psychosis, anxiety, depression, etc. because underlying concepts referring to mental states may differ.
- For some, counselling is an unknown concept and problems may be dealt with by talking to elders or group discussions.
- The western model of counselling, where concrete advice or feedback is not given, may be considered unhelpful.
- Minor mental health problems may be accommodated within the family and are not seen as requiring help.
- There may be different notions of politeness, i.e. body language, modes of speech, presentation of oneself, different attitudes to ages (equals wisdom), eye contact, body contact, etc.

When asylum seekers approach healthcare organisations they may initially focus on physical symptoms, thereby leading to misunderstandings and misdiagnosis.

Some asylum seekers/refugees may link mental health to the spiritual world – for example, the Somali beliefs about each individual's genie that can interfere with daily life if its needs are not acknowledged and met.

Professionals may have little understanding of the real experiences and events that asylum seekers/refugees describe, resulting in a diagnosis of PTSD which overshadows their current problems and stresses.

Specific services for asylum seekers, refugees and the victims of torture are discussed.

Weblink Medical Foundation for the Care of Victims of Torture – www.torturecare.org.uk

Communication with patients from other cultures

Bhui K, Bhugra D 2004 Communication with patients from other cultures: the place of explanatory models. Advances in Psychiatric Treatment 10: 474–478

Explanatory models represent the position from which patients may express distress. They can govern how patients interpret a psychiatric explanation of their problems. It is the process of exploring with the patient their identity, and the explanatory model ensures improved understanding and informs the successful negotiation of different world views. Symbols can be more reliably understood than language.

Drenan G, Swarz L 2002 The paradoxical use of interpreting in psychiatry. Social Science and Medicine 54: 1853–1866

- Psychiatric practice in multilingual settings involves various people acting as interpreters.
- The use of interpreters can lead to different conclusions about the significance of expressions of distress – for example, whether they are culturally grounded and normal or whether they indicate psychopathology.

Williams B, Healy D 2001 Perceptions of illness causation among new referrals to a community mental health team: explanatory model or exploratory map? Social Science and Medicine 53: 465–476

- Explanatory models are not fixed and stable representations but fluctuate and are recruited in a context-dependent manner.

American Psychiatric Association 2002 Cultural assessment in clinical psychiatry. American Psychiatric Publishing, Washington, DC

Box 6.1

Assessing depression in migrants

- Assess sadness, joylessness, hopelessness, lack of energy, poor concentration
- Look for biological symptoms such as loss of sleep and libido, and variations of appetite
- Assess the reasons for migration, preparation and the actual act of migrating
- Ascertain aspirations and achievements
- Ascertain social support and peer group contacts
- Assess negative life events, feelings of loss and grief
- Assess self-esteem and self-confidence
- Assess whether any social skills deficit is present
- Assess the degree of culture shock
- Assess cultural identity

Table 6.1 Aetiological model of common mental disorders and migration: vulnerability factors predispose individuals to common mental disorders after migration

Vulnerability factors	Protective factors
Premigration	
Biological and psychological factors	Psychological factors such as resilience
Social skills deficit	Higher socioeconomic status
Forced migration	Preparation and adequate run-in time
Persecution	
Migration	
Negative life events	Strong cultural and ethnic identity
Bereavement	Social support and social networks
Postmigration	
Culture shock	Resilience
Culture conflict	Social support
Discrepancy between achievement and expectation	

Cultural formulations were introduced into DSM-IV in an attempt to make diagnostic practice more culturally appropriate, relevant and representative.

The five elements of cultural formulation are:

- the cultural identity of the individual
- cultural explanations of the individual's illness
- the influence of the patient's psychosocial environment and level of functioning within it
- cultural elements in the patient–professional relationship
- the use of cultural assessment in deciding diagnosis and care.

Shiori T, Someya T, Helmests D et al 1999 Misinterpretation of facial expression: a cross-cultural study. Psychiatry and Clinical Neuroscience 53: 45–50

- International research which showed that a finite number of emotions are recognised in all societies and cultures – surprise, disgust, fear, anger, contempt, happiness and sadness.
- Accurate recognition of these emotional states varies with culture and observer.

Depression in migrants and ethnic minorities

Bhugra D, Ayonrinde O 2004 Depression in migrants and ethnic minorities. Advances in Psychiatric Treatment 10: 13–17

Migration can place an individual under considerable stress. Depression is not consistently found to be a common sequel to migration. In schizophrenia it has been argued that schizotypal personality disorder is associated with migration and subsequent psychosis, but no similar model has been identified for depression in migrants. Most epidemiological studies have used European or North American assessment instruments, which may not identify cases of 'non-western' depression (Box 6.1).

The initial stresses of the act of migration are replaced by the stresses of living in an alien culture, thus the stage at which data are collected can affect results. Mismatched aspirations and achievements can also produce stress. If achievements do not match aspirations then the individuals are open to low mood, a sense of alienation and a sense of failure (Table 6.1).

Murphy HBM, Wittkower ED, Chance N 1967 Cross cultural inquiry into the symptomatology of depression: preliminary report. International Journal of Social Psychiatry 13: 6–15

- Reported that psychiatrists in 30 countries found varying prevalence of depressive symptoms such as identified fatigue, loss of appetite, loss of sexual interest, weight loss and self-accusatory ideas.

Jablensky A, Sartorius N, Gulbinat W et al 1981 Characteristics of depressive patients contacting psychiatric services in four cultures. A report from the WHO collaborative study on the assessment of depressive disorders. Acta Psychiatrica Scandinavica 63: 367–383

- In a five centre, cross-cultural study the core symptoms of depression were found to be sadness, joylessness, anxiety, tension, lack of energy, loss of interest, poor concentration and ideas of insufficiency, inadequacy and worthlessness.

Cochrane R 1977 Mental illness in immigrants to England and Wales. Social Psychiatry 12: 25–35

- Reported that rates of admission to psychiatric hospitals in England and Wales were nearly twice as high among immigrants compared with native groups.
- After standardisation for age and gender, studies showed much higher admission rates for Irish and West Indian immigrants than for those from India or Pakistan.

Cochrane R 1983 The social causation of mental illness. Longman, London

- Subsequently attributed some of the discrepancy in these rates to selective migration, ambivalent relationships and adjustment to culture.

Bhugra D 2003 Migration and depression. Acta Psychiatrica Scandinavica (Suppl) 418: 67–73

- The presence and expression of guilt, somatic symptoms and shame in migrants can depend on their culture of origin.
- Depressive manifestations can be overlooked.
- The time elapsed since migration is important.
- The period immediately after migration is a time of vulnerability, as is the period 5–7 years later, when individuals have settled down but not fulfilled their aspirations.

Table 6.2 Weekly prevalence of depressive neurosis

	Males (%)	**Females (%)**
White	2.7	4.8
Irish	5.8	6.8
African-Caribbean	5.6	6.4
Indian	2.5	3.2
Pakistani	3.8	2.9
Bangladeshi	1.6	2.2

Ward E 1967 Some observations of the underlying dynamics of conflict in a foreign student. Journal of the American College of Health 10: 430–440

- Identified a foreign student syndrome including increased hospital admission, non-specific somatic complaints, a passive withdrawn interaction style and an unkempt appearance.

Furnham, A 1961 Adjustment of sojourners. In: Kim YY, Gudykunst WB (eds) Cross-cultural adaptation. Sage, Newbury, CA

Identified psychological problems in students:
- British students   14%
- Iraqi, Iranian, Nigerian   28%
- Turkish, Egyptian   22%
- Indian subcontinent   18%

Babiker I, Cox J, Miller P 1980 The measurement of cultural distance and its relationship to medical consultations, symptomatology and examination performance of overseas students at Edinburgh University. Social Psychiatry and Psychiatric Epidemiology 15: 109–116

- Noted that increased rates of medical consultations and symptoms were associated with greater distance from country/culture of origin.
- Health services were seen as an approachable haven.

Nazroo J 1997 Ethnicity and mental health. PSI, London

Migrants had lower rates of depression:
- The lower rates of depression in migrants did not occur in Pakistani groups.
- Those who were fluent in English reported the same rates of depression as their British counterparts.

The weekly prevalence of depressive neurosis using the clinical interview schedule (revised version) is outlined in Table 6.2.

Sproston K, Nazroo J 2002 Ethnic minority psychiatric illness rates (EMPIRIC) – Quantitative Report. A survey carried out on behalf of the Department of Health by the National Centre for Social Research and the Department of Epidemiology and Public Health at the Royal Free and University College Medical School. DH, London

- Irish migrants had the highest prevalence of common mental disorders (although only 10% of Irish men with any ICD-10 diagnosis met the criteria for a depressive episode).
- Differences across ethnic groups were not statistically significant.
- Among the Indian and Pakistani groups, common mental disorders were more prevalent in women than

in men; however, rates were also high among those who were born in England or migrated here at an early age.

Bochner S 1986 Coping with unfamiliar cultures. Australian Journal of Psychology 38: 347–358

- Suggests that two modes of cultural contact govern the reaction of people to unfamiliar cultures.
- These are the adjustment to and reflective learning in the new culture.
- Exaggerated deculturation occurs when individuals exposed to another culture reject both the old and new cultures and retreat into one of their own.
- Marginal syndrome occurs when individuals vacillate between their old and new cultures.

Furnham A, Bocher S 1986 Culture shock. Routledge, London

- Having an external locus of control has been shown to be related to poor mental health and a lack of adaptation.
- Individuals who accept their fate may also be able to accept their stresses.
- Eight theoretical constructs for adjustment postmigration were suggested and included:
  - movement as loss
  - fatalism
  - selective migration
  - expectations
  - negative life events
  - social support
  - social skills deficit
  - clash of values with the new culture.

Oberg K 1960 Culture shock: adjustment to new culture environments. Practical Anthropology 7: 177–182

Discussed six aspects to culture shock:
- Strain
- Sense of loss or feelings of deprivation
- Rejection by members of the new culture
- Role expectation and role confusion
- Surprise, anxiety and indignation
- Feelings of impotence.

Gilbert P, Allan S 1998 The role of defeat and entrapment (arrested flight) in depression: an exploration of an evolutionary view. Psychological Medicine 28: 585–598

- Proposed that important cognitive factors for depression are social rank, defeat and a sense of entrapment.
- If the pathway to flight is blocked for personal or social reasons, the sense of entrapment may be more significant.

- Arrested flight involves suppression of explorative behaviour, submissive postures, isolation and severely restricted movement.

Definition

Acculturation – the process by which a minority group assimilates cultural values and beliefs of a majority community, whether voluntary or forced.

Culture conflict – the sense of tension experienced by people from a minority culture – for example, the children of immigrant parents, when the parents' culture and values compete with the majority culture in which the children spend a significant part of the day. This can cause increased alienation and isolation, with the children belonging to neither culture.

Culture shock – sudden unpleasant feelings that violate an individual's expectations of the new culture and cause them to value their own culture negatively.

Exaggerated deculturation – individuals exposed to another culture may reject both the old and new cultures and retreat into one of their own.

Marginal syndrome – individuals may vacillate between the old and new cultures.

Weblink EMPIRIC Report – www.dh.gov.uk/assetRoot /04/02/40/34/04024034.pdf
See also the 'General topics' section in Chapter 2 (Affective disorders), pages 28 and 30.

The health of survivors of torture and organised violence

Burnett A, Peel M 2001 The health of survivors of torture and organised violence. British Medical Journal 322: 606–609

The physical effects are discussed, including fractures, soft tissue injury, head injuries with or without subsequent epilepsy, hearing loss and the sequelae of sexual violence.

Sexual health screening should be sensitively discussed. The possibility of rape or sexual violence should also be considered in men.

Emotional distress may be expressed with physical symptoms such as sleep disturbance, fatigue and pain. These symptoms can last up to 2 years. Realistic and supportive management is preferable to medication and additional adverse effects.

Difficulties of diagnosis across cultures are discussed; in particular, that a refugee may meet the criteria for PTSD but continues to function and manage their life. In that instance a psychiatric diagnosis may not be valid or helpful.

Amnesty International 2000 Annual Report 2000. Amnesty International, London

- Torture was the basis for the application in 8.4% (approximately 6000 people) of those seeking asylum in the UK in 1999.
- This is likely to be an underestimate due to underreporting.

Burnett A 1999 Guidelines for healthworkers providing care for Kosovan refugees. Medical Foundation for the Care of Victims of Torture and DH, London

- Refugees can exhibit symptoms of anxiety, depression, guilt and shame due to past experiences and adjustment to their new situation.

Watters C 1998 The mental health needs of refugees and asylum seekers: key issues in research and service development. In: Nicholson F (ed.) Current issues of asylum law and policy. Ashgate, Aldershot, pp 282–297

- A diagnosis of post-traumatic stress disorder can overshadow the trauma that a refugee suffers in their new country in terms of isolation, hostility, violence and racism.

Bracken P, Giller J, Summerfield D 1995 Psychological response to war and atrocity: the limitations of current concepts. Social Science and Medicine 40: 1073–1082

- Recovery is linked with establishing social networks, achieving economic independence and making contact with appropriate cultural institutions.
- A psychiatric diagnosis may disempower and further add to stigma.

Definition

Torture is any act by which severe pain or suffering, whether physical or mental, is intentionally inflicted on a person for such purposes as:

- obtaining from him or a third person information or a confession
- punishing him for an act that he or a third person has committed or is suspected of having committed
- or intimidating or coercing him or a third person
- or for any reason based on discrimination of any kind

when such pain or suffering is inflicted by or at the instigation of a public official acting in an official capacity. (*Source:* United Nations.)

Organised violence – that which has a political motive.

Weblink Amnesty International – www.web.amnesty.org.

See also the 'General topics' section in Chapter 23 (Post-traumatic stress disorder), page 367.

Health needs of asylum seekers and refugees

Burnett A, Peel M 2001 Health needs of asylum seekers and refugees. British Medical Journal 322: 544–547

Physical illnesses include hepatitis, malaria, HIV/AIDS and tuberculosis. Parasitic disease also occurs. Health screening of refugees on arrival in a country may not be done. Refugees' expectations of the health service will be affected by their experiences in their home country. They may not have an established primary care system and may expect referral to secondary care for all health needs. Departments for communicable disease often take responsibility for the health of refugees. This is stigmatising.

Good communication is important and helps to establish trust. The use of interpreters is helpful. Sensitive information may not be discussed if interpreters are family members or if an interpreter is not trusted. Culturally sensitive health services should be provided. This should include the gender of interpreters and health staff. Domestic violence should be considered. Symptoms of psychological distress are common but may not equate with psychiatric illness.

Connelly J, Schweiger M 2000 The health risks of the UK's new Asylum Act. British Medical Journal 321: 5–6

- Asylum seekers in the UK are faced with poverty, dependence and a lack of cohesive social support.

Carey Wood J, Duke K, Karn V, Marshall T 1995 The settlement of refugees in Britain. Home Office Research Study 141. HMSO, London

- One in six refugees in the UK has a physical health problem that impacts on their life.
- Two-thirds of refugees in the UK have suffered from anxiety or depression.

Brent and Harrow Health Authority 1995 Brent and Harrow Refugee survey. Brent and Harrow Health Authority, London

- Depression, anxiety, panic attacks or agoraphobia occur.

Acheson D 1998 Independent inquiry into inequalities in health. The Stationery Office, London

- Social isolation and poverty have further effects on mental health.

Shackman J, Reynolds J 1996 Working with refugees and torture survivors: help for the helpers. In: Heller T, Reynolds J, Gomm R, Pattison S (eds) Mental health matters: a reader. Macmillan/Open University, London

- Improvements are seen as refugees adjust, are reunited with their families and take up educational and employment opportunities.

Cienfuegos AJ, Monelli C 1983 The testimony of political repression as a therapeutic instrument. American Journal of Orthopsychiatry 53: 43–51

- In some, but not all, cases it can be therapeutic for refugees to tell their story.

Evelyn Oldfield Unit 1997 Guidelines for providers of counselling training to refugees and guidelines for refugee community organizations providing counselling. Refugee Mental Health Forum, London

- Counselling which is culturally sensitive can be beneficial.
- The training of members of refugee committees in counselling skills can be helpful.

Praxis 1998 Hosting: an innovative scheme to meet the emergency accommodation needs of asylum seekers. Crisis, London

- Refugee community organisations can reduce isolation by providing support, information and advocacy services.

Gorst-Unsworth C, Goldenberg E 1998 Psychological sequelae of torture and organized violence suffered by refugees from Iraq. Trauma-related factors compared to social factors in exile. British Journal of Psychiatry 172: 90–94

- In this study of Iraqi asylum seekers in London, depression was more closely linked with poor social support than with a history of torture.

Watters C 1998 The mental health needs of refugees and asylum seekers: key issues in research and service development. In: Nicholson F (ed.) Current issues of asylum law and policy. Ashgate, Aldershot

- The best mental health outcomes are achieved in those who form links and friendships with people from their own country and from their host country.

Wallace T 1990 Refugee women: their perspectives and our responses. Oxfam, Oxford

- Women are particularly vulnerable to physical assault, sexual harassment and rape.
- Their experiences may not be taken seriously.

Ferron S, Morgan J, O'Reilly M 2000 Hygiene promotion – a practical manual for relief and development. CARE International and Intermediate Technology Publications, London

- Women may be the most seriously affected by displacement.
- Women often take responsibility for education and cultural cohesion in a community; these are important factors in adjustment.
- Women may not be involved in training and employment programmes.
- Women have domestic responsibilities that can leave them in a vulnerable position.

Gammell H, Ndahiro A, Nicholas N, Windsor J 1993 Refugees (political asylum seekers): service provision and access to the NHS. Newham Health Authority and Newham Healthcare, London

- Women are less likely to be literate or speak English.
- They are more likely to report problems with health and depression.
- Refugee women are less likely to attend health and screening programmes.
- In one study, only 5% of women aged over 50 had had breast screening and only 53% had had a cervical smear.

Melzak S, Kasabova S 1999 Working with children and adolescents from Kosovo. Medical Foundation for the Care of Victims of Torture, London

- For refugee children the greatest benefit is achieved by becoming part of the local school community, by learning and by making friends.

Management of psychiatric inpatient violence: patient ethnicity and use of medication, restraint and seclusion

Gudjonsson GH, Rabe-Hesketh S, Szmukler G 2004 Management of psychiatric in-patient violence: patient ethnicity and use of medication, restraint and seclusion. British Journal of Psychiatry 184: 258–262

Significant ethnic differences have been found on a forensic unit in the management of psychiatric patients after a violent incident. It has been established that patients of Afro-Caribbean background are more likely to be arrested, imprisoned and detained in a psychiatric hospital following offending behaviour. There is little research regarding the influence of ethnicity.

Aims

This study hypothesised that ethnic differences would be found in the management of patients after a violent incident.

Such differences may be explained by variables such as age, gender, the nature of the incident, the extent of injuries inflicted, Mental Health Act 1983 status and staff perceptions of the patient's disturbance and potential danger.

Method

- 1515 violent incidents occurring over a 3-year period on 14 different general wards were examined.
- Three management outcomes were considered:
  - medication
  - restraint
  - seclusion.

Results

- Black patients were more likely to be given emergency medication and secluded after violent incidents than white patients.
- These differences were not significant when confounding factors were corrected for.
- Black patients were as likely to be physically restrained. Differences disappeared when the odds ratio was adjusted for other variables.
- Racial 'stereotyping' was unlikely to have played a major direct role in determining nurses' responses.

> Davies S, Thornicroft G, Leese M et al 1996 Ethnic differences in risk of compulsory psychiatric admission among representative cases of psychosis in London. British Medical Journal 312: 534–537

- A South London study.
- Examined the ethnic differences in compulsory psychiatric admission to hospital.
- Black Caribbean and black African patients were overrepresented and this was not related to psychiatric diagnosis and sociodemographic differences.

> Gudjonsson GH, Rabe-Hesketh S, Wilson C 2000 Violent incidents on a medium secure unit over a 17 year period. Journal of Forensic Psychiatry 10: 249–263

- Black patients are treated differently following an untoward incident.

See also the 'General topics' section in Chapter 12 (General psychiatry), pages 177 and 186.

What brings asylum seekers to the UK?

> Burnett A 2001 What brings asylum seekers to the United Kingdom? British Medical Journal 322: 485–488

- The majority of asylum seekers in the UK are single men under 40.
- The asylum process is lengthy, complex and highly stressful.
- The policy of fining airline and transport companies for carrying people without the correct documentation has meant that it is virtually impossible to enter the country as a legal asylum seeker. It may also mean that there are people who are unable to flee to a place of safety.
- Dispersal to allocated accommodation across the UK means that refugees may be isolated within areas where they are bullied or harassed. Those who move nearer to their families lose their access to vouchers and financial support. They may also face the problems associated with being homeless.

Definitions

Asylum seeker – asylum claim submitted, awaiting Home Office decision.

Exceptional leave to remain (ELR) – the Home Office accepts there are strong reasons why the person should not return to their country of origin and grants the right to stay in Britain for 4 years. Expected to return if the home country situation improves. Ineligible for family reunion.

Indefinite leave to remain (ILR) – given permanent residence in Britain indefinitely. Eligible for family reunion only if able to support family without recourse to public funding.

Refugee – any person who 'owing to well-founded fear of being persecuted for reasons of race, religion, nationality, membership of a particular social group or political opinion, is outside of his nationality and is unable to or, owing to such fear, is unwilling to return to it'. (Source: Geneva Convention 1951.)

Refugee status – accepted as a refugee under the Geneva Convention. Given leave to remain in the UK for 4 years, and can then apply for settled status. Eligible for family reunion for one spouse and all children under 18 years.

Refusal – the person has a right of appeal, within strict time limits.

Working with patients with religious beliefs

> Dein S 2004 Working with patients with religious beliefs. Advances in Psychiatric Treatment 10: 287–295

A rejecting attitude towards psychiatry is common to many religious groups, for many reasons. For example, the stigma of mental illness may affect the marriage prospects of members of religious communities. Patients may perceive doctors as failing to understand their religious beliefs and at worse as ridiculing their beliefs. Consequently patients may have little faith in medical professionals. It may be necessary to use a 'culture broker' – someone from the same religious group as the patient who acts as the patient's advocate.

Common religious problems that may be a focus of clinical attention include questioning and loss of faith, change of religious denomination, conversion to a new religion and intensification of adherence to the beliefs and practices of one's own faith. These problems should be distinguished from functional psychiatric disorders, although they may lead to psychiatric illness. Their resolution generally requires referral to religious professionals, such as a chaplain or someone influential in a religious organisation.

Hospital chaplains in the UK receive some training in mental health through the College of Health Care Chaplains. They may provide help with religious problems such as discussion of the relation between sin and mental illness, provision of absolution and prayer for patients. They can provide guidelines relating to the 'normality' of religious beliefs.

Neeleman J, Lewis G 1994 Religious identity and comfort beliefs in three groups of psychiatric patients and a group of medical controls. International Journal of Social Psychiatry 40: 124–134

- Psychiatrists are often far less religious than their patients.

Keating AM, Fretz BR 1990 Christians' anticipations about counsellors in response to counsellors' descriptions. Journal of Counselling Psychology 37: 293–296

- There is evidence that religious individuals are less satisfied with a non-religious clinician than with a religious one.

American Psychiatric Association Task Force 1975 Psychiatrists' viewpoints on religion and their services to religious institutions and the ministry. American Psychiatric Association, Washington, DC

- The general public and psychiatric patients report themselves to be more religious and to attend church more regularly than mental health professionals.

Cox J 1996 Psychiatry and religion: a general psychiatrists' perspective. In: Bhugra D (ed.) Psychiatry and religion: context, consensus and controversy. Routledge, London, p 158

- If mental health services in a multicultural society are to become more responsive to 'user' needs, then eliciting this 'religious history' with any linked spiritual meanings should be a routine component of a psychiatric assessment and of preparing a more culturally sensitive 'care plan'.

Batson CD, Ventis WL 1993 The religious experience: a social, psychological perspective. Oxford University Press, New York; Pargament KI, Brant CR 1998 Religion and coping. In: Koenig HG (ed.) Handbook of religion and mental health. Academic Press, San Diego, CA

- Recent attempts at empirical assessments of the relationships between religion, spirituality and mental health suggest that religion may actually promote better mental health.
- Work is limited to Christianity and Judaism.

Peterson EA, Nelson K 1987 How to meet your clients' spiritual needs. Journal of Psychosocial Nursing 25: 34–39

- Some patients describe problems as spiritual rather than religious.
- Spiritual problems generally mean a transcendent relationship between the person and the 'higher being' – 'a quality that goes beyond a specific religious affiliation'.

Greenberg D, Witzum E 2001 Sanity and sanctity: mental health work among the ultra orthodox in Jerusalem. Yale University Press, New Haven, CT

- In many religious groups psychiatry and psychology are considered suspect – they both dismiss dogma and God's existence.
- Mental health professionals may become angered by patients with religious beliefs, arguing that they are 'primitive' and detrimental to their health.
- Mental health professionals may react to these emotions in a number of ways:
  - with excessive curiosity about the patient's religious beliefs and practices
  - by ignoring cultural influences or tensions and treating the patient as though they belong to their own cultural group
  - by behaving aggressively towards the patient, becoming angry when the patient refuses to comply with treatment or accept the psychiatrist's formulation.
- This study also undertook a review of the prevalence of obsessive–compulsive disorder in a variety of cultural backgrounds.
- Religious background was not found to be a causative factor in this disorder.

Richardson JT 1985 Psychological and psychiatric studies and new religions. In: Brown LB (ed.) Advances in the psychology of religion. Pergamon, Oxford; Barker E 1996 New religious movements: a practical introduction. HMSO, London

- There is little evidence that belonging to a new religious movement or cult is generally detrimental to mental health.
- Leaving a religious movement (often by forcible removal) may result in a number of problems.
- Problems can include agitation, panic attacks, nightmares and repetitive chanting.
- These symptoms collectively are called 'information disease'.

Bogart G 1992 Separation from a spiritual teacher. Journal of Personal Psychology 24: 1–21

- When a member of a spiritual group separates from their leader, psychological symptoms can include agitation, low mood and nightmares.

Hay D 1987 Exploring inner space, 2nd edn. Penguin, Harmondsworth

- Mystical experiences are common in the UK and the USA, with about a third of people reporting them at some stage of their lives.
- Such experiences include feelings of unity with the universe and ecstatic states associated with universal love.
- Such experiences are transient but they may have long-term effects on function.
- The aetiology of mystical experiences is varied.
- Aetiology includes states which are drug induced, occur during meditation or pathological states (e.g. with temporal lobe epilepsy or psychosis).

Clarke I 2001 Psychosis and spirituality. Exploring the new frontier. Whurr, Gateshead

- Criteria such as negative effect on life functioning, loss of volition and loss of insight occur in psychosis but not in mystical states.

Basford TK 1990 Near death experience: an annotated bibliography. Garland, New York; Fenwick P, Fenwick E 1995 The truth in the light. Headline, London

- The near death experience is not attributable to mental disorder.
- Anger, depression and isolation may occur following this experience.
- Generally individuals report beneficial side effects, including positive attitude and value changes and some personality transformation.

Littlewood R, Lipsedge R 1981 Some social and phenomenological characteristics of psychotic immigrants. Psychological Medicine 11: 289–302

- A UK study of schizophrenia.
- Up to 45% of black immigrants had religious delusions compared with 14% of white UK-born patients.

Scarnatie R, Madrey M, Wise A 1991 Religious beliefs and practices among the most dangerous psychiatric inmates. Forensic Reports 4: 1–16

- A study of psychiatric inmates in an American penal institution.
- Over half of the most dangerous inmates had religious delusions.

Lewis CA 1998 Cleanliness is next to godliness: religiosity and obsessiveness. Journal of Religion and Health 37: 49–61

- Religiosity is associated with obsessional traits but not with obsessional neurosis.

Definitions

Religion – adherence to and beliefs and practices of an organised church or religious institution. (*Source:* Shafranske E, Maloney H 1990 Clinical psychologists' religious and spiritual orientations and their practice of psychotherapy. Psychotherapy 27: 72–78.)

Weblink Information Network Focus on Religious Movements (INFORM): a voluntary organisation that provides information about religious movements and that can recommend access to counselling services – www.inform.ac/infmain.html.

Policy and legislation

Delivering race equality in mental health care

Department of Health 2005 Delivering race equality in mental health care. An action plan for reform inside and outside services and the Government's response to the independent inquiry into the death of David Bennett. DH, London. Online. Available: www.dh.gov.uk/assetRoot/04/10/07/75/04100775.pdf [†]

A 5-year action plan for reducing inequalities in black and minority ethnic patients' mental health care. This includes their access to, experience of, and outcomes from mental health services.

The report includes the government response to the recommendations made by the inquiry into the death of David Bennett.

[†] Crown copyright. Reproduced with permission.

It draws on three recent publications:

- Inside outside: improving mental health services for black and minority ethnic communities in England
- Delivering race equality: a framework for action
- The independent inquiry into the death of David Bennett.

The basic framework for the programme is built on three principles:

- More appropriate and responsive services: achieved through action to develop organisations and the workforce, to improve clinical services and to improve services for specific groups, such as older people, asylum seekers and refugees, and children
- Community engagement: delivered through healthier communities and by action to engage communities in planning services, supported by 500 new community development workers
- Better information: from improved monitoring of ethnicity, better dissemination of information and good practice, and improved knowledge about effective services. This will include a new regular census of mental health patients.

It is envisaged that this document will support implementation of the Race Relations Act (2000) and that by 2010 there will be:

- less fear of mental health services among BME communities and service users
- increased satisfaction with service
- a reduction in the rate of admission of people from BME communities to psychiatric inpatient units
- a reduction in the disproportionate rates of compulsory detention of BME service users in inpatient units
- fewer violent incidents that are secondary to inadequate treatment of mental illness
- a reduction in the seclusion in BME groups
- the prevention of deaths in mental health services following physical intervention
- more BME service users reaching self-reported states of recovery
- a reduction in the ethnic disparities found in prison populations
- a more balanced range of effective therapies, such as peer support services and psychotherapeutic and counselling treatments, as well as pharmacological interventions that are culturally appropriate and effective
- a more active role for the BME communities and BME service users in the training of professionals, in the development of mental health policy, and in the planning and provision of services
- a workforce and organisation capable of delivering appropriate and responsive mental health services to BME communities.

Inside outside: improving mental health services for black and minority ethnic communities in England

Department of Health 2003 Inside outside: improving mental health services for black and minority ethnic communities in England. DH, London. Online. Available: www.dh.gov.uk/assetRoot/04/01/94/52/04019452.pdf[†]

The 1999 National Service Framework for Mental Health recognised that ethnic minorities were not well served by mental health services. This document reports on the proposals for the Department of Health developed by the Mental Health Taskforce. These aim to make mental health services appropriate to a multicultural society. It is reported that minority ethnic groups experience mental health services as coercive, institutionally racist and possessing a tendency to override individual needs with organisational requirements.

The three basic strategic objectives are:

- to reduce and eliminate ethnic inequalities in mental health service, experience and outcome
- to develop a mental health workforce that is capable of delivering effective mental health services to a multicultural population
- to enhance or build capacity within black and minority communities and the voluntary sector for dealing with mental health and mental ill-health.

A number of standards are set out. These include:

- Standard One: Mental Health Promotion
- Standard Two: Primary Care
- Standard Three: Access to Services
- Standards Four and Five: Effective Services for People with Severe Mental Illness
- Standard Six: Caring about Carers
- Standard Seven: Preventing Suicide.

Specific proposals include:

- ensuring language access for persons who prefer a language other than English
- statutory mental health providers working collaboratively with the local voluntary sector in developing and sustaining a variety of service models to meet the needs of minority ethnic groups
- audit of use of psychotropic medication and Mental Health Act legislation in terms of ethnicity
- improving research governance in relation to ethnicity and cultural diversity.

Eating disorders

7

Chapter contents

Ethical issues

Consent in relation to the treatment of eating disorders

Honig P, Jaffa T 2000 Consent in relation to the treatment of eating disorders. Opinion and debate. Psychiatry Bulletin 24: 409–411

Gaining consent and managing times when consent is not given are fundamental to the treatment of those with eating disorders. This is most easily illustrated with regard to anorexia nervosa as this is more likely life threatening. Ambivalence is understandable as the treatment and the illness pull the patient in opposite directions.

Consent

Achieving clarity surrounding consent has three functions:
- to protect the patient's rights
- to encourage professionals to remain within legal frameworks and to respect patient rights
- to promote a collaborative approach to management.

Maximising consent relies on:
- imparting information – to allow patients and their families to make decisions that will aid recovery
- working with motivation – consent should be seen as an ongoing process which is tied to motivation. The balance between wishing to recover and wanting to remain ill will fluctuate with time.

The key issues of this approach include:
- establishing a relationship
- working on motivational issues for one difficulty at a time, eventually compiling a motivational profile that informs treatment
- matching intervention to the stage of motivation
- family work
- supporting the ideas generated by families where possible to encourage cohesive and consistent treatment.

When consent to treatment is not achievable

1. An adult who has the ability to understand choices regarding the illness and treatment offered but refuses to consent to treatment.

   Approach:
   - Ensure the patient has all the information.
   - Involve family and significant others.
   - Check exactly what the patient is not consenting to (may just be one aspect).
   - Check if their wishes may therefore be feasible.
   - Decide how urgent the treatment is.
   - If not life threatening, it may be that refusal can be accepted and the motivational–collaborative approach is acceptable.
   - If intervention is urgent, then the Mental Health Act can be used.

   Mental Health Act Commission (Guidance Note 3; 1997):
   - Clarifies that anorexia nervosa is a mental disorder under the terms of the Act and that compulsory feeding may be a medical treatment in this case.

Department of Health 1999 Reform of the Mental Health Act 1983: proposals for consultation. The Stationery Office, London

- Also proposes that 'feeding contrary to the will of the patient' should be considered 'specified treatment'.

2. A child under 18 years who has the ability to understand choices regarding the illness and treatment offered but refuses to consent to treatment can be treated under the Children Act 1989 with parental consent even if they understand the issues but refuse consent.

3. A child under 18 years who is unable to understand the nature of treatment and the consequences of refusing it can be treated with parental consent, under common law.

Approach:

- Continue to attempt to enhance the patient's level of competence.
- Legal advice should be sought as to whether to proceed with treatment under the Children Act.
- The Children Act ensures the patient's views are considered formally whilst protecting the treating professional from accusations of assault.
- There is less stigma attached to the use of the Children Act.
- The Children Act may be more appropriate with younger children.
- The Mental Health Act has the advantage that safeguards offered by the Act are in place.
- The Mental Health Act may be more appropriate with adolescents.
- Previous detention under the Mental Health Act can limit travel and emigration applications.

Strober M, Freeman R, Morrell W 1997 The long term course of severe anorexia nervosa in adolescents: survival analysis of recovery, relapse and outcome predictors over 10–15 years in a prospective study. Eating Disorders 22: 339–360

- The authors suggest that it is helpful to provide information about the natural course of the illness.
- The information should be matched to motivational stages.

See also the 'Ethical issues' section in Chapter 9 (Ethical issues), page 125.

General topics

The aetiology of eating disorders

Collier DA, Treasure JL 2004 The aetiology of eating disorders. British Journal of Psychiatry 185: 363–365

Anorexia nervosa has classically been seen as a syndrome with cultural and social origins rather than a developmental or biological disorder.

Lasegne formalised the concept of a non-specific, environmentally responsive neurosis occurring in women and springing from a dysfunctional family system. In the late 1970s, bulimia was described as an 'ominous' variant of anorexia.

Cultural explanations have included society's preoccupation with being thin and more recently gender dynamics involving power and self-determination. Twin and family studies have shown genetic components in the aetiology.

It seems that anorexia, bulimia and obesity are best seen as heterogeneous disorders with complex multifactorial aetiology. The aetiology includes genetics, environmental factors and social factors. Diagnostic classifications may overemphasise certain features of eating disorders, such as the fear of fatness which is absent in many cases.

Distinct diagnostic syndromes may mask differences between the heterogeneous groups – for example, binge eating not only occurs in bulimia nervosa, it may also be a feature of anorexia nervosa and obesity.

Fairburn CG, Harrison PJ 2003 Eating disorders. Lancet 361: 407–416

- The diagnosis is unstable, with clinical features changing over time.
- Patients often switch between anorexia and bulimia.
- Depression and anxiety are common comorbid disorders.
- There are common and distinct risk factors for the two disorders which cause methodological difficulties in research.

Keel PK, Fichter M, Quadflieg N et al 2004 Application of a latent class analysis to empirically define eating disorder phenotypes. Archives of General Psychiatry 61: 192–200

- Family studies.
- Identified four types of eating disorder:
  - restricting anorexia nervosa, with obsessive–compulsive symptoms
  - restricting anorexia nervosa, without obsessive–compulsive symptoms
  - combination of purging anorexia and bulimia nervosa
  - bulimia nervosa with self-induced vomiting.

Anderluh MB, Tchanturia K, Rabe-Hesketh S et al 2003 Childhood obsessive–compulsive personality traits in adult women with eating disorders: defining a broader eating disorder phenotype. American Journal of Psychiatry 160: 242–247

- Found childhood perfectionism appears to be a strong risk factor for adult eating disorder.

Vervaet M, van Heeringen C, Audenaert K 2004 Personality-related characteristics in restricting versus binging and purging eating disordered patients. Comprehensive Psychiatry 45: 37–43

- Those with both constrained (anorexic) and disinhibited (bulimic) eating share the personality trait of high harm avoidance.
- Novelty seeking is related to bulimia only as in exploratory excitability, impulsivity and extravagance.

Devlin B, Bacanu SA, Klump KL et al 2002 Linkage analysis of anorexia nervosa incorporating behavioural covariates. Human Molecular Genetics 11: 689–696

- Compulsivity and obsessionality are linked with anorexia nervosa.
- Including obsessionality in the behavioural phenotype of anorexia nervosa may be a powerful tool for genetic linkage analysis.

Tchanturia K, Anderluh B, Morris RG et al 2004 Cognitive flexibility in anorexia and bulimia nervosa. Journal of the International Neuropsychological Society 10: 513–520

- Compulsivity may be linked to perceptual and cognitive inflexibility which is demonstrated by those with anorexia nervosa in the acute state, and perhaps also after recovery.
- This appears to be associated with childhood obsessive–compulsive traits.
- These are familial traits not shared by people with bulimia nervosa.
- Inflexibility may be an endophenotype, linked to constrained eating.

Kaye WH, Frank GK, Meltzer CC et al 2001 Altered serotonin 2A receptor activity in women who have recovered from bulimia nervosa. American Journal of Psychiatry 158: 1152–1155

- Abnormal levels of 5HT1A have been found in recovered patients, with different diagnostic groups showing differing alterations.
- The fact that abnormalities persist after recovery suggests that serotonin function may be a trait marker for eating disorders.

Bulik CM, Sullivan PF, Wade TD et al 2000 Twin studies of eating disorders: a review. International Journal of Eating Disorders 27: 1–20

- Eating disorders have a genetic component.
- Genetics and environment contribute fairly equally to the disorder.
- Many traits related to eating disorders have a heritable component, e.g.

  - binge eating
  - self-induced vomiting
  - drive for thinness
  - dietary restriction
  - disinhibition.

Grice DE, Halmi KA, Fitcher MM et al 2002 Evidence for a susceptibility gene for anorexia nervosa on chromosome 1. American Journal of Human Genetics 70: 787–792

- Identified chromosome 1p34 with linkage analysis of pedigrees with at least one pair of relatives with restrictive anorexia nervosa.

Devlin B, Bacanu SA, Klump KL et al 2002 Linkage analysis of anorexia nervosa incorporating behaviour covariates. Human Molecular Genetics 11: 689–696

- The drive for thinness and obsessionality tracked most closely with anorexia nervosa.
- There were novel genetic loci on chromosome 1 for composite measure and chromosome 13 for drive for thinness.

Bulik CM, Devlin B, Bacanu SA et al 2003 Significant linkage on chromosome 10p in families with bulimia nervosa. American Journal of Human Genetics 72: 200–207

- Bulimia nervosa, with self-induced vomiting, has been linked to chromosome 10.
- This provides evidence for the hypothesis that bulimia nervosa is a distinct phenotype.
- This position is also a known locus for obesity, consistent with the elevated family history of obesity seen in those with bulimia nervosa.

Ribases M, Gratacos M, Fernandez-Aranda F et al 2004 Association of BDNF with anorexia, bulimia and age of onset of weight loss in six European populations. Human Molecular Genetics 13: 1205–1212

- Brain drive neurotrophic factor (BDNF) has also been implicated as a susceptibility gene for anorexia nervosa. This protein is involved in hypothalamus-regulated feeding behaviour as well as the regulation of serotonin levels.
- A multicentre European study showed that polymorphism in this gene increases susceptibility to all eating disorders, perhaps with the involvement of the affective component.

See also articles on bulimia, below.

Bulimia nervosa – 25 years on

Palmer R 2004 Bulimia nervosa: 25 years on. British Journal of Psychiatry 185: 447–448

Bulimia appeared in DSM-III. It required only binge eating for the diagnosis. Since then it has been re-named bulimia nervosa and has more in-depth criteria. The ICD criteria resemble those described by Russell. It has hierarchical weight over anorexia nervosa – even if weight is low. This differs from DSM-IV where such people would fit within the criteria for anorexia nervosa, subtype binge/purging.

Since Russell's paper in 1979 (see below) there has been a significant rise in the diagnosis of bulimia nervosa. The rapidity of this rise suggests psychosocial factors are central. This does not mean, however, that there is no genetic predisposition. It may be that alterations in the environment may expose a previously masked genetic vulnerability.

Classification systems do not cover the breadth of disorders. Further study and observation are suggested.

Russell GFM 1979 Bulimia nervosa: an ominous variant of anorexia nervosa. Psychological Medicine 9: 429–448

- Coined the term bulimia nervosa.
- It was described as an 'ominous variant of anorexia nervosa'.

Fairbairn CG, Belgin SJ 1990 Studies of the epidemiology of bulimia nervosa. American Journal of Psychiatry 147: 401–408

- Estimated that bulimia nervosa was a disorder affecting 1 in 10 women in the western world.

Fairbairn CG, Marcus MD, Wilson GT 1993 Cognitive–behavioural therapy for binge eating and bulimia nervosa: a comprehensive treatment manual. In: Fairburn CG, Wilson GT (eds) Binge eating: nature, assessment and treatment. Guilford, New York, pp 361–404

- Investigated treatment with CBT for bulimia nervosa.
- Concluded that CBT is beneficial in the treatment of bulimia nervosa.
- CBT is associated with full remission of symptoms in up to 50% of cases.
- Lesser degrees of improvement were found in other patients.

Fairbairn CG 1997 Interpersonal psychotherapy for bulimia nervosa. In: Garner DM, Garfinkel PE (eds) Handbook of treatment for eating disorders, 2nd edn. Guildford, New York, pp 278–294

- Interpersonal therapy (IPT) is also effective in the treatment of bulimia nervosa.
- It has a slower response rate than that for CBT.

Shrober M, Bulik CM 2002 Genetic epidemiology of eating disorders. In: Fairburn CG, Brownell KD (eds) Eating disorders and obesity: a comprehensive handbook. Guildford, New York

- Suggested that the genetic predisposition for both bulimia nervosa and anorexia nervosa is shared.

Nasser M 1997 Culture and weight consciousness. Routledge, London

- Found that bulimia nervosa (seen predominantly as a disorder of western and urban populations) is being increasingly seen in the more affluent, urban and westernised sections across the world.

Treatment – Psychopharmacology

Antidepressants versus placebo for people with bulimia nervosa

Bacaltchuk J, Hay P 2003 Antidepressants versus placebo for people with bulimia nervosa **(Cochrane Review)**. In: The Cochrane Library, Issue 4. CD003391. Update Software, Oxford

- 19 trials compared antidepressants (TCAs, SSRIs, MAOIs and others) with placebo.
- The results were similar for the different groups in terms of efficacy.
- Treatment with a single antidepressant produced a greater overall remission rate (NNT 4; mean duration of treatment = 9 weeks).
- However, those treated with antidepressants were more likely to drop out due to adverse events, TCAs in particular.
- Fluoxetine was less likely to cause people to drop out.
- It was not possible to distinguish between antidepressant and antibulimic effects.

Antidepressants versus psychological treatments and their combination for bulimia nervosa

Bacaltchuk J, Hay P, Trefiglio R 2001 Antidepressants versus psychological treatments and their combination for bulimia nervosa **(Cochrane Review)**. In: The Cochrane Library, Issue 4. CD003385. Update Software, Oxford

- Five trials compared antidepressants with psychological treatments:
  - patients receiving antidepressants had a remission rate of 20%
  - those receiving psychological treatments had a remission rate of 39%

- the antidepressant group had greater numbers of dropouts (NNH 4, over a 17.5-week treatment period).
- Five trials compared antidepressants with combination treatment (antidepressants and psychological treatments):
  - the antidepressant group had a remission rate of 23%
  - the combination therapy group had a remission rate of 42%.
- Seven trials compared psychological treatments and combination therapy:
  - psychological treatment led to a remission rate of 36%
  - combination therapy led to a remission rate of 49%
  - more people left from the combination treatment arm (NNH 7).

The only statistically significant result was that combination treatments were more effective than single psychotherapy.

Treatment – Psychological Therapies

Individual psychotherapy in the outpatient treatment of adults with anorexia nervosa

Hay P, Bacaltchuk J, Claudino A, Ben-Tovin D, Yong PY 2003 Individual psychotherapy in the outpatient treatment of adults with anorexia nervosa **(Cochrane Review)**. In: The Cochrane Library, Issue 4. CD003909. Update Software, Oxford

- Six small trials were identified, including two involving children and adolescents.
- Two trials suggested that 'treatment as usual' may be less effective than a specific psychotherapy.
- One study had dietary advice as the control intervention. There was a 100% non-completion rate in this group.
- Further study is urgently required.

Interventions for preventing eating disorders in children and adolescents

Pratt BM, Woolfenden SR 2002 Interventions for preventing eating disorders in children and adolescents **(Cochrane Review)**. In: The Cochrane Library, Issue 2. CD002891. Update Software, Oxford

- Out of eight pooled comparisons, only one statistically significant effect was noted. This was a reduction in the internalisation or acceptance of societal ideas relating to appearance at 3- and 6-month follow-up.
- The clinical significance of this is unclear.
- There was insufficient evidence regarding the efficacy of any of the prevention programmes.
- There was no suggestion that any of them caused harm.

Psychotherapy for bulimia nervosa and bingeing

Hay PJ, Bacaltchuk J, Stefano S 2004 Psychotherapy for bulimia nervosa and bingeing **(Cochrane Review)**. In: The Cochrane Library, Issue 3. CD000562. Update Software, Oxford

- Trials were of variable quality and often with small sample sizes.
- The results showed that CBT, and particularly CBT-BN, were efficacious in the treatment of people with bulimia nervosa and, to a lesser extent, related eating disorders.
- This applied in group and individual settings.
- Interpersonal psychotherapy was also effective, particularly in the longer term.
- Self-help approaches showed some effect, although modest when the therapy was applied without guidance ('pure' self-help).
- Psychotherapy alone is unlikely, however, to have an impact on body weight in people with bulimia nervosa and related eating disorders.

Guidelines

Royal College of Psychiatrists guidelines for the nutritional management of anorexia nervosa

Royal College of Psychiatrists 2005 Guidelines for the nutritional management of anorexia nervosa. Council Report CR130. Royal College of Psychiatrists, London

In people with anorexia nervosa, nutritional management is central to their treatment.

There is little evidence on the practice of nutritional intervention. Current practice is largely based on clinical experience. There is little guidance on malnutrition specific to anorexia nervosa.

This document provides a series of provisional recommendations. It is kept under review as new knowledge becomes available.

Nutritional interventions ought to be approached within the overall psychological context. Competent cellular function is required before body composition, the ultimate goal, can be corrected.

Dietary history

A dietary history, performed ideally by a dietitian, identifies:

- specific deficiencies of protein, fatty acids and micronutrients
- information on fluid intake
- consumption of alcohol and caffeine
- smoking
- use of vitamins
- measurement of weight and height.

Specific biochemical and metabolic problems

- Hypokalaemia – usually the result of self-induced vomiting and/or laxative misuse. Can be refractory secondary to low magnesium or calcium levels.
- Hyponatraemia – may be caused by diarrhoea and vomiting, diuretic abuse or excess water intake.
- Folic acid deficiency.
- Vitamin B12 deficiency – especially if avoiding animal-derived foods.
- Iron supplements (can be dangerous too early in refeeding).
- Zinc deficiency – can results in altered taste and a variety of neuropsychiatric symptoms.

Refeeding

- Patients should be monitored closely.
- There is risk of biochemical, cardiovascular and fluid balance problems.
- Patients at particular risk include:
  - those with very low weight
  - those who have had previous biochemical abnormalities or purge
  - those with other medical conditions.
- Electrolyte alterations are most likely to occur in the first 2 weeks.
- The increased carbohydrate metabolism that occurs with refeeding can deplete the already low thiamine levels and there is a risk of hypophosphataemia.
- Abnormal liver function tests – common, usually self-limiting.

- Delayed gastric emptying results in the sensation of fullness and bloating.
- Small meals and low dose metoclopramide can be helpful.

Weight gain

- With chronic starvation the daily energy requirement is reduced so weight gain is possible with a relatively low intake.
- Weight gain of 0.5–1 kg a week is viewed as optimum and 2200–2500 kcal per day should achieve this.
- Gain will be quicker at the start of refeeding and slow as the metabolic rate and exercise levels increase over time.
- Vegan diets present a problem in that they do not provide adequate phosphate or energy.
- Vegetarian diets pose no such difficulties.
- Those who have induced vomiting recently or abused laxatives commonly develop peripheral oedema – up to several kilograms – which must be differentiated from cardiac failure.
- There is no consensus on how a target weight is decided upon but this is generally determined at the start of treatment. Often it is set at a body mass index of 19–20, the minimum healthy weight.
- Some suggest that ultrasound confirmation of ovarian maturity as a marker of adequate weight restoration is useful.

Enteral feeding

- Limited role but may be required.
- Nasogastric is preferred but nasojejunal can be helpful where delayed gastric emptying is a problem.
- Phosphate supplements are required if the person is severely emaciated.
- Vitamin B and C supplements are advocated prior to refeeding and additional minerals may be required.
- Patients should be observed for hyperglycaemia.

Children and adolescents

- Children differ physiologically and psychologically from adults.
- Their nutritional management cannot be separated from other aspects.
- Units must be age appropriate and have staff experienced in all modalities of patient care.
- Adolescents should ideally be treated in different settings.
- Younger people cause more concern as they dehydrate more quickly; emaciation also has a faster onset.

- BMI gives less useful information in children and adolescents and is not a reliable marker of fat, protein or carbohydrate changes.
- Growth and height will be stunted if anorexia nervosa develops before growth is completed.
- Anorexia nervosa can exist with steady weight if it occurs during an expected growth spurt.
- Enteral feeding is obviously essential if the risk of death is imminent.

Recommendations

- Patients with anorexia nervosa should have a dietary assessment.
- Formal nutritional assessment should be completed on admission, with unit policies on these procedures.
- Full physical assessment is required.
- Blood tests should be comprehensive and abnormalities should be referred to experts.
- Refeeding should start slowly.
- Weight gain of 0.5–1 kg per week is recommended.
- Early stages of refeeding pose risks and patients should be closely monitored.
- Micronutrient supplements are recommended for both inpatients and outpatients.
- Oral thiamine is recommended with rapid weight gain.
- Enteral feeding should be administered only by experienced teams.
- This should be administered slowly using an isotonic 1 kcal/ml (4.2 kJ/ml) standard formula delivered by fine-bore nasogastric tube.
- Give parenteral B and C vitamins prior to enteral feeding as well as additional phosphate and possible mineral supplement.
- Written protocols are recommended for dietary advice when using enteral feeding.
- In outpatients, weight gain should not be more than 0.5 kg per week; serum electrolytes should be closely monitored if weight gain is more than 0.3 kg per week.
- If the illness is chronic, slow but safe weight gain can be aimed for, with quality of life being maximised and admission avoided if possible.
- Care should be taken to protect the cultural and religious practices of the patient unless treatment is threatened.
- Children and adolescents should be treated in a service that is age appropriate.
- It should be borne in mind that monitoring BMI in children and adolescents is not as reliable as in adults.
- Expected weight should appreciate premorbid weight and height and parental weight and height.
- Target weight should be reviewed regularly, taking into account the growth of the patient.

- Pubertal development should be maintained if possible within two standard deviations of the norms for age.

See also the 'Guidelines' section in Chapter 21 (Physical health), page 315.

Eating disorders: core interventions in the treatment and management of anorexia nervosa, bulimia nervosa and related eating disorders. NICE Clinical Guideline 9*

Care across all conditions

Assessment and coordination of care

- Assessment of people with eating disorders should be comprehensive and include physical, psychological and social needs, and a comprehensive assessment of risk to self. [C]
- The level of risk to the patient's mental and physical health should be monitored as treatment progresses because it may increase – for example, following weight gain or at times of transition between services in cases of anorexia nervosa. [C]
- For people with eating disorders presenting in primary care, GPs should take responsibility for the initial assessment and the initial coordination of care. This includes the determination of the need for emergency medical or psychiatric assessment. [C]
- Where management is shared between primary and secondary care, there should be clear agreement among individual healthcare professionals on the responsibility for monitoring patients with eating disorders. This agreement should be in writing (where appropriate using the care programme approach) and should be shared with the patient and, where appropriate, their family and carers. [C]

Providing good information and support

- Patients and, where appropriate, carers should be provided with education and information on the nature, course and treatment of eating disorders. [C]
- In addition to the provision of information, family and carers may be informed of self-help groups and support groups, and offered the opportunity to participate in such groups where they exist. [C]
- Healthcare professionals should acknowledge that many people with eating disorders are ambivalent about treatment. Healthcare professionals should also recognise the consequent demands and challenges this presents. [C]

Getting help early

- People with eating disorders seeking help should be assessed and receive treatment at the earliest opportunity. [C]

- Early treatment is particularly important for those with or at risk of severe emaciation and such patients should be prioritised for treatment. [**C**]

Management of physical aspects
- Where laxative abuse is present, patients should be advised to gradually reduce laxative use and informed that laxative use does not significantly reduce calorie absorption. [**C**]
- Treatment of both subthreshold and clinical cases of an eating disorder in people with diabetes is essential because of the greatly increased physical risk in this group. [**C**]
- People with type 1 diabetes and an eating disorder should have intensive regular physical monitoring because they are at high risk of retinopathy and other complications. [**C**]
- Pregnant women with eating disorders require careful monitoring throughout the pregnancy and in the postpartum period. [**C**]
- Patients with an eating disorder who are vomiting should have regular dental reviews. [**C**]
- Patients with an eating disorder who are vomiting should be given appropriate advice on dental hygiene, which should include avoiding brushing after vomiting, rinsing with a non-acid mouthwash after vomiting and reducing an acid oral environment (e.g. limiting acidic foods). [**C**]
- Healthcare professionals should advise people with eating disorders and osteoporosis or related bone disorders to refrain from physical activities that significantly increase the likelihood of falls. [**C**]

Additional considerations for children and adolescents
- Family members, including siblings, should normally be included in the treatment of children and adolescents with eating disorders. Interventions may include sharing of information, advice on behavioural management and facilitating communication. [**C**]
- In children and adolescents with eating disorders, growth and development should be closely monitored. Where development is delayed or growth is stunted despite adequate nutrition, paediatric advice should be sought. [**C**]
- Healthcare professionals assessing children and adolescents with eating disorders should be alert to indicators of abuse (emotional, physical and sexual) and should remain so throughout treatment. [**C**]
- The right to confidentiality of children and adolescents with eating disorders should be respected. [**C**]
- Healthcare professionals working with children and adolescents with eating disorders should familiarise themselves with national guidelines and their employers' policies in the area of confidentiality. [**C**]

Identification and screening of eating disorders in primary care and non-mental health settings
- Target groups for screening should include young women with low body mass index (BMI) compared with age norms, patients consulting with weight concerns who are not overweight, women with menstrual disturbances or amenorrhoea, patients with gastrointestinal symptoms, patients with physical signs of starvation or repeated vomiting, and children with poor growth. [**C**]
- When screening for eating disorders, one or two simple questions should be considered for use with specific target groups (e.g. 'Do you think you have an eating problem?' and 'Do you worry excessively about your weight?'). [**C**]
- Young people with type 1 diabetes and poor treatment adherence should be screened and assessed for the presence of an eating disorder. [**C**]

Anorexia nervosa

Assessment and management of anorexia nervosa in primary care

- In anorexia nervosa, although weight and BMI are important indicators they should not be considered the sole indicators of physical risk (as they are unreliable in adults and especially in children). [**C**]
- In assessing whether a person has anorexia nervosa, attention should be paid to the overall clinical assessment (repeated over time), including rate of weight loss, growth rates in children, objective physical signs and appropriate laboratory tests. [**C**]
- Patients with enduring anorexia nervosa not under the care of a secondary care service should be offered an annual physical and mental health review by their GP. [**C**]

Psychological interventions for anorexia nervosa

The delivery of psychological interventions should be accompanied by regular monitoring of a patient's physical state including weight and specific indicators of increased physical risk.

Common elements of the psychological treatment of anorexia nervosa
- Therapies to be considered for the psychological treatment of anorexia nervosa include cognitive analytic therapy (CAT), cognitive behaviour therapy (CBT), interpersonal psychotherapy (IPT), focal psychodynamic therapy and family interventions focused explicitly on eating disorders. [**C**]
- Patients and, where appropriate, carer preference should be taken into account in deciding which psychological treatment is to be offered. [**C**]

- The aims of psychological treatment should be to reduce risk, to encourage weight gain and healthy eating, to reduce other symptoms related to an eating disorder, and to facilitate psychological and physical recovery. [C]

Outpatient psychological treatments in first episode and later episodes

- Most people with anorexia nervosa should be managed on an outpatient basis, with psychological treatment (with physical monitoring) provided by a healthcare professional competent to give it and to assess the physical risk of people with eating disorders. [C]
- Outpatient psychological treatment for aneroxia nervosa should normally be of at least 6 months' duration. [C]
- For patients with anorexia nervosa, if during outpatient psychological treatment there is significant deterioration, or the completion of an adequate course of outpatient psychological treatment does not lead to any significant improvement, more intensive forms of treatment (e.g. a move from individual therapy to combined individual and family work, or day-care or inpatient care) should be considered. [C]
- Dietary counselling should not be provided as the sole treatment for anorexia nervosa. [C]

Psychological aspects of inpatient care

- For inpatients with anorexia nervosa, a structured symptom-focused treatment regime with the expectation of weight gain should be provided in order to achieve weight restoration. It is important to monitor the patient's physical status carefully during refeeding. [C]
- Psychological treatment should be provided which has a focus both on eating behaviour and attitudes to weight and shape, and on wider psychosocial issues with the expectation of weight gain. [C]
- Rigid inpatient behaviour modification programmes should not be used in the management of anorexia nervosa. [C]

Post-hospitalisation psychological treatment

- Following inpatient weight restoration, people with anorexia nervosa should be offered outpatient psychological treatment that focuses both on eating behaviour and attitudes to weight and shape, and on wider psychosocial issues, with regular monitoring of both physical and psychological risk. [C]
- The length of outpatient psychological treatment and physical monitoring following inpatient weight restoration should typically be at least 12 months. [C]

Additional consideration for children and adolescents with anorexia nervosa

- Family interventions that directly address the eating disorder should be offered to children and adolescents with anorexia nervosa. [B]
- Children and adolescents with anorexia nervosa should be offered individual appointments with a healthcare professional separate from those with their family members or carers. [C]
- The therapeutic involvement of siblings and other family members should be considered in all cases because of the effects of anorexia nervosa on other family members. [C]
- In children and adolescents with anorexia nervosa, the need for inpatient treatment and the need for urgent weight restoration should be balanced alongside the educational and social needs of the young person. [C]

Pharmacological interventions for anorexia nervosa

There is a very limited evidence base for the pharmacological treatment of anorexia nervosa. A range of drugs may be used in the treatment of comorbid conditions but caution should be exercised in their use, given the physical vulnerability of many people with anorexia nervosa.

- Medication should not be used as the sole or primary treatment for anorexia nervosa. [C]
- Caution should be exercised in the use of medication for comorbid conditions such as depressive or obsessive–compulsive features as they may resolve with weight gain alone. [C]
- When medication is used to treat people with anorexia nervosa, the side effects of drug treatment (in particular, cardiac side effects) should be carefully considered and discussed with the patient because of the compromised cardiovascular function of many people with anorexia nervosa. [C]
- Healthcare professionals should be aware of the risk of drugs that prolong the QTc interval on the ECG; for example, antipsychotics, tricyclic antidepressants, macrolide antibiotics, and some antihistamines. In patients with anorexia nervosa at risk of cardiac complications, the prescription of drugs with side effects that may compromise cardiac functioning should be avoided. [C]
- If the prescription of medication that may compromise cardiac functioning is essential, ECG monitoring should be undertaken. [C]
- All patients with a diagnosis of anorexia nervosa should have an alert placed in their prescribing record concerning the risk of side effects. [C]

Physical management of anorexia nervosa

Anorexia nervosa carries considerable risk of serious physical morbidity. Awareness of the risk, careful monitoring and, where appropriate, close liaison with an experienced physician are important in the management of the physical complications of anorexia nervosa.

Managing weight gain

- In most patients with anorexia nervosa, an average weekly weight gain of 0.5-1 kg in inpatient settings and 0.5 kg in outpatient settings should be an aim of treatment. This requires about 3500 to 7000 extra calories a week. [C]

- Regular physical monitoring, and in some cases treatment with a multivitamin/multimineral supplement in oral form, is recommended for people with anorexia nervosa during both inpatient and outpatient weight restoration. [C]
- Total parenteral nutrition should not be used for people with anorexia nervosa, unless there is significant gastrointestinal dysfunction. [C]

Managing risk

- Healthcare professionals should monitor physical risk in patients with anorexia nervosa. If this leads to the identification of increased physical risk, the frequency of the monitoring and nature of the investigations should be adjusted accordingly. [C]
- People with anorexia nervosa and their carers should be informed if the risk to their physical health is high. [C]
- The involvement of a physician or paediatrician with expertise in the treatment of medically at-risk patients with anorexia nervosa should be considered for all individuals who are medically at risk. [C]
- Pregnant women with either current or remitted anorexia nervosa should be considered for more intensive prenatal care to ensure adequate prenatal nutrition and fetal development. [C]
- Oestrogen administration should not be used to treat bone density problems in children and adolescents as this may lead to premature fusion of the epiphyses. [C]
- Whenever possible patients should be engaged and treated before reaching severe emaciation. This requires both early identification and intervention. Effective monitoring and engagement of patients at severely low weight, or with falling weight, should be a priority. [C]

Feeding against the will of the patient

- Feeding against the will of the patient should be an intervention of last resort in the care and management of anorexia nervosa. [C]
- Feeding against the will of the patient is a highly specialised procedure requiring expertise in the care and management of those with severe eating diasorders and the physical complications associated with it. This should only be done in the context of the Mental Health Act 1983 or Children Act 1989. [C]
- When making the decision to feed against the will of the patient, the legal basis for any such action must be clear. [C]

Service interventions for anorexia nervosa

This section considers those aspects of the service system relevant to the treatment and management of anorexia nervosa.

- Most people with anorexia nervosa should be treated on an outpatient basis. [C]

- Inpatient treatment or day patient treatment should be considered for people with anorexia nervosa whose disorder has not improved with appropriate outpatient treatment, or for whom there is a significant risk of suicide or severe self-harm. [C]
- Inpatient treatment should be considered for people with anorexia nervosa whose disorder is associated with high or moderate physical risk. [C]
- Where inpatient management is required for people with anorexia nervosa, this should be provided within reasonable travelling distance to enable the involvement of relatives and carers in treatment, to maintain social and occupational links and to avoid difficulty in transition between primary and secondary care services. This is particularly important in the treatment of children and adolescents. [C]
- People with anorexia nervosa requiring inpatient treatment should be admitted to a setting that can provide the skilled implementation of refeeding with careful physical monitoring (particularly in the first few days of refeeding), in combination with psychosocial interventions. [C]
- Healthcare professionals without specialist experience of eating disorders, or in situations of uncertainty, should consider seeking advice from an appropriate specialist when contemplating a compulsory admission for a patient with anorexia nervosa, regardless of the age of the patient. [C]
- Healthcare professionals managing patients with anorexia nervosa, especially those with the binge–purging sub type, should be aware of the increased risk of self-harm and suicide, particularly at times of transition between services or service settings. [C]

Additional considerations for children and adolescents

- Healthcare professionals should ensure that children and adolescents with anorexia nervosa who have reached a healthy weight have the increased energy and necessary nutrients available in their diet to support further growth and development. [C]
- In the nutritional management of children and adolescents with anorexia nervosa, carers should be included in any dietary education or meal planning. [C]
- Admission of children and adolescents with anorexia nervosa should be to age-appropriate facilities (with the potential for separate children and adolescent services), which have the capacity to provide appropriate educational and related activities. [C]
- Where a young person with anorexia nervosa refuses treatment that is deemed essential, consideration should be given to the use of the Mental Health Act 1983 or the right of those with parental responsibility to override the young person's refusal. [C]

- Relying indefinitely on parental consent to treatment should be avoided. It is recommended that the legal basis under which treatment is being carried out should be recorded in the patient's case notes, and this is particularly important in the case of children and adolescents. [C]
- For children and adolescents with anorexia nervosa, where issues of consent to treatment are highlighted, healthcare professionals should consider seeking a second opinion from an eating disorders specialist. [C]
- If the patient with anorexia nervosa and those with parental responsibility refuse treatment, and treatment is deemed to be essential, legal advice should be sought in order to consider proceedings under the Children Act 1989. [C]

Bulimia nervosa

Psychological interventions for bulimia nervosa

- As a possible first step, patients with bulimia nervosa should be encouraged to follow an evidence-based self-help programme. [B]
- Healthcare professionals should consider providing direct encouragement and support to patients undertaking an evidence-based self-help programme as this may improve outcomes. This may be sufficient treatment for a limited subset of patients. [B]
- Cognitive behaviour therapy for bulimia nervosa (CBT-BN), a specifically adapted form of CBT, should be offered to adults with bulimia nervosa. The course of treatment should be for 16–20 sessions over 4–5 months. [A]
- When people with bulimia nervosa have not responded to or do not want CBT, other psychological treatments should be considered. [B]
- Interpersonal psychotherapy should be considered as an alternative to CBT, but patients should be informed it takes 8–12 months to achieve results comparable with cognitive behaviour therapy. [B]

Pharmacological interventions for bulimia nervosa

- As an alternative or additional first step to using an evidence-based self-help programme, adults with bulimia nervosa may be offered a trial of an antidepressant drug. [B]
- Patients should be informed that antidepressant drugs can reduce the frequency of binge eating and purging, but the long term effects are unknown. Any beneficial effects will be rapidly apparent. [B]
- Selective serotonin reuptake inhibitors (SSRIs) (specifically fluoxetine) are the drugs of first choice for the treatment of bulimia nervosa in terms of acceptability, tolerability and reduction of symptoms. [C]
- For people with bulimia nervosa, the effective dose of fluoxetine is higher than for depression (60 mg daily). [C]
- No drugs, other than antidepressants, are recommended for the treatment of bulimia nervosa. [B]

Management of physical aspects of bulimia nervosa

Patients with bulimia nervosa can experience physical problems as a result of a range of behaviours associated with the condition. Awareness of the risks and careful monitoring should be a concern of all healthcare professionals working with people with this disorder.

- Patients with bulimia nervosa who are vomitting frequently or taking large quantities of laxatives (especially if they are also underweight) should have their fluid and electrolyte balance assessed. [C]
- When electrolyte disturbance is detected, it is usually sufficient to focus on eliminating the behaviour responsible. In the small proportion of cases where supplementation is required to restore electrolyte balance, oral rather than intravenous administration is recommended, unless there are problems with gastrointestinal absorption. [C]

Service interventions for bulimia nervosa

The great majority of patients with bulimia nervosa can be treated as outpatients. There is a very limited role for the inpatient treatment of bulimia nervosa. This is primarily concerned with the management of suicide risk or severe self-harm.

- The great majority of patients with bulimia nervosa should be treated in an outpatient setting. [C]
- For patients with bulimia nervosa who are at risk of suicide or severe self-harm, admission as an inpatient or day patient, or the provision of more intensive outpatient care, should be considered. [C]
- Psychiatric admission for people with bulimia nervosa should normally be undertaken in a setting with experience of managing this disorder. [C]
- Healthcare professionals should be aware that patients with bulimia nervosa who have poor impulse control, notably substance misuse, may be less likely to respond to a standard programme of treatment. As a consequence treatment should be adapted to the problems presented. [C]

Additional considerations for children and adolescents

- Adolescents with bulimia nervosa may be treated with CBT-BN adapted as needed to suit their age, circumstances and level of development, and including the family as appropriate. [C]

Atypical disorders including binge eating disorder

General treatment of atypical eating disorders

- In the absence of evidence to guide the management of atypical eating disorders (also known as eating disorders not otherwise specified) other than binge eating disorder, it is recommended that the clinician considers following the guidance on the treatment of the eating problem that most closely resembles the individual patient's eating disorder. [C]

Psychological treatments for binge eating disorder

- As a possible first step, patients with binge eating disorder should be encouraged to follow an evidence-based self-help programme. [B]
- Healthcare professionals should consider providing direct encouragement and support to patients undertaking an evidence-based self-help programme as this may improve outcomes. This may be sufficient treatment for a limited subset of patients. [B]
- Cognitive behaviour therapy for binge eating disorder (CBT-BED), a specifically adapted form of CBT, should be offered to adults with binge eating disorder. [A]
- Other psychological treatments (interpersonal psychotherapy for binge eating disorder and modified dialectical behaviour therapy) may be offered to adults with persistent binge eating disorder. [B]
- Patients should be informed that all psychological treatments for binge eating disorder have a limited effect on body weight. [A]
- When providing psychological treatments for patients with binge eating disorder, consideration should be given to the provision of concurrent or consecutive interventions focusing on the management of any comorbid obesity. [C]
- Suitably adapted psychological treatments should be offered to adolescents with persistent binge eating disorder. [C]

Pharmacological interventions for binge eating disorder

- As an alternative or additional first step to using an evidence-based self-help programme, consideration should be given to offering a trial of an SSRI antidepressant drug to patients with binge eating disorder. [B]
- Patients with binge eating disorders should be informed that SSRIs can reduce binge eating, but the long-term effects are unknown. Antidepressant drug treatment may be sufficient treatment for a limited subset of patients. [B]

A, B and C indicate grades of recommendation (see Appendix II for full details). * Reproduced with permission from the National Institute for Health and Clinical Excellence, London.

Education and training

8

Chapter contents

General topics

Appraisal and revalidation of consultant psychiatrists

Roy D 2004 Appraisal and revalidation of consultant psychiatrists in the NHS. A report from the Special Committee on Clinical Governance. Psychiatric Bulletin 28: 387–390

'A steer' to help psychiatrists with appraisal, job planning and revalidation.

The GMC proposes a revalidation process to maintain a doctor's licence to practise where revalidation is achieved through satisfactory appraisal documentation.

The new consultant contract requires consultants to achieve a satisfactory appraisal and contribute towards the job planning process. The appraisee should keep an up-to-date folder and prepare a personal development plan prior to appraisal by a consultant colleague.

Subjects to be covered at appraisal include:
- good medical care
- serious untoward incidents
- complaints
- performance indicators and outcome measures
- record of CPD
- relationships with colleagues, patients and carers
- teaching
- health and probity
- management.

Weblink Royal College of Psychiatrists – http://pb.rcpsych. org/cgi/content/full/28/10/387.

How to make journal clubs more interesting

Swift G 2004 How to make journal clubs more interesting. Advances in Psychiatric Treatment 10: 67–72

The majority of training rotations include a journal club, relevant to the critical review paper of the MRCPsych Part II examination. Agreed goals may enhance the learning experience. There is no single ideal format. Journal clubs promote evidence-based practice and teaching critical appraisal. They also fulfil requirements for continuing professional development. Where psychiatric services are spread over a large geographical area the journal club may promote peer contact. It is unlikely that journal clubs encourage participants to read more. There are well-designed studies to investigate the impact of journal clubs on patient outcomes.

No research has looked at the contribution of particular journal club formats to success in the critical review paper in Part II of the MRCPsych examination. It may be preferable to have a senior trainee as the journal club leader as the journal club may be less inhibiting and more relevant to the needs of colleagues. The group leader should ensure that the boundaries of the group are clear in terms of timing, holidays, preparation, etc. and that the environment is conducive.

It is suggested that there should be consideration as to who should fund the provision of food, particularly in view of the recent discussions regarding sponsorship from pharmaceutical companies. Journal clubs directed at the critical review paper of the MRCPsych Part II may be enthusiastically received by trainees, but may be repetitive for permanent staff. Presentation of journals in a structured way can help with the consistent identification of methodological flaws. Trainees and consultants may be reluctant to attend if they are not confident in their critical appraisal skills. Journal clubs with an evidence-based format may be more relevant in terms of clinical practice because it focuses on a topic rather than on a single paper. Alternative journal clubs that use a more creative approach, including videos, book reviews, story telling, etc. were not seen as an easy option, but led to improved recall.

Parkes J, Hyde C, Deeks J et al 2001 Teaching critical appraisal skills in health care settings **(Cochrane Review)**. In: The Cochrane Library, Issue 3. Update Software, Oxford

- Journal clubs probably do improve knowledge of biostatistics and clinical epidemiology.
- The evidence base is small.

Heiligman PM, Wollitzer OW 1987 A survey of journal clubs in US family practice residencies. Journal of Medical Education 62: 928–931

- Having a designated leader correlates with effectiveness.
- Essential attributes of a facilitator include an interest in medical education and a belief that the club has an important role in that process.

Sidorov J 1995 How are internal medicine journal clubs organised and what makes them successful? Archives of Internal Medicine 155: 1193–1197

- Longevity and high levels of attendance are associated with the provision of food and mandatory attendance.

Van Derwood JG, Tietze PE, Nagy MC 1991 Journal clubs in family practice residency programs in the southeast. South Medical Journal 84: 483–487

- Enthusiastic support from the programme director is associated with attendance rates.
- Attendance was highest when the programme director rated the educational value of the club as 'vital' and lowest when it was rated as 'having no educational value'.

Cramer JS, Mahony MC 2001 Introducing evidence-based medicine to the journal club, using a structured pre- and post-test: a cohort study. BMC Medical Education 1(1): Epub

Suggested the following format for a family medicine journal club:
- Over the course of a year, a written test consisting of about 10 questions was given to participants before and after each club meeting.
- The director of the club set the questions, which were based on critical appraisal of the papers to be discussed.

- This allowed ongoing assessment of performance and learning.
- This format did not require the paper to have been read in advance, and more closely mimics exam conditions.

Coomarasamy A, Latthe P, Papaioannou S et al 2001 Critical appraisal in clinical practice: sometimes irrelevant, occasionally invalid. Journal of the Royal Society of Medicine 94: 573–577

- In a study of an obstetrics and gynaecology journal club it was found that 11 of 55 consecutive appraisals missed the article most relevant to the clinical question.

Modernising medical careers

Department of Health 2003 Modernising medical careers. The response of the four UK Health Ministers to the consultation on 'Unfinished Business: Proposals for reform of the Senior House Officer grade'. DH, London

This report is the ministerial response to proposed changes in postgraduate training.

In 2002, Sir Liam Donaldson, Chief Medical Officer for England, proposed changes to postgraduate medical education in *Unfinished Business*. He noted that half of all SHO posts were short term and were not integrated into a training scheme. Variable selection and training standards prevailed. Time spent in the grade did not correlate with training requirements.

The proposals from *Unfinished Business* were:
- a 2-year foundation programme to develop core, generic clinical skills, with rotation to specialties to aid career choice
- a subsequent time-limited basic specialist training programme, resulting in accreditation as a specialist or general practitioner
- assessment to be competency based and involve RITAs
- Royal College examinations to retain a vital (if somewhat undefined) role in training.

The proposals would result in earlier completion of training and greater access to CCSTs or equivalents for career grade staff.

Modernising Medical Careers largely endorsed the proposals, as follows:
- After the first foundation year, trainees should fulfil the requirements for full registration as detailed in *Good Medical Practice* (GMC 1995).
- Summative assessment would inform.
- Year 2 of foundation training would expose trainees to a variety of specialist experience.
- Trainees who are undecided about their career path would benefit from the variety of experience.
- Trainees with firm career aims could undertake training in their chosen specialty, which may count as Certificate of Completion of Training (CCT) relevant training.

- Trainees will then compete for access to basic specialist training with competency-based assessment.
- After award of the CCT some consultants may undergo further training leading to 'deep specialisation'.

Weblink Scottish Executive – www.mmc.scot.nhs.uk/documents/ModernisingMedicalCareers.pdf.

New ways of working for psychiatrists

Department of Health 2005 New ways of working for psychiatrists: enhancing effective, person-centred services through new ways of working in multidisciplinary and multi-agency contexts. Care Services Improvement Partnership, London. Online. Available: www.baat.org/270394A_Psychiatry_report.pdf

The report of a national steering group aiming to help mental health services make the most of their psychiatric staff in the face of increased demands and ongoing workforce challenges.

Recommendations

- Emphasis on a consultative role for consultant psychiatrists within multidisciplinary teams.
- Distributing leadership and responsibility across teams to allow consultants to concentrate on more complex cases.
- Raising profiles of social workers, pharmacists, primary care workers and other allied health professionals within teams, including supplementary and independent prescribing.

The next steps – the future shape of foundation, specialist and general practice training programmes

Department of Health 2004 The Next Steps – The Future Shape of Foundation, Specialist and General Practice Training Programmes. Online. Available: www.mmc.nhs.uk/download_files/The-next-steps.pdf

Modernising Medical Careers in 2003 set out proposals for the provision of care in the UK by trained as opposed to trainee doctors. This document expands on some of the previous reforms.

- The role of the PMETB is emphasised. It will be the sole authority for deciding whether training undertaken as a second year foundation trainee can count towards a CCT.
- Consideration of the Working Time Directive.
- The need for 'robust' governance of foundation programmes is raised.
- Discusses in more detail the entry and exit from training at various stages.

POEM: Patient-oriented evidence that matters

Smith R 2002 POEM: Patient-oriented evidence that matters [editorial]. British Medical Journal 325: 983

There are three criteria for a POEM (patient-oriented evidence that matters):

1. It addresses a question that doctors encounter.
2. It measures outcomes that doctors and their patients care about:
   - symptoms
   - morbidity
   - quality of life
   - mortality.
3. It has potential to change the ways doctors practice.

- *Example*: POEM risk of suicide in bipolar disorder is least with lithium.
- *Question*: What drug used in the treatment of bipolar disorder is most effective for reducing risk of suicide?
- *Reference*: Goodwin FK, Fireman B, Simon GE et al 2003 Suicide risk in bipolar disorder during treatment with lithium and divalproex. Journal of the American Medical Association 290: 1467–1473.

Background

Lithium is used in the treatment of bipolar disorder with the increase in use of anticonvulsants. There is consistent evidence to suggest that lithium reduces suicide rates.

Method

- A retrospective cohort study.
- The rates of completed suicide were compared in patients receiving lithium, carbamazepine and divalproex treatment.
- The mean follow-up period was 3 years.
- Suicide deaths were identified from health plan mortality records and death certificate reports.

Results

- The risk of suicide was 2.7 times higher during treatment with divalproex than with lithium.
- Rates for non-fatal suicide were also higher with divalproex.
- Patients taking carbamazepine were found more likely to be hospitalised for suicide attempts although the power is low.
- The risk of suicide seems to be lower with lithium than divalproex and carbamazepine.
- More reliable evidence could be obtained from prospective randomised trials that compare the drugs head to head.
- The level of evidence of this study is IIb.

Postgraduate Medical Education and Training Board

Postgraduate Medical Education and Training Board 2004 PMETB – The first three years. PMETB, London. Online. Available: www.pmetb.org.uk/media/pdf/0/b/PMETB_the_first_three_years_(2004).pdf

A description of the background, function and future aims of the Postgraduate Medical Education and Training Board, a statutory body that became fully operational in September 2005. It arose from the government's desire to modernise medical institutions and maintain independent self-regulation whilst increasing public involvement.

This single organisation will be responsible for postgraduate medical training as opposed to the diverse collection of institutions which had evolved over previous centuries. It is hoped that this will result in greater transparency, consistency and improved quality assurance.

It will address challenges in service provision and training caused by workforce pressures. It will balance this with the public's desire to be treated by experienced specialists. Other aims will include improved international recruitment and a rationalisation of inspection processes in the NHS.

Psychiatry as a career choice compared with other specialities

Rajagopal S, Singh Rehill K, Goodfrey E 2004 Psychiatry as a career choice compared with other specialities: a survey of medical students. Psychiatric Bulletin 28: 444–446

This study aimed to establish the attitudes of UK medical students to psychiatry as a career option. Previous research has shown that medical students display a number of negative attitudes towards psychiatry as a specialty.

Method

- Students at a London medical school were given a questionnaire to complete.

Results

- Psychiatry remains unpopular.
- It was the least sought after specialty and was viewed as boring, unscientific, stressful, frustrating and unenjoyable.
- A family history of mental illness is positively associated with choosing psychiatry.
- Personal history of psychiatric illness was not a significant factor.

Discussion

- Recruitment in psychiatry remains an issue that could be addressed by education programmes organised by the Royal College of Psychiatrists.

Furnham AF 1986 Medical students' beliefs about 9 different specialities. British Medical Journal (Clinical Research Edition) 293: 1607–1610

- Medical students perceive psychiatry as having the lowest status of all the specialties.

Eagle PF, Marcos LR 1980 Factors in medical students' choice of psychiatry. American Journal of Psychiatry 137: 423–427

- The negative attitudes of medical students about psychiatry as a medical specialty extend to the psychiatrists.
- They were described as emotionally unstable, confused and lower in competence than surgeons and physicians.

Storer D 2002 Recruiting and retaining psychiatrists. British Journal of Psychiatry 180: 296–297

- Found the number of medical students wanting to become psychiatrists is significantly lower than the number required to serve the population.

Royal College of Psychiatrists 2002 Annual census of psychiatric staffing 2001. Occasional Paper OP54. Royal College of Psychiatrists, London

- 12% of consultant posts remain vacant and recruitment continues to be problematic.

Tomorrow's doctors

General Medical Council 2003 Tomorrow's doctors. Recommendations on undergraduate medical education. GMC, London. Online. Available: www.gmc-uk.org/education/undergraduate/tomdoc.pdf

This document superseded the 1993 guidance of the same title and set out the characteristics of the kind of graduate the GMC believes that medical schools should produce.

Recommendations

- Early introduction of undergraduates to principles set out in *Good Medical Practice* (GMC 1995).
- Clear appropriate standards for students and medical schools.
- Detailed curricula and assessments.
- Core curricula supported by student-selected topics.
- Factual information to be kept to the minimum required.
- More emphasis on skills, especially communication skills, self-directed learning and critical appraisal of evidence.
- Awareness of importance of public safety and rights.

- List of basic medical procedures that graduates should be able to perform.
- Universities to support struggling/concerning students, but also to identify risks to the public and manage appropriately.

User and carer involvement

Livingstone G, Cooper C 2004 User and carer involvement. Advances in Psychiatric Treatment 10: 85–92

Patients' role in training has generally been a passive one. National policy has emphasised the importance of user and carer involvement in mental health services at a variety of levels. A number of bodies exist to ensure that patients and carers are involved with both the academic and the clinical side of health care – The Patients' Forum, INVOLVE (previously Consumers in NHS Research) and the Commission for Patient and Public Involvement in Health. Some users and carers feel they could and should play an active part in teaching as they have a unique understanding of their own illness and the experience of being in the healthcare system.

Training, practice and research usually define expertise. Patients' expertise is defined by experience, and this different perspective gives them a unique role in teaching. There is a move away from using patients to educate towards the use of actors. There are differences in the two models of training: one prioritises the need to standardise, so that all learners see the same range and pattern of illnesses; the other emphasises the need to see real patients who react in a non-standard way.

Patient involvement could be increased in specific educational situations to include the teaching of communication skills and the role of questioners using the problem-based learning concept. Patients usually reported benefit from involvement through learning more about themselves and through personal satisfaction, empowerment and increased confidence.

After involvement of users in training, participants were significantly more positive towards users generally and showed greater awareness of stigmatising factors of mental illness.

There is a role for users and carers in teaching psychiatric trainees, including training in interview skills and contributions to the MRCPsych course. There is the potential to employ users in an educational role and a small number of academic posts already exist. This raises issues in terms of appropriate training and standards and the need for accurate and appropriate content.

User organisations have a major role in health promotion, including running training courses on topics such as listening and counselling skills. There is a lack of information regarding the involvement of those from ethnic minorities in mental health training, either users or carers.

Voluntary organisations are leading proponents of user training. Although there has been some resistance from professional groups, evaluation shows that service user involvement in training has a positive impact.

Wood J, Wilson-Barnett J 1999 The influence of user involvement on the learning of mental health nursing students. NT Research 4: 257–270

- Nursing students who had more and earlier exposure to user involvement showed more empathy, used less jargon and had a more individualised approach to patients.

Walters K, Buszewicz M, Russell J et al 2003 Teaching as therapy: cross sectional and qualitative evaluation of patients' experiences of undergraduate psychiatry teaching in the community. British Medical Journal 326: 740–750

- Conducted a questionnaire and an in-depth interview study with patients, medical students and general practitioner tutors involved in a teaching programme.
- The general practitioner recruited patients who were well and asked them if they would agree to a student interviewing them, usually at home, with the aim of teaching the students about psychiatric illness and the process of recovery.
- All groups interviewed suggested that there were direct benefits to the patients taking part, such as empowerment and raised self-esteem.
- A few patients found the interviews distressing, and research is needed to identify characteristics that would allow patients who might be distressed to be distinguished from those who would benefit.

Wass V, Jones R, Van der Vleuten CPM 2001 Standardized or real patients to test clinical competence? The long case revisited. Medical Education 35: 321–329

- The use of 'long cases' was neither more nor less reliable than using the objective standardized clinical examination in a final year qualifying undergraduate clinical examination.

Whys and hows of patient-based teaching

Doshi M, Brown N 2005 Whys and hows of patient-based teaching. Advances in Psychiatric Treatment 11: 223–231

Patient-based teaching in psychiatry can include trainees shadowing trainers, assessing patients and feeding back and presenting cases to the clinical team. Trainers can use direct observation and video interviews to observe trainee performance. This article discusses the provision of patient-based teaching.

Kneebone D, Scott W, Darzi A et al 2004 Simulation and clinical practice: strengthening the relationship. Medical Education 38: 1095–1102

- Concluded that there is evidence that learning skills using simulated patients does not match real-life practice.

Spencer J 2003 ABC of learning and teaching in medicine: learning and teaching in the clinical environment. British Medical Journal 326: 591–594

- The teaching of clinical skills using real patients is lifelike and relevant to future working practice.

Hartley S, Gill D, Walters K et al 2003 Teaching medical students in primary and secondary care. Oxford University Press, Oxford

- Patient-based learning allows trainees to learn in context and shows increased recall of learning.

Dent JA 2001 Hospital wards. In: Dent JA, Harden M (eds) Practical guide for medical teachers. Churchill Livingstone, Edinburgh, pp 98–108

- Trainees can generalise skills learned from one patient to other patients with similar or different problems.
- Trainees can also learn from observing an experienced clinician's approach with real patients.

Ferenchick G, Simpson D, Blackman J et al 1997 Strategies for efficient and effective teaching in the ambulatory care setting. Academic Medicine 72: 277–280

- Another advantage of patient-based learning is that the trainee can receive direct feedback from the patient.

Cox K 1993 Planning bedside teaching – 1. Overview. Medical Journal of Australia 158: 280–282

- Found that clinical teaching using inpatients is often on an ad hoc basis with poor supervision.
- It is also affected by the range of cases available.
- Only some parts of the curriculum can be taught by patient-based teaching alone.

Ramani S 2003 Twelve tips to improve bedside teaching. Medical Teacher 25: 112–115

- Patient-based teaching need not be directed by the availability of cases.
- With careful planning on the part of the trainer the curriculum can be systematically covered.

Kolb DA 1984 Experiential learning: experience as the source of learning and development. Prentice Hall, Englewood Cliffs, NJ

- Described four steps in experiential learning:
  - the concrete experience
  - reflective observations
  - abstract conceptualisation
  - active experimentation.
- Thus direct experience and subsequent reflection teach new skills that can be generalised and later tested in new situations.

Policy and Legislation

The European Working Time Directive

Department of Health 2004 The European Working Time Directive. DH, London. Online. Available: www.dh.gov. uk/PolicyAndGuidance/HumanResourcesAndTraining

The EWTD is a directive from the Council of the European Union. It acts to protect the health and safety of workers in the European Union.

It sets out minimum requirements with regard to working hours, rest periods, annual leave and arrangements for people who work at night.

The directive was enacted in UK Law as the Working Time Regulations and came into effect in 1998.

The main features are:
- a maximum of 48 hours per week
- 11 hours continuous rest in 24 hours
- 24 hours continuous rest in 7 days (or 48 hours in 14 days)
- 20-minute break in work periods over 6 hours
- 4 weeks' annual leave
- A maximum of 8 hours' work in 24 hours on average for people who work at night.

The UK Working Time Regulations are UK health and safety legislation. Contracts that require trainee doctors to work outside these regulations are illegal. There is some provision to apply for a variation within the regulations or by collective agreement (a derogation). For junior doctors the UK has derogated from the minimum daily rest requirements set out by the EWTD so that junior doctors are entitled to 'compensatory' rest equivalent to that which is lost when the ideal daily rate is not achieved.

The SiMAP judgement

This case, brought to the European Court of Justice on behalf of a group of Spanish doctors, led to a ruling that all the hours which a resident spent on call would count as working time. Whilst the ruling is specific to this particular case, it follows that a similar interpretation of working time should apply in the UK.

Ethical issues

Chapter contents

Ethical issues

Advance refusals of treatment

Department of Health 2001 Advance refusals of treatment. Reference guide to consent for examination or treatment. DH, London

Patients may have a 'living will' or 'advance directive' specifying how they would like to be treated in the case of future incapacity. While professionals cannot be required by such directives to provide particular treatments (which might be inappropriate), case law is now clear that an advance refusal of treatment which is valid and applicable to subsequent circumstances in which the patient lacks capacity is legally binding. An advance refusal is valid if made voluntarily by an appropriately informed person with capacity. Failure to respect such an advance refusal can result in legal action against the practitioner.

If there is doubt about the validity of an advance refusal, a ruling should be sought from the court. It is not legally necessary for the refusal to be made in writing or formally witnessed, although such measures add evidentiary weight to the validity of the refusal. A health professional may not override a valid and applicable advance refusal on the grounds of the professional's personal conscientious objection to such a refusal.

Although the issue has not yet come before a court, it has been suggested that as a matter of public policy individuals should not be able to refuse in advance measures which are essential to keep a patient comfortable. This is sometimes referred to as 'basic' or 'essential' care, and includes keeping the patient warm and clean and free from distressing symptoms such as breathlessness, vomiting and severe pain. However, some patients may prefer to tolerate some discomfort if this means they remain more alert and able to respond to family and friends.

However, although basic/essential care would include the offer of oral nutrition and hydration, it would not cover force feeding an adult or the use of artificial nutrition and hydration. The courts have recognised that a competent individual has the right to choose to go on a 'hunger strike', although this may be qualified if the person has a mental disorder. Towards the end of such a period an individual is likely to lose capacity (become incompetent) and the courts have stated that if the individual has, whilst competent, expressed the desire to refuse food until death supervenes, the person cannot be force fed or fed artificially when incompetent. If the person is refusing food as a result of mental disorder and is detained under the Mental Health Act 1983, different considerations may apply and more specialist guidance should be consulted.

Assisted suicide

Huxtable R 2004 Assisted suicide [editorial]. British Medical Journal 328: 1088–1089

Background

Existing legislation regarding assisted suicide is complex and unclear. The Suicide Act 1961 legislates for a maximum prison sentence of 14 years for aiding suicide. There have been recent investigations of a retired GP, Patrick Kneen, who is also the chairman of the Voluntary Euthanasia Society. This followed allegations that he conspired to assist the suicide of a friend and may have intended to provide him with sleeping tablets. Dr Kneen and his wife were both investigated, but neither was charged.

Other topical issues include the case of 'leaving the pills' for which no health professional has been prosecuted. One case was overthrown as the judge said that providing the option was 'not enough'. Death tourism is increasingly an issue.

House of Lords 2004 Select Committee on Assisted Dying for the Terminally Ill Bill. First Report 2004. Online. Available: www.publications.parliament.uk/pa/ld200304/ldbills/017/2004017.pdf

This Bill provides for a competent and terminally ill person (major) who is suffering unbearably to request either assisted suicide or voluntary euthanasia. It describes the necessary procedures, which would include examination by a competent physician to confirm that the patient would die of natural causes within a set time period (maximum period of a few months). On confirmation of this, the patient must sign a written declaration of intent. Thereafter the patient may receive within 14 days the means to take their own life or voluntary euthanasia.

R (on the application of Pretty) v DPP [2002] 1 FLR 268 (House of Lords). Application no. 2346/02 Pretty v UK (2002) 35 EHRR 1 (European Court of Human Rights)

*   Mrs Pretty suffered from motor neurone disease and sought clarification that her husband would not be charged should he assist in her suicide.
*   The UK courts and the European Court of Human Rights 'denied that the right to life encompassed a right to choose the timing and manner of one's death'.
*   The preservation of life and protection of the vulnerable were key issues.

Probation for parents who watched their daughter die. Independent 18 November 1989, p 3

*   Sara Johnstone, who had motor neurone disease, took an overdose. Her parents were not involved in assisting with this. At her request they did not summon assistance. They were later convicted of assisting in her suicide. They were found to be guilty of 'purely negative conduct'.
*   This ruling is contradictory when the principles of the Assisted Dying for the Terminally Ill Bill are considered, in particular the aim for compassionate treatment.

Re B (Adult refusal of Medical Treatment) [2002] 2 All ER 449

*   Ms B was ventilator dependent.
*   The Court of Appeal confirmed the common law right of a competent patient to refuse medical treatment, even if in exercising this right the patient's death would result.
*   A competent refusal was accepted.
*   This is in contradiction with the case of Sara above.

The Clunis Inquiry

Court C 1994 Clunis Inquiry cites 'catalogue of failures'. British Medical Journal News 308: 613

Christopher Clunis was a patient with schizophrenia who had been discharged from hospital. He stabbed and killed a musician, Jonathon Zito, at a London underground station.

The inquiry team, chaired by Jean Ritchie QC, reported that it was a 'catalogue of failure and missed opportunity'. The blame was found to lie between psychiatrists, social workers, the Crown Prosecution Service and the probation service. It was noted that as his mental state deteriorated, so too did the level of care that he received. Eight days before the murder he had been found wandering the streets with a screwdriver and a bread knife.

Specific concerns were:

*   the lack of prompt response from the police
*   that his history of violence was not assessed by his doctors, psychiatric nurses or social workers
*   a lack of resources.

The report suggested that a special supervision group be set up to cover the most difficult and disturbed patients nationwide. Such patients would be cared for by specialist teams. The names of patients would be entered on a special register. New funds would be sourced for their care. It was estimated that between 3000 and 4000 patients would fulfil the criteria.

Such patients would have two of the following criteria:

*   They had been detained more than once
*   A history of violence or persistent offending
*   A lack of response to treatment by general psychiatric services
*   Homelessness.

Further recommendations included:

*   a supervised discharge order to allow patients to be recalled should they fail to comply with treatment
*   the proviso that mental health teams should not hand over care when a patient moves until they are satisfied that the new team has clearly taken responsibility for them.

The team stated that the current government policy of care in the community is 'beneficial to the vast majority of people who suffer from mental illness'.

Dancing with the devil? Psychiatry's relationship with the pharmaceutical industry

Shooter M 2005 Dancing with the devil? A personal view of psychiatry's relationship with the pharmaceutical industry [editorial]. Psychiatric Bulletin 29: 81–83

Answered suggestions that psychiatrists are 'pill pushers' who are in the keep of drug companies by stressing that medication can be of benefit to patients. Furthermore, pharmaceutical companies had invested significant amounts of money with benefits for patients, regardless of the actual aim.

The view that medication is overprescribed may reflect the fact that it is widely available in comparison with psychological and other treatments. There are expectations on psychiatrists to provide a quick, medical cure. Social unhappiness may be medicalised. Psychiatrists may use medication as the form of treatment with which they are most familiar. Health professionals may wish to provide holistic, in-depth treatment packages but this may be impossible in normal clinical settings.

Psychiatrists may receive incentives or be 'used' by pharmaceutical companies in a number of ways, from flights to international conferences to free advertising (drug names on pens, cups, etc.) of products. Pharmaceutical sponsorship of trials can lead to biased results.

Shooter MS 2003 The patient's perspective on medicines in mental illness. British Medical Journal 327: 824–826

- Patients are not given good information.
- Minimisation of side effects, some of which can have fatal consequences, leads to a loss of trust in medical professionals.
- This is further compounded if patients believe that medication is being overprescribed, both in real terms and in comparison to other forms of help.

Rose D 2003 Collaborative research between users and professionals: peaks and pitfalls. Psychiatric Bulletin 27: 404–406

- It may be helpful to focus on the subjective views of patients and not on the results from science-based trials.

Department of Health 2001 Treatment choices in psychological therapies and counselling. Evidence-based clinical practice guidelines. The Stationery Office, London

- Psychological therapies are not uniformly or widely available and therapists are poorly trained.

Boardman J 2003 Work, employment and psychiatric disability. Advances in Psychiatric Treatment 9: 327–334

- There is insufficient focus on obtaining employment, housing or vocational rehabilitation.
- These factors are vital to the well-being of severely mentally ill patients.

Healy D, Thase ME 2003 Is academic psychiatry for sale? British Journal of Psychiatry 182: 388–391

- Wrote that 90% of JAMA authors have had dealings with a drug company.

Comment

- The College has published good practice recommendations for the interaction between psychiatrists and pharmaceutical companies –www.rcpsych.ac.uk.
- Pharmaceutical companies must also act within the recommendations of their own professional body.

Healing ourselves: ethical issues in the care of sick doctors

Adshead G 2005 Healing ourselves: ethical issues in the care of sick doctors. Advances in Psychiatric Treatment 11: 330–337

There are issues which arise during the assessment and treatment of doctor-patients that occur during the assessment and treatment of non-doctor-patients. These include issues of confidentiality with regard to collaborative history from the family and to communication with employers. There should be appropriate discussion with the doctor-patient regarding the limits of confidentiality and the doctor's duties in disclosure in situations of risk.

Doctors requiring inpatient treatment, whether formal or informal, may receive preferential treatment, with out-of-area placement to protect their professional identity. Other patients do not receive such treatment. Furthermore, this may increase the perception of stigma and shame.

The aim of treatment for doctor-patients may not be clear. It may be difficult to distinguish between treatment to make the patient safer rather than better. An example given is when abstinence is achieved by patients with substance misuse problems whilst there are ongoing underlying emotional problems. It can be difficult to decide when a return to work is appropriate, especially if there is pressure from the patient and/or workplace for a return to work.

Psychological and psychodynamic theories regarding care-giving styles are also discussed.

Baldwin P, Dodd M, Wrate R 1997 Young doctors' health: how do working conditions affect attitudes, health and performance? Social Science and Medicine 45: 35–40

- Doctors have higher rates of somatic and social dysfunction.

Hardy GE, Shapiro D, Borrill C 1997 Fatigue in the workforce of national health trusts: levels of symptomatology and links with minor psychiatric disorder, demographic, occupational and work factors. Journal of Psychosomatic Research 43: 83–92

- Doctors have increased levels of fatigue compared to the general population.

Graham J, Ramirez A 1997 Mental health of hospital consultants. Journal of Psychosomatic Research 43: 227–231

- There are higher levels of psychiatric illness in those who practise medicine.

Hawton K, Clements A, Sakarovitch C et al 2001 Suicide in doctors. Journal of Epidemiology and Community Health 55: 296–300

- This study concluded that the well-documented increase in rates of suicide in doctors is due to depression and substance misuse.

There are different types of mental ill-health in doctors. Physical illness (e.g. cancer, epilepsy) can have psychological effects on the doctor's identity and practice. Psychiatric and psychological conditions may affect an individual's fitness to practise – for example, depression, bipolar illness and substance misuse. Stress and burnout can lead to work, family, life and compassion failure. There are also problems specific to psychiatrists. These include stigma, hypocrisy, anxiety, the lack of an evidence base in psychiatry and an increased risk of psychiatric problems.

Rout U 1999 Job stress among general practitioners and nurses in primary care in England. Psychological Reports 85: 981–986

- Stress is high in hospital doctors and general practitioners.

Bogg J, Gibbs T, Bundred P 2001 Training, job demands and mental health of pre-registration house officers. Medical Education 35: 590–595

- Junior doctors and female doctors are particularly at risk of stress.

McManus IC, Winder B, Gordon D 2002 The causal links between stress and burnout in a longitudinal study of UK doctors. Lancet 350: 2089–2090

- Found a relationship between stress and burnout.
- In doctors the diagnosis of burnout may be preferable to that of depression as there is less stigma.
- There is clear overlap between the diagnoses of burnout, depression and anxiety.

Guthrie E, Tattan T, Williams E et al 1999 Sources of stress, psychological distress and burnout in psychiatrists. Comparison of junior doctors, senior registrars and consultants. Psychiatric Bulletin 23: 207–212

- The rate of stress is high in psychiatric doctors and junior staff in particular.
- There is a relationship between stress, fear of exposure and working in stressful and violent disciplines, such as emergency departments and residential forensic psychiatry.

Baldwin P, Dodd M, Wrate R 1997 Young doctors' health: health and health behaviour. Social Science and Medicine 45: 41–44

- Doctors are not good patients and this starts early in their career with self-medication and self-management.
- One in three junior doctors had no general practitioner.

Tattersall A, Bennett P, Pugh S 1999 Stress and coping in hospital doctors. Stress Medicine 15: 109–113

- Doctors can fall into a vicious circle when they are ill.
- Responses to illness can include wishful thinking and emotional distancing, which may be beneficial in the short term.
- In the long term, however, such responses can decrease the likelihood that doctors will acknowledge that they are ill and that their illness is impacting on their work.

Mukherjee R, Fialho A, Wijetunge A et al 2002 The stigmatisation of psychiatric illness: the attitudes of medical students and doctors in a London teaching hospital. Psychiatric Bulletin 26: 178–181

- Doctors are no less affected by the stigma of mental illness than the rest of the population.

There are a number of ethical issues that face psychiatrists when they assess and treat doctors who are ill. The psychiatrist must remain impartial and not be swayed by personal reactions. In particular the outcome of the assessment may lead to a sick doctor being unable to work and in some circumstances absolute confidentiality cannot be guaranteed. The treating psychiatrist has a duty to report a poorly performing doctor, with or without that doctor's permission if necessary. Sick doctors may wish to receive treatment out of area or via private services to protect their identity. It may be difficult to find the balance between employment as an important support structure during treatment and recovery and a doctor-patient's fitness to work.

The following factors can contribute to work stress in doctors:

- Treatment and care of patients, particularly complex cases
- Insufficient clinical time
- Professional isolation
- Intensive contact with very ill patients
- Conflicts within clinical teams
- Lack of autonomy

- Increasingly high expectations from the public
- Role conflict between work and family
- Long hours
- Little family time.

Brooke D 1997 Impairment in the medical and legal professions. Journal of Psychosomatic Research 43: 27–34

- Self-help groups are beneficial in doctors with addiction problems.
- There may be difficulty, however, in accessing these due to financial constraints.
- Such groups are generally only available in the private sector and private medical insurance may not cover such costs.

Paice E, Rutter H, Wetherall M et al 2002 Stressful incidents, stress and coping strategies in the pre-registration house officer year. Medical Education 36: 56–65

Occupational interventions that improve mental health include:
- more support for junior staff
- more time for discussion
- less tolerance of sleep deprivation
- strategies to balance work and family life.

Thompson W, Cupples M, Sibbett C et al 2001 Challenge of culture, conscience and contract to general practitioners' care of their own health. British Medical Journal 323: 728–731

- This study of general practitioners found that doctors need to present an image of perfect health to colleagues and patients.

Definition

Burnout – a syndrome characterised by symptoms of emotional exhaustion, depersonalisation and low personal achievement. (*Source:* McManus et al 2002, as above.)

Weblinks

Doctors' SupportLine –www.doctorssupport.org.

National Clinical Assessment Service –www.ncas.npsa. nhs.uk.

Information, consent and perceived coercion: patients' perspectives on ECT

Rose DS, Wykes TH, Bindman JP, Fleischmann PS 2005 Information, consent and perceived coercion: patients' perspectives on electroconvulsive therapy. British Journal of Psychiatry 186: 54–59

In England and Wales there are special common law safeguards for patients voluntarily undergoing ECT. There are safeguards under both current and proposed legislation for those receiving compulsory treatment.

Consent is only valid if the patient has been adequately informed of the risk and benefits and freely chooses to undergo treatment.

Method

- A systematic review of studies of the retrospective views of patients about informed consent and perceived coercion.

Results

- 17 previous studies were included.
- There were differences in the studies and the questions asked were not always directly comparable.
- None of the 12 studies gave a consistent picture.
- 45–55% of respondents reported that they were given adequate explanation of ECT.
- The objective knowledge of ECT was examined by four studies – the proportion of respondents who had basic knowledge of ECT was low (e.g. few seemed to know convulsion was involved).
- Testimony data suggest that:
  - some felt pressured into ECT
  - insufficient information was provided
  - there was a lack of information
  - patients felt helpless
  - some people felt coerced because of threats of the Mental Health Act.
- Four studies asked if patients had sufficient information about side effects:
  - Some patients believed that side effect profiles were downplayed.
  - Over half of the comments were specifically linked to the possible side effects of long-term memory loss.
- Only two studies looked at ECT given using legal powers.

Discussion

- Approximately half of those undergoing ECT did not feel they had received sufficient information.
- Patients who felt they had full knowledge ranged from 7 to 16%.
- One-third felt they had been coerced into treatment.
- The testimonies are less likely to be representative as biases exist – for example, in the decision to put a testimony on the internet.
- The proposed legislation will introduce the safeguard that the decision regarding compulsion to have ECT will be made by the mental health tribunals rather than with a second opinion.
- There is growing interest in perceived coercion. It is argued that legal compulsion is not the only kind of coercion that recipients of mental health services experience.

- ECT has special status under English law as the procedure of obtaining informed consent must be recorded.
- Despite patients signing a consent form, many still felt coerced, suggesting that this as a safeguard is ineffective in a proportion of cases.
- There was some evidence that people felt they had no choice about having ECT, with some studies more explicit than others – the Mind study indicated a significantly higher proportion of patients felt they had no choice.

Pedler M 2000 Shock treatment: a survey of people's experience of electro-convulsive therapy (ECT). Mind, London

- ECT is still regarded as a controversial treatment by many.

National Institute for Clinical Excellence 2003 Guidance on use of electro-convulsive therapy (ECT). NICE, London

- NICE recently recommended improvements to the procedures of consent to ECT.

Malcolm K 1999 Patients' perceptions and knowledge of electroconvulsive therapy. Psychiatric Bulletin 13: 161–165

- Patients treated formally were likely to be less knowledgeable about ECT than those receiving informal treatment.
- They were more likely to be unhappy with information provision.

Psychiatry and the pharmaceutical industry

Moncrieff J, Hopker S, Thomas P 2005 Psychiatry and the pharmaceutical industry: who pays the piper? Psychiatric Bulletin 29: 84–85

A perspective from the Critical Psychiatry Network

Psychiatry is vulnerable to the pharmaceutical industry because there can be blurring of boundaries between normality and illness. There can be implications with regard to research.

Psychiatrists must endeavour to remain independent for the sake of the patients, the public and their reputation. It is suggested that the profession needs to examine the ethics of drug company gifts and the subsidy of CME. Local level subsidies should be eliminated so that trainees are not influenced. The College should have a register of members' interests and blind trusts should be set up as an alternative to direct sponsorship. Psychiatrists should also have to declare in monetary terms how much they received from drug companies each year.

Considerations

- Drug companies exert influence on patients, carers, society and prescribers.
- Patients are led to believe that pharmacological treatments are the solution, resulting in disillusionment and disappointment when this is not the case.
- Drug company information conveys and reinforces the message that mental disorders are caused by chemical imbalances.
- The government has cut expenditure on research.
- The pharmaceutical industry is funding and conducting an increasing proportion of research on medical drugs – becoming increasingly influential in determining the perception of psychiatry and the treatments available.

National Institute for Clinical Excellence 2003 Depression: core interventions in management of depression in primary and secondary care. NICE, London

- Questions the value of prescribing antidepressants for widespread unhappiness.

Moynihan R, Health I, Henry D 2002 Selling sickness: the pharmaceutical industry and disease-mongering. British Medical Journal 324: 886–891

- The pharmaceutical industry may encourage the medicalisation of social and personal problems.

Safer DJ 2002 Design and reporting modifications in industry sponsored comparative psychopharmacology trials. Journal of Nervous and Mental Disease 190: 583–592; Melander H, Ahlqvist-Rastad I, Meijer G et al 2003 Evidence b(i)ased medicine – selective reporting from studies sponsored by the pharmaceutical industry: review of studies in new drug applications. British Medical Journal 326: 1171–1173

- There is empirical evidence showing that results can be manipulated in favour of the pharmaceutical company's drug, depending on trial design, conduct and reporting of results.

Moncrieff J, Crawford M 2001 British psychiatry in the twentieth century – observations from a psychiatric journal. Social Science and Medicine 53: 1171–1173

- Psychiatry has been inclined to favour biological methods of mental disorder with physical treatments as a means of bolstering credibility and the claim of authority in the management of mental disorder.

Boyd EA, Bero LA 2000 Assessing faculty financial relationships with industry. Journal of the American Medical Association 284: 2209–2214

- Documents the links between individuals and institutions with the industry.
- The industry is also increasingly sponsoring aspects of service provision within the NHS.

> Healy D 2003 Conspiracy of consensus. Mental Health Today November: 27–30

- NICE has been criticised for allowing the industry to exert an overly strong influence on the process of guideline development, the result being that some guidelines reflect market interests.

Weblink Good psychiatric practice: interim guidance on the relationship between psychiatrists and commercial sponsors and the sponsorship of College activities (Royal College of Psychiatrists Council Report 117) – www.rcpsych.ac.uk/members/currentissues/goodpsychiatricpractice.aspx

Withdrawing and withholding life-prolonging treatment

> Department of Health 2001 Reference guide to consent for examination or treatment: children and young people, DH, London[†]

General principles

The same legal principles apply to withdrawing and withholding life-prolonging treatment as apply to any other medical intervention. However, the gravity and sensitivity of these decisions are such that the assessment of capacity and of best interests is particularly important. Sometimes decisions will need to be made immediately – for example whether it is appropriate to attempt resuscitation after severe trauma. When more time is available and the patient is an adult or child without capacity, all those concerned with the care of the patient – relatives, partners, friends, carers and the multidisciplinary team – can potentially make a contribution to the assessment. The discussions and the basis for decisions should be recorded in the notes.

Legally, the use of artificial nutrition and hydration (ANH) constitutes medical treatment. Thus the legal principles which apply to the use of ANH are the same as those which apply to all other medical treatments such as medication or ventilation. The courts have confirmed that the current case law in this area is compatible with the Human Rights Act 1998.

There is an important distinction between withdrawing or withholding treatment which is of no clinical benefit to the patient or is not in the patient's best interests, and taking a deliberate action to end the patient's life. A deliberate action which is intended to cause death is unlawful. Equally, there is no lawful justification for continuing treatment which is not in an incompetent patient's best interests.

[†] Crown copyright. Reproduced with permission.

Adults and children with capacity

Except in circumstances governed by the Mental Health Act 1983, if an adult with the capacity to make the decision refuses treatment, or requests that it be withdrawn, practitioners must comply with the patient's decision.

However, if a child with capacity makes such a request, this may be overridden, either by a person with parental responsibility or by the courts. Moreover, the courts consider that to take a decision which may result in the individual's death requires a very high level of understanding, so that many young people who would have the capacity to take other decisions about their medical care would lack the capacity to make such a grave decision.

Refusal by a child with capacity must always be taken very seriously, even though legally it is possible to override their objections. It is not a legal requirement to continue a child's life-prolonging treatment in all circumstances. For example, where the child is suffering an illness where the likelihood of survival even with treatment is poor, and treatment will pose a significant burden on the child, it may not be in the best interests of the child to continue treatment.

Adults and children lacking capacity

If a child lacks capacity it is still good practice to involve the child as far as is possible and appropriate in the decision. The decision to withdraw or withhold life-prolonging treatment must be founded on the welfare of the child. If there is disagreement between those with parental responsibility for the child and the clinical team concerning the appropriate course of action, a ruling should be sought from the court.

If an adult lacks capacity, and has not made an advance refusal of treatment which is valid and applicable to the circumstances, the decision must be based on the best interests of the adult, again involving the patient as far as possible.

The BMA has suggested that extra safeguards should be followed before a decision to withhold or withdraw ANH is made: that a senior clinician not otherwise involved in the patient's care should formally review the case; that the details of cases where ANH has been withdrawn should later be made available for clinical audit; and, where the patient is in PVS or a state closely resembling PVS, that legal advice should be sought. Further, the courts have stated that it is good practice for court approval to be sought before ANH is withdrawn from patients in PVS.

General topics

The Bournewood case

Mr L is a 49-year-old man with autistic-spectrum disorder. He has no verbal communication and limited understanding.

He was found to be incapable of giving or withholding consent to medical treatment. In 1997 he was admitted to Bournewood Hospital as an informal patient. Admission was viewed to be in his best interests and with necessity. It was intended that he would be detained under the Mental Health Act if he tried to leave.

Mr L brought legal proceedings against the hospital management, claiming that in effect he had been held unlawfully. The case was heard by the High Court, Court of Appeal and also the House of Lords before making it to the European Court of Human Rights.

The High Court found that Mr L was not detained and that he was treated in his best interests and with the common law principle of necessity.

The Court of Appeal disagreed. It found that Mr L was detained. Only capable patients may be admitted to hospital informally and only if this is with consent. Incapable patients must be admitted under the appropriate mental health legislation.

Thereafter Mr L was detained under the Mental Health Act 1983. He was discharged 5 months later.

The House of Lords found against the Court of Appeal and said that Mr L was not detained. Any detention would have been in his best interests and therefore lawful under the common law of necessity.

Having failed in the House of Lords, the case went to the European Court of Human Rights. The decision made by the European Court of Human Rights was published on 5 October 2004. It stated that a patient can be said to be detained in a mental hospital even though he has never been prevented from leaving it. Article 5 of the European Convention on Human Rights – the right to liberty – applies in these circumstances, i.e. where patients are confined to hospital under the common law doctrine of necessity, Article 5 is breached.

Weblinks

The European Court of Human Rights –www.echr.coe.int.

The Royal College of Psychiatrists: response to the Bournewood Consultation –www.rcpsych.ac.uk/pressparliament/collegeresponses/bournwoodresponse.aspx.

See also the 'Ethical issues' section in Chapter 14 (Learning Disabilities Psychiatry), page 215.

Re C (Adult: Refusal of Medical treatment) [1994] 1 WLR 290

* C was an adult inpatient at Broadmoor Mental Hospital.
* He had chronic schizophrenia with the delusional belief that he was a world renowned doctor.
* He had gangrene of his leg.
* His physicians believed that amputation of his leg was necessary to save his life.
* C refused treatment.

* He was found capable of passing the three-stage test for capacity.
* His delusional beliefs were not found to make him incapable of making a decision about his medical treatment.
* He did not have the amputation and survived.

The three-stage test of capacity requires the patient to be able to:

1. understand information relevant to the decision about treatment
2. believe in that information
3. weigh the information in the balance when arriving at a choice.

Chatterton v Gerson (1981) 1 ALL ER 257

* Mrs Chatterton suffered intractable pain as a result of a trapped nerve following a hernia operation.
* Dr Gerson, a pain specialist, performed an operation to relieve the pain, which resulted in permanent immobility of her right leg.
* Mrs Chatterton claimed that she should have been informed of the risks and claimed battery.
* It was held that she had been informed in broad terms of the nature of the procedure, i.e. she had been informed and consented to an operation of her right leg.
* The fact she may not have been informed of the risks of paralysis could not amount to battery but any claim would have to be made in terms of negligence.

Devi v West Midlands RHA (1980) C.L.Y. 687

* This woman gave consent to a uterine repair.
* A hysterectomy was performed.
* The surgeon was found liable to battery as there was no information given regarding the nature of the operation.
* Battery refers to any non-consensual touching.

Gillick v West Norfolk and Wisbech Area Health Authority and Another (1986) AC 112

* Mrs Gillick began a nationwide petition against the DHSS regarding contraception for under-16s.
* Mrs Gillick sought a declaration from the High Court that none of her five daughters (ages ranged from 1 to 13) could receive advice or prescription of contraceptive medication.

- She was ruled against.
- In 1985 the Law Lords ruled that it was lawful for doctors to prescribe the contraceptive pill for those under 16 without parental consent in exceptional circumstances.
- Lord Scarman found that for a child to be competent they must be able to understand the implications on health in both the short and long term.
- If a minor has sufficient intelligence and understanding to enable him/her to understand the treatment and implications of treatment, then he/she is 'Gillick competent'.
- Gillick competence means that the patient can consent to treatment.
- Refusal of treatment may be treated differently.

See also the 'Ethical issues' section in Chapter 5 (Child and Adolescent Psychiatry), page 69.

Re F (mental patient sterilisation) [1990] 2 AC 1 (sterilisation for contraceptive purposes)

- The House of Lords considered whether it was in the best interests of an incompetent adult female patient to be sterilised to prevent her becoming pregnant.
- It was found that 'in the case of unconscious or incompetent adults a doctor will not be acting unlawfully if he or she acts in the patient's best interests'.
- Furthermore, 'the operation or treatment will be in their best interest if, but only if, it is carried out in order to save their lives, or to ensure improvement or prevent deterioration in their physical or mental health'.

Re M (child: refusal of medical treatment) [1992] 2 FLR 1097

- M was a competent 15 year old who sustained acute heart failure and required a transplant.
- She stated she did not wish to receive someone else's heart, did not wish to take medicine for the rest of her life and so refused to give consent.
- It was declared in her best interests to have the transplant.
- M ultimately consented to the treatment.
- Should she not have consented to treatment then it is clear that treatment would have been declared lawful.

See also the 'Ethical issues' section in Chapter 5 (Child and Adolescent Psychiatry), page 69.

Re MB (Medical Treatment) [1997] 2 FLR 426

- MB was a pregnant woman who did not wish to have a caesarean section.
- The caesarean section was considered necessary for the 'distressed fetus'.
- The Court of Appeal found that: 'A person lacks capacity if some impairment or disturbance of mental functioning renders the person unable to make a decision whether to consent to or refuse treatment.'
- Capacity regarding medical treatment requires that a person can:
  - understand the information
  - weigh up the information
  - retain the information
  - come to a decision
  - communicate their decision.

Weblink Official Solicitor's Practice Note on Declaratory Proceedings – www.officialsolicitor.gov.uk/docs/practice_note_medicalandwelfare.doc.

Re Y (Adult patient) (Transplant: Bone Marrow) (1996) 35 BMLR 111

- Y was 25 years old, severely mentally and physically handicapped.
- She lived in a nursing home but had a close relationship with her family.
- One of her sisters had leukaemia and required a bone marrow transplant.
- Y was the only suitable donor.
- The court considered it was in Y's best interests to donate bone marrow to her sister.
- There was no therapeutic medical benefit to Y.
- There was minimal risk to Y from the procedure.
- The court considered it was in Y's emotional, social and psychological best interests to provide the transplant.
- Should Y's sister die then Y's mother would no longer be able to visit her due to the social situation.

Tarasoff v Regents of the University of California in 1976 (17. Cal. 3d 425 – July 1, 1976. S.F. No. 23042)

Prosenjit Poddar was an Indian graduate student at the University of California. He and a fellow student, Tatiana Tarasoff, went on a couple of dates. He believed they had a special relationship and was unhappy that Tatiana was in the company of other men. He became depressed and began to attend the University Student Health Service psychologist. He disclosed to the psychologist that he intended to get a gun and shoot TT. The psychologist wrote to the campus police requesting that Poddar be taken to a psychiatric hospital. The campus police interviewed PP and did not believe him to be dangerous. He was released on the promise that he would stay away from TT. When the Health Service psychologist returned from holiday he decided that the original letter to the police be destroyed and no further action taken. TT spent the summer in Brazil with her aunt. During this time PP moved in with her brother. When she returned from holiday he stalked her and later stabbed her to death.

Tatiana's parents sued the campus police, the University Health Service and the Regents of the University of California for failing to warn them and their daughter that she was in danger. The initial trial court dismissed the case because it felt there was no cause of action. Prior to Tarasoff, a doctor had a duty to a patient but not to a third party. The Appeals Court supported the dismissal.

Tarasoff I decision: Duty to warn

- An appeal was then made to the California Supreme Court.
- They found for TT's family.
- The court held that a therapist bears a duty to use reasonable care to give threatened persons such warnings as are essential to avert foreseeable danger arising from a patient's condition.

Tarasoff II decision: Duty to protect

- 'The protective privilege ends where the public peril begins.'
- The trial court was then instructed to hear the case against the police and employees of the university.
- The same case was thus re-heard in 1976.
- The court stated that: 'When a therapist determines that his patient presents a serious danger of violence to another, he incurs an obligation to use reasonable care to protect the intended victim against such danger. This discharge of duty may require the therapist to take one or more of various steps. Thus, it may call for him to warn the intended victim, to notify the police, or to take whatever steps are reasonably necessary under the circumstances.'
- The defendants argued that psychiatrists are unable to accurately predict violence. The response from the court was that therapists do not need to provide a perfect performance 'but only to exercise that reasonable degree of skilled care ordinarily possessed by members of their profession under similar circumstances'.

The case was settled out of court for a significant sum. PP served 4 years of a 5-year sentence for manslaughter. His case was later overturned on technicalities (faulty jury instructions on diminished capacity). A second trial was not heard and PP returned to India.

Policy and Legislation

Confidentiality: NHS code of practice

Department of Health 2003 Confidentiality: NHS code of practice. DH, London[†]

A duty of confidence arises when one person discloses information to another (e.g. patient to clinician) in circumstances where it is reasonable to expect that the information will be held in confidence. It:

- is a legal obligation that is derived from case law
- is a requirement established within professional codes of conduct
- must be included within NHS employment contracts as a specific requirement linked to disciplinary procedures.

The confidentiality model

This model outlines the requirements that must be met in order to provide patients with a confidential service. Record holders must inform patients of the intended use of their information, and give them the choice to give or withhold their consent as well as protecting their identifiable information from unwarranted disclosures.

The four main requirements are:

- *Protect* – look after the patient's information
- *Inform* – ensure that patients are aware of how their information is used
- *Provide choice* – allow patients to decide whether their information can be disclosed or used in particular ways

and, in support of these requirements:

- *Improve* – always look for better ways to protect, inform and provide choice.

Common law of confidentiality

This is not codified in an Act of Parliament but built up from case law where practice has been established by individual judgments. The key principle is that information confided should not be used or disclosed further, except as originally understood by the confider, or with their subsequent permission. Although judgments have established that confidentiality can be breached 'in the public interest', these have centred on case-by-case consideration of exceptional circumstances.

Human Rights Act 1998 (HRA98)

Article 8 of the HRA98 establishes a right to 'respect for private and family life'. This underscores the duty to protect the privacy of individuals and preserve the confidentiality of their health records. Current understanding is that

---

compliance with the Data Protection Act 1998 and the common law of confidentiality should satisfy HRA98 requirements.

Common law and disclosure in the public interest

The key principle of the duty of confidence is that information confided should not be used or disclosed further in identifiable form, except as originally understood by the confider, or with their subsequent permission.

There are exceptions to the duty of confidence that may make the use or disclosure of confidential information appropriate. Statute law requires or permits the disclosure of confidential patient information in certain circumstances, and the courts may also order disclosures. Case law has also established that confidentiality can be breached where there is an overriding public interest.

In the 'public interest'/to protect the public

Under common law, staff are permitted to disclose personal information in order to prevent and support detection, investigation and punishment of serious crime and/or to prevent abuse or serious harm to others where they judge, on a case-by-case basis, that the public good that would be achieved by the disclosure outweighs both the obligation of confidentiality to the individual patient concerned and the broader public interest in the provision of a confidential service.

Whoever authorises disclosure must make a record of any such circumstances, so that there is clear evidence of the reasoning used and the circumstances prevailing. Disclosures in the public interest should also be proportionate and limited to the relevant details. It may be necessary to justify such disclosures to the courts or to regulatory bodies, and a clear record of the decision-making process and the advice sought is in the interests of both staff and the organisations in which they work.

Wherever possible, the issue of disclosure should be discussed with the individual concerned and consent sought. Where this is not forthcoming, the individual should be told of any decision to disclose against their wishes. This will not be possible in certain circumstances – for example, where the likelihood of a violent response is significant or where informing a potential suspect in a criminal investigation might allow them to evade custody, destroy evidence or disrupt an investigation.

Each case must be considered on its merits. Decisions will sometimes be finely balanced and staff may find it difficult to make a judgement. It may be necessary to seek legal or other specialist advice (e.g. from professional, regulatory or indemnifying bodies) or to await or seek a court order. Staff need to know who and where to turn to for advice in such circumstances.

Weblink Department of Health – www.dh.gov.uk.

Guidelines

Good psychiatric practice: confidentiality and information sharing

Royal College of Psychiatrists 2005 Good psychiatric practice: confidentiality and information sharing. Council Report CR133. RCP, London

Doctors have an ethical duty to keep patient information confidential. The sharing of patient-identifiable information is, by definition, disclosure. Doctors have a duty of confidentiality to their patient. Confidentiality and privacy are legal concepts. Doctors also have moral and legal obligations within the broader social context. Therefore, doctors also have a duty to inform their patients that, in exceptional circumstances (usually where there might be harm to others), the duty to confidentiality may be overridden. Disclosure may then occur without patient consent. Doctors need not inform their patients that they intend to disclose information if that disclosure would prejudice the reason for disclosure.

For there to be a breach in confidentiality, three elements are required:
* Information is shared in circumstances that create an obligation of confidentiality, such as a private consultation
* Information is private
* Unauthorised disclosure is harmful to the patient.

Disclosure of confidential information can occur in the following circumstances:
* Where the patient gives consent to disclosure
* Where disclosure is in the public interest
* Where it is required by statute or on the order of a court.

Recommendations

* Patients and carers should be provided with relevant information about how their information is used.
* Such information should be accessible and provided in a number of forms, including the use of interpreting services if necessary.
* Patients should be made aware of the spread of information within and between primary and secondary care.
* Consent to disclosures outwith the NHS should be sought.
* The spread of information between patients and carers should be explicitly discussed and their wishes clarified.
* Patients should receive copies of letters about them, unless the letter contains information regarding a third party or if it would be harmful to the patient.

- Appointment letters should be marked as confidential and only opened by the addressee.
- The spread of information within the multidisciplinary team should be explained to patients.
- In inpatient settings it is the duty of the consultant to ensure that members of the clinical team are aware of the duty of confidentiality and the specific professional codes.
- Patient-identifiable information should not usually be shared with other agencies (social services, non-statutory services, etc.) without explicit consent.
- Members of the CPA meetings should understand that the medical duty of confidentiality is imposed.
- Guidelines regarding the spread of information should be developed by services and should include intra- and interagency working.
- If a doctor is asked to provide a written report about a patient, then the content of that report should be discussed with the patient and consent to the disclosure sought.

Weblinks

British Medical Association. Confidentiality and disclosure of health information – www.bma.org.uk/ap.nsf/Content/Confidentialitydisclosure.

General Medical Council. Confidentiality: protecting and providing information – www.gmc-uk.org/guidance/library/confidentiality.asp.

Royal College of Psychiatrists – www.rcpsych.ac.uk.

GMC guidelines on provision of information on consent

Patients have the right to information about their condition and the treatment options available to them. The amount of information will vary according to factors such as the nature of the condition, the complexity of the treatment, the risks associated with the treatment or procedure, and the patient's own wishes.

Doctors should be sensitive to each individual patient's needs, views and beliefs. Doctors should be honest, accurate and thorough in their replies to a patient's questions. Information should only be withheld if it would be harmful to the patient. This implies serious harm as opposed to upset or distress. The patient may require the following information before they can consider consent with regard to treatment:

- Diagnosis and prognosis
- Prognosis without treatment
- Role of further investigations if the diagnosis is not clear
- Treatment and management options, including the option not to treat
- Purpose of proposed investigation or treatment
- Details of the procedures or therapies involved in investigation and treatment, including subsidiary treatment

- Preparations on the part of the patient
- Details of common adverse effects occurring during or after treatment
- Explanations of the likely benefits and the probabilities of success for each treatment option, with discussion of any serious or frequently occurring risks or resulting lifestyle changes
- Advice on whether the proposed intervention is experimental
- How and when the patient's condition and any side effects will be monitored or reassessed
- Name of the doctor with overall responsibility
- Whether doctors in training/students will be involved
- Ability of the patient to change their mind at any time
- Availability of a second opinion
- Any costs or charges incurred by the patient.

Weblink   General Medical Council –www.gmc-uk.org.

British Medical Association 2003 The consent tool kit, 2nd edn. BMA, London. Online. Available: www.bma.org.uk/ap.nsf/Content/consenttk2

The tool kit consists of a series of cards relating to specific areas of consent such as providing treatment to children, consent and research, obtaining consent for teaching purposes, assessing competence and determining best interests.

Medical rules for drivers

Driver and Vehicle Licensing Centre 2006 Medical rules for drivers: at a glance booklet. DVLA, Swansea. Online. Available: www.dvla.gov.uk/at_a_glance/content.htm

This publication summarises the national medical guidelines of fitness to drive. It is only accurate at the time of publication.

It is for guidance only. While it provides some idea of the anticipated outcome of a medical enquiry, the specific medical factors of each case will be considered before an individual licensing decision is reached.

Notification to DVLA

It is the duty of the licence holder or licence applicant to notify the DVLA of any medical condition that may affect safe driving. On occasions, however, there are circumstances in which the licence holder cannot, or will not do so.

The GMC has issued clear guidelines applicable to such circumstances, which state:

> The DVLA is legally responsible for deciding if a person is medically unfit to drive. They need to know when driving licence holders have a condition, which may, now or in the future, affect their safety as a driver.

Therefore, where a patient has such a condition, you should:

- make sure that the patient understands that the condition may impair their ability to drive. If a patient is incapable of understanding this advice (e.g. because of dementia), you should inform the DVLA immediately
- explain to the patient that they have a legal duty to inform the DVLA about the condition.

If a patient refuses to accept the diagnosis or the effect of the condition on their ability to drive, you can suggest that they seek a second opinion, and make appropriate arrangements for the patient to do so. You should advise the patient not to drive until the second opinion has been obtained.

If the patient continues to drive when they are not fit to do so, you should make every reasonable effort to persuade them to stop. This may include telling their next of kin. If they agree you may do so.

If you do not manage to persuade the patient to stop driving, or you are given or find evidence that a patient is continuing to drive contrary to advice, you should disclose relevant medical information immediately, in confidence, to the medical adviser at the DVLA.

Before giving information to the DVLA you should try to inform the patient of your decision to do so. Once the DVLA has been informed, you should also write to the patient to confirm that a disclosure has been made.

Weblink General Medical Council – www.gmc-uk.org/guidance/library/confidentiality.asp.

See also the 'Guidelines' section in Chapter 12 (General psychiatry), page 200.

At-a-glance: Chapter 1 – Neurological disorders

Disorder	Group 1 entitlement ODL–car,m/cycle	Group 2 entitlement VOC–LGV/PCV
1. EPILEPSY Epileptic attacks are the most frequent medical cause of collapse at the wheel. **NB**: If, within a 24-hour period, more than one epileptic attack occurs, these are treated as a 'single event' for the purpose of applying the epilepsy regulations. Epilepsy includes all events, major, minor and auras.	**THE EPILEPSY REGULATIONS APPLY** Provided a licence holder/applicant is able to satisfy the regulations, a 3-year licence will normally be issued. Till 70 restored if seizure free for 7 years with medication if necessary in the absence of any other disqualifying condition.	Regulations require a driver to remain free of epileptic attacks for at least 10 years without anticonvulsant medication in that time.
2. FIRST EPILEPTIC SEIZURE/ SOLITARY FIT **Also see under:** 1. Fits associated with misuse of alcohol or misuse of drugs whether prescribed or illicit. 2. Neurosurgical conditions.	**One year off driving with medical review before restarting driving.** Till 70 restored provided no further attack and otherwise well. (Special consideration **may** be given when the epileptic attack is associated with certain clearly identified non-recurring **provoking cause**.)	Following a first unprovoked seizure, drivers must demonstrate 10 years' freedom from further seizures, without anticonvulsant medication in that time. 1. Following a solitary seizure associated with either alcohol or substance misuse or prescribed medication, a 5-year period free of further seizures, without anticonvulsant medication in that time, is required. If there are recurrent seizures, the epilepsy regulations apply.

Neurological disorders (cont'd)

Disorder	Group 1 entitlement ODL–car,m/cycle	Group 2 entitlement VOC–LGV/PCV
3. **CHRONIC NEUROLOGICAL DISORDERS** e.g. Parkinson's disease, multiple sclerosis, muscle and movement disorders including motor neurone disease, likely to affect vehicle control because of impairment of coordination and muscle power. See also driving assessment for disabled drivers.	Providing medical assessment confirms that driving performance is not impaired, can be licensed. A short period licence may be required. Should the driver require a restriction to certain controls, the laws requires this to be specified on the licence.	Recommended refusal or revocation if condition is progressive or disabling. If driving would not be impaired and condition stable, can be considered for licensing subject to satisfactory reports and annual review.
4. **CEREBROVASCULAR DISEASE**: including stroke due to occlusive vascular disease, spontaneous intracerebral haemorrhage, TIA and amaurosis fugax.	**Must not drive for at least 1 month.** May resume driving after this time if the clinical recovery is satisfactory. There is no need to notify DVLA **unless** there is residual neurological deficit 1 month after the episode; in particular, visual field defects, cognitive defects and impaired limb function. Minor limb weakness alone will not require notification unless restriction to certain types of vehicle or vehicles with adapted controls is needed. Adaptations may be able to overcome severe physical impairment. A driver experiencing multiple TIAs over a short period of time may require 3 months' freedom from further attacks before resuming driving and should notify DVLA. Epileptic attacks occuring at the time of a stroke/TIA or in the ensuing 24 hours may be treated as provoked for licensing purposes in the absence of any previous seizure history or previous cerebral pathology. Seizures occurring at the time of cortical vein thrombosis require 6 months' freedom from attacks before resuming driving.	Recommended refusal/ revocation for at least 12 months following a stroke or TIA. Can be considered for licensing after this period if there is a full and complete recovery and there are no other significant risk factors. Licensing will also be subject to satisfactory medical reports including exercise ECG testing.

Neurological disorders (cont'd)

Disorder	Group 1 entitlement ODL–car,m/cycle	Group 2 entitlement VOC–LGV/PCV
5. **EPILEPSY/EPILEPTIC SEIZURES** General guidance for **ALL** has neurosurgical conditions if associated with epilepsy or epileptic seizures.	In all cases where epilepsy has been diagnosed the *epilepsy regulations must apply*. These cases will include all cases of single seizure where a primary cerebral cause is present and the liability to recurrence cannot be excluded. An exception may be made when seizures occur **at the time** of an acute head injury or intracranial surgery.	In all cases where a 'liability to epileptic seizures' either primary or secondary has been diagnosed the specific *epilepsy regulation for this group must apply*. The only exception is a seizure occuring immediately at the time of the acute head injury or intracranial surgery, and not thereafter and/or where no liability to seizure has been demonstrated. Following head injury or intracranial surgery, the epilepsy risk must fall to 2% per annum or less before returning to vocational driving.

At-a-glance: Chapter 4 – Psychiatric disorders

Disorder	Group 1 entitlement ODL–car,m/cycle	Group 2 entitlement VOC–LGV/PCV
1. **ANXIETY OR DEPRESSION** (without significant memory or concentration problems, agitation, behavioural disturbance or suicidal thoughts)	**DVLA need not be notified** and driving may continue.	Very minor short-lived illnesses need not be notified to DVLA.
MORE SEVERE ANXIETY STATES OR DEPRESSIVE ILLNESSES (with significant memory or concentration problems, agitation, behavioural disturbance or suicidal thoughts) **NB**: For cases which also involve persistent misuse of or dependency on alcohol/drugs, please refer to the appropriate section of Chapter 5. Where psychiatric illness has been associated with substance misuse, continuing misuse is not acceptable for licensing.	**Driving should cease** pending the outcome of medical enquiry. A period of stability depending upon the circumstances will be required before driving can be resumed. Particularly dangerous are those who may attempt suicide at the wheel.	Driving may be permitted when the person is well and stable for a period of 6 months. Medication must not cause side effects which would interfere with alertness or concentration. Driving is usually permitted if the anxiety or depression is long-standing, but maintained symptom-free on doses of psychotropic medication which do not impair. DVLA may require psychiatric reports. **NB**: It is the illness rather than the medication, which is of prime importance.

Psychiatric disorders (cont'd)

Disorder	Group 1 entitlement ODL–car,m/cycle	Group 2 entitlement VOC–LGV/PCV
2. **ACUTE PSYCHOTIC DISORDERS OF ANY TYPE** **NB**: For cases which also involve persistent misuse of or dependency on alcohol/drugs, please refer to the appropriate section of Chapter 5. Where psychiatric illness has been associated with substance misuse, continuing misuse is not acceptable for licensing.	**Driving must cease** during the acute illness. Re-licensing can be considered when all of the following conditions can be satisfied: a) Has remained well and stable for at least 3 months. b) Is compliant with treatment. c) Is free from adverse effects of medication which would impair driving. d) Subject to a favourable specialist report. Drivers who have a history of instability and/or poor compliance will require a longer period off driving.	**Driving must cease** pending the outcome of medical enquiry. It is normally a requirement that the person should be well and stable for 3 years (i.e. to have experienced a good level of functional recovery with insight into their illness and to be fully adherent to the agreed treatment plan, including engagement with the medical services) before driving can be resumed. In line with good practice, attempts should be made to achieve the minimum effective antipsychotic dose; tolerability should be optimal and not associated with any deficits (e.g. in alertness, concentration and motor performance) that might impair driving ability. Where in patients with established illness the history suggests a likelihood of relapse, the risk should be appraised as low (either in the treated or untreated state). DVLA will normally require a consultant report that specifically addressess the relevant issues above before the license can be considered.
3. **HYPOMANIA/MANIA** **NB**: For cases which also involve persistent misuse of or dependency on alcohol/drugs, please refer to the appropriate section of Chapter 5. Where psychiatric illness has been associated with substance misuse, continuing misuse is not acceptable for licensing.	**Driving must cease** during the acute illness. Following an **isolated episode**, re-licensing can be reconsidered when **all** the following conditions can be satisfied: a) Has remained well and stable for at least 3 months. b) Is compliant with treatment. c) Has regained insight. d) Is free from adverse effects of medication which would impair driving. e) Subject to a favourable specialist report.	**Driving must cease** pending the outcome of medical enquiry. It is normally a requirement that the person should be well and stable for 3 years (i.e. to have experienced a good level of functional recovery with insight into their illness and to be fully adherent to the agreed treatment plan, including engagement with the medical services) before driving can be resumed. In

Psychiatric disorders (cont'd)

Disorder	Group 1 entitlement ODL–car,m/cycle	Group 2 entitlement VOC–LGV/PCV
	REPEATED CHANGES OF MOOD: Hypomania or mania are particularly dangerous to driving when there are repeated changes of mood. Therefore, when there have been four or more episodes of mood swing within the previous 12 months, at least **6 months**, stability will be required under condition (a), in addition to satisfying conditions (b) to (e).	line with good practice, attempts should be made to achieve the minimum effective dose of psychotropic medication; tolerability should be optimal and not associated with any deficits (e.g. in alertness, concentration and motor performance) that might impair driving ability. Where in patients with established illness the history suggests a likelihood of relapse, the risk should be appraised as low (either in the treated or untreated state). DVLA will normally require a consultant report that specifically addresses the relevant issues above before the licence can be considered.
4. **CHRONIC SCHIZOPHRENIA and other chronic psychoses** **NB**: For cases which also involve persistent misuse of or dependency on alcohol/drugs, please refer to the appropriate section of Chapter 5. Where psychiatric illness has been associated with substance misuse, continuing misuse is not acceptable for licensing.	The driver must satisfy **all** the following conditions: a) Stable behaviour for at least 3 months. b) Is adequately compliant with treatment. c) Remains free from adverse effects of medication which impair driving. d) Subject to a favourable specialist report. **Continuing symptoms**: Even with limited insight, these do not necessarily preclude licensing. symptoms should be unlikely to cause significant concentration problems, memory impairment or distraction whilst driving. Particularly dangerous are those drivers whose psychotic symptoms relate to other road users.	**Driving must cease** pending the outcome of medical enquiry. It is normally a requirement that the person should be well and stable for 3 years (i.e. to have experienced a good level of functional recovery with insight into their illness and to be fully adherent to the agreed treatment plan, including engagement with the medical services) before driving can be resumed. In line with good practice, attempts should be made to achieve the minimum effective antipsychotic dose; tolerability should be optimal and not associated with any deficits (e.g. in alertness, concentration and motor

Psychiatric disorders (cont'd)

Disorder	Group 1 entitlement ODL–car,m/cycle	Group 2 entitlement VOC–LGV/PCV
		performance) that might impair driving ability. Where in patients with established illness the history suggests a likelihood of relapse, the risk should be appraised as low (either in the treated or untreated state). DVLA will normally require a consultant report that specifically addresses the relevant issues above before the licence can be considered.
5. **DEMENTIA OR ANY ORGANIC BRAIN SYNDROME**	It is extremely difficult to assess driving ability in those with dementia. Those who have poor short-term memory, disorientation, lack of insight and judgement are almost certainly not fit to drive. The variable presentations and rates of progression are acknowledged. Disorders of attention will also cause impairment. A decision regarding fitness to drive is usually based on medical reports. In early dementia when sufficient skills are retained and progression is slow, a licence may be issued subject to annual review. A formal driving assessment may be necessary.	Refuse or revoke licence.
6. **LEARNING DISABILITY** Severely below average general intellectual functioning accompanied by significant limitations in adaptive functioning in at least two of the following areas: communication, self-care, home-living, social/ interpersonal skills, use of community resources, self-direction, functional academic skills, work, leisure, health and safety.	Severe learning disability is not compatible with driving and the licence application must be refused. In milder forms, provided there are no other relevant problems, it may be possible to hold a licence, but it will be necessary to demonstrate adequate functional ability at the wheel.	Recommended permanent refusal or revocation if severe. Minor degrees of learning disability when the condition is stable with no medical or psychiatric complications may be compatible with the holding of a licence.

Psychiatric disorders (cont'd)

Disorder	Group 1 entitlement ODL–car,m/cycle	Group 2 entitlement VOC–LGV/PCV
7. DEVELOPMENT DISORDERS (includes Asperger's syndrome, autism, severe communication disorders and attention deficit hyperactivity disorder).	A diagnosis of any of these conditions is not in itself a bar to licensing. Factors such as impulsivity, lack of awareness of the impact of own behaviours on self or others need to be considered.	Continuing minor symptomatology may be compatible with licensing. Cases will be considered on an individual basis.
8. BEHAVIOUR DISORDERS (includes post head injury syndrome, personality disorders, and non-epileptic seizure disorder).	If seriously disturbed (e.g. violent behaviour or alcohol abuse and likely to be a source of danger at the wheels), licence would be revoked or the application refused. Licence will be issued after medical reports confirm that behavioural disturbances have been satisfactorily controlled.	Recommended refusal or revocation if associated with serious behaviour disturbance likely to make the individual a source of danger at the wheel. If psychiatric reports confirm stability, then consideration would be given to restoration of the licence.

Important note

Psychiatric conditions not normally requiring notification (e.g. eating disorders) or those conditions which do not fit neatly into the aforementioned classification will need to be reported to the DVLA if causing impairment of consciousness or symptoms that will either distract from the task of driving or prevent the driver from operating the controls of the vehicle safely. The patient should be advised to declare both the condition and the symptoms of concern.

Severe mental disorder is a prescribed disability for the purposes of Section 92 of the Road Traffic Act 1988. Regulations define 'severe mental disorder' as including mental illness, arrested or incomplete development of the mind, psychopathic disorder or severe impairment of intelligence or social functioning. The standards must reflect not only the need for an improvement in the mental state, but also a period of stability, such that the risk of relapse can be assessed should the patient fail to recognise any deterioration.

Medication

Section 4 of the Road Traffic Act 1988 does not differentiate between illicit or prescribed drugs. Therefore, any person who is driving or attempting to drive on the public highway or other public place whilst unfit due to any drug is liable to prosecution.

All drugs acting on the central nervous system can impair alertness, concentration and driving performance. This is particularly so at initiation of treatment or soon after, and when dosage is being increased. Driving must cease if adversely affected.

The older tricyclic antidepressants can have pronounced cholinergic and antihistaminic effects which may impair driving. The more modern antidepressants may have fewer adverse effects. These considerations need to be taken into account when planning the treatment of a patient who is a professional driver.

Antipsychotic drugs, including the depot preparations, can cause motor or extrapyramidal effects as well as sedation or poor concentration, which may, either alone or in combination, be sufficient to impair driving. Careful clinical assessment is required.

The epileptogenic potential of medication should be considered, particularly when patients are professional drivers.

Benzodiazepines are the most likely psychotropic medication to impair driving performance, particularly the long-acting compounds. Alcohol will potentiate the effects.

Doctors have a duty of care to advise their patients of the potential dangers of adverse effects from medication and interactions with other substances, especially alcohol.

Drivers with psychiatric illnesses are often safer when well and on regular psychotropic medication than when they are ill. Inadequate treatment or irregular compliance may render a driver impaired by both the illness and the mediation.

At-a-glance: Chapter 5 – Drug and alcohol misuse and dependency

Alcohol problems	Group 1 entitlement ODL–car, m/cycle	Group 2 entitlement VOC–LGV/PCV
1. ALCOHOL MISUSE There is no single definition which embraces all the variables in this condition but the following is offered as a guide: 'A state which because of consumption of alcohol, causes disturbance of behaviour, related disease or other consequences, likely to cause the patient, their family or society harm now, or in the future, and which may or may not be associated with dependency.' Reference to ICD-10 F10.1 is relevant.	Persistent alcohol misuse, confirmed by medical enquiry and/or by evidence of otherwise unexplained abnormal blood markers, requires licence revocation or refusal until a minimum 6-month period of controlled drinking or abstinence has been attained, with normalisation of blood parameters. Patient recommended to seek advice from medical or other sources during the period off the road.	Persistent alcohol misuse, confirmed by medical enquiry and/or by evidence of otherwise unexplained abnormal blood markers, requires revocation or refusal of a vocational licence until at least 1-year period of abstinence or controlled drinking has been attained, with normalisation of blood parameters. Patient recommended to seek advice from medical or other sources during the period off the road.
2. ALCOHOL DEPENDENCY "A cluster of behavioural, cognitive and physiological phenomena that develop after repeated alcohol use and which include a strong desire to take alcohol, difficulties in controlling its use, persistence in its use despite harmful consequences, with evidence of increased tolerance and sometimes a physical withdrawal state." Indicators may include a history of withdrawal symptoms, of tolerance, of detoxification(s) and/or alcohol-related fits. Reference to ICD-10 **F10.2-F10.7 inclusive** is relevant.	Alcohol dependency, confirmed by medical enquiry, requires licence revocation or refusal until a 1-year period free from alcohol problems has been attained. Abstinence will normally be required, with normalisation of blood parameters, if relevant. **LICENCE RESTORATION** Will require satisfactory medical reports from own doctor(s) and may require independent medical examination and blood tests, arranged by DVLA. Consultant support/referral may be necessary. See also under "Alcohol related seizures".	Vocational licensing will not be granted where there is a history of alcohol dependency within the past 3 years. **LICENCE RESTORATION** Will require satisfactory medical reports from own doctor(s) and may require independent medical examination and blood tests, arranged by DVLA. Consultant support/referral may be necessary. See also under "Alcohol related seizures".

Drug and alcohol misuse and dependency (cont'd)

Alcohol problems	Group 1 entitlement ODL–car, m/cycle	Group 2 entitlement VOC–LGV/PCV
3. **ALCOHOL-RELATED SEIZURE(S)**	Following a solitary alcohol-related seizure, a licence will be revoked or refused for a minimum 1-year period from the date of the event. Where more than one seizure has occurred, consideration under the Epilepsy Regulations will be necessary. Medical enquiry will be required before licence restoration to confirm appropriate period free from persistent alcohol misuse and/or dependency. Independent medical assessment with blood analysis and consultant reports will normally be necessary.	Following a **solitary** alcohol-related seizure, a licence will be revoked or refused for a minimum **5-year** period from the date of the event. Licence restoration thereafter requires: a) No underlying cerebral structural abnormality b) Off antiepileptic medication for at least 5 years c) Maintained abstinence from alcohol if previously dependent d) Review by an addiction specialist and neurological opinion. Where **more than one seizure** has occurred or there is an underlying cerebral structural abnormality, the **Vocational Epilepsy Regulations** apply.
4. **ALCOHOL-RELATED DISORDERS** e.g. hepatic cirrhosis with neuropsychiatric impairment, psychosis	**Driving should cease.** Licence normally recommended to be refused/revoked until there is satisfactory recovery and is able to satisfy all other relevant medical standards.	Licence recommended to be refused/revoked.

High Risk Offender Scheme

This scheme relates to drivers convicted of certain drink/driving offences and meeting any of the following:
- One disqualification for driving, or being in charge of a vehicle, when the level of alcohol in the body equalled or exceeded:
  - 87.5 micrograms per 100 millilitres of breath, or
  - 200 milligrams per 100 millilitres of blood, or
  - 267.5 milligrams per 100 millilitres of urine.
- Two disqualifications within the space of 10 years for drinking and driving, or being in charge of a vehicle whilst under the influence of alcohol.
- One disqualification for refusing/failing to supply a specimen for analysis.

DVLA will be notified of such offenders by the courts.

When an application for licence reinstatement is made, an independent medical examination will be conducted, which includes a questionnaire, serum AST, ALT, GGT and MCV assay and may include further assessments as indicated. If favourable, a 'Till 70' licence is restored for Group 1 and a recommendation can be made regarding the issue of a Group 2 licence.

If a High Risk Offender has a previous history of alcohol dependency or persistent misuse, but has satisfactory examination and blood tests, a short period licence is issued for ordinary and vocational entitlement but dependent on their ability to meet the standard as specified.

A High Risk Offender found to have a current history of alcohol misuse/dependency and/or an unexplained abnormal blood test analysis will have the application refused.

Drug and alcohol misuse and dependency (cont'd)

Drug problems	Group 1 entitlement	Group 2 entitlement
5. DRUG MISUSE AND DEPENDENCY Reference to **ICD-10 F10.1-F10.7** inclusive is relevant.		
Cannabis amfetamines Ecstasy and other psychoactive substances, including LSD and hallucinogens	Persistent use of, or dependency on these substances, confirmed by medical enquiry, will lead to licence refusal or revocation for a minimum **6 month** period free of such use has been attained. Independent medical assessment and urine screen arranged by DVLA, may be required.	Persistent use of, or **dependency on** these substances, will lead to refusal or revocation of a vocational licence for a minimum 1-year period free of such use has been attained. Independent medical assessment and urine screen arranged by DVLA, **will normally** be required.
Heroin Morphine Methadone* Cocaine	Persistent use of, or dependency on these substances, confirmed by medical enquiry, will lead to licence refusal or revocation for a minimum **1-year** period free of such use has been attained. Independent medical assessment and urine screen arranged by DVLA, may be required. In addition, favourable consultant or specialist report **may** be required on reapplication. *Applicants or drivers **complying fully with a** consultant-supervised oral methadone maintenance programme may be licensed, subject to favourable assessment and, normally, annual medical review. Applicants or drivers on an oral **buprenorphine** programme may be considered applying the same criteria. There should be no evidence of continuing use of other substances, including cannabis.	Persistent use of, or dependency on these substances, will require revocation or refusal of a vocational licence until a minimum **3-year** period free of such use has been attained. Independent medical assessment and urine screen arranged by DVLA, will normally be required. In addition, favourable consultant or specialist report will be required before relicensing. *Applicants or drivers complying fully with a consultant-supervised oral methadone maintenance programme may be considered for an annual review licence once a **minimum 3-year** period of stability on the maintenance programme has been established, with favourable random urine tests and assessment. Expert Panel advice will be required in each case.

Drug and alcohol misuse and dependency (cont'd)

Drug problems	Group 1 entitlement	Group 2 entitlement
Benzodiazepines The non-prescribed use of these drugs and/or the use of supratherapeutic dosage, whether in a substance withdrawal/maintenance programme or otherwise, constitutes misuse/dependency for licensing purposes. The prescribed use of these drugs at therapeutic doses (*BNF*), without evidence of impairment, does not amount to misuse/dependency for licensing purposes (although clinically dependence may exist).	Persistent misuse of, or dependency on these substances, confirmed by medical enquiry, will lead to licence refusal or revocation until a minimum 1-year period free of such use has been attained. Independent medical assessment and urine screen arranged by DVLA, may be required. In addition, favourable consultant or specialist report may be required on reapplication.	Persistent misuse of, or dependency on these substances, will require revocation or refusal of a vocational licence for a minimum 3-year period. Independent medical assessment and urine screen arranged by DVLA, **will normally** be required. In addition, favourable consultant or specialist report will be required before relicensing.
Multiple substance misuse and/or dependency–including misuse with alcohol–is incompatible with licensing fitness		
6. **SEIZURE(S) ASSOCIATED WITH DRUG MISUSE/DEPENDENCY**	Following a **solitary** seizure associated with drug misuse or dependency a licence will be refused or revoked for a minimum **1-year** period from the date of the event. Where more than one seizure has occurred, consideration under the Epilepsy Regulations will be necessary. Medical enquiry will be required before licence restoration to confirm appropriate period free from persistent drug misuse and/or dependency. Independent medical assessment with urine analysis and consultant reports will normally be necessary.	Following a **solitary** seizure associated with drug misuse or dependency, a licence will be revoked or refused for a minimum **5-year** period from the date of the event. Licence restoration thereafter requires: a) No underlying cerebral structural abnormality b) Off antiepileptic medication for at least 5 years c) Maintained abstinence from drugs if previously dependent d) Review by an addiction specialist and neurological opinion.

Drug and alcohol misuse and dependency (cont'd)

Drug problems	Group 1 entitlement	Group 2 entitlement
		Where **more than one seizure** has occurred or there is an underlying cerebral structural abnormality, the **Vocational Epilepsy Regulations** apply.

NB: A person who has been re-licensed following persistent drug misuse or dependency must be advised as part of their after-care that if their condition recurs they should cease driving and notify DVLA Medical Branch.

At-a-glance: Chapter 8 – Miscellaneous conditions

Impairment of cognitive function (e.g. post stroke, post head injury, early dementia)

There is no single or simple marker for assessment of impaired cognitive function although the ability to manage day-to-day living satisfactorily is a possible yardstick of cognitive competence. In-car assessments, on the road with a valid licence, are an invaluable method of ensuring that there are no features present liable to cause the patient to be a source of danger – for example, visual attention, easy distractibility, and difficulty performing multiple tasks. In addition, it is important that reaction time, memory, concentration and confidence are adequate and do not show impairment likely to affect driving performance.

Cognitive disability – Group 2

- Impairment of cognitive functioning is not usually compatible with the driving of these vehicles.
- Mild cognitive disability may be compatible with safe driving and individual assessment will be required.

Reference guide to consent for examination or treatment

Department of Health 2001 Reference guide to consent for examination or treatment. DH, London

It is a general legal and ethical principle that valid consent must be obtained before starting treatment or physical investigation, or providing personal care, for a patient. This principle reflects the right of patients to determine what happens to their bodies. A health professional who does not respect this principle may be liable both to legal action by the patient and action by their professional body.

While there is no English statute setting out the general principles of consent, case law ('common law') has established that touching a patient without valid consent may constitute the civil or criminal offence of battery.

Valid consent

For consent to be valid, it must be given voluntarily by an appropriately informed person (the patient or, where relevant, someone with parental responsibility for a patient under the age of 18) who has the capacity to consent to the intervention in question. Acquiescence where the person does not know what the intervention entails is not 'consent'.

Capacity

For a person to have capacity, they must be able to comprehend and retain information material to the decision, especially as to the consequences of having or not having the intervention in question, and must be able to use and weigh this information in the decision-making process.

Adults are presumed to have capacity, but where any doubt exists the health professional should assess the capacity of the patient to take the decision in question. Patients may have capacity to consent to some interventions but not to others. A patient's capacity to understand may be temporarily affected by factors such as confusion, panic, shock, fatigue or medication.

The patient is entitled to make a decision based on their religious belief or value system, even if it is perceived by others to be irrational, as long as the patient understands what is entailed in their decision. However, if the decision is based on a misperception of reality, as opposed to an unusual value system – for example a patient who, despite the obvious evidence, denies that his foot is gangrenous, or a patient with anorexia nervosa who is unable to comprehend her failing physical condition – then the patient may not be able to comprehend and make use of the relevant information and hence may lack capacity to make the decision in question.

Health professionals should take all reasonable steps to facilitate communication with the patient, using interpreters or communication aids as appropriate.

Many people with learning disabilities have the capacity to consent if time is spent explaining to the individual the issues in simple language, using visual aids and signing if necessary.

Where appropriate, those who know the patient well, including their family, carers and staff from professional or voluntary support services, may be able to advise on the best ways to communicate with the person.

Voluntary consent

To be valid, consent must be given voluntarily and freely, without pressure or undue influence being exerted on the patient either to accept or refuse treatment.

When patients are seen and treated in environments where involuntary detention may be an issue, such as prisons and mental hospitals, there is a potential for treatment offers to be perceived coercively, whether or not this is the case. Coercion invalidates consent and care must be taken to ensure that the patient makes a decision freely. Coercion should be distinguished from providing the patient with appropriate reassurance concerning their treatment, or pointing out the potential benefits of treatment for the patient's health. However, threats such as withdrawal of any privileges or loss of remission of sentence for refusing consent, or using such matters to induce consent, are not acceptable.

Sufficient information

To give valid consent the patient needs to understand in broad terms the nature and purpose of the procedure. Any misrepresentation of these elements will invalidate consent. Where relevant, information about anaesthesia should be given as well as information about the procedure itself.

The requirements of the legal duty to inform patients have been significantly developed in case law. In 1985, the House of Lords decided in the Sidaway case (Sidaway v Board of Governors of the Bethlem Royal Hospital [1985] AC 871) that the legal standard to be used when deciding whether adequate information had been given to a patient should be the same as that used when judging whether a doctor had been negligent in their treatment or care of a patient: a doctor would not be considered negligent if their practice conformed to that of a responsible body of medical opinion held by practitioners skilled in the field in question (known as the 'Bolam Test') (Bolam v Friern Hospital Management Committee [1957] 2 All ER 118). Whether the duty of care had been satisfied was therefore primarily a matter of medical opinion. However, Sidaway also stated that it was open to the courts to decide that information about a particular risk was so obviously necessary that it would be negligent not to provide it, even if a 'responsible body' of medical opinion would not have done so.

The General Medical Council has gone further, stating in guidance that doctors should do their best to find out about patients' individual needs and priorities when providing information about treatment options.

Self-harm

Cases of self-harm present a particular difficulty for health professionals. Where the patient is able to communicate, an assessment of their mental capacity should be made as a matter of urgency. If the patient is judged not to be competent, they may be treated on the basis of temporary incapacity. Similarly, patients who have attempted suicide and are unconscious should be given emergency treatment if any doubt exists as to either their intentions or their capacity when they took the decision to attempt suicide.

Competent patients do have the right to refuse life-sustaining treatment (other than treatment for mental disorder under the Mental Health Act 1983), both at the time it is offered and in the future. If a competent patient has harmed themselves and refuses treatment, a psychiatric assessment should be obtained. If the use of the Mental Health Act 1983 is not appropriate, then their refusal must be respected. Similarly, if practitioners have good reason to believe that a patient genuinely intended to end their life and was competent when they took that decision, and are satisfied that the Mental Health Act is not applicable, then treatment should not be forced upon the patient although clearly attempts should be made to encourage them to accept help.

Adults without capacity

General principles Under English law, no one is able to give consent to the examination or treatment of an adult who is unable to give consent for themselves (an 'incapable' adult). Therefore, parents, relatives or members of the healthcare team cannot consent on behalf of such an adult. However, in certain circumstances, it will be lawful to carry out such examinations or treatment.

A key principle concerning treatment of the incapable adult is that of the person's best interests. 'Best interests' are not confined to best medical interests: case law has established that other factors which may need to be taken into account include the patient's values and preferences when competent, their psychological health, well-being, quality of life, relationships with family or other carers, spiritual and religious welfare and their own financial interests. It is good practice for the healthcare team to involve those close to the patient in order to find out about the patient's values and preferences before loss of capacity, unless the patient has previously made clear that particular individuals should not be involved.

Where there is doubt about an individual's capacity or best interests, the High Court can give a ruling on these matters and on the lawfulness or unlawfulness of a proposed procedure.

Temporary incapacity An adult who usually has capacity may become temporarily incapable – for example while under a general anaesthetic or sedation, or after a road traffic accident. Unless a valid advance refusal of treatment is applicable to the circumstances, the law permits interventions to be made which are necessary and no more than is reasonably required in the patient's best interests pending the recovery of capacity. This will include, but is not limited to, routine procedures such as washing and assistance with feeding. If a medical intervention is thought to be in the patient's best interests but can be delayed until the patient recovers capacity and can consent to (or refuse) the intervention, it must be delayed until that time.

Permanent or long-standing incapacity Where the adult's incapacity is permanent or likely to be long-standing, it will be lawful to carry out any procedure which is in the 'best interests' of the adult. The House of Lords has suggested that action taken to 'preserve the life, health or well-being' of a patient will be in their best interests, and subsequent court judgments have emphasised that a patient's best interests go beyond their best medical interests, to include much wider welfare considerations.

Referral to court

The courts have identified certain circumstances when referral should be made to them for a ruling on lawfulness before a procedure is undertaken. These are:

* sterilisation for contraceptive purposes
* donation of regenerative tissue such as bone marrow
* withdrawal of nutrition and hydration from a patient in a persistent vegetative state
* when there is doubt as to the patient's capacity or best interests.

Forensic psychiatry

10

Chapter contents

General topics

Aspects of morbid jealousy

Kingham M, Gordon H 2004 Aspects of morbid jealousy. Advances in Psychiatric Treatment 10: 207–215

The prevalence of morbid jealousy is unknown. It is regarded as a rare disorder. There are no community studies of prevalence. The most commonly cited forms of psychopathology of morbid jealousy are delusions, obsessions and overvalued ideas. Comorbidity is common, including personality disorder, mental illness and substance misuse.

Vauhkonen K 1968 On the pathogenesis of morbid jealousy. Acta Scandinavica Supplementum 202: 2–261

- Morbidly jealous individuals interpret conclusive evidence of infidelity from irrelevant occurrences.
- They refuse to change their beliefs even in the face of conflicting information.
- They tend to accuse the partner of infidelity with many others.

Shepherd M 1961 Morbid jealousy: some clinical and social aspects of a psychiatric symptom. Journal of Mental Science 107: 688–704

- Morbid jealousy should be considered a descriptive term for the disorders resulting from a number of psychopathologies within separate psychiatric diagnoses.
- Economic depression has been associated with an increased incidence of delusional jealousy.

- Alcohol misuse has a well-recognised association with morbid jealousy.
- This author viewed alcohol as exacerbating rather than being the primary cause of the jealousy.
- Amfetamine and cocaine use can give rise to delusions of infidelity that may persist after intoxication ceases.
- Aggressive challenging of the partner may be followed by intense remorse during which suicidal action may occur.
- If morbid jealousy is refractory to treatment, geographical separation may be all that is effective.

Mullen PE 1990 Morbid jealousy and the delusion of infidelity. In: Bluglass R, Bowden P (eds) Principles and practice of forensic psychiatry. Churchill Livingstone, London, pp 823–834

- Considered morbid jealousy to be associated with four features:
  - An underlying mental disorder emerges before or with the jealousy
  - The features of the underlying disorder coexist with the jealousy
  - The course of morbid jealousy closely relates to that of the underlying disorder
  - The jealousy has no basis in reality.
- Obsessional disorder as the core of morbid jealousy is rare.
- Violence may occur in any relationship marred by jealousy, although the risk may be greater in morbid jealousy.

Mullen PE, Mack LH 1985 Jealousy, pathological jealousy and aggression. In: Farrington DP, Gunn J (eds) Aggression and dangerousness. Wiley, London, pp 103–126

- Depression was present in more than half of the patients in this study of morbid jealousy.

- 15% of the individuals had an associated organic psycho-syndrome.
- More than half of the morbidly jealous individuals physically assaulted their partner.
- None of the assaultative individuals had come to the attention of the criminal justice system.
- Morbidly jealous men were more likely to attack their partners than were morbidly jealous women.
- Men tend to inflict more serious injuries.
- The lower rates of physical harm caused by women may be due to underreporting.

Marazziti D, Di Nasso E, Masala I et al 2003 Normal and obsessional jealousy: a study of a population of young adults. European Psychiatry 18: 106–111

- Found that in distinguishing normal from obsessional jealousy, the following are more extreme in obsessional jealousy:
  - time consumed by jealous concerns
  - difficulty in ignoring the concerns
  - impaired relationships
  - limitations placed on the partner's freedom
  - checking on the partner's activities.

Dutton DG 1994 Behavioural and affective correlates of borderline personality organisation in wife assaulters. International Journal of Criminal Justice and Behaviour 17: 26–38

- Borderline personality organisation is an important potential predisposing condition in any form of morbid jealousy.
- It may be especially so in individuals with a paranoid personality, which gives rise to overvalued ideas of infidelity.

Michael A, Mirza S, Mirza KAH et al 1995 Morbid jealousy in alcoholism. British Journal of Psychiatry 167: 668–672

- Morbid jealousy was present in 34% of men recruited from alcohol treatment services.
- Given the prevalence of harmful and dependent use of alcohol in the UK, these figures suggest that morbid jealousy is not rare.
- 65 of 71 male subjects were described as developing morbid jealousy following, and presumably secondary to, alcohol dependence.

Pillai K, Kraya N 2000 Psychostimulants, adult attention deficit and hyperactivity disorder and morbid jealousy. Australian and New Zealand Journal of Psychiatry 34: 160–163

- One case report described a man who developed morbid jealousy after receiving dexamphetamine for adult attention deficit hyperactivity disorder.

Mooney HB 1965 Pathologic jealousy and psycho-chemotherapy. British Journal of Psychiatry 111: 1023–1042

- In a UK population, 20% of morbidly jealous individuals had made suicide attempts.
- 14% of morbidly jealous individuals were considered to have made 'homicidal attempts'.
- The majority of homicidal attempts were made against the accused's partner.
- Delusions of infidelity, whether occurring alone or in the context of schizophrenia, may respond to antipsychotic medication.
- One-third of the patients were considered to have made significant improvement.
- Patients with psychotic disorders had a poorer prognosis.

West DJ 1965 Murder followed by suicide. Heinemann, London

- Where jealousy gives rise to fatal violence against the partner, this may be followed by suicide.

Dell S 1984 Murder into manslaughter. Oxford University Press, Oxford

- Concluded that amorous jealousy/possessiveness accounted for 17% of all cases of homicide in the UK.

Mowat RR 1966 Morbid jealousy and murder. Tavistock, London

- Reported on 110 morbidly jealous subjects who had killed or committed serious assaults and been admitted to a forensic psychiatric facility.
- In 94 cases the victim had been the partner.
- Seven out of 110 victims of homicide or serious assault were supposed paramours.

Mirrlees-Black C 1999 Findings from a new British crime survey self-completion questionnaire. The Stationery Office, London

- British crime survey.
- Domestic violence is a common result of jealousy.
- 23% of women and 15% of men have been physically assaulted by their partners.
- Domestic violence is associated with an increased risk of death at the hands of the perpetrator.

Silva JA, Ferrari MM, Leong GB et al 1998 The dangerousness of persons with delusional jealousy. Journal of the American Academy of Psychiatry and the Law 26: 607–623

- A sample of 20 individuals with delusional jealousy, 19 of whom were male.
- 13 individuals had threatened to kill their spouse because of alleged infidelity.
- Nine had actually attacked their spouse.
- Overall, 12 had harmed their spouse, three using a weapon.
- The presence of paranoid delusions and command hallucinations to injure the spouse were associated with violence.
- Individuals with delusional jealousy who perpetrate violence may be driven directly by psychotic phenomena.
- Alcohol consumption was also associated with a higher risk of assault.
- More than 50% of the alleged paramours were known to the subject; however, no serious threats of harm or incidents of violence were made against them.

Byrne A, Yatham LN 1989 Pimozide in pathological jealousy. British Journal of Psychiatry 155: 249–251

- Delusions of infidelity, whether occurring alone or in the context of schizophrenia, may respond to antipsychotic medication.

Stein DJ, Hollander E, Josephson SC 1994 Serotonin uptake blockers for the treatment of obsessional jealousy. Journal of Clinical Psychiatry 55: 30–33

- Obsessional jealousy may respond to selective serotonin reuptake inhibitors.

Dolan M, Bishay N 1996 The effectiveness of cognitive therapy in the treatment of non-psychotic morbid jealousy. British Journal of Psychiatry 168: 588–593

- Cognitive therapy is effective in morbid jealousy, mainly when obsessions are prominent.

Mullen PE, Pathe M, Purcell R 2000 Stalkers and their victims. Cambridge University Press, Cambridge

- Among stalkers, those who have had a prior relationship with the victim may be most likely to act violently against them.

Scott P 1977 Assessing dangerousness in criminals. British Journal of Psychiatry 131: 127–142

- The possibility that morbid jealousy will recur is significant.
- Scott reported a number of second homicides due to morbid jealousy following discharge from prison or release from special hospital after years of apparent well-being.

Definition

Jealousy – feeling or showing resentment towards a person one thinks of as a rival.

Morbid jealousy – a range of irrational thoughts and emotions, together with associated unacceptable or extreme behaviour, in which the dominant theme is a preoccupation with a partner's sexual unfaithfulness based on unfounded evidence.

Association between stalking, victimisation and psychiatric morbidity

Purcell R, Pathe M, Mullen PE 2005 Association between stalking, victimisation and psychiatric morbidity in a random community sample. British Journal of Psychiatry 187: 416–420

Stalking is a prevalent social problem. It may affect up to 10% of adults at some point in their lives. It can lead to significant morbidity in its victims, including anxiety disorders, depressive disorder, suicidation and post-traumatic stress disorder.

Method

- An Australian community sample.
- Examined psychiatric symptomatology in a representative community sample of stalking victims versus a control group that had never experienced harassment.
- 1844 surveys examining the experience of harassment and current mental health were completed.
- The sample was divided into subjects sustaining brief harassment, protracted stalking and the control group.
- All respondents completed the General Health Questionnaire and the Impact of Events Scale.

Results

- Rates of caseness on the GHQ-28 were higher in the stalked group (36.4%) than the group experiencing brief harassment (21.9%) and the control group (19.3%).
- Stalking that persists beyond a 2-week period is associated with high rates of persistent anxiety, depression and post-traumatic stress symptoms.
- A significant minority consider suicide as a means of managing their ongoing distress and harassment.
- Psychiatric morbidity did not differ with recency of victimisation.
- 34.1% still met caseness 1 year after the end of the stalking.
- In a significant minority of victims, stalking victimisation is associated with psychiatric morbidity that may persist long after it has ceased.

- Recognition of the immediate and long-term impact of stalking is necessary to assist victims and help alleviate distress and long-term disability.

Purcell R, Pathe M, Mullen PE 2004 Stalking. Defining and prosecuting a new category of offending. International Journal of Law and Psychiatry 27: 157–169

- In keeping with legal definitions of stalking, respondents who acknowledged two or more intrusions that induced fear were broadly classed as victims.
- Short-lived harassment is intense but usually does not last more that 2 weeks.
- If it continues for longer periods than this it is likely to continue for months. In this case the victim is more likely to be known to the perpetrator and the stalking may involve various methods of pursuit.

Dangerous people with severe personality disorder

Mullen P 1999 Dangerous people with severe personality disorder. British Medical Journal 319: 1146–1147

This paper comments on the report from the Department of Health on *Managing Dangerous People with Severe Personality Disorder*. The author suggests the 'British proposals for managing them are glaringly wrong – and unethical'.

The government's *Framework for the Future* proposes legal powers for the indefinite detention of people with dangerous severe personality disorder. Psychiatrists are to be employed to better identify people with dangerous severe personality disorder and to develop 'approaches to detention and management'. Research will be established to support development of policy and practice. The proposals make a point of insisting that 'indeterminate detention will be authorised only on the basis of evidence from an intensive specialist assessment'.

Mullen suggests that people with personality disorders attract little interest from mental health professionals and even less from those who provide the funding. Clinical experience, however, suggests that we can improve, if not cure, these disorders, even if research has failed to identify the best approaches. In addition, those people with a severe personality disorder are not inevitably likely to seriously offend, despite being overrepresented amongst recidivist offenders.

Crime and violence are clearly major political issues

In England and Wales, section 2 of the Crimes (Sentencing) Act already provides discretionary life sentences for those convicted a second time of a serious violent or sexual offence. The courts are hesitant to impose this but it would appear that the hope is that if the courts are provided with medical evidence that offenders have dangerous severe personality disorders, they will be more inclined to impose such sentences.

The government's proposals masquerade as extensions of mental health but are in fact proposals for preventative detention, not too far removed from the dangerous offender and sexual predator laws in North America.

It is suggested that there should be financial provision for the treatment of individuals with personality disorder within mental health services. This would reduce the morbidity and mortality as well as contributing to community safety.

Kury H, Ferdinand T 1999 Public opinion and punitivity. International Journal of Law and Psychiatry 22: 373–392

- Surveys indicate growing public support for more punitive approaches to offenders.

Heilbrun K, Ogloff JRP, Picarello K 1999 Dangerous offender statutes in the United States and Canada: implications for risk assessment. International Journal of Law and Psychiatry 22: 393–415

- Probability of future offending is most effectively predicted by past offending.

Quinsey VL, Harris GT, Rice ME, Cormier CA 1998 Violent offenders: appraising and managing risk. American Psychological Association, Washington, DC; Steadman HJ, Mulvey E, Monahan J et al 1998 Violence by people discharged from acute psychiatric inpatient facilities and by others in the same neighborhoods. Archives of General Psychiatry 55: 393–401

- Discuss violence by people discharged from acute psychiatric inpatient facilities and by others in the same neighbourhoods.
- Variables such as substance abuse or a history of being abused as a child, have significant, if less consistent, associations with increased rates of future violence.
- Mental health variables contribute little to such predictive characteristics.

Eastman N 1999 Public health psychiatry or crime prevention? British Medical Journal 318: 549–551

- The aim to encourage judges to impose discretionary life sentences circumventing the European Convention on Human Rights.
- The ECHR prohibits preventative detention except in those of unsound mind.

Weblink Department of Health 1999 Managing dangerous people with severe personality disorder. Home Office,

London – www.archive.official-documents.co.uk/document/cm50/5016-ii/5016ii04.htm

Dangerous severe personality disorder

Feeney A 2003 Dangerous severe personality disorder. Advances in Psychiatric Treatment 9: 349–358

The draft Mental Health Bill published in June 2002 was widely criticised, with particular concerns about the possible detention of those with personality disorders solely for the protection of the general public.

There are concerns that a single group of high-risk individuals is responsible for a disproportionate number of violent and sexual crimes. It is estimated 30 prisoners are released every month with histories that cause significant concern.

There is no proven link between severity of personality disorder and dangerousness.

It has been suggested that because psychopathy is a rare condition there is more chance of false positives rather than false negatives when screening. There is also the potential for spurious associations between high PCL-R scores and previous offending since the PCL-R rates offending behaviour.

Legislation in England and Wales already provides a number of options for prolonged detention to protect the public. Conviction of life is mandatory for murder and discretionary life sentences are available when the crime is deemed serious enough; however, only 2% of those eligible for such discretionary sentences have been given them. Automatic life sentences are given when a person commits a second serious offence. The courts also have the power to order a 'hospital direction'. There is also provision for passing sentences longer than usual for those who are felt to pose an ongoing risk on an indefinite basis.

In the USA, 16 states use the sexual predator law. This prevents the release of inmates who are about to complete their criminal sentence but are deemed to be at high risk of re-offending if released. Thirty-eight states use the death penalty for first-degree murder. The prosecution can submit actuarial risk assessments in order to predict the risk of re-offending to the presiding judge. If an inmate is deemed to be insane, they cannot be executed and are transferred to hospital for treatment until deemed fit enough for transfer back and execution on recovery. In Canada they have a dangerous offender order, an intermediate prison sentence, for those who have a greater than 50% chance of re-offending after a 10-year sentence. Few are released for this order. South Africa has a similar policy.

The concept of dangerousness has been superseded by assessment of risk. Psychiatrists are unable to control most of the factors that influence dangerousness and there is little evidence that treating personality disorder would reduce dangerousness levels. There is an unrealistic expectation that psychiatrists can predict risk and therefore protect society.

DSPD services carry extreme stigma. This is not in line with the National Service Framework principle that 'health and social services should combat discrimination against individuals and groups with mental heath problems and promote their social inclusion'. There is no reciprocity, with the person deriving no benefit to their loss of freedom. Furthermore, the obligation of the service to share information may alienate the target group even more, which in turn can increase the risk.

Straw J 1999 Severe personality disorders. Hansard (UK Parliamentary Reports, House of Commons, London). 15 February, pp 601–613

- Stated that psychiatrists were 'writing off' the individuals with personality disorder by selecting only the treatable ones for admission.
- In his original personal statement, Jack Straw said that those identified with having a dangerous and severe personality disorder should not be written off as untreatable and that they must have the best possible chance of becoming safe, so as to be returned to the community, whenever possible.
- '...there is, however, a group of dangerous and severely personality disordered individuals from whom the public at present are not properly protected...there should be new legislative powers for the indeterminate, but renewable detention of dangerously personality disordered individuals. These powers will apply whether or not someone was before the courts for an offence.'

Department of Health 2002 Reforming the Mental Health Act: a White Paper. Part II: High risk patients. The Stationery Office, London

- Termed high-risk individuals as dangerous and severely personality disordered (DSPD).

Farnham F, James D 2001 Dangerousness and dangerous law. Lancet 358: 1926

- Stated that 'DSPD' is a neologism.
- The term is without legal or medical status.

Department of Health 2002 The draft Mental Health Bill: Clause 6(4). The Stationery Office, London

- DSPD is not mentioned in the draft Bill.
- The Bill does contain the scope to detain 'those who pose a substantial risk of harm to others'.

Rozenberg J 2001 Law chief to call to lock up child sex suspects. Daily Telegraph, 27 December

- Discussed the Lord Chief Justice Woolf debate on Radio 4 (The Today Programme).
- He called for a form of protective custody for 'a very small minority of people'.
- He stated that this may be an infringement of the rights of the individual.
- The rights of the people who would be offended against in the future must be considered.

Prichard J 1835 A treatise on insanity and other disorders affecting the mind. Gilbert and Piper, London

- Outlined moral insanity and described a condition which is the recognisable forerunner to the modern concept of dissocial personality disorder.
- Characteristics include:
  - moral derangement (emotional or psychological)
  - loss of self-control
  - abnormal temper, emotions and habits
  - abnormal inclinations, likings and attachments
  - normal 'intellect'
  - rational but incapable of decency
  - no delusions or hallucinations.

Checkley H 1941 The mask of sanity. CV Mosby, St Louis

- Theorised that those who suffer from psychopathy appear sane but have a profound disorder in their thinking.
- Described psychopathy as involving abnormalities in interpersonal, affective and behavioural symptoms (Box 10.1).

Hare R, Cooke D, Clark D, Grann M et al 2000 Psychopathy and the predictive validity of the PCL-R: an international perspective. Behavioural Sciences and Law 18: 623–645

- Individuals who score over 30 on the PCL-R have a higher rate of recidivism.

Singleton N, Meltzer H, Gartward R 1998 Psychiatric morbidity among prisoners in England and Wales. Office for National Statistics, London

- A survey of penal institutions in England and Wales.
- Criteria for personality disorder were met by:
  - 78% of male remand prisoners
  - 64% of sentenced male prisoners
  - 50% of female prisoners.

Hare R, Cooke D, Hart S 1999 Psychopathy and sadistic personality disorder. In: Milton T, Blaney P, Davis R (eds) Oxford textbook of psychopathology. Oxford University Press, Oxford

- Argued that individuals with psychopathy know right from wrong.

Box 10.1

Psychopathological abnormalities

Interpersonal
- Superficially charming
- Grandiose
- Egocentric
- Manipulative

Affective
- Shallow, labile emotions
- Lack of empathy
- Lack of guilt
- Little subjective distress

Behavioural
- Impulsive
- Irresponsible
- Prone to boredom
- Lack of long-term goals
- Prone to breaking rules

- They should not be treated as if they are ill.

Department of Health and The Home Office 1994 Report of the Department of Health and Home Office Working Group on Psychopathic Disorder. DH, London

- Individuals suffering from psychopathic disorder are unaware that their actions are wrong and therefore should not be blamed for them.

Lewis G, Appelby L 1988 Personality disorder: the patients psychiatrists dislike. British Journal of Psychiatry 153: 44–49

- Recognised ambivalence from psychiatrists towards those with personality disorder.
- Non-engagement with these individuals has been commonplace using the treatability clause within the Mental Health Act.

Gunn J 2000 Future directions for treatment in forensic psychiatry. British Journal of Psychiatry 176: 332–338

- Concluded that individuals with personality disorder who are not treated by mental health services often end up with involvement from the criminal justice system, which is ill-equipped to deal with them.

Fallon P, Burglass R, Edwards B et al 1996 Report of the Committee of Inquiry into the Personality Disorder Unit, Ashworth Special Hospital (2 vols and Executive Summary) (Cm 4194 1 and 2). The Stationery Office, London

- The Fallon report suggested that people with personality disorder get reviewable sentences.
- These would not require a psychiatrist to sanction the extension of the sentence.
- A survey found that approximately 63% of forensic psychiatrists supported this move.

Dolan B, Coid J 1993 Psychopathic and antisocial people with severe personality disorders. Treatment and research issues. Gaskell, London

- Henderson Hospital has the best evidence for successful treatment in personality disorder.
- It functioned as a therapeutic community.

Norton K 1992 Personality disordered individuals: the Henderson Hospital model of treatment. Criminal Behaviour and Mental Health 2: 180–191

Described the features of the Henderson Hospital:
- Voluntary nature of the programme
- Discharge if the patient does not engage
- Clear hierarchy and a set of rules which promotes self-responsibility for one's own actions and understanding of the actions of others
- Limited time period of treatment.

Wong S, Gordon A 2001 The violence risk scale. Forensic Update 67, October

- Violence risk scale being trialled at Broadmoor – a pilot scheme.
- Incorporates six static and 20 dynamic risk factors.
- Thought to be useful for tracking progress.
- This is important given the proposals stating that people will not be released until the public risk has been reduced to an acceptable level.

Tyrer P, Merson S, Onyett S et al 1994 The effect of personality disorder on clinical outcome, social networks and adjustment: a controlled trial of psychiatric emergencies. Psychological Medicine 24: 731–740

- The use of the term 'severe personality disorder' differs markedly from its original definition.
- Neither DSM-IV nor ICD-10 has a way of recording the severity of personality disorder.
- The term DSPD was originally coined by the government but is now used for the programme designed to serve those with severe personality disorder.

Buchanan A, Lesse M 2001 Detection of people with severe personality disorders: a systematic review. Lancet 358: 1955–1959

- Reviewed studies dating back to 1970, looking at sensitivity and specificity as tools to measure 'dangerousness'.
- They found that six people needed to be detained in order to prevent one offence.

Legal dilemma

The government has claimed that DSPD programmes are fully compliant with the Human Rights Act 1998.

Gunn M, Holland T 2002 Some thoughts on the proposed Mental Health Act. Journal of Mental Health Law December: 367

- Proposed legislation would allow detention of unconvicted individuals with personality disorder if they were deemed at significant risk of future serious offending.
- It is argued here that this would be a serious breach of the individual's rights under Article 5 of the Human Rights Act (prohibition of unlawful detention).

Dangerous Severe Personality Disorder Programme

Prompting for the DSPD programme came mainly from the high profile case of Michael Stone. In 1996 MS killed Megan and Lin Russell, the wife and daughter of a local GP, and attacked their other daughter, Josie. This attack occurred years after his personality disorder was deemed untreatable.

Following collaboration between the Home Office, HM Prison Service and the Department of Health, a new service has been developed which aims to deliver new mental health services for people who are or have been considered dangerous as a result of severe personality disorder. The programme is included in the government's manifesto. The pilot programme is now underway.

Features

- To protect the public from some of the most dangerous people in society.
- To provide appropriate and effective services to improve mental health outcomes, enabling positive progress.
- Supporting public protection throughout the development of pilot treatment services for dangerous offenders whose offending is linked to severe personality disorder.
- Aimed at people who have committed a violent and/or sexual crime and have been detained under the criminal justice system or current mental health legislation.
- Works with some of the most difficult and dangerous persons in society. Therefore the challenges include assessment, treatment and management as well as

the delivery of effective services and the longer term prospects of reducing the risk of re-offending.

- Pilot programme is currently set up in prisons and special hospitals.
- Programmes are in progress in Broadmoor and Rampton Hospitals, and Frankland and Whitemoor prisons, with a total of 300 beds available.
- Assessment and treatment programmes are under active development.

Weblink DSPD programme – www.dspdprogramme.gov.uk.

Detention of people with dangerous severe personality disorders

Buchanan A, Lesse M 2001 Detention of people with dangerous severe personality disorders: a systematic review. Lancet 358: 1955–1959

This paper comments on government proposals to reduce the risks posed by people with 'dangerous' severe personality disorders (DSPD), including the legal framework of indeterminate detention.

This review aimed to establish the degree to which those operating the framework will be able to predict which people act violently in the future.

Method

- Reviewed published reports in which the accuracy of a clinical judgement or a statistically derived prediction of dangerousness was validated in adults in the community. Calculated the sensitivity and specificity of the procedures used in each study.
- They applied them to purported base rates of violence in those with DSPD.

Results

- Included 23 studies.
- 21 studies were used to calculate sensitivity and specificity.
- Six people would have to be detained in order to prevent one violent attack.
- It is likely that in practice the number of people requiring detention is higher than that reported.

Intimate partner violence

Ferris LE 2004 Intimate partner violence [editorial]. British Medical Journal 328: 595–596

Intimate partner violence is a major public health and human rights issue. There are only limited evaluations of interventions. Until it is clear whether interventions are beneficial or harmful, doubt will remain as to the need for psychiatric intervention.

Intimate partner violence can be identified in two ways:
- universal screening method
- diagnostic method (case identification based on specific signs and symptoms).

The latter method is preferred for its focus on time and resources for people in immediate need of help. It is clear that if intimate partner violence is identified, a risk assessment needs to be carried out immediately. Referral to victim support seems the logical pathway, especially if shelter and counselling are required. These interventions have not been critically evaluated despite their widespread implementation. There is, however, scope for further research. In the interim, doctors should be referring patients to one or more interventions against intimate partner violence based on the perceived needs of the patients.

World Health Organization 2003 The WHO multi-country study on women's health and domestic violence against women. WHO, Geneva. Online. Available: www.who.int/gender/violence/multicoubtry

- Are currently investigating rates of international prevalence, determinates and consequences of domestic violence.

Ramsay J, Richardson J, Carter YH et al 2002 Should health professionals screen women for domestic violence? A systematic review. British Medical Journal 325: 314–326

- The diagnostic method is preferred, given the lack of evidence on universal screening.

Hegarty K, Gunn J, Chondros P et al 2004 Association between depression and abuse by partners of women attending general practice: descriptive, cross sectional survey. British Medical Journal 328: 621–624

- Clinicians should be mindful of mental health conditions, particularly depression, which is strongly associated with intimate partner violence.
- Evidence exists for the effectiveness of screening and treating depression.

Heise L, Garcia-Moreno C 2002 Violence by intimate partners. In: Krug EG, Dahlberg LL, Mercy JA, Zwi AB, Lozano R (eds) World report on violence and health. World Health Organization, Geneva, pp 87–122

- Found the evidence regarding legal remedies such as mandatory arrest or court restraining orders conflicting.

Gondolf EW, Jones AS 2001 The program effect of batterer programs in three cities. Violence Victims 16: 693–704

- A large multisite study from the US.
- Found that there were moderate effects on levels of recidivism in a study of abuser treatment programmes.
- The dropout rate was high.

> Home Office Research, Development and Statistics Directorate, Policing and Reducing Crime Unit 1999 Reducing domestic violence…what works? Outreach and advocacy approaches. Home Office, London. Online. Available: www.homeoffice.gov.uk/docs/brief.html

- Community-based outreach programmes in both the UK and Australia have shown good results in dealing with individuals and families.

Measurement of risk by a community forensic mental health team

> Dowsett J 2005 Measurement of risk by a community forensic mental health team. Psychiatric Bulletin 29: 9–12

Aim

To evaluate the predictive validity of the HCR-20 risk assessment instrument in an inner city forensic team.

Method

- Cases were evaluated and followed up (average of 2.5 years) to collect information on recidivism.
- Patients were being treated by a medium secure unit (MSU) aftercare service which manages patients discharged from hospital.
- The study collected comprehensive clinical and offending data on patients of the community forensic team.
- Case notes were reviewed and the patients' keyworkers interviewed.
- Information on risk was collected using the HCR-20.
- The PCL-R was also completed in two-thirds of cases.
- Recidivism data (after risk assessment) were collected from file review and community review meetings.

Results

- 47 patients were included.
- The majority of cases were African–Caribbean men and around one-third were on Home Office restriction orders.
- Most patients had a psychotic illness and were on neuroleptic medication, with around half on atypical neuroleptics.
- Nearly all the patients had a history of violence.
- About 1 in 10 had committed homicide.

- Severity of previous offending was illustrated by the high numbers registering at least one instance of risk behaviour in the Eastman and Bellamy system (admission to secure services schedule).

HCR-20 results

- All historical risk factors for this patient sample are above average in the HCR-20 scoring framework.
- Patients had high scores on clinical risk factors of lack of insight and negative attitudes.
- The striking thing about risk (R) is the high level of access to destabilisers.

Recidivism data

- Over the follow-up period, eight patients were charged or convicted of a new offence, all of which were violence offences.
- Comparing their HCR-20 score with the remainder of the sample showed a significant result.

Discussion

- The community forensic patients had high levels of serious offending, with many having severe mental illness as well as personality disorder.
- The HCR-20 was easy to execute. The clinical and risk scales suggest that insight is often limited in this group and that access to destabilisers (e.g. substances, weapons and potential victims) is a problem.
- The patients who re-offended all had HCR-20 scores significantly higher than the mean for the sample. It therefore seems to be a useful instrument for stratifying risk within community forensic settings.
- A minority of these offences took place in the context of a deteriorating mental state. It is therefore suggested that the criminogenic factors should be taken into more consideration in mentally disordered offenders and targeted more effectively.

Relationship between forensic and generic services

- One patient subgroup (all scored under 15 on HCR-20) had been stable for some years without relapse. Were it not for the history of very serious past offences or due to restriction orders, their care could be transferred back to generic services.
- Another patient subgroup (scores between 15 and 28) relapsed frequently but could be treated within general wards at those times. They may be disadvantaged by not being looked after by a local generic service.
- The third group for whom mental health issues was only a small part of the problem would benefit from a multifaceted approach targeting criminality,

supervising placement and working with substance misuse, poor anger management and specific psychological approaches.

See also Rating scales, page 168.

Mental disorder in prisons

Birmingham L 2004 Mental disorder in prisons [editorial]. Psychiatric Bulletin 28: 393–397

Major reform of prison healthcare provision requires the NHS to have a far greater role in treating mental health problems in this population. It is anticipated that the NHS will assume full responsibility for prison health care. Psychiatrists will have greater roles – addictions and child and adolescent psychiatry in particular.

Health Advisory Committee for the Prison Service 1997 The provision of mental health care in prisons. Prison Service, London

- Stated that prisoners were entitled to the same range and quality of NHS services as the general public.

Home Office 2003 World prison population list, 4th edn. Home Office, London

- The prison population in England and Wales is 72,500.
- The number of people in English prisons has increased by 50% in the past decade.

Fazel S, Danesh J 2002 Serious mental disorder in 23,000 prisoners: a systematic review of 62 surveys. Lancet 359: 545–550

- Around one in seven prisoners has a psychotic illness or major depression.
- Approximately half of all male prisoners and one in five women have an antisocial personality disorder.
- This is substantially higher than in community samples.

Maden A, Taylor CJA, Brooke D et al 1995 Mental disorder in remand prisoners. Home Office, London

- Confirmed that mental disorder is particularly prevalent among prisoners.
- The highest levels of morbidity are present in prisoners on remand and women populations.
- Mental disorder, which includes substance misuse, is found in:
  - 37% of sentenced males
  - 63% of men on remand
  - 57% of sentenced women
  - 76% of women on remand.

- Multiple diagnoses are common, with approximately a quarter of men and a third of women on remand receiving two or more diagnoses.
- Demonstrated significant levels of unmet mental health treatment needs among remand prisoners in particular.

Singleton N, Meltzer H, Gatward R 1998 Psychiatric morbidity among prisoners in England and Wales. Office for National Statistics, London

- Conducted a large prison survey on behalf of the Office for National Statistics.
- Representative sample of approximately 3000 prisoners from all penal establishments in England and Wales.
- Found mental disorder in each category to be much higher than in the general population.
- Rates of psychotic disorder fell in young offender institutions (10% in adult versus 3% in young males).
- Among women, rates of psychotic disorder were highest for women holding offences of violence and lowest for those with drug charges.
- Antisocial personality disorder was the most prevalent diagnosis in each of the four prisoner subgroups.
- The second most common disorder was paranoid personality disorder in men and borderline personality disorder in women.
- Neurotic symptoms were common – sleep problems, worry, fatigue, depression and irritability.
- The most frequently used drugs in prison were heroin and cannabis.
- Rates for multiple disorders were particularly high in remand prisoners.
- Two-thirds of sentenced prisoners and three-quarters of remand prisoners who showed evidence of functional psychosis were found to have three or four other disorders. Found:
  - 18% of male sentenced prisoners
  - 21% of male remand prisoners
  - 40% of all women had sought/received help for emotional or mental problems in the preceding year.
- 22% of women remand prisoners said they had been admitted to a psychiatric hospital at some stage in their life.
- Prisoners with psychosis were the most likely to have been refused help, prior to imprisonment.
- Found that male prisoners on remand who are psychotic are more likely to be locked up longer than other prisoners.

Harty M, Tighe J, Lesse M et al 2003 Inverse care for mentally ill prisoners: unmet needs in forensic mental health services. Journal of Forensic Psychology and Psychiatry 14: 600–614

- Prisoners were more likely to have a chaotic lifestyle.
- They had characteristics of:
  - frequent changes of accommodation
  - homelessness
  - substance use.
- Many of them had no previous contact with mental health services.

Isherwood S, Parrott J 2002 Audit of transfers under the Mental Health Act from prison – the impact of organisational change. Psychiatric Bulletin 26: 368–370

- Found lengthy delays in transferring prisoners to hospital, most frequently due to lack of psychiatric beds.

Birmingham L, Mason D, Grubin D 1996 Prevalence of mental disorder in remand prisoners: consecutive case study. British Medical Journal 313: 1521–1524

- 26% of men were found to have a mental disorder.
- 62% had substance misuse disorders.
- 5% have a diagnosis of psychosis.
- Psychotic people were no more likely than individuals with another mental disorder to have any mental state abnormality detected.

Parsons S, Walker L, Grubin D 2001 Prevalence of mental disorder in female remand prisoners. Journal of Forensic Psychiatry 164: 55–61

- 29% of women were found to have a mental disorder on reception.
- 11% of this group had psychosis.
- Standard health screening measures in reception were cursory and ineffective.
- The screening devices missed three-quarters of those thought to be suffering from a mental illness.
- Only one in four patients identified by researchers as having a psychotic illness were picked up at reception.

Coid J 1988 Mentally abnormal prisoners on remand – rejected or accepted by the NHS? British Medical Journal 296: 1779–1782

- Some prisoners who would benefit from hospital treatment are overlooked as they are perceived to be too disturbed, dangerous or as criminals who are unsuitable for treatment.

Birmingham L, Mason D, Grubin D 1998 A follow up study of mentally disordered men remanded to prison. Criminal Behaviour and Mental Health 8: 202–213

- Mentally ill prisoners receive no treatment or aftercare when released from prison as their treatment needs are not identified.

Nurse J, Woodcock P, Ormsby J 2003 Influence of environmental factors on mental health within prisons: focus group study. British Medical Journal 327: 480–485

- Found that prisoners have long periods of isolation with little mental stimulation contributing to poor mental health, frustration and anger as well as anxiety.

Coid J, Petruckevitch A, Bebbington P et al 2003 Psychiatric morbidity in prisons and solitary cellular confinement, I: disciplinary segregation. Journal of Forensic Psychiatry and Psychology 14: 298–319

- Those who reported being placed in solitary confinement in prison were more likely to have an extensive history of previous psychiatric treatment and a diagnosis of schizophrenia or depression.

Reed J, Lyne M 1997 The quality of healthcare in prison: results of a year's programme of semi-structured inspections. British Medical Journal 315: 1420–1424

- Reed found that few of the prisons he inspected provided health care broadly equivalent to NHS care.

Mental illness in people who kill strangers

Shaw J, Amos T, Hunt I et al 2004 Mental illness in people who kill strangers. A longitudinal study and national clinical survey. British Medical Journal 328: 734–737

- A longitudinal study and national clinical survey.
- Measured the changes over time in the frequency of homicides committed by strangers.
- Aimed to evaluate the personal and clinical characteristics of people who commit stranger homicides.

Secretary of State 2001 Criminal Statistics England and Wales 2000: statistics relating to crime and criminal proceedings for the year 2000. The Stationery Office, London

- This study accessed the homicide index – collated using the information on all homicides from all police forces in England and Wales.
- Over the past 30 years the number of homicides has increased.
- Stranger homicides increased four-fold between 1967 and 1997.
- Stranger homicides increased two-fold as a proportion of all homicides.

- Homicides as a whole almost doubled in the same time period.
- There was no increase in the number of patients put on a hospital order as a result of any type of homicide.
- The proportion of homicides leading to hospital order has decreased.
- In the study period, 22% of the total homicides were stranger homicides.
- Perpetrators were predominantly male, especially when strangers were killed.
- Psychiatric reports were obtained in 1168 (73%) of homicides, including 234 (65%) of stranger homicide.
- Those committing stranger homicide were more likely to:
  - have a history of drug misuse, and
  - alcohol and drugs were more likely to have contributed to the offence.
- Those committing stranger homocide were less likely to:
  - have a history of mental disorder
  - symptoms of mental disorder
  - previous contact with mental health services.
- Of 234 total stranger homicides:
  - 37 had prior contact with mental health services
  - 10 had a diagnosis of schizophrenia
  - two patients with schizophrenia had been in contact with services in the previous week
  - eight people with schizophrenia had been in contact with services in the year prior to the offence.

Thornicroft G, Strathdee G 1994 How many psychiatric beds? British Medical Journal 308: 816–819

- While the number of homicides has increased, the number of psychiatric beds in the UK has more than halved.
- Some cases of homicide have been reported as failures of community care.

Preventing crime by people with schizophrenic disorders

Hodkins S, Muller-Isberner R 2004 Preventing crime by people with schizophrenic disorders: the role of psychiatric services. British Journal of Psychiatry 185: 245–250

Preventative interventions would need to consider when offending begins, when people with schizophrenia who commit crime present to mental health services and what their particular problems are.

Aims

This study attempted to identify opportunities for interventions to prevent offending among men with schizophrenia by tracking their histories of offending and admissions to hospital.

Three hypotheses were examined:
- Had men with schizophrenia who had committed crimes warranting admission to forensic settings previously been in general psychiatric hospitals?
- What proportion of men with schizophrenia treated in general settings have a record of criminality?
- Were there problems evident on admission to general psychiatric settings that indicated the need for treatments and services designed to prevent criminality?

Method

- A comparison was made between patients discharged from forensic psychiatric hospitals in four countries.
- The majority of subjects were male and had a diagnosis of schizophrenia, schizoaffective disorder or schizophreniform disorder.
- 232 men with schizophreniform disorders recently discharged from psychiatric hospitals were included.
- Information was gathered from interview with the patient, medical and criminal records and a named family member.
- Violent crimes were defined as all offences causing physical harm, threats of violence or harassment, all types of sexual aggression, illegal possession of firearms or explosives and all kinds of forcible confinement, arson and robbery.

Results

- Patients who had committed their first crime before admission to general psychiatric services:
  - were in general 5 years older than those who had no criminal record
  - were older on first admission
  - had a history of behavioural difficulties in childhood or adolescence
  - had a history of substance misuse prior to age 18
  - had a history of alcohol abuse or dependence at first admission
  - had a diagnosis of antisocial personality disorder.
- Features predictive of crime were:
  - antisocial personality disorder – over six times increase in risk
  - institutionalised prior to the age of 18 – increased risk by 2.89 times
  - alcohol abuse or dependence at first admission – increased risk by 4.06 times.
- Those who had committed a crime prior to first admission to a psychiatric hospital had a higher score than those with no criminal history for the deficient affective experience score from the PCL-R (4.3 versus 2.63).

Discussion

- 78% of patients in the forensic hospital had been admitted to a general hospital prior to committing the offence which resulted them being admitted to the forensic hospital.
- 24% of the general psychiatric patients had committed a crime.
- 14% of the general population had committed a crime prior to first admission compared to 40% of the patients being discharged from the forensic hospital.
- A large number of these were receiving care at the time of their offending which the authors suggest compels us to develop policies and procedures to identify patients engaging in antisocial and criminal behaviours and provide them with interventions to prevent such behaviours.
- The repeated finding is that it is more common for men who develop schizophrenia than those who do not to display early-onset stable patterns of antisocial behaviour, suggesting that there is a link. The link, however, remains poorly understood at this time.

Bonta J, Law M, Hanson K 1998 The prediction of criminal and violent recidivism among mentally disordered offenders: a meta-analysis. Psychological Bulletin 123: 123–142

- Past criminality is the best predictor of future criminality.

Moffitt TE 1993 Adolescent-limited and life-course persistent antisocial behaviour: a developmental taxonomy. Psychological Review 100: 674–701

- Prospective, longitudinal study based in a number of countries.
- Approximately 5% of males display antisocial behaviour from early childhood which escalates in severity with age, until criminal offending begins during adolescence.

Moffitt TE, Caspi A 2002 Childhood predictors differentiate life-course persistent and adolescence-limited antisocial pathways among males and females. Development and Psychopathology 13: 355–375

- The subjects (male) met criteria for conduct disorder in childhood/adolescence and for antisocial personality disorder in adulthood.

Armstrong T, Costello EJ 2002 Community studies on adolescent substance use, abuse or dependence and psychiatric comorbidity. Journal of Consulting and Clinical Psychology 70: 1224–1239

- Those with conduct disorder who are exposed to drugs display an earlier onset of substance misuse, which is, in turn, associated with persistence.

King VL, Kidorf MS, Stoller KB et al 2001 Influence of antisocial personality subtypes on drug abuse treatment response. Journal of Nervous and Mental Disease 189: 593–601

- The presence of antisocial personality disorder is associated with a poor response to substance misuse interventions, irrespective of a diagnosis of schizophrenia.

Arsneault L, Cannon M, Witton J et al 2004 Causal association between cannabis and psychosis: examination of the evidence. British Journal of Psychiatry 184: 110–117

- Prospective studies have shown that cannabis increases the incidence of schizophrenia in those with a genetic predisposition.

Hodkins S, Cote G 1993 The criminality of mentally disordered offenders. Criminal Justice and Behaviour 28: 115–129

- Men with antisocial personality traits are similar in age at first crime and types and frequencies of crime whether or not they have concurrent schizophrenia.

See also the 'General topics' section in Chapter 26 (Schizophrenia), page 378.

Psychiatric aspects of the assessment and treatment of sex offenders

Gordon H, Grubin D 2004 Psychiatric aspects of the assessment and treatment of sex offenders. Advances in Psychiatric Treatment 10: 73–80

The number of offences committed often exceeds that registered in the criminal record. There is little published evidence to indicate whether psychodynamic psychotherapy (group or individual) can reduce recidivism, even when there is improved insight and understanding. The role of the psychiatrist can be unclear, particularly when there is no evidence of mental illness per se. The psychiatrist may be seen not only as a treatment provider, but also as a public protector. In reality, treatment must serve both functions, and should be delivered by a multiagency team. Ethical issues arise in trial methodology in terms of having an untreated control group and with regard to gaining consent.

Home Office 2003 MAPPA guidance: multi-agency public protection arrangements. National Probation Directorate, London

- For adult sex offenders in the community, the role of multi-agency public protection panels (MAPPPs) is of primary importance.

- Established under the Criminal Justice and Court Services Act 2000, these panels started to operate formally from April 2001 throughout England and Wales.
- They involve close liaison between police and probation services, and ensure that arrangements are in place to assess and manage the risks posed by sexual and violent offenders.
- They provide a framework for interagency working with social services departments, housing authorities, youth offending teams, mental health trusts and organisations representing a mental health trust on a MAPPP, or in relation to a patient under their care. Issues of confidentiality may arise.

Grubin D, Gunn J 1991 The imprisoned rapist and rape. HMSO, London

- Most sex offenders do not have a major mental illness.

Smith AD, Taylor PJ 1999 Serious sex offending against women by men with schizophrenia: relationship of illness and psychotic symptoms to offending. British Journal of Psychiatry 174: 233–237

- People with schizophrenia or related psychosis may commit sex offences or show abnormal sexual behaviour.
- This may be related to the psychosis itself.

Craissati J, Hodes P 1992 Mentally ill sex offenders: the experience of a regional secure unit. British Journal of Psychiatry 161: 846–849

- People with schizophrenia or related psychosis may commit sex offences or show abnormal sexual behaviour.
- This may be related to disinhibition secondary to the psychosis.

Smith AD 1999 Aggressive sexual fantasy in men with schizophrenia who commit contact sex offences against women. Journal of Forensic Psychiatry 10: 538–552

- People with schizophrenia or related psychosis may commit sex offences or show abnormal sexual behaviour.
- This may be related to the presence of deviant sexual fantasies.

Brockman B, Bluglass R 1996 A general psychiatric approach to sexual deviation. In: Rosen I (ed.) Sexual deviation, 3rd edn. Oxford University Press, Oxford, pp 1–42

- Affective disorder is not usually associated with serious sexual offending.

- Patients with hypomania may behave in a sexually disinhibited manner, leading to offences ranging from indecent exposure to indecent assault.

Kafka MP, Prentky R 1992 Fluoxetine treatment of non-paraphilic sexual addictions and paraphilias in men. Journal of Clinical Psychiatry 53: 351–358

- Patients with paraphilias not infrequently have a comorbid history of dysthymia or depression.

Hucker S, Langevin R, Dickey R et al 1998 Cerebral damage and dysfunction in sexually aggressive men. Annals of Sex Research 1: 33–47

- Sexual offending may be associated with organic brain damage.

Walker N, McCabe S 1973 Crime and insanity in England: new solutions and new problems. Edinburgh University Press, Edinburgh

- Sexual offending may be associated with learning disability.

Williams LM, Finkelhor D 1990 The characteristics of incestuous fathers: a review of recent studies. In: Marshall WL, Laws DR, Barbaree HE (eds) The handbook of sexual assault: issues, theories and treatment of the offender. Plenum Press, New York, pp 231–255

- Sexual offending may be associated with substance misuse.

Reiss D, Grubin D, Meux C 1996 Young 'psychopaths' in special hospital: treatment and outcome. British Journal of Psychiatry 168: 99–104

- Sexual offending may be associated with personality disorder.

Templemann TL, Stinnett RD 1991 Patterns of sexual arousal and history in a 'normal' sample of young men. Archives of Sexual Behaviour 10: 137–150

- Sexually deviant fantasies and related deviant behaviour are also common in the non-offending population.
- Only in a proportion of sex offenders are paraphilias found.

Baker M, White T 2002 Sex offenders in high-security care in Scotland. Journal of Forensic Psychiatry 13: 285–297

- In the assessment of sex offenders and in cases of mental illness, evaluation should determine when deviant fantasies developed.

- It is important to ascertain whether they were already present or developed with or during the course of the illness.

Thornton D 2002 Constructing and testing a framework for dynamic risk assessment. Sexual Abuse: a Journal of Research and Treatment 14: 139–153

- The sex offender treatment programme in England and Wales has categorised the psychological characteristics associated with sexual offending into four domains:
  - Sexual interests (including sexual preoccupation, as well as sexual preference for children or violence)
  - Distorted attitudes and beliefs (so-called cognitive distortions, and beliefs supportive of rape)
  - Socioaffective management (e.g. emotional regulation and intimacy problems)
  - Self-management (e.g. poor problem-solving abilities, lifestyle impulsiveness).

Hanson RK, Bussiere MT 1998 Predictors of sexual offender recidivism: a meta-analysis. Department of the Solicitor General, Ottawa

- Denial of offending and lack of victim empathy are factors which relate to engagement in treatment.
- Denial of re-offending and lack of victim empathy have not been shown to predict re-offending.
- Risk of sex offence recidivism is associated with plethysmographic evidence of response to paedophilic stimuli.

Hanson RK, Harris AJR 2000 Where should we intervene? Dynamic predictors of sexual offence recidivism. Criminal Justice and Behaviour 27: 6–35

- Divided dynamic risk factors into two categories:
  - stable factors, such as an offender's attitudes or ability to 'regulate' his sexual and more general behaviour
  - fluctuating factors, such as cooperation and access to victims.

Barker JG, Howell RJ 1992 The plethysmograph: a review of recent literature. Bulletin of the American Academy of Psychiatry and Law 20: 13–25

- Penile plethysmography provides an objective measure of sexual arousal.

Rice ME, Harris GT, Quinsey VL 1990 A follow up of rapists assessed in a maximum security psychiatric facility. Journal of Interpersonal Violence 5: 435–448

- Risk of sex offence recidivism is associated with plethysmographic evidence of response to non-sexual violence.

Simon WT, Schouten PGW 1993 The plethysmograph reconsidered: comments on Barker and Howell. Bulletin of the American Academy of Psychiatry and Law 21: 505–512

- There are methodological difficulties relating to the use of plethysmographic tests.
- These include difficulties in the standardisation of the method, limited control data for normal populations, and the ability of people taking the test to fake non-arousal by various means.

Launay G 1999 The phallometric assessment of sex offenders: an update. Criminal Behaviour and Mental Health 9: 254–274

- Phallometry can provide useful information, particularly in terms of identifying focuses for treatment.

Abel GG, Lawry SS, Karlstrom E et al 1994 Screening tests for paedophilia. Criminal Justice and Behaviour 21: 115–131

- Devised a method of assessing sex offenders without the intrusiveness of penile plethysmography.
- The method comprises a questionnaire about sexual thoughts, fantasies and behaviour, and a computerised assessment of gaze times at slides depicting a range of prepubescent, teenage and adult males and females, and scenes suggesting paraphilias.
- The assessment was found to be most accurate with 'child molesters' who prefer pubescent boys.

English K 1998 The containment approach: an aggressive strategy for the community management of adult sex offenders. Psychology, Public Policy and Law 4: 218–235

- The polygraph test can be an effective tool when used in the context of treatment or supervision following conviction.
- It can be an effective means of overcoming denial and detecting when offenders are engaging in high-risk behaviours that might lead to re-offending.

Grubin D 2003 The role of the polygraph in the assessment and management of risk in sex offenders in the community. In: Matravers A (ed.) Sex offenders in the community. William Publishing, Cullompton

- Polygraphy is based on autonomic nervous system responses associated with the anxiety of deception.
- False-positive rates are approximately 10% and false-negative rates are approximately 20%, but need more accurate assessment.
- For those already convicted of sexual offences, the detection of lies is probably less relevant than the technique's ability to facilitate disclosures.

Marshall WL, Anderson D, Fernandez YM 1999 Cognitive behavioural treatment of sexual offenders. Wiley, Chichester

- Cognitive behavioural therapy for sex offenders aims to assist the offender take responsibility for the behaviour leading to the offence.
- It also develops cognitive and behavioural controls to enable the offender to avoid or escape the re-offending.

Ortmann J 1980 The treatment of sexual offenders: castration and anti-hormone therapy. International Journal of Law and Psychiatry 3: 443–451

- Surgical castration is now a historic treatment only, although studies showed a considerable reduction in sexual recidivism.

Bradford JMW 1988 Organic treatment for the male sexual offender. Annals of the New York Academy of Sciences 528: 193–202

- Cyproterone acetate resulted in a significant reduction of plasma testosterone concentration and level of sexual arousal measured by penile plethysmography.
- It led to a reduction in the self-reported frequencies of masturbation, sexual tension and sexual fantasies.

Meyer WJ, Cole C, Emory E 1992 Depo Provera treatment for sex offending behaviour: an evaluation of outcome. Bulletin of the American Academy of Psychiatry and Law 20: 249–259

- A study of 40 men, most of whom were paedophiles.
- Compared treatment with medroxyprogesterone (periods of 6 months to 12 years) with group and individual psychotherapies.
- The control group had refused drug treatment but received psychotherapy.
- 18% of the drug treatment group re-offended, rising to 35% after it was discontinued. This compared with 55% of those in the control group.

Rosler A, Witztum E 1998 Treatment of men with paraphilia with a long acting analogue of gonadotrophin releasing hormone. New England Journal of Medicine 338: 416–422

- An Israeli uncontrolled study of 30 men with paraphilias treated in the community. Treatment with the long acting GnRH agonist analogue triptorelin continued for up to 42 months.
- Treatment was associated with complete abolition of self-reported deviant sexual fantasies, urges and behaviour.

Rosler A, Witztum E 2000 Pharmacotherapy of paraphilias in the next millennium. Behavioural Sciences and the Law 18: 43–56

- The GnRH analogues cause side effects associated with reduced androgen secretion.
- These include a reduction in bone mineral density which requires monitoring.

Sterkmans P, Geerts F 1992 Is benperidol the specific drug for the treatment of excessive and disinhibited sexual behaviour? Acta Neurologica et Psychiatrica Belgica 66: 1030–1040

- Benperidol is sometimes used to control sexually inappropriate behaviour in psychotic patients.
- The effects of benperidol on such behaviour are unreliable and unsupported by evidence.

Greenberg DM, Bradford JMW 1997 Treatment of the paraphilic disorders: a review of the role of the selective serotonin reuptake inhibitors. Sexual Abuse: a Journal of Research and Treatment 9: 349–360

- SSRIs may be beneficial in the treatment of paraphilias.
- Mechanisms proposed include a reduction in obsessive–compulsive behaviour, elevation of mood, lowering of impulsivity, lessening of anxiety and facilitation of non-paraphilic arousal.
- Further study is required.

Psychopathic personality in young people

Dolan M 2004 Psychopathic personality in young people. Advances in Psychiatric Treatment 10: 466–473

Whilst conduct disorder, antisocial personality disorder and psychopathy are terms often used interchangeably, there are significant differences between them and their associated correlates. Conduct disorder and antisocial personality disorder primarily focus on behavioural problems. Psychopathy (as described by Hare) emphasises deficits in affective and interpersonal functioning. The estimated prevalence of adult psychopathy in the general population is 1%, rising to between 15 and 25% in incarcerated groups. Impairments in executive (prefrontal) dysfunction are implicated in the aetiology of conduct disorder and psychopathy.

There have been no studies of the stability of psychopathic traits across the younger age range or of prevalence of psychopathy in the juvenile general population. Although the callous–emotional and interpersonal aspects of psychopathy share some features with the pervasive developmental disorders, no study has specifically addressed the relationship between them. No studies have been done of the presence of comorbid disruptive behavioural disorders.

Psychopathy may be as important a moderator of treatment outcome in adolescents as it is in adults. As yet there have been no risk prediction studies in children with psychopathic traits and none of the adolescent studies has examined which (if any) of the callous–unemotional or behavioural factors of the psychopathy subscales contribute most to predictive accuracy.

Instruments developed for assessing psychopathy in child and adolescent populations require further validation in a variety of populations and settings before they can be used with confidence in the prediction of risk and, hence, sentence planning in the criminal justice system.

At present there is no general agreement on whether or not psychopathy exists in childhood and adolescence. Longitudinal studies demonstrating the stability of psychopathic traits over the lifespan and evidence that the same aetiological factors contribute to this disorder at all ages are required.

Hare RD 1998 Psychopathy, affect and behaviour. In: Cooke D, Forth A, Hare R (eds) Psychopathy: theory, research and implications for society. Kluwer, Dordrecht, pp 108–139

- There are high rates of antisocial personality disorder (50–80%) in prison populations.
- Only 20% of these individuals meet Hare's criteria for psychopathy.

Cooke DJ, Michie C 2001 Refining the construct of psychopathy: towards a hierarchical model. Psychological Assessment 13: 171–188

- Proposed a three-factor structure which includes:
  - an arrogant, deceitful interpersonal style, involving dishonesty, manipulation, grandiosity and glibness
  - defective emotional experience, involving lack of remorse, poor empathy, shallow emotions and a lack of responsibility for one's own actions
  - behavioural manifestations of impulsiveness and sensation seeking.

Forth AE, Burke HC 1998 Psychopathy in adolescence: assessment, violence and developmental precursors. In: Cooke D, Forth A, Hare R (eds) Psychopathy: theory, research and implications for society. Kluwer, Dordrecht, pp 205–230

- The development of conduct disorder and psychopathy are associated with family background variables including parental rejection, inconsistent discipline and abuse.
- Delinquent offenders with pronounced psychopathic traits have an earlier onset of offending and commit more crimes than non-psychopathic criminal youth.

- Psychopathy scores have been found to correlate significantly with the severity of conduct problems, antisocial behaviour and delinquency in adolescents.
- There were rates of psychopathy of 3.5% in young people in community care, 12% in those on probation and 28.3% in those incarcerated, which is higher than that reported in adult samples.
- These higher rates may relate to higher ratings on items relating to impulsivity and irresponsibility in younger samples.

Moffitt TE, Henry B 1994 Neuropsychological studies of juvenile delinquency and violence: a review. In: Milner JS (ed.) Neuropsychology of aggression. Kluwer Academic, Norwell, pp 131–140

- Children with conduct disorder, particularly those with repeated violent behaviour, exhibit neuropsychological deficits.

Raine A 1993 The psychopathology of crime: criminal behaviour as a clinical disorder. Academic Press, San Diego, CA

- Children with conduct disorder have reduced levels of arousal.

Kochanska G 1993 Towards a synthesis of parental socialisation and child temperament in early development of conscience. Child Development 64: 228–240

- Suggested that behavioural inhibition is critical in the development of conscience in young children.
- Low fear children do not respond to the type of socialisation (gentle, non-power, assertive discipline) that led to conscience development in more fearful children.

Frick PJ 2002 Juvenile psychopathy from a developmental perspective: implications for construct development and use in forensic assessments. Law and Human Behaviour 26: 247–253

- The existence and assessment of psychopathy in children and adolescents is a contentious issue.
- The author suggests that diagnosis presents no more of a challenge than any other measure of psychopathology in children and adolescents.
- Psychopathy assessment in juveniles may be a means of early detection and intervention in high risk groups.

Myers WC, Burker RC, Harris HE 1995 Adolescent psychopathy in relation to delinquent behaviours, conduct disorder and personality disorder. Journal of Forensic Sciences 40: 436–440

- Delinquent offenders with pronounced psychopathic traits re-offend more often than non-psychopathic criminal youth.

Spain SE, Douglas KS, Poythress NG et al 2004 The relationship between psychopathic features, violence and treatment outcomes: the comparison of three youth measures of psychopathic features. Behavioural Sciences and the Law 22: 85–102

- Delinquent offenders with pronounced psychopathic traits offend more violently than non-psychopathic criminal youth.

Rogers R, Johansen J, Chang JJ et al 1997 Predictors of adolescent psychopathy: oppositional and conduct-disordered symptoms. Journal of the American Academy of Psychiatry and the Law 25: 261–271

- Found modest correlation between psychopathy scores and ratings of non-compliance with treatment in 81 adolescent inpatients.

O'Neill M, Lidz V, Heilbrun K 2003 Adolescents with psychopathic characteristics in a substance-abusing cohort. Treatment process and outcomes. Law and Human Behaviour 27: 299–313

- Reported that psychopathy score was negatively correlated with attendance rates, quality of participation and clinical improvement in adolescents in a substance misuse treatment programme.

Definition

Psychopathy – a personality disorder characterised by a constellation of interpersonal, affective and behavioural characteristics. (*Source:* Hare RD 1998 Psychopathy, affect and behaviour. In: Cooke D, Forth A, Hare R (eds) Psychopathy: theory, research and implications for society. Kluwer, Dordrecht, pp 105–139.)

See also the 'General topics' section in Chapter 5 (Child and adolescent psychiatry), page 73.

Rates of mental disorder in people convicted of homicide

Shaw J, Hunt I, Flynn S 2006 Rates of mental disorder in people convicted of homicide. National clinical survey. British Journal of Psychiatry 188: 143–147

Previous studies examining the relationships between homicide and mental illness have varied in their use of diagnostic criteria.

Method

- A national clinical survey of people convicted of homicide carried out as part of the National Confidential Inquiry into Suicide and Homicide by People with Mental Illness.
- 1594 people were identified in England and Wales between 1996 and 1999.
- Aimed to measure the rate of mental disorder in people convicted of homicide using the following variables:
  - lifetime diagnosis
  - mental illness at time of the offence
  - contact with psychiatric services
  - diminished responsibility verdict
  - hospital disposal.
- The relationship between definitions, verdict and outcome in court were also examined.

Results

- 34% of people convicted of homicide had a mental disorder.
- The most common diagnoses were personality disorder, alcohol dependence and drug dependence.
- The majority of people convicted of homicide had had no contact with psychiatric services.
- 5% of people convicted had a lifetime prevalence of schizophrenia.
- 10% of patients had symptoms of psychiatric illness at the time of the offence.
- 9% of people had a diminished responsibility verdict.
- 7% of people had a hospital disposal.
- Most people with schizophrenia had a diminished responsibility verdict and/or a hospital disposal.
- Hospital orders were associated with severe mental illness and psychotic symptoms.

Should psychiatrists protect the public?

Coid J, Maden J 2003 Should psychiatrists protect the public? A new risk reduction strategy, supporting criminal justice, could be effective. British Medical Journal 326: 406–407

Proposed changes in mental health legislation regarding high risk patients with an emphasis on public protection has provoked outcry among psychiatrists. There are concerns that preventative legislation is being hidden within a medical legislative framework and that this is contrary to human rights legislation.

There are two main issues to consider:
- Is the health service equipped to play a leader's role in public protection?

- Does the Home Office public protection agenda fit with the principles underpinning the Department of Health strategy for mental health?

The authors propose that the criminal justice system takes the lead, with psychiatry adding a supporting role. Offending rates are not influenced by psychiatric interventions as mental health is only one of main contributing problems. There is scope for a contributory role in risk reduction. Future focus should be on a hybrid where the criminal legislation predominates and there is less reliance on mental health.

Mental Health Law Subcommittee 2001 Response to the government's White Paper 'Reforming the Mental Health Act'. Royal College of Psychiatrists, London

- The College has stated that intervention from psychiatrists should be for the benefit of the patient.
- Public protection should be secondary.

Department of Health and Home Office 2000 Reforming the Mental Health Act. Part I: the new legal framework. Part II: High risk patients. The Stationery Office, London

- The proposed MHA shows less focus on previous restrictions on detention.
- Whether a condition is treatable will no longer present a barrier.
- Tribunals will preserve the rights of patients at the expense of increased bureaucracy.
- It appears that psychiatrists will remain the gatekeepers to poorly resourced services, with secure services remaining inadequate.
- The Department of Health continues to use the term 'personality disorders' with reference to psychopathy.
- There is therefore the risk of medicalisation of offending, with blurring of the boundaries between mental health and criminal justice.

Scottish Executive 2000 Report of the committee on serious violent and sexual offenders. Scottish Executive, Edinburgh

- Scotland has developed different proposals
- Psychopathic individuals should be imprisoned if their offences warrant it and discretionary life sentences can address any persistent risk.
- Currently such sentences are only used in 2% of cases that would be eligible.
- Psychiatrists could have an advisory role.
- The courts should continue to decide on the appropriate disposal of high risk offenders.
- Psychological services must be enhanced.
- There should be legislation enabling movement between prison and secure hospitals.

- Forensic services could be expanded to enable them to provide support to police and probation services in the community.
- Multiagency protection panels should be the first port of call for referrals for future mental health assessment under the new legislation.
- At present the resources are not sufficient to provide mental health services to more than a handful of such panels.

Policy and Legislation

Justice for all

Criminal Justice System 2002 Justice for all. A White Paper. The Stationery Office, London[†]

This White Paper announced a programme of reform for the Criminal Justice System and outlined a long-term strategy that aims to modernise all aspects of the CJS from detection and rehabilitation of offenders to crime reduction.

Proposals include:
- a better deal for victims and witnesses
- fairer, more effective trials
- consistent sentencing
- more effective punishment and rehabilitation
- joined-up working – which includes the Crown Prosecution Service, the police and court administration.

The goal is for safe, strong communities. This will be addressed via:
- tough action on antisocial behaviour, hard drugs and violent crime
- rebalancing the CJS in favour of the victim
- giving the police and prosecution the tools to bring more criminals to justice.

The Paper states that the majority of crime is committed by a relatively small number of persistent offenders. There are weaknesses in the current system, with too few criminals being brought to justice, too many defendants who offend on bail, too much delay in bringing them to trial, too many guilty go unconvicted and too many who go without the sentence that they and society need.

Where a defendant is convicted, there will be actions to:
- ensure a focus on custody of dangerous, serious and seriously persistent offenders and those who consistently breach community sentences
- ensure that dangerous, violent and sexual offenders can be kept in custody for as long as they present a risk to the public

[†] Crown copyright. Reproduced with permission.

- ensure tough, more intensive community sentences with multiple conditions such as tagging, reparation, drug treatment and testing to deny liberty, rehabilitate the offender and protect the public
- ensure more uniformity in sentencing through a new Sentencing Guidelines Council
- enable courts to offer drug treatment as part of a community sentence for juveniles
- introduce a new sentence of Custody Minus – community supervision backed by automatic return to custody if the offender fails to comply with the conditions of their sentence
- introduce a new sentence of Custody Plus – to ensure that short sentence prisoners are properly supervised and supported after release
- introduce intermittent custody to enable use of weekend or night-time custody for low risk offenders.

Sentences for violent and sexual offenders

The government is determined to ensure that the public is properly protected from dangerous and sexual offenders. They recognise that this issue is of critical importance to the public and are determined to implement a range of proposals to address the fear many people have of being attacked, the anxiety faced by parents about the safety of their children, and to ensure that communities can live together without fear and distrust.

The Paper states that the government will overhaul sentences for violent and dangerous offenders and ensure that on release there are rigorous and ongoing supervision and public protection measures.

The government states that they will ensure that the public are adequately protected from those offenders whose offences do not currently attract a maximum penalty of life imprisonment but who are nevertheless assessed as dangerous. They believe that such offenders should remain in custody until their risks are considered manageable in the community. For this reason an indeterminate sentence for sexual and violent offenders who have been assessed and considered dangerous is proposed. The offender would be required to serve a minimum term and would then remain in prison beyond this time, until the Parole Board was completely satisfied that the risk had sufficiently diminished for that person to be released and supervised in the community. The offender could remain on licence for the rest of their life.

Plans to deal with dangerous people with severe personality disorder are already in place. Revisions to mental health legislation in the recently published Mental Health Bill will make it possible to detain individuals for as long as their disorder means that they continue to present a risk to the public, subject to review by a Mental Health Tribunal.

The government is considering a new Order to provide protection against dangerous and violent offenders, similar to the existing Sex Offenders Order. This will ensure that the police will have the right tools to manage such offenders in the community and deal with them effectively if they believe that the public is at risk of serious harm.

Policies on the protection of the public and punishment must always be the domain of Parliament and will be kept under review to ensure that this important principle is maintained, along with Parliament's duty and right to adequately protect the public it serves.

There will be a focus on:

- violent crime
- reducing domestic violence
- tackling street crime
- racist crime
- vehicle crime
- domestic burglary
- tackling antisocial behaviour
- building safer communities
- tackling drugs
- children and young people.

Antisocial behaviour

This refers to a collection of behaviours including threatening and intimidating people, vandalism and abandoning cars.

Antisocial Behaviour Orders have been created which prohibit individuals from certain acts or from entering particular areas, and often include prohibitions on inciting or encouraging others to commit specified antisocial acts.

For less severe behaviours, a more informal Acceptable Behaviour Contract may be appropriate.

Weblink Criminal Justice System for England and Wales –www.cjsonline.gov.uk.

Report of the Committee on Serious Violent and Sexual Offenders

Scottish Executive 2000 Report of the Committee on Serious Violent and Sexual Offenders (Chairman: Lord MacLean). Scottish Executive, Edinburgh. Online. Available: www.scotland.gov.uk/maclean/docs/svso-00.asp[†]

The MacLean Committee on Serious Violent and Sexual Offenders was established in March 1999.

Its remit was:

> To consider experience in Scotland and elsewhere and to make proposals for the sentencing disposals for, and the future management and treatment of, serious sexual and violent offenders who may present a continuing danger to the public, in particular:

- to consider whether the current legislative framework matches the present level of knowledge of the subject, provides the courts with an appropriate range of options and affords the general public adequate protection from these offenders
- to compare practice, diagnosis and treatment with that elsewhere, to build on current expertise and research to inform the development of a medical protocol to respond to the needs of personality disordered offenders
- to specify the services required by this group of offenders and the means of delivery
- to consider the question of release/discharge into the community and service needs in the community for supervising those offenders.

Definition

The concern of the Committee is reducing the continuing risk to the public from serious violent and sexual crime. Such offenders are not best identified solely in terms of the particular offence for which they are convicted, or a particular characteristic such as personality disorder. It is possible to identify, by structured assessment, offenders who present particularly high risks to the safety of the public. Such offenders are referred to as 'high risk offenders' throughout the report.

Risk assessment

- Formalised risk assessment should be used to a greater degree throughout the criminal justice process, based on best available evidence.
- Risk assessment methods have become available in recent years which have improved the ability to predict risk of future violence.
- Structured clinical judgement, which takes into account historical factors shown empirically to have a bearing on risk, together with individual significant factors, should continue to be developed.

Risk Management Authority

This body would have three roles in relation to risk assessment and risk management:
- policy
- standard-setting
- operational management.

Sentencing

The range of current sentencing options is adequate for the majority of offenders.

A new sentence, based on risk, is required for high risk offenders. The sentence would remain in force for the offender's entire life. This is the Order for Lifelong Restriction.

Order for Lifelong Restriction

This sentence would:
- be imposed if a person was found by the High Court to be a high risk offender following an accredited risk assessment
- be lifelong
- begin with a custodial sentence, the minimum length of which would be based on punishment for the index offence, and which would continue for an indeterminate period established by the offender's level of ongoing risk
- be based on close supervision upon release, the nature of which would also be based upon risk
- be based on swift and predictable recall to custody at any time if licence conditions are breached.

The option to impose an OLR would only be available in the High Court.

Offenders with mental disorders

Some high risk offenders suffer from mental disorders. Their offending may (wholly or in part) or may not be related to their mental disorder.

As with non-mentally disordered offenders, a thorough assessment of risk is required in the case of potential high risk offenders. However, there is also a need to thoroughly assess mental state over a period of months to decide on the appropriate disposal.

An interim hospital order, lasting a maximum of 12 months, should be imposed in all cases where:
- the offender is an appropriate candidate for assessment to determine whether they meet the statutory criteria for the imposition of an OLR, *but*
- there is evidence that the offender may be suffering from a mental disorder for which treatment is appropriate.

If an offender is high risk and suffers from a mental disorder that meets the criteria for compulsory detention, the sentence should be an OLR together with a hospital direction. If an offender is high risk but does not meet the statutory criteria for such detention, the sentence should be an OLR.

If a person who is mentally disordered is found insane in bar of trial or acquitted on the grounds of insanity and is found to be a high risk offender, the disposal should be a hospital order with restrictions.

Designated Life Tribunal

Decisions on release and recall to prison of high risk offenders serving OLRs would be the responsibility of the Parole Board, acting through a Designated Life Tribunal. Such decisions would be informed by the risk assessment and management plan. The Designated Life Tribunal should have a new power to order a future release date, dependent on progress.

Offenders with personality disorder

The Committee's recommendations are based on the importance of the identification and management of high risk offenders, whether personality disordered or not. It has, however, considered the issue of personality disorder, particularly severe antisocial personality disorder, its relationship with serious offending, and its management and treatment.

There are many types of personality disorder, the majority of which are not related to an increased likelihood of offending.

The type and degree of personality disorder most closely linked to offending is severe personality disorder. It is not known how many serious violent or sexual offenders have severe personality disorder. However, among Scotland's total sentenced male prison population it has been estimated that 6–8% have severe antisocial personality disorder.

'Medical protocol'

It is not appropriate to develop a 'medical protocol' for serious offenders with personality disorder. Consideration should be given to the development of national guidelines for personality disorder in general by the Scottish Intercollegiate Guidelines Network.

Modern mental health models of care sit uneasily with the management of challenging, manipulative offenders with severe antisocial personality disorder.

Present understanding does not support compulsory hospitalisation and medical treatment for severe antisocial personality disorder. Compulsory admissions to hospital based on personality disorder are presently extremely rare in Scotland. Serious violent or sexual offenders with personality disorders and no other mental disorders should continue, in the main, to serve prison sentences rather than be sent to hospital.

Treatment – Psychological Therapies

Family and parenting interventions in children and adolescents with conduct disorder

Woolfenden SR, Williams K, Peat J 2001 Family and parenting interventions in children and adolescents with conduct disorder and delinquency aged 10–17 (Cochrane Review). In: The Cochrane Library, Issue 2. CD003015. Update Software, Oxford

- Eight trials were suitable for inclusion ($n = 749$).
- Results showed that family and parenting interventions for juvenile delinquents and their families lead to significant reductions in time spent in institutions.
- There was also a significant reduction in re-arrest rates and in the rate of re-arrest at 1–3 years.
- However, there was marked heterogeneity in the results.
- No significant difference was found for psychosocial outcomes such as family functioning and child/ adolescent behaviour.

See also the 'Treatment – Psychological therapies' section in Chapter 5 (Child and adolescent psychiatry), page 78.

Interventions for learning disabled sex offenders

Ashman L, Duggan L 2002 Interventions for learning disabled sex offenders **(Cochrane Review)**. In: The Cochrane Library, Issue 2. CD003682. Update Software, Oxford

- No randomised controlled trial evidence was found regarding the use of interventions for learning disabled sex offenders.

Management for people with disorders of sexual preferences and for convicted sexual offenders

White P, Bradley C, Ferriter M, Hatzipetrou L 1998 Management for people with disorders of sexual preferences and for convicted sexual offenders **(Cochrane Review)**. In: The Cochrane Library, Issue 4. CD000251. Update Software, Oxford

- This area lacks a strong evidence base.
- A single trial found that medroxyprogesterone acetate given alongside imaginal desensitisation was no better than imaginal desensitisation alone in the treatment of problematic/anomalous sexual behaviour and desire.
- A relapse prevention programme showed a trend towards reduction in non-sexual violent crimes while having no effect on sex offending levels.
- A large pragmatic trial investigated the effects of group therapy on rates of recidivism in sex offenders and showed no beneficial effects.

Psychodynamic lessons in risk assessment and management

Doctor R 2004 Psychodynamic lessons in risk assessment and management. Advances in Psychiatric Treatment 10: 267–276

Highlights the two conceptual approaches to risk assessment and management – the actuarial and the clinical.

Actuarial approach

- Details facts about the patient from history as well as current presentation.
- A formula is then used to weight the facts and predict the chance of future risk.
- One of the problems is that these judgements are subjective clinical judgements.

Clinical approach

- The more reliable approach.
- Assessment of risk following clinical assessment of the individual.
- Focus on depth and breadth of clinical experience.

Psychodynamic approaches can be helpful in enabling the patient to become aware of their own mind and its function. It is thought that although such an approach may initially be distressing, it could eventually lead to a healthier and more stable internal reality which would subsequently reduce the risk of violent behaviour. Using psychodynamic methods the inner world of the patient is explored, within an environment that is safe. Using conscious countertransference can in most cases be controlled and can be extremely useful in recognising the person's personality and way of interacting with others.

Often the level of risk can be underestimated by the professional as the person with a dangerous/psychotic state of mind tends to minimise or rationalise their behaviour. Patients with personality disorders can often make us feel manipulated and provoked, making the professional feel hostile, rejecting and abusive. It is therefore very important to recognise and tolerate unbearable psychic pain; in fact, failure to recognise the unconscious communications of the patient can lead to inadequate assessment and even the chance of escalating violence.

A psychodynamic approach can present alternative ways of examining the patient's mind and how past violence resides in that mind. It is also useful in identifying why certain patients cannot summon the defences to prevent the discharge of violent impulses. It must be remembered that environment also has effects. Psychoanalytical approaches are particularly useful when dealing with paraphilias and borderline states.

Patients with both of these disorders operate a paradox which means that a distorted and misrepresented reality is created. In borderline states, attempts are made to reconcile contradictory ideas that can no longer exist as separate entities, with aggression and violence resulting if the solution is inadequate to contain the internal conflict.

People in the 'borderline position' can therefore misinterpret reality, despite not being psychotic, and therefore live in an unreal world with illusion and fantasy.

Hinshelwood RD 1999 The difficult patient. The role for 'scientific psychiatry' in understanding patients with chronic schizophrenia or severe personality disorder. British Journal of Psychiatry 174: 187–190

- Talks of a 'scientific attitude'.
- Defines workers as retreating emotionally from the difficult and potentially violent patient.
- This may, in fact, encourage the psychotic patient's removal or usual rapport with others.

Bion WR 1957 Differentiation of the psychotic from non-psychotic personalities. In: Second thoughts: selected papers on psychoanalysis. Jason Aronson, New York, pp 43–46

- Described two parts of the mind:
  - a non-psychotic part, capable of reflective thinking
  - a psychotic part, which is more primitive and results from a hatred of psychic reality.
- As far as possible patients will present the non-psychotic part which can then lead to a potential underestimation of the risks.

Gelder M, Gath D, Mayou R et al 1998 Oxford textbook of psychiatry, 3rd edn. Oxford University Press, Oxford

- 90% of psychotic patients present with a lack of insight which translates to denial and rationalisation.

Freud S 1955 Neurosis and psychosis. In: Strachey J (ed. and trans.) Standard edition of the complete works of Sigmund Freud, Vol. 23. Hogarth Press, London, pp 195–204

- Psychotic patients seek refuge in an unreal state as they cannot tolerate either their inner or external world.
- The refuge is reinforced by secret beliefs disguised in perversions.
- If they can maintain a psychic homoeostasis they can function reasonably well.
- When there is a threat to this equilibrium they often attend for treatment.

Glasser M 1979 Some aspects of the role of aggression in the perversions. In: Rosen I (ed.) Sexual deviation. Oxford University Press, Oxford

- Describes the core complex of paraphilias.
- This is the interrelationship between feelings, ideas and attitudes that stems from early experiences.
- There is also the persistence of primitive levels of functioning.
- In males he suggests that a longing to be close to mother is ultimately dangerous and leads to the loss of self.
- The conflict of the wish to merge with mother and the fear of complete loss of self can create a claustrophobic

feeling in the consulting room and almost invariably the patient acts out, classically, by missing sessions.

- Aggression is also a component of the core complex.
- The ego attempts to resolve the vicious circle of dangers and conflicts by the use of sexualisation, with aggression potentially becoming sadistic.
- Destruction is converted to a desire to hurt and control.
- In sadistic sexual crimes the understanding of a person as a separate and real object decreases and can even be completely lost.

Minne C 2003 A psychoanalytic aspect to the risk containment of dangerous patients treated in high security hospitals. In: Doctor R (ed.) Dangerous patients: a psychodynamic approach to risk assessment and management. Karnac, London

- Talks about the role of the psychotherapist in the management of dangerous patients.
- Suggested potential roles are:
  - monitoring the internal state of the patient and therefore the level of risk
  - supervising other team members – for example, to discuss splitting, which is extremely common in these cases
  - improving awareness of the unconscious processes at work.
- Minne also suggests that professionals be aware of the new-found appreciation that the patient's own mind can be assaultative to their internal world.
- Conflict may arise between confidentiality with regard to the patient and the need to share information with the patient.
- Patients should be empowered and enabled to share information themselves. If this is not possible, the proposed sharing of information should be discussed with the patient first.

Psychological interventions for those who have sexually offended or are at risk of offending

Kenworthy T, Adams CE, Bilby C, Brooks-Gordon D, Fenton M 2003 Psychological interventions for those who have sexually offended or are at risk of **(Cochrane Review)**. In: The Cochrane Library, Issue 4. CD004858. Update Software, Oxford

- Nine RCTS of over 500 males with follow-up of over a decade were included.
- CBT (group therapy) may reduce re-offending rates at 1 year for child molesters compared with standard care (NNT 6).

- A trial comparing psychodynamic group therapy with no treatment for 231 men guilty of paedophilia, exhibitionism or sexual assault found that re-arrest over 10 years was greater for the treatment group, but this was not statistically significant.

Assessment Tools and Rating Scales

Historical, Clinical, Risk-20 (HCR-20)

Webster CD, Douglas KS, Eaves D et al 1997 HCR-20: assessing risk of violence (version 2). Mental Health Law, Policy Institute, Simon Fraser University, Vancouver, BC

- The original HCR-20 was modified following initial clinical trials.
- Intended for use with civil and forensic psychiatric and criminal justice populations.
- 20 items including the Hare PCL-SV.
- 10 historical variables.
- Five clinical variables.
- Five risk management factors.
- Each item is scored:
  - not present (0)
  - possibly present (1)
  - definitely present (2)
- Yields a total score out of 40.

Psychopathy Checklist-Revised (PCL-R)

Hare RD 1991 Manual for the Hare Psychopathy Checklist-Revised. Multi-Health Systems, Toronto, Canada

- 20-item rating scale, each item rated 0 (does not apply) to 2 (definitely applies).
- Designed to measure traits of personality disorder.
- Items:
  - Glibness/superficial charm
  - Grandiose sense of self-worth
  - Need for stimulation/proneness to boredom
  - Pathological lying
  - Conning/manipulative
  - Lack of remorse or guilt
  - Shallow affect
  - Callous/lack of empathy
  - Parasitic lifestyle
  - Poor behavioural control
  - Promiscuous sexual behaviour
  - Early behavioural problems

- Lack of realistic, long-term goals
- Impulsivity
- Irresponsibility
- Failure to accept responsibility for own actions
- Many short-term marital relationships
- Juvenile delinquency
- Revocation of conditional release
- Criminal versatility.
- Scored on the basis of both semi-structured and collateral information.
- Validated in adult male correctional and forensic psychiatric populations.
- Research has shown that it is a reasonable predictor of violence across diverse populations.
- It is a tool to identify psychopathy – not a risk assessment tool.

Psychopathy Checklist-Screening version (PCL-SV)

> Hart SD, Cox DN, Hare RD 1995 The Hare Psychopathy Checklist – screening version (PCL-SV). Multi-Health Systems, Toronto, Canada

- 12-item abbreviated tool designed to screen for the possible presence of psychopathy.
- Based on a subset of the PCL-R, it is particularly well suited for community samples.
- If the score is suggestive of psychopathy, a full PCL-R is completed.

Sexual Violence Risk-20 (SVR-20)

> Boer DP, Hart SD, Kropp PR et al 1997 Manual for sexual violence risk-20: professional guidelines for assessing risk of sexual violence. British Columbia Institute on Family Violence, Vancouver, BC

- 20-item guide for assessing risk of violence in sex offenders.
- 11 items deal with psychosocial adjustment.
- Seven items deal with sexual offences.
- Two items deal with future plans.
- Each item is scored:
  - definitely not present   **N**
  - possibly present   **P**
  - definitely present   **Y**
- Mainly used to help structure clinical assessments.

Static 99

> Hanson RK, Thornton D 1999 Static 99. Solicitor General of Canada, Ottawa, Ontario

- 10-item actuarial tool designed to assess the long-term potential for sexual recidivism among adult male sex offenders.
- Incorporates RRASOR (Rapid Risk Assessment for Sex Offender Recidivism, 4-item screening instrument) factors.
- Used predominantly within the correctional system.

RRASOR items

- Prior sexual charges or convictions
- Victim gender
- Age
- Relationship to victim.

Additional to RRASOR items

- Prior sentencing dates
- Non-contact offences
- Index non-sexual violence
- Prior non-sexual violence
- Stranger victim
- Single.

Violence Risk Appraisal Guide (VRAG)

> Harris GT, Rice ME 1993 Actuarial assessment of risk among sex offenders. Annals of the New York Academy of Sciences 989: 198–210

- 12-item actuarial scale which has been widely used to predict the risk of violence within a specific time frame following the release of violent mentally disordered offenders.
- Developed at the Penetanguishene Mental Health Centre.
- Uses clinical records, particularly psychosocial history, as the basis for scoring.
- Incorporates the PCL-R in the calculation of risk.

Gender

General Topics

Do men need special services?

Kennedy H 2001 Do men need special services? Advances in Psychiatric Treatment 7: 93–99

It is well recognised that males have higher rates of developmental and conduct disorders, a higher prevalence of addiction problems (predominant in prison populations) and have a rising suicide rate in younger men. Epidemiological studies note the higher prevalence of depression and anxiety disorders in women and some studies suggest that severe mental illness is as common in males and as it is females. It could be argued that the differences in figures for suicide rates and the prevalence of mental illness may reflect flaws in epidemiological screening instruments rather than real differences.

Historically, many services have been separated by gender and while education establishments and military services etc. have moved towards integration, prisons and high secure hospitals have tended to maintain segregation. This may reflect a male preponderance in these services or segregation due to perceived risk. It is likely that mixed gender services are more therapeutic. Only a small proportion of men need to be within an all-male environment in order to ensure the safety of any women.

Professionals should consider unrecognised morbidity that may account for the apparent epidemiological gap between suicide and psychiatric disorder rates for men and women. These might include distorted grief reactions, rage attacks, attachment disorders and paraphilias. Alternatives include disorders of habit and impulse related to addictions, such as repetitive self-harm, pathological gambling and kleptomania.

Specialist treatment services for men would address disorders that occur only or most commonly in men in a manner that is acceptable and accessible. Consideration of the adverse effects of medication for patients with severe and enduring mental illness should be addressed. Impotence, loss of assertiveness, loss of self-confidence and loss of energy due to sedation can impact on compliance and the therapeutic relationship.

Redman S, Webb GR, Hennrikus DJ et al 1991 The effects of gender on diagnosis of psychological disturbance. Journal of Behavioural Medicine 14: 527–540

- Mental illness is more likely to go unrecognised in men, particularly in primary care.

Office for National Statistics 1998 Psychiatric morbidity among prisoners in England and Wales. The Stationery Office, London

- Men with severe mental illness, addictions and affective disorders are overrepresented in forensic populations when compared with the general population.
- This includes court diversion schemes, prison populations and secure facilities.
- The mental health problems of these men had not been recognised by primary care or mental health services.
- The consequences of illness can lead to criminalisation.

Humphries MS, Johnstone EC, MacMillan JF et al 1992 Dangerous behaviour preceding first admissions for schizophrenia. British Journal of Psychiatry 161: 501–505

- Found that the first presentation of severe mental illness in many cases is to the police or to the criminal justice system.

Drever F, Bunting J 1997 Patterns and trends in male mortality. In: Drever F, Whitehead M (eds) Health inequalities. The Stationery Office, London

- Suicide in young men in inner cities is rising at a time when rates for suicide in other groups are falling.
- Suggests that services are not recognising these individuals.

Boardman AP 1987 The General Health Questionnaire and the detection of emotional disorder by general practitioners. A replicated study. British Journal of Psychiatry 151: 373–381

- Men prefer to disclose symptoms of mental illness to female general practitioners.

Oriel KA, Fleming MF 1998 Screening men for partner violence in a primary care setting. A new strategy for detecting domestic violence. Journal of Family Practice 46: 493–498

- Little is known about the long-term sequelae of physical and sexual abuse in males.
- Men who are violent to their partners are more likely to have been abused themselves in childhood, to have a depressive disorder and to be heavy users of alcohol.

King MB 1990 Male rape. British Medical Journal 302: 179

- Sexual assault is not reported or recognised in men as it is in women, despite the fact that the long-term sequelae can be just as severe.

Fava GA, Anderson K, Rosenbaum JF 1990 'Anger attacks': possible variants of panic and major depressive disorders. American Journal of Psychiatry 147: 867–870

- The equivalence between panic and rage in terms of psychopharmacology and physiology is noted.
- Men are more likely to display anger or rage.
- Women are more likely to display fear or panic.
- Both behaviours impact on the family system.
- For men, domestic demands may be met and a powerful image established.
- For women, control can be established via dependence on the family system.

Needs of women patients with mental illness

Ramsay R, Welch S, Youard E 2001 Needs of women patients with mental illness. Advances in Psychiatric Treatment 7: 85–92

There are differences in the prevalence rates for specific psychiatric disorders in women and differences in how they present and how they are managed. Instruments to measure the needs of individual patients are generally not gender specific. Differences may reflect the cultural norms in the way that men and women communicate and interact with services. They may also reflect the attitudes and behaviour of health professionals around gender differences.

Gaps and deficiencies in services are noted for women with eating disorders, women-only services for those who have been physically or sexually abused, and women requiring medium secure forensic placement. Mothers who distrust services, perhaps because they fear their children may be taken in to care, may not seek professional help. This may also be true for young and inexperienced mothers. Single teenage mothers may be particularly vulnerable.

Long-term sequelae of abuse, childhood sexual abuse, domestic violence and rape should be considered. The benefits and difficulties of gaining employment are important. Minority groups may have specific problems. This can include a double stigma in lesbian and bisexual women with mental illness and the cultural barriers to gaining psychiatric services for women from different ethnic backgrounds. The number of women living alone increases with age. The psychosocial and employment history of older women may not be viewed as relevant and they may be labelled as being a generic old lady.

Johnson S, Buszewicz M 1996 Women's mental illness. In: Abel K, Buszewicz M, Davidson S et al (eds) Planning community mental health services for women. A multiprofessional handbook. Routledge, London, pp 6–19

- There are links between neurotic disorders and social factors.
- Research into the possibility of social factors as a cause for the gender differences in the rates of psychiatric illness has been prompted by the higher levels of anxiety and depression in women.
- General practitioners are more likely to refer men to secondary care.

Castle DJ, Murray RM 1991 The neurodevelopmental basis of sex differences in schizophrenia. Psychological Medicine 21: 565–575

- This study attributed gender differences in schizophrenia to aetiological factors.
- Men are more likely to have a neurodevelopmental form of the illness and women a stronger genetic component.

Gold JH 1998 Gender differences in psychiatric illness and treatments. Journal of Nervous and Mental Disease 186: 769–775

- There are differences in the response to drug treatment due to hormonal differences.

- Oestrogen could potentiate the effects of neuroleptic medications so that women require a lower dose.

Goldberg D, Huxley P 1992 Common mental disorders. Routledge, London

- Women are more likely than men to present to their general practitioner with physical and psychological complaints.

Department of Health 2000 In-patients formally detained in hospitals under the Mental Health Act 1983 and other legislation, England: 1988–89 to 1998–99. DH, London

- In 1991/1992 the number of men detained under the Mental Health Act became higher than the number of women detained for the first time.
- Between 1988/89 and 1998/99 the number of women being detained increased but the rate of increase was higher for men.

Perkins RE, Rowland LA 1991 Sex differences in service usage in long-term psychiatric care. Are women adequately served? British Journal of Psychiatry 158(10): 75–79

- Older women with severe and enduring mental illness who are looked after by continuing care services receive less intensive input than their male counterparts.
- Women account for a higher proportion of those in day services for people with a low level of function than men.

Potts MK, Burnam MA, Wells KB 1991 Gender differences in depression detection: a comparison of clinician diagnosis and standardized assessment. Psychological Assessment 3: 609–615

- Male and female doctors were more likely to diagnose depression in women in a group of patients who all met the diagnostic criteria for depression.

Cooper H, Arber S, Fee I et al 1999 The influence of social support and social capital on health. Health Education Authority, London

- The health of women is more closely linked to social environment than the health of men.

Millar J 1992 State, family and personal responsibility: the changing balance for lone mothers in the UK. In: Ungerson C, Kember M (eds) Women and social policy, 2nd edn. Macmillan, Basingstoke, pp 146–162

- Britain has a lone parent family rate of 17%, which is among the highest in Europe.

Pound A, Abel K 1996 Motherhood and mental illness. In: Abel K, Buszewicz M, Davidson S et al (eds) Planning community mental health services for women. A multiprofessional handbook. Routledge, London, pp 20–35

- Women who had poor experiences of parenting can find it difficult to receive practical help with child care and social support when they become parents themselves.

Nicholson J, Geller JL, Fisher WH et al 1993 State policies and programs that address the needs of mentally ill mothers in the public sector. Hospital and Community Psychiatry 44: 484–489

- Health professionals involved with mothers with severe mental illness may not see themselves as having a role with regard to parenting issues.
- Child care issues may be viewed as a matter for social services.

Aruffo JF, Coverdale JH, Chacko RC et al 1990 Knowledge about AIDS among women psychiatric outpatients. Hospital and Community Psychiatry 41: 326–328

- Unplanned pregnancies can arise due to a lack of understanding regarding contraception in women with mental illness.

Franklin BJ 1998 Forms and functions: assessing housing need in the community care context. Health and Social Care in the Community 6: 420–428

- There is a lack of planning regarding the needs of communities with respect to housing and in particular the need for appropriate housing for homeless women with psychiatric illness.

Marshall M, Reed JL 1992 Psychiatric morbidity in homeless women. British Journal of Psychiatry 160: 761–768

- Homeless women have:
  - better social support networks than homeless men
  - lower levels of substance misuse
  - higher levels of psychiatric illness.

Definition

Health care need – the population's ability to benefit from healthcare. (*Source:* Stevens A, Rafferty J 1994 Health care needs assessment: the epidemiologically based needs assessment reviews. Radcliffe Medical Press, Oxford.)

Psychiatric services for women

Kohen D 2001 Psychiatric services for women. Advances in Psychiatric Treatment 7: 328–334

There are arguments for and against the provision of specialised psychiatric services for women. Specialist treatment may lead to segregation and a belief that general psychiatrists do not have a role in their treatment. On the other hand, there is evidence that specific needs of women can be neglected. These include mental illness in pregnant women and mothers, domestic violence and child abuse, vulnerability, stigma and victimisation.

Comorbid illness and the way in which psychiatric illness presents are also important issues. The differences between genders in the course of schizophrenia and bipolar disorders are well established, as are differences in the risk of developing side effects with psychotropic medication. Eating disorders occur predominantly in women.

When planning psychiatric services for women a number of factors should be considered. These include demographic variables (birth rates, rates of single parenthood and ethnic mix), deprivation indices and statistical information on the prevalence of deliberate self-harm, domestic violence and sexual abuse.

The provision of women-specific psychiatric services in the community can begin within an established general community team on a keyworker basis. This team can liaise with general services, gather information regarding unmet needs and offer advice and education on gender-specific issues such as pregnancy, breast feeding and mothering. Establishing links with other organisations will also be a function of the team and may include ethnic women's organisations and organisations for mental health. Specific organisations may include MIND, the Association for Postnatal Illness and the National Childbirth Trust.

Meltzer H, Gill B, Petticrew M et al 1995 The prevalence of psychiatric morbidity among adults living in private households. Office of Population Censuses and Surveys of Psychiatric Morbidity in Great Britain. Report I. HMSO, London

- The prevalence of a number of disorders is higher in women.
- These include depression, dysthymia, seasonal affective disorder, generalised anxiety disorders, panic attacks, phobias and deliberate self-harm.

Kessler RC, McGonagle KA, Zhao S et al 1994 Lifetime and 12 months prevalence of DSM-III-R psychiatric disorders in the United States. Archives of General Psychiatry 51: 8–19

- The lifetime prevalence of major depression in women is almost twice that in men.
- Depression occurs in more than one in five women.

Maden T 1996 A psychiatric profile in female prison population. In: Women, prisons and psychiatry. Butterworth-Heinemann, Oxford

- There are more than 3000 women in British prisons, over half of whom would warrant a psychiatric diagnosis.

Angermeyer MC, Kuhn L, Goldstein JM 1990 Gender and the course of schizophrenia in treated outcomes. Schizophrenia Bulletin 16: 293–307

- Women with severe and enduring mental illness have lower levels of rehospitalisation and a shorter length of inpatient stay than men.

Vaughn CE, Snyder KS, Jones S et al 1984 Family factors in schizophrenia relapse. Replication in California of British research on expressed emotion. Archives of General Psychiatry 41: 1169–1177

- Women with severe and enduring mental illness are less sensitive and respond less to expressed emotion.

Kohen D 1999 Specialised in-patient psychiatric services for women. Psychiatric Bulletin 23: 31–33

- A number of single gender acute psychiatric wards exist where motherhood is an important aspect of assessment.
- Difficulties arise due to a lack of cohesion between inpatient and community services.

Fenton W, Mosher L, Herrell J et al 1998 Randomised trial of general hospital and residential alternative care for patients with severe and persistent mental illness. American Journal of Psychiatry 155: 516–522

- The commonest community facilities for women with severe and enduring mental illness tend to be hostels.
- There is increasing occurrence of community treatment of acute mental illness and increasing numbers of women-only community placements.

Royal College of Psychiatrists 1992 Report of the General Psychiatry Section Working Party on post-natal illness. Psychiatric Bulletin 16: 519–522

- Inappropriate use of mother and baby units and difficulties in establishing guidelines for their use have led ultimately to bed closures.

Violence in women with psychosis

Dean K, Walsh E, Moran P et al 2006 Violence in women with psychosis in the community: prospective study. British Journal of Psychiatry 188: 264–270

There have been few studies of gender and violence for patients living in the community. Previous research has noted associations between violence in people with psychotic illness and substance misuse, non-compliance with medication, personality disorder and active psychotic symptoms.

Method

- 304 women with chronic psychosis who live in the community were studied.
- The rates of physical assault carried out by this group were studied prospectively over a 2-year period.
- Demographic and clinical factors were recorded as potential predictors of assault.
- Information was collected by interview, case note review and a number of assessment tools and rating scales.
- The criminal records of patients were obtained from the British Home Office.

Results

- The rate of assault over the 2-year period was 17%.
- Associations were found between carrying out an assault and:
  - previous violence
  - non-violent convictions
  - victimisation
  - being of African–Caribbean ethnic origin
  - cluster B personality disorder
  - high levels of unmet need.
- Almost one in five of the population studied carried out an assault during the 2-year period.

See also the 'General topics' section in Chapter 26 (Schizophrenia), page 378.

Policy and Legislation

Safety, privacy and dignity in mental health units

NHS Executive 2000 Safety, privacy and dignity in mental health units. Guidance on mixed sex accommodation for mental health services. NHS Executive, Leeds[†]

NHS Trusts need to ensure that all patients are protected from physical, psychological or sexual harm while they are being treated in mental health facilities, and to recognise that the needs of male and female patients may be different.

Mixed sex accommodation is to be phased out and eliminated in 95% of health authority areas by 2002.

[†] Crown copyright. Reproduced with permission.

Ward environment and culture

Assessment

- The initial assessment of each patient's needs should include consideration of the risk of the patient being abused, or of abusing others. Staff should find out if the patient would prefer to stay in a single-sex or mixed environment.
- Assessment should aim to identify at an early stage any patients who may be predatory or likely to abuse or offend. This may require proactive management to prevent inappropriate/unwanted behaviour. Similarly, patients at risk of self-harm should be identified.
- Risk assessment and management should be a continuous prominent feature of care plans. They should identify patients who are known to be vulnerable because of their illness or likely behaviour. Individual strategies may need to be developed for vulnerable patients – for example, where patients may be sexually disinhibited because of their illness.

Support

- Women patients should have access to a female member of staff at all times, and an escort of the same gender should always be available (particularly in secure psychiatric facilities when a patient poses a risk of escaping). Staff carrying out physical examinations should either be of the same sex or there should be a same sex chaperone present. Women should have access to appropriate toiletries and sanitary protection.
- Where possible, women patients should have the opportunity to associate together in women-only lounge areas, if they so wish, and take part in women-only therapy groups and social activities. This should apply particularly in units where women patients are in the minority (e.g. in some secure settings).
- Patients should be given access to local organisations, advocacy projects, and religious and cultural groups from their own ethnic community. Voluntary organisations and/or local user groups should be involved in planning, evaluating and monitoring of services.
- Women should have access, where possible, to a female doctor for physical health care, if they so wish.
- Patients should be given clear information on how to raise concerns and to whom.

Security

- If restraint is used, a member of staff of the same sex should be present as soon as possible.
- Single rooms are helpful in promoting privacy, but there should be an overarching, fail-safe system for entry into rooms if staff are concerned about patients' security. It is important that an assessment is made of the patient's vulnerability to self-harm and/or suicide before placing any patient in single room accommodation.
- Toilet and bathing facilities should be clearly labelled in a way that can be understood by patients from minority ethnic groups and those with visual or cognitive impairment. They should be designated male or female

and located in separate areas, close to male/female sleeping areas.

Supervision

* Ward managers should ensure that there is appropriate observation of all women patients who have been assessed as being at risk or vulnerable to sexual exploitation by men. Similarly, ward managers should ensure that patients who are regarded as a risk to others are appropriately supervised. Women patients and vulnerable men should have appropriate staff supervision at night to make them feel safe.

Patients with special needs

Older people

* Older people, especially women, tend to find mixed sex accommodation less acceptable than younger people.
* Older people may be more sensitive to mixing with members of the opposite sex, and less willing to voice any complaints.
* Arrangements also need to take account of any physical frailty. Older people with disabilities are more likely to require assistance with intimate personal care so there

needs to be sufficient staff of appropriate gender for these care tasks.

* Disinhibition and inappropriate sexual behaviour are common features of dementia so units for such patients need both space to move about but also sufficient rooms to allow privacy.

Children and young people

* There is specific guidance available regarding facilities for children and young people.
* Where, exceptionally, children or adolescents have to be admitted to adult wards, separate written guidance is to be drawn up that takes account of any special risks to them or needs they may have arising from their age and/or illness.

Mothers and babies

* Mother and baby units should be self-contained and separate from the general psychiatric ward. Health visiting staff or, where appropriate, midwifery staff attend the mother and baby in hospital. Where opportunities arise as a result of refurbishment or the design of new facilities, consideration must be given to providing accommodation that has the flexibility to meet individual needs.

General psychiatry

12

General topics

Assessing violence risk in general adult psychiatry

Higgins N, Watts D, Bindman J, Slade M, Thornicroft G 2005 Assessing violence risk in general adult psychiatry. Psychiatric Bulletin 29: 131–133

Aims

- To investigate current practice in assessment of risk of harm to others in general adult psychiatry services.
- To review risk assessment documentation in use.

Method

- Two consultant psychiatrists from each of 66 trusts in England were randomly selected.
- They were sent a brief, semi-structured interview regarding risk assessment documentation, training and local guidelines.

Results

- The responses suggest that most trusts have standard risk forms incorporating the assessment of violence.
- Around half of the trusts provide training for the use of their standard risk assessments.
- Almost half of consultants had not attended training.
- There was striking variation in the risk assessment forms, both in content and complexity.
- Structured narrative sections seemed to combine the best elements of actuarial and clinical risk assessment,

allowing the focus of inquiry to be directed and for the risk factors to be seen in context.
- The rationale behind scoring or grading systems to summarise findings was not clear. Scores may be reproducible and seem scientific, but their validity is questionable.
- There was often a lack of direction noted in how to interpret the results.
- A narrative summation was thought to be useful in collating what is known about the patient, allowing the balancing of risk and mitigating factors.
- Around half the forms did not include a plan for managing risk.
- Although clinical management plans are detailed elsewhere in CPA documentation, they are not specific to risk.
- There is wide variation in risk assessment tools across the country.
- There is a need for consensus with regard to what risk assessment should entail in general psychiatry.

See also the 'General topics' section in Chapter 10 (Forensic psychiatry), pages 153, 155-157 and 162.

The beginning of the end for the Kraepelinian dichotomy

Craddock N, Owen MJ 2005 The beginning of the end for the Kraepelinian dichotomy. British Journal of Psychiatry 186: 364–366

The Kraepelinian dichotomy is the term used to describe the long-held assumption that schizophrenia and bipolar disorder are distinct entities, with separate underlying disease processes and treatments. However, many individuals with severe psychiatric illness have concurrent mood and psychotic symptoms. There may not be a clear biological distinction between the two disorders. Molecular genetic studies are beginning to challenge and may soon contradict the traditional dichotomous view.

Kraepelin used clinical features, outcome and family history in the absence of laboratory tests, as do modern operational classifications. The fact that the disorders tend to breed true gave weight to the argument in favour of a biological distinction. The disorders also have different clinical features and outcomes.

The dichotomous view has formed the basis of the operational diagnostic criteria. This has added rigour and reproducibility to psychiatric research.

Recent findings are compatible with a model of functional psychosis in which susceptibility to a spectrum of clinical phenotypes is under the influence of overlapping sets of genes, which – in addition to environmental factors – determine the individual's expression of illness.

A multidimensional approach would allow the overlap of functional psychosis, bipolar disorder and other disorders. The writers argue for changes in classification to benefit patients and to increase the professional standing of psychiatry. Patients want a clear and unambiguous diagnosis but psychiatrists may be reluctant to arrive at a diagnosis prematurely. A spectrum classification may enable clinicians to provide a clearer diagnosis.

Spectrum disorders such as 'psychosis spectrum illness' or 'mood reality disorder' are suggested with the understanding that specific tests and a period of observation may be required to clarify the likely course of illness and response to treatment.

Crow TJ 1990 The continuum of psychosis and its genetic origins. The sixty-fifth Maudsley lecture. British Journal of Psychiatry 156: 788–797

- The categorical approach should be abandoned.
- A dimensional or continuous formulation is favoured.
- There are insufficient robust scientific data.
- There are difficulties in applying dimensional classifications in clinical practice and research.

Craddock N, O'Donovan MC, Owen MJ 2005 Genetics of schizophrenia and bipolar disorder: dissecting of psychosis. Journal of Medical Genetics 42: 193–204

- Family studies suggest overlap between schizophrenia and bipolar illness.
- There is also an overlap between schizophrenia, bipolar disorder and schizoaffective disorder.
- A twin study which did not use hierarchical classification systems demonstrated an overlap in the genetic susceptibility to mania and schizophrenia.

- It confirmed that there are genes specific to the two prototypal disorders.
- Genes have been identified which seem to confer risk of both schizophrenia and bipolar disorder.
- 13q is implicated in both. DISC1 (disrupted in schizophrenia 1) is interrupted in a family in which both schizophrenia and bipolar disorder co-segregate with a chromosomal translocation.

Cardno AG, Rijsdijk FV, Sham PC et al 2002 A twin study of genetic relationships between psychotic symptoms. American Journal of Psychiatry 159: 539–545

- There is evidence for genes that confer susceptibility to both disorders.

Berrettini W 2003 Evidence for shared susceptibility in bipolar disorder and schizophrenia. American Journal of Medical Genetics 123: 59–64

- Systematic, whole genome linkage studies of schizophrenia and bipolar disorder have implicated some chromosomal regions in common, consistent with the shared susceptibility genes.
- Recent research suggests that schizophrenia, schizoaffective disorder and bipolar disorder might be associated with polymorphism in this gene.

Children of adults with severe mental illness

Cowling V, Luk EL, Mileshkin C, Birleson P 2004 Children of adults with severe mental illness: mental health, health seeking and service use. Psychiatric Bulletin 28: 43–46

It is recognised that the children of parents with mental health problems could be targeted in the prevention and early intervention of mental health problems. There is a lack of research in this area.

Aim

- To establish the prevalence of childhood mental health problems in children of parents registered with area mental health services in Australia.

Method

- 128 dependent children (aged 2 months to 18 years) of 61 parent-patients were identified.
- Parents had a range of psychiatric disorders and were being treated by an area mental health service.
- Demographic information was collected with the Strengths and Difficulties Questionnaire (SDQ).

- Service use was calculated from the Service Utilisation Questionnaire.
- The help-seeking questionnaire assessed the presence and type of perceived barriers to seeking help.

Results

- Parents reported that 61% of children had difficulty with mental health.
- The severity of children's illness was recorded as minor for 38 children, definite for 17 children and severe for 7 children.
- In 60% of these, the difficulties were rated as having a severe impact on the family and the child.
- 37 of the 61 parents reported reluctance to seek help in the past year.
- Parents that did seek help sought it from a variety of services – the GP most commonly and then the school guidance teacher.

Prevalence of children with mental health problems

- Data on 101 children were analysed.
- Children in the study had 2.5 times the rate of mental health problems compared with the community norm.
- Emotional problems, peer relationship problems and conduct problems were noted.
- Although almost all of the children with mental health problems (defined by the SDQ) in this study attended at least one clinical service, 63% of parents reported a reluctance to seek help in the preceding 12 months for their child's behaviour.

Limitations

- Lack of objective information on diagnosis for children or parents.
- People with severe illness were excluded.

Oates M 1997 Patients as parents: the risk to children. British Journal of Psychiatry 170 (Suppl 32): 22–27

- Children of parents with mental illness may be exposed to considerable psychosocial and genetic risks.

Najman JM, Williams GM, Nikles J et al 2000 Mother's mental illness and child behaviour problems: cause–effect association or observation bias? Journal of the American Academy of Child and Adolescent Psychiatry 39: 592–602

- Anxious or depressed mothers reported more cases of disturbance in their children than mentally healthy parents or the children themselves.

See also the 'General topics' section in Chapter 5 (Child and adolescent psychiatry), page 72.

Clinical guidelines in mental health

Kendall T, Pilling S, Whittington C et al 2005 Clinical guidelines in mental health II: a guide to making NICE guidelines. Psychiatric Bulletin 29: 3–9

Clinical guidelines and the development process for NICE guidelines by the National Collaborating Centre for Mental Health (NCCMH) are discussed. NICE clinical practice guidelines are evidence based. Their development follows a predetermined, internationally agreed method that aims to determine which treatments have the best evidence of effectiveness. They assess which patients and which disorders benefit from treatment. They appraise the evidence in a systematic, critical and unbiased way (Box 12.1).

International guidelines on guideline development can be found at www.agreecollaboration.org
See also Appendices I and II for information on guidelines, levels of recommendation, etc.

How the environment affects mental health

Rutter M 2005 How the environment affects mental health. British Journal of Psychiatry 187: 4–6

For many years there was an assumption that the statistical associations between risky environments and mental disorders represented the operation of environmentally mediated causal pathways.

This is challenged by three considerations:
- Psychosocial researchers recognise the need to differentiate between 'risk indicators' and risk mediators – for example, the risk for antisocial behaviour associated with broken homes is not due to the break-up itself but the associated discord and conflict.
- There is a two-way interaction between parent and child which requires longitudinal research to determine the direction of the causal arrow.
- Twin and adoptee studies showed that, even though risks were due to an environmental feature, the risks might nevertheless be genetically mediated in part.

The distinction between shared and non-shared environmental effects has hindered progress due to the way they have been interpreted. The presumption has been that family-wide influences have little effect on either psychological development or risk of psychopathological disorder. The distinction is in fact solely concerned with whether the environmental influences tend to make siblings similar or different. Shared and non-shared experience varies according to the type of psychopathology, so that effects are more pertinent to antisocial behaviour than depression.

Box 12.1

Developmental process for a NICE guideline

1. Guideline commissioned.
2. A Guideline Development Group (GDG) is created, including members from:
   - the Department of Health
   - the National Collaborating Centre for Mental Health (NCCMH), funded by NICE
   - national stakeholder organisations, e.g.
     – drug companies
     – professional organisations
     – user and carer groups.
   Members of the GDG collaborate to agree the limits of the guideline.
3. The GDG chair is appointed by NCCMH.
   - The chair has wide experience in the relevant field. The chair is supported by at least one national expert from each treatment modality (e.g. psychological services).
   - Primary care is also usually represented. Two service users and a carer are also involved to help the GDG. Clinicians with a good grasp of evidence-based practice are also recruited.
4. The GDG decide what questions the guideline should answer, with scientific, health economic and technical support from the NCCMH. Each question must establish PICO:
   - **P** the service user **P**opulation
   - **I** the **I**ntervention
   - **C** the service or **C**are with which the intervention is to be compared
   - **O** the **O**utcomes against which the intervention and comparator will be compared.
5. A systematic review of randomised controlled trials is undertaken.
   - Evidence is searched electronically, with hand searching for completeness.
   - Studies of low quality can be excluded after independent review.
6. A meta-analysis is undertaken.
   - The high quality evidence is then loaded into Review Manager for meta-analysis. This pools the data on larger numbers than would be found in a single RCT, making the evidence more reliable.
   - The pooled data is shown as forest plots.
7. Developing evidence statements.
   - These are developed using the same PICO pattern as the clinical questions.
   - Each evidence statement is allocated a grade, adapted from an internationally agreed protocol.
   - These are probabilistic statements that indicate the likelihood that a treatment will alter the outcomes for a particular population of people when compared to another intervention or control condition.
   - The key issues are whether the difference in outcomes is statistically significant and whether that difference is clinically valuable.
   - If no RCT evidence is available, then lower levels of evidence may be used in the guideline.
8. Developing clinical recommendations.
   - This involves the GDG taking a broad view of all the possible comparative outcomes for a treatment, including side effects and acceptability of treatment.
   - Recommendations are all graded according to their evidential score.
9. Developing good practice points.
   - These cover the areas of practice where evidence is unlikely to be forthcoming or where value-based recommendations are deemed desirable by the GDG.
10. Integrating the recommendations and developing the NICE guideline.
    - When the GDG has agreed all the recommendations, a series of care pathways are developed, tracing the routes and contexts within which service users and carers could receive treatment within the NHS.
    - Recommendations can then be inserted into the care pathways at the most appropriate points. This integrated care pathway forms the NICE guideline for that condition.
11. Consultation process with subsequent revision of the guideline.

Plomin R, Rutter M 2005 Environmentally mediated risks for psychopathology: research strategies and findings. Journal of the American Academy of Child and Adolescent Psychiatry (in press)

- Twin and adoptee strategies have produced good evidence of the reality and importance of environmentally mediated risks for psychological and psychopathological outcomes.
- A key influence that has been highlighted recently is genetically influenced vulnerability to (or protection against) environmental risk.

- Changes in environment and associated variables and risks lead to a number of suggestions:
  - environmental influences operate within the normal range and not just in relation to extreme environments
  - environmental effects impact on middle childhood and adulthood as well as infancy
  - environmentally mediated risks include prenatal influences (e.g. maternal drug and alcohol use and severe maternal stress) as well as postnatal physical influences (e.g. acquired brain injury and heavy cannabis use in adolescence)
  - with all the known physical and psychological risk factors, there is a huge individual variation in response, with some succumbing, some resilient and some even appearing strengthened.

Plomin R, Daniels, D 1987 Why are children in the same family so different from one another? Behavioural and Brain Sciences 10: 1–16

- The authors argued that environmental differences among families are of little consequence.
- Attention should be focused on child-specific environmental influences.

Collishaw S, Maughan B, Goodman R et al 2004 Time trends in adolescent mental health. Journal of Child Psychology and Psychiatry 45: 1350–1362

- Over the past 50 years there has been a substantial rise in the rate of many types of mental disorder in young people.
- The exact cause remains unclear but the environmental factors involved require urgent investigation.

Jones PB, Fung WLA 2005 Ethnicity and mental health: the example of schizophrenia in the African–Caribbean population in Europe. In: Rutter M, Tienda M (eds) Ethnicity and causal mechanisms. Cambridge University Press, Cambridge.

- The same applies to the higher levels of schizophrenia in individuals of Caribbean origin compared with ethnically similar individuals living in the West Indies or with white people living in the UK.
- Research challenges are still to be met. In particular these are:
  - the need for a better understanding of the types of environmental influence that have major risk effects
  - the identification of the origins of environmental risk factors and whether they lie in gene–environment correlations, so that genetic factors have their impact on behaviours that shape or select environments and thereby influence the likelihood of experiencing stress or adversity, societal elements or personal experiences

- the determination of changes in the organism that provide the basis for the persistence of environmental effects on psychological functioning or psychopathology. There is evidence to support the view that gene expression can be affected by environmental factors, not through effects on genes sequences but through effects on gene expression.

Rutter M 2006 The psychological effects of early institutional rearing. In: Marshall P, Fox N (eds) The development of social engagement: neurobiological perspectives. Oxford University Press, New York

- Environment affects the programming of brain development, first shown with respect to vision (which led to a Nobel Prize for Hubel and Wiesel) as well as neuroendocrine structure and functioning, and through such effects may influence brain development.
- Experiences may affect patterns of interpersonal interaction that become influential through their role in shaping later environments. In addition, people have to appraise experiencing, i.e. what happens to people influences their mental concepts and models of self and their environment.

Definitions

Risk indicators – indexed risk but did not cause it.

Risk mediators – features involved in the actual risk processes leading to mental disorder.

Impact of compulsory detention on admission rates

Kisely SR, Jianguo X, Preston NJ 2004 Impact of compulsory community treatment on admission rates. Survival analysis using linked mental health and offender databases. British Journal of Psychiatry 184: 432–438

The effects of compulsory community treatment for psychiatric patients and the subsequent decrease in admission rates is controversial.

Aims

This Australian study aimed to:
- compare the readmission rate of patients receiving compulsory community treatment with two control groups
- examine sociodemographic factors, clinical features, previous psychiatric history and forensic history
- examine whether community treatment orders (CTOs) reduce admission rates.

Method

- Survival analysis of CTO cases and controls was performed for three linked clinical settings in Western Australia.
- Information came from the Police Offenders' Database, Mental Health Information System record of all inpatients, outpatients and community contacts and the Mental Health Review Board database of all involuntary treatment in the state.
- A linked database, which records all public and private discharges, transfers to another facility and deaths, was used.
- Offender databases were also used.

Results

- 265 people who received compulsory community treatment between November 1997 and November 1998 were identified.
- This is equivalent to 15 per 100,000 of the general population.
- 15% were placed on a CTO in the community and the remainder discharged from hospital on a CTO.
- Cases were matched with two control groups: matched controls and consecutive (matched on date of discharge) controls
- Two-thirds of all subjects were admitted to hospital in the subsequent year.
- The risk of admission was significantly higher in the CTO group.
- There was no difference in admission rates between the two control groups.
- Other risk factors for readmission were:
  - being of aboriginal descent
  - younger age
  - lifetime single status
  - psychiatric comorbidity in the previous year
  - personality disorder
  - shorter psychiatric history
  - previous inpatient health service use.
- Place of residence, diagnosis and involuntary status, gender, educational level, work status and forensic history were not predictive factors.
- CTOs alone do not reduce admissions.

Impact of psychiatric disturbance on identifying psychiatric disorder in relatives

Coelho HF, Cooper PJ, Murray L 2006 Impact of psychiatric disturbance on identifying psychiatric disorder in relatives: study of mothers and daughters. British Journal of Psychiatry 188: 288–289

Previous research has concluded that collecting the psychiatric history of family members may not be accurate and may be influenced by the psychiatric history of the person reporting the said family history.

Method

- 115 women were included in a family aggregation study of generalised social phobia and generalised anxiety disorder.
- Data were recorded about the presence of mood disorder, anxiety disorder and alcohol dependence in the women.
- These women and their mothers were assessed with the SCID-1.
- The women were interviewed regarding the psychiatric histories of their mothers.

Results

- Daughters with anxiety disorders were no more likely to report anxiety symptoms in their mothers than daughters without an anxiety disorder.
- Daughters with a history of mood disorder or alcohol dependence had a lower threshold for reporting these disorders in their mothers.

IQ and mental disorder in young men

Mortensen EL, Sorensen HJ, Jensen HH et al 2005 IQ and mental disorder in young men. British Journal of Psychiatry 187: 407–415

Most research to date on IQ and risk of mental disorder has focused on schizophrenia, with evidence from a number of international studies of an association between schizophrenia and lower IQ. Studies examining other psychiatric disorders and IQ are limited.

Method

- A prospective 20-year study.
- Data are taken from the Copenhagen Perinatal Cohort on IQ in early adulthood.
- Data are collected on the risk of hospitalisation for a range of psychiatric disorders.
- Only males were included.
- Only hospital attendances were examined.

Results

- Low IQ was significantly associated with:
  - schizophreniform psychoses
  - other psychotic disorders
  - adjustment disorders

- personality disorders
- alcohol and substance use disorders.
- After adjustment for comorbidity, only the association between low IQ and non-psychotic disorders remained significant.
- The higher the IQ test score, the longer the average time until first admission.
- Mood disorders and neuroses were not significantly related to low IQ scores.
- Low IQ may be a consequence of mental disorder or a causal factor.

Clinical implications

- The mean IQ score for psychiatric patients is relatively low and evaluation of cognitive function should be an integral part of assessment.
- In individual patients, poor cognitive function does not necessarily reflect effects of mental disorders and may rather suggest a low premorbid IQ.

David AS, Malmberg A, Brand L et al 1997 IQ and risk for schizophrenia: a population based cohort study. Psychological Medicine 27: 1311–1323

- Lower IQ was positively associated with schizophrenia.
- Low IQ was also associated with non-schizophrenic disorders.

Zammit S, Allebeck P, Davis AS et al 2004 A longitudinal study of pre-morbid IQ score and risk of developing schizophrenia, bipolar disorder, severe depression and other nonaffective psychoses. Archives of General Psychiatry 61: 354–360

- A study of Swedish conscripts.
- Severe depression is associated with low IQ.

Weiser M, Reichenberg A, Rabinowitz J et al 2004 Cognitive performance of male adolescents is lower than controls across psychiatric disorders: a population-based study. Acta Psychiatrica Scandinavica 110: 471–475

- Provided evidence that most diagnostic categories are associated with low IQ in male adolescents.

Length of hospitalisation for people with severe mental illness

Johnstone P, Zolese G 1999 Length of hospitalization for people with severe mental illness (**Cochrane Review**). In: The Cochrane Library, Issue 2. CD000384. Update Software, Oxford

- Five RCTs were included.
- Patients admitted for planned short stay had no more readmissions, no more losses to follow-up and were more successfully discharged on time compared to long-stay or standard care patients.
- There was some evidence that short-stay patients were no more likely to leave hospital early and had a greater chance of being employed.
- Further study is required to look at mental, social and family outcomes, including user satisfaction, deaths, violence, criminal behaviour and costs.

Limits of psychiatry

Double D 2002 The limits of psychiatry. British Medical Journal 324: 900–904

The biomedical model of care can encourage the belief that medication is a cure-all. It has been suggested that biological and psychological considerations are also important. It can be helpful to acknowledge the uncertainties of clinical practice. The cultural role of psychiatry is more obvious than in the rest of medicine because of its historical and current role in social control. It was only after the Mental Health Treatment Act 1930 that voluntary treatment became an option in Britain.

The author discusses his scepticism about the expansion of psychiatry over the past 50 years, including:
- the rise in expectations of solutions to mental health problems
- the legitimacy of psychiatric interventions for social and personal problems
- the development of psychiatry based on a biomedical model leading to drug treatment being seen as the answer for multiple problems
- the refocusing of psychiatry on the patient as a person, emphasising the uncertainty in the practice.

The number of psychiatric beds has reduced and yet the activity of mental health services has increased. Antidepressant prescription has more than doubled in the past 7 years. The number of consultant psychiatrists has more than doubled over the past 22 years. As the availability of psychiatric services increases, the boundaries of psychiatric disorder increase. Everyday problems can be medicalised. An example might be the increase in medication for children with hyperactivity disorders which means that there is less of a focus on family and social issues.

Singleton N, Meltzer H, Gartward R 1998 Psychiatric morbidity among prisoners in England and Wales. The Stationery Office, London

- The number of psychiatric beds has decreased.

- The number of people in prison with a mental disorder has risen.
- The proportion of mental health problems is higher in women than in men.

Richman A, Barry A 1985 More and more is less and less. The myth of massive psychiatric need. British Journal of Psychiatry 146: 164–168

- As more resources are provided, more resources are perceived to be needed, with the subsequent understandable disillusionment of staff.

Meltzer H, Gill B, Pettigrew M, Hinds K 1996 The prevalence of psychiatric morbidity among adults living in private households. OPCS surveys of psychiatric morbidity in Great Britain, Report No. 1. HMSO, London

- The largest epidemiological study of the prevalence of psychiatric disorders conducted in the UK.
- 12.3% of men and 19.5% of women are found to have a neurotic disorder in a given week.

Zito JM, Safer DJ, dosReis S et al 2000 Trends in prescribing of psychotropic medication in preschoolers. Journal of the American Medical Association 283: 1025–1030

- The diagnosis of ADHD has increased dramatically in recent years.
- This has led to an increase in the prescription of stimulants in the US.

Wender PH 1998 Attention-deficit hyperactivity disorder in adults. Psychiatric Clinics of North America 21: 761–774

- Suggest that adult ADHD is the most common undiagnosed chronic psychiatric condition in adults.

Charlton BG 1998 Psychopharmacology and the human condition. Journal of the Royal Society of Medicine 91: 699–701

- Concluded that SSRIs have been used and promoted as lifestyle drugs, with their use approved for multiple conditions.

Rosenhan DL 1973 On being sane in insane places. Science 179: 250–258

- Classic study in which 'pseudo-patients' employed by the experimenter gained admission to different hospitals.
- Each presented with a single complaint – hearing a voice saying 'empty', 'hollow' or 'thud'.
- On admission they stopped simulating any symptoms.
- All patients received a psychiatric diagnosis, predominantly schizophrenia.
- Rosenhan concluded that diagnosis is subjective and does not reflect patient characteristics.

- Staff were informed of the experiment after the study.
- They were warned that more 'pseudo-patients' may present.
- No patients did re-present; however, staff suspected up to 10% of subsequent patients of being 'pseudo-patients'.

Klerman GL 1978 The evolution of a scientific nosology. In: Shershow JC (ed.) Schizophrenia: science and practice. Harvard University Press, Cambridge, MA

Aspects of a neo-Kraepelinian approach:
- Psychiatry is a branch of general medicine
- Psychiatry should be based on science
- Psychiatry treats those who are unwell and require treatment
- It is possible to delineate between the normal and the sick
- Mental illness exists and it is the role of scientists to find causes, diagnosis and treatment
- There should be a focus on the biological aspects of psychiatric conditions
- Diagnosis and classifications should be explicit and intentional
- There should be robust coding of diagnoses to enable research and they should be taught at medical school
- Statistics should be employed to improve the validity and reliability of the diagnoses.

Wilson M 1993 DSM-III and the transformation of American psychiatry: a history. American Journal of Psychiatry 150: 399–410

Assumptions of Meyer's biopsychological model:
- The boundaries between illness and normality are fluid because normal people can become ill if exposed to sufficient stress or trauma
- There is a continuum of severity from neurosis through to psychosis
- Psychic conflict and a noxious environment causes mental illness
- Doctors have an opportunity to redefine their roles and responsibilities with postmodernity.

Weblink The Critical Psychiatry Network, dedicated to forming a constructive framework for renewing mental health policy without polarising psychiatry and being against psychiatry – www.criticalpsychiatry.co.uk

Personality and comorbidity of common psychiatric disorders

Khan AA, Jacobson KC, Gardner CO et al 2005 Personality and comorbidity of common psychiatric disorders. British Journal of Psychiatry 186: 190–196

The co-occurrence of psychiatric and personality disorders has been consistently reported.

This study examines the association of variation in personality traits of neuroticism, extraversion and novelty seeking, and comorbidity among eight psychiatric disorders:

- major depression
- generalised anxiety disorder (GAD)
- panic disorder
- any phobia
- alcohol dependence
- drug dependence
- antisocial personality disorder
- conduct disorder.

It examines levels of comorbidity among psychiatric disorders explained by individual personality dimensions.

Method

- 7588 individual twins were assessed from a population-based twin registry.
- The outcome measures were the common psychiatric disorders above.
- The following subgroups were assessed:
  - internalising disorders (depression, anxiety, panic and phobias)
  - externalising disorders (drug and alcohol dependence, antisocial personality and conduct disorders)
  - personality dimensions of neuroticism, extraversion and novelty seeking.
- The proportion of comorbidity explained by each personality dimension was calculated using structural equation modelling.

Results

- High scores on neuroticism significantly increased the chance of all the disorders examined.
- For each standard deviation increase in neuroticism, the highest risk increase was for GAD and the lowest for conduct disorder.
- Novelty seeking was most strongly associated with externalising disorders such as substance dependence, antisocial personality disorder and conduct disorder.
- Internalising disorders were more prevalent in females with externalising disorders than in males.
- Age was positively associated with internalising disorders and the reverse was true of age and externalising disorders.
- The relationship between neuroticism and alcohol dependence was significantly stronger in females than in males.
- On average, neuroticism accounted for 26% of comorbidity among the disorders included.

- The results were consistent with previous findings which suggest that neuroticism is a potential general underlying vulnerability factor for psychopathology.
- High novelty seeking increased the risk for externalising disorders significantly.
- High novelty seeking accounted for the largest proportion of comorbidity between externalising disorders.
- There was no relationship between high novelty seeking and internalising disorders.
- Neuroticism was comparable to novelty seeking with regard to comorbidity of externalising disorders.

Kendler KS, Neale MC, Kessler RC et al 1993 A longitudinal twin study of personality and major depression in women. Archives of General Psychiatry 50: 853–862

- Comorbidity between major depression and GAD (and to a lesser extent major depression and alcohol dependence) largely results from common genetic factors.
- 50% of the genetic liability for major depression was the same as neuroticism.

It is reasonable to hypothesise that there may be a common genetic liability between personality and comorbid psychiatric disorders that lends itself to further research. *See also the 'General topics' section in Chapter 19 (Personality disorders), page 287.*

Psychiatric comorbidity

Maj M 2005 'Psychiatric comorbidity': an artefact of current diagnostic systems? British Journal of Psychiatry 186: 182–184

The term 'comorbidity' was first used in medicine by Feinstein in 1970 to denote cases in which a 'distinct additional clinical entity' occurred during the clinical course of a patient having an index disease. The term has become used in psychiatry to indicate that the patient has either a psychiatric and a medical diagnosis or two or more psychiatric diagnoses.

The increase in recent times is in part a consequence of the use of standardised diagnostic interviews which identify several clinical aspects extending beyond the primary diagnosis. The emergence of psychiatric comorbidity has been to some extent a by-product of some specific features of current diagnostic systems. It is suggested that this may, in fact, be detrimental as the complex clinical condition may split into several pieces, making polypharmacy common and making diagnosis more unreliable as clinicians focus their attention on one or other of the different 'pieces'.

A contributing factor is that a symptom cannot appear in more than one disorder – for example, DSM does not allow anxiety to be recorded within the depression criteria. The proliferation of diagnostic categories in recent classifications has been an additional determination of the proliferation of the phenomenon. The limited number of hierarchical rules also makes 'comorbidity' more prolific. Another relevant feature is that the current diagnostic systems are based on operational diagnostic criteria. Traditional clinical descriptions tended to offer a differential diagnosis, whereas the current operational definitions encourage multiple diagnoses.

Kessler RC, McConagle KA, Zhao S et al 1994 Lifetime and 12-month prevalence of DSM-III-R psychiatric disorders in the United States: results from the National Comorbidity Survey. Archives of General Psychiatry 51: 8–19

- 51% of patients with a diagnosis of depression had at least one concomitant ('comorbid') anxiety when assessed in the US National Comorbidity Survey.

Wittchen H-U, Nelson CB, Lachner G 1998 Prevalence of mental disorders and psychological impairments in adolescents and young adults. Psychological Medicine 28: 109–126

- 48.6% had comorbidity in the Early Developmental Stages of Psychopathology Study.

Andrews G, Slade T, Issakidis C 2002 Deconstructing current comorbidity: data from the Australian National Survey of Mental Health and Well-Being. British Journal of Psychiatry 181: 306–314

- 21% of people in Australia with a mental disorder met the criteria for three or more concomitant ('comorbid') disorders.

Poverty, social inequality and mental health

Murali V, Oyebode F 2004 Poverty, social inequality and mental health. Advances in Psychiatric Treatment 10: 216–224

Poverty is a multidimensional phenomenon, encompassing inability to satisfy basic needs, lack of control over resources, lack of education and poor health. The lowest income groups are more likely to suffer negative effects of 'risky' behaviour than their less poor counterparts. People in lower socioeconomic classes, because of their life circumstances, are exposed to more stressors, with fewer resources to manage them. Poverty is associated with many long-term problems, such as poor health and increased mortality, school failure, crime and substance misuse.

Epidemiological studies have demonstrated an inverse relationship between mental illness and social class.

Psychiatric disorders have consistently been shown to be more common among people in lower social classes. The relationship between low socioeconomic status and personality disorders has not been extensively studied. There is some evidence that personality disorders are more frequent among single individuals from lower socioeconomic classes in inner cities.

World Health Organization 1995 Bridging the gaps. WHO, Geneva

- The world's most ruthless killer and the greatest cause of suffering on earth is extreme poverty.

Townsend P 1979 Poverty in the United Kingdom. Penguin, London

- There is a marked difference between absolute and relative poverty. Even in countries where families generally have access to sufficient resources to maintain life, many are living in disadvantageous circumstances with poor housing and diet, and amenities that do not live up to the expectation of society in general.

Smith GD, Bartly M, Blane D 1990 The Black Report on socioeconomic inequalities in health: 10 years on. British Medical Journal 301: 373–377

- The financial gap between the wealthy and the poor in the UK is not diminishing.
- The differences in health between social classes I and V are increasing.

Wilkinson RG 1996 Unhealthy societies: the afflictions of inequality. Routledge, London

- People who live in deprived communities, where there is underinvestment in the social and physical infrastructure, experience poor health, resulting in higher mortality for those of lower socioeconomic class.
- The effects of income inequality cause stress, frustration and family disruption, which then increase the rates of crime, homicide and violence.

Kaplan GA, Haan MN, Syme S et al 1987 Socio-economic status and health. In: Amler RW, Dull HB (eds) Closing the gap: the burden of unnecessary illness. Oxford University Press, New York, pp 125–129

- Described the inverse association between socioeconomic level and risk of disease.

Subsequent statistical research into the growth of health inequalities in England and Wales is outlined in Table 12.1.

Langner TS, Michael ST 1963 Life stress and mental health. Collier-Macmillan, London

Table 12.1 Standardised mortality rates per 100, 000 for men aged 20–64 years in England and Wales: comparison of years 1970–72 and 1991–93

Social class	1970–72	1991–93
I Professional	500	280
II Managerial	526	300
III-N Skilled (non-manual)	637	426
III-M Skilled (manual)	683	493
IV Partly skilled	721	492
V Unskilled	897	806
All classes	624	419

- Poverty can be both a determinant and a consequence of poor mental health.
- There was a direct relationship between the experience of poverty and high rates of emotional disturbance.
- There is differential availability and use of treatment modes and facilities by different social classes.

Meltzer H, Gill B, Petticrew M et al 1995 OPCS (Office of Population Censuses and Surveys). Surveys of psychiatric morbidity in Great Britain. HMSO, London

- Employment status was a major factor in relation to the differences in prevalence rates of all psychiatric disorders in adults.
- Unemployment was associated with:
  - a significantly increased odds ratio of psychiatric disorders compared with the reference group
  - a four-fold increase in the odds of drug dependence after controlling for other socioeconomic variables
  - a three-fold increase in the odds of phobia and functional psychosis
  - twice the odds of depressive episode, generalised anxiety disorder and obsessive–compulsive disorder
  - an increase in the odds of mixed anxiety and depressive disorder by more than two-thirds.

Argyle M 1994 The psychology of social class. Routledge, London

- The highest prevalence of psychosis in men and women is found in social class V.
- It is unclear if this relates to social causation or to social drift.

Goldberg EM, Morrison SL 1963 Schizophrenia and social class. British Journal of Psychiatry 109: 785–802

- The social class distribution of the fathers of patients with schizophrenia did not deviate from that of the general population.
- The excess of low socioeconomic status among people with schizophrenia was mainly attributable to individuals who had drifted down the occupational and social scale prior to the onset of psychosis.

Mulvany F, O'Callaghan E, Takei N et al 2001 Effect of social class at birth on risk and presentation of schizophrenia: a case-control study. British Medical Journal 323: 1398–1401

- Low social class at birth was not associated with increased risk of schizophrenia.

Brown AS, Susser ES, Jandorf L et al 2000 Social class of origin and cardinal symptoms of schizophrenic disorders over the early illness course. Social Psychiatry and Psychiatric Epidemiology 35: 53–60

- Studied the relationship between social class of origin and cardinal symptoms of schizophrenic disorders over the course of early illness.
- People with schizophrenia from upper or middle class had lower levels of hallucinations and delusions.
- People with schizophrenia from lower social class were older at first contact with psychiatric services.
- It may be that people from lower social classes find it difficult to access services, or that they are more tolerant and accepting of the behavioural aspects of the disorder.
- People from higher social classes might be better informed about mental illness and seek treatment earlier.

Dohrenwend BP, Levav I, Shrout PE et al 1992 Socioeconomic status and psychiatric disorders: the causation–selection issue. Science 255: 946–952

- Low socioeconomic status is associated with high prevalence of mood disorders.

Murphy JM, Oliver DC, Monson RR et al 1991 Depression and anxiety in relation to social status: a perspective epidemiological study. Archives of General Psychiatry 48: 223–229

- Longitudinal research in Stirling County indicated that during the 1950s and 1960s the prevalence of depression was significantly and persistently higher in the low socioeconomic status population than in other socioeconomic status levels.
- There was a trend for prior depression to be associated with subsequent downward mobility which may reflect the disabling aspects of the illness.

Eisemann M 1996 Social class and social mobility in depressed patients. Acta Psychiatrica Scandinavica 73: 399–402

- Patients with major depressive disorder or bipolar depression were more 'downwardly mobile' than people with neurotic depression.

Department of Health 1999a The National Confidential Enquiry into suicide and homicide by people with mental illness. DH, London

- The majority of people who had completed suicide were either unemployed or had a long-term illness.

Gunnell DJ, Peters TJ, Kammerling RM et al 1995 Relation between parasuicide, suicide, psychiatric admissions and socio-economic deprivation. British Medical Journal 311: 226–230

- There was a strong association between suicide, parasuicide and socioeconomic deprivation.

Kennedy HG, Iveson RC, Hill O 1999 Violence, homicide and suicide: strong correlation and wide variation across districts. British Journal of Psychiatry 175: 462–466

- Homicide and suicide occur more frequently in highly populated, deprived areas.

Crawford MJ, Price M 1999 Increasing rates of suicide in young men in England during the 1980s: the importance of social context. Social Science and Medicine 49: 1419–1423

- Noted increasing rates of suicide in young unemployed men living in conditions of extreme social deprivation.

Marzuk PM, Tardiff K, Leon AC et al 1997 Poverty and fatal accidental drug overdoses of cocaine and opiates in New York City: an ecological study. American Journal of Drug and Alcohol Abuse 23: 221–228

- The mortality rates of overdoses involving cocaine and opiates are significantly associated with poverty status.

Harrison L, Gardiner E 1999 Do the rich really die young? Alcohol-related mortality and social class in Great Britain, 1988–94. Addiction 94: 1871–1880

- Social class is a risk factor for alcohol-related mortality, which is also linked to social structural factors such as poverty, disadvantage and social class.
- Alcohol-related mortality rates are higher for men in the manual occupations than in the non-manual occupations.
- Alcohol-related mortality is also age related.

- Men between 25 and 39 in the unskilled manual class are 10–20 times more likely to die from alcohol-related causes than those in the professional class.
- Men aged 55–64 years in the unskilled manual class are approximately 2.5–4 times more likely to die than their professional counterparts.
- Younger women in the manual classes are more likely to die from alcohol-related causes, but among older women it is those in the professional class that have the greater mortality.

Hans SL 1999 Demographic and psychosocial characteristics of substance-abusing pregnant women. Clinical Perinatology 26: 55–74

- Black women and poorer women are more likely to use illicit substances, particularly cocaine.
- White women and better educated women are more likely to use alcohol.

Lynam DR, Caspi A, Moffitt TE et al 2000 The interaction between impulsivity and neighbourhood context on offending: the effects of impulsivity are stronger in poorer neighbourhoods. Journal of Abnormal Psychology 109: 563–574

- Low family income and poor housing predict official and self-reported juvenile and adult offending.
- The relationship between poverty and criminality is complex and continuous.
- The interaction between impulsivity and neighbourhood on criminal activities indicates that the effects of impulsivity are stronger in poorer neighbourhoods than in better-off ones.

Farrington DP 1995 The development of offending and antisocial behaviour from childhood: key finding from the Cambridge Study in Delinquent Development. Journal of Child Psychology and Psychiatry 36: 929–964

- In the Cambridge Study in Delinquent Development, an unstable job record at the age of 18 years was an important independent predictor of young men's convictions between the ages of 21 and 25.
- Having an unskilled manual job record at the age of 18 was an independent predictor of adult social dysfunction and antisocial personality at the age of 32.
- Between the ages of 15 and 18, young males were convicted at a higher rate when they were unemployed than when they were employed, suggesting unemployment is associated with crime. This may reflect financial need.
- One of the most important childhood predictors of delinquency was poverty.

Department of Health 1999b Saving lives: our healthier nation. The Stationery Office, London

- Children in the poorest households are three times more likely to have a mental illness than children in the best-off households.

Duncan GJ, Brooks-Gunn J (eds) 1997 Consequences of growing up poor. Russell Sage, New York

- Poverty and social disadvantage are most strongly associated with deficits in children's cognitive skills and educational achievements.

Kaplan GA, Turrell G, Lynch JW et al 2001 Childhood socioeconomic position and cognitive function in adulthood. International Journal of Epidemiology 30: 256–263

- Studied childhood socioeconomic position and cognitive function in adulthood.
- Higher socioeconomic position and greater educational attainment in childhood are associated with cognitive function in adulthood.
- Both mothers and fathers contribute to their offspring's formative cognitive development and later-life cognitive ability.

Pagani L, Boulerice B, Vitaro F et al 1999 Effects of poverty on academic failure and delinquency in boys: a change and process model approach. Journal of Child Psychology and Psychiatry 40: 1209–1219

- Poverty was found to have an effect on both academic failure and extreme delinquency after controlling for maternal education and early childhood behaviour.

The rediscovery of recovery

Roberts G, Wolfson P 2004 The rediscovery of recovery: open to all. Advances in Psychiatric Treatment 10: 37–49

It can be assumed that people with severe mental illness do not recover, leading to low expectations which erode hope and collude with chronicity.

Service users are redefining their roles and are developing a model in which people can recover without or in spite of the help of doctors.

Recovery is a potentially unifying and collaborative goal. Recovery literature often characterises psychiatrists as risk averse and driven by a prescribing, relapse-prevention and maintenance model of care which fosters dependence. This has been termed warehousing.

The measurement of recovery is at an early stage. There remains a need to combine relevant subjective accounts with reproducible objective measures. Being met with hope and optimism, especially at the initial contact, is significant in patients' accounts of recovery. Many patients associate being well with giving up medication, even when there are adverse, and sometimes repetitive, consequences. A negotiating stance, in which risks can be taken within safe parameters and lessons learned from experience, is helpful. It needs to be acknowledged that it is possible for some to recover and stay well without medication, but there is no reliable way of knowing who will remain well.

Stopping medication is probably the most common cause of relapse. Prompt access to services and the role of the hospital in a crisis are important, but on resolution service users may well want to break contact again. Recovery should allow for ethnicity and diversity, taking into account patients' personal beliefs.

The recovery movement centres on an outward, pro-recovery approach, offering a broad, inclusive, humanistic philosophy that could unite professionals, service users and others in the collaborative project of working for better lives for those who experience severe mental health problems. Some service users have felt threatened by a robustly expressed recovery model, feeling that they cannot recover and attempts to do so will only invite failure. Other service users feel that their lives have been so blighted that there is nothing to return to, and have created a new lifestyle based on that premiss.

Some professionals are worried that redefining recovery as open to all, even in the presence of chronic illness, risks generating false hope and colluding with denial. There are also concerns regarding what will happen to current services and that if recovery is expected, then what will happen to those services which currently provide ongoing support to people with chronic mental illness.

Anthony WA 1993 Recovery from mental illness: the guiding vision of the mental health service system in the 1990s. Psychological Rehabilitation Journal 16: 11–23

- Interest in 'recovery' has evolved from both the physical disability movement and deinstitutionalisation within psychiatry, creating a new vision for mental health services in the US during the 1990s.
- Effective service development must be based on what people in recovery have found to be helpful or valuable, but this is significantly different from what is currently found in standard psychiatric textbooks.

Allott P, Loganathan L, Fulford KWM 2002 Discovering hope for recovery from a British perspective. In: Lurie S, McCubbin M, Dallaire B (eds) International innovations in community mental health [special issue]. Canadian Journal of Community Mental Health 21(3)

- The UK developments in recovery have been traced to antidiscriminatory and disability legislation, the growth of consumerism and broad initiatives in support of the Department of Health's expert patients programme.

National Institute for Clinical Excellence 2002 Schizophrenia: core interventions in the treatment and management of schizophrenia in primary and secondary care. Clinical Guideline 1. NICE, London. Online. Available: www.nice.org.uk/pdf/CG1NICEguideline.pdf

Focus on a user-led perspective, the aims of which include:
- discussing preferences and recording advance directives
- offering help in an atmosphere of hope and optimism
- fostering a collaborative working relationship
- acknowledging that the service user's preferences are central
- acknowledging that parents have the right to be fully informed and share in decision making
- encouraging patients to write an account of their illness in their notes
- recording treatment preferences
- assessment of current occupational status and future potential
- comprehensive care coordination
- engaging with patients in a kind and constructive partnership
- giving patients choice following the provision of clear and intelligible information and a full discussion.

Ohio Department of Mental Health 2003 Ohio Mental Health Recovery and Consumer Outcomes Initiative 2003. Online. Available: www.mh.state.oh.us/oper/outcomes/outcomes.index.html

The most important recovery-orientated practices identified by service users are:
- Encourage my independent thinking
- Treat me in a way that helps my recovery process
- Treat me as an equal in planning my services
- Give me the freedom to make my own mistakes
- Treat me like they believe I can shape my own future
- Listen to me and believe what I say
- Look at and recognise my abilities
- Work with me to find the resources or services I need
- Be available to talk to me when I need to talk to someone
- Teach me about the medications I am taking.

Harding CM, Brooks GW, Asolaga T et al 1987 The Vermont longitudinal study of persons with severe mental illness. 1: Methodological study sample and overall status 32 years later. American Journal of Psychiatry 144: 718–726

- Long-term study of patients with severe and chronic mental illness.
- Patients were found to be significantly improved or recovered.
- Recovery meant on no medication, working, relating to family and friends, integrated into the community and behaviour such that there was no evidence of previous illness.
- Selection bias and the unusual comprehensiveness of the patients' treatment prevent generalisation.

Warner R 1994 Recovery from schizophrenia: psychiatry and political economy, 2nd edn. Routledge, New York

- A review of 85 studies, from the past 100 years, of recovery from schizophrenia.
- A clear picture of long-term outcome has not emerged.
- The lack of a clear picture was attributed to the limited validity of schizophrenia as a diagnostic entity.

Harrison G, Hopper K, Craig T et al 2001 Recovery from psychotic illness: a 15- and 25-year international follow up study. British Journal of Psychiatry 178: 506–517

- A study of 1633 participants from 14 culturally diverse areas.
- Patients were reviewed 15 and 25 years after diagnosis.
- The results were in line with previous studies.
- Global outcomes at 15 years and 25 years were favourable for over half of all people.
- There was evidence of a 'late recovery' effect, which supported the case for therapeutic optimism.

Ralph RO, Lambert D, Kidder KA 2002 The recovery perspective and evidence-based practice for people with serious mental illness: a guideline developed for the Behavioural Health Recovery Management Project. Center for Psychiatric Rehabilitation, University of **Chicago**

- It is a largely non-medical assertion that medical practice is governed by 'the medical model'.
- Non-medical recovery literature yields a strong and clear view that psychiatric thought and practice are almost entirely hostage to the medical model.
- The model is often depicted as narrowly focused on disease, treatment and biological reductionism with an evidence basis.
- Recovery models have a broader, person-centred focus, based upon evidence largely composed of personal narrative and the views of 'experts by experience'.

Repper J, Perkins R 2003 Social inclusion and recovery. Baillière Tindall, London

- Empowerment is a core dynamic in promoting recovery.

- Dimensions of hope-inspiring relationships include:
  - valuing people as human beings
  - acceptance and understanding
  - believing in the person's abilities and potential
  - attending to people's abilities and interests
  - accepting failures and setbacks as part of the recovery process
  - accepting that the future is uncertain
  - finding ways of sustaining our own hope and guarding against despair
  - accepting that we must learn and benefit from experience.

McGorry PD 1992 The concept of recovery and secondary prevention in psychotic disorders. Australian and New Zealand Journal of Psychiatry 26: 3–17

- Explanations of illness should take into account the patient's readiness to accept them.
- Denial of illness can result from premature discussions.

Roberts GA 2000 Narrative and severe mental illness: what places do stories have in an evidence based world? Advances in Psychiatric Treatment 6: 432–441

- If symptoms carry significant meaning for individuals, then their presence and absence are both significant.
- The process of recovery may be accompanied by complex losses and powerful realisations.

Deegan P 1996 Recovery as a journey of the heart. Psychiatric Rehabilitation Journal 19: 91–97

- Professionals must embrace the concept of the dignity of risk and the right of failure if they are to be supportive to patients.

Copeland ME 2002 Overview of WRAP: Wellness Recovery Action Plan. Mental Health Recovery Newsletter 3: 1–9

- One of the most popular and well-established recovery tools.
- It begins by helping patients to equip themselves with 'personal wellness tools'.
- This involves identifying actions, thoughts and behaviours that, from personal experience, are associated with staying well and reducing symptoms.
- These are written into a plan which includes daily triggers and how to avoid them, warning signs and how to respond to them, and a crisis plan.

Butterworth R, Dean J 2000 Putting the missing rungs into the vocational ladder. Life in the Day 4: 5–9

- A survey of mental health service users in the Bristol area.
- Less than half of the participants were engaged in any form of occupational activity.
- In 1997 a Work Development Team was created.

- Since then over 200 people have returned to full-time employment.
- A job retention service also exists.

Davidson L, Strauss J 1992 Sense of self in recovery from severe mental illness. British Journal of Medical Psychology 65: 131–145

- A key correlate of favourable long-term outcome in schizophrenia is the patient's ability to differentiate themselves from their diagnosis.
- Other important features are a sense of intact, healthy self, separate from the illness experience.

Leibrich J 1999 A gift of stories: discovering how to deal with mental illness. University of Otago Press, Dunedin

- An anthology of personal recovery stories.
- The exchange of meanings and stories by people with severe mental illness can significantly influence their experience.
- They are helpful in redefining yourself as 'in recovery' as opposed to being 'chronically ill'.

Definition

Recovery involves a deeply personal, unique process of changing one's attitudes, values, feelings, goals, skills and roles. It is a way of living a satisfying, hopeful, and contributing life even with limitations caused by the illness. Recovery involves the development of new meaning and purpose in one's life as one grows beyond the catastrophic effects of mental illness. (*Source:* Anthony WA 1993 Recovery from mental illness: the guiding vision of the mental health service system in the 1990s. Psychosocial Rehabilitation Journal 24: 159–168.)

Weblinks

Department of Health's Expert Patient Programme – www lmca.org.uk/docs/expert.htm

Long-term Medical Conditions Alliance (LMCA) – www. lmca.org.uk

Manic Depression Fellowship's self-help resources – www. mdf.org.uk

New Zealand Mental Health Commission – www.mhc.govt. nz

Rethink's self-management project – www.rethink. org/living_with_mental_illness/recovery_and_self_ management/index.html

Survivors Network (UK) – www.healthy-life-styles.com

Root cause analysis of untoward incidents in mental health services

Neal LA, Watson D, Hicks T et al 2004 Root cause analysis applied to the investigation of serious untoward incidents in mental health services. Psychiatric Bulletin 28: 75–77

There is growing international concern that health services worldwide have underestimated harm or injury experienced by patients as a result of medical error and adverse events in healthcare settings.

Department of Health 2001 Building a safer NHS for patients. DH, London

- This publication showcased the government's plans for promoting patient safety.
- The guidance details the methods for investigating every homicide (and some suicides) by patients in current or recent contact with mental health services.
- The plan incorporates the development of the technique of root cause analysis (RCA) within the NHS.
- This process was initially used in industry to identify causal or systems factors in serious adverse events.
- There is no prescribed method for RCA in mental health services.

Gitlow H, Oppenheim A, Oppenheim R 1995 Quality management: tools and methods for improvement. Irwin, Burr Ridge, IL

- Root cause analysis is a business-derived term.
- It is an integral part of a group of problem-solving techniques of total quality management with overarching concepts, the ultimate aim of which is continuous quality improvement.
- It has been described as a structured investigation aiming to identify the true cause of a problem and the actions necessary to eliminate it.

Andersen B, Fagerhaug T 2000 Root cause analysis: simplified tools and techniques. ASQ Quality Press, Milwaukee, WI

- The causes of untoward events in large organisations are often complex but the 'root cause' can set the cause-and-effect chain in motion.

Rose N 2000 Six years' experience in Oxford: review of serious incidents. Psychiatric Bulletin 24: 243–246

- Described in detail a method of conducting internal investigations in mental health services, on which the RCA should be built.
- Contributory factors listed include:
  - institutional
  - organisational
  - task or process
  - team
  - individual
  - equipment and resources
  - patient.

- The name is a misnomer in that the fundamental or root cause may not be found and the process may focus on interrelated issues which may be improved.

Hawkins SA, Hastie R 1990 Hindsight: biased judgements of past events after the outcomes are known. Psychological Bulletin 107: 311–327

- Talked about 'hindsight bias' which includes speculating on what might have been the outcome if a different course of action had been taken.

Reiss D 2001 Counterfactuals and inquiries after homicide. Journal of Forensic Psychiatry 12: 169–181

- Considered that conclusions drawn from hindsight bias may be meaningless and called it 'counterfactual bias'.

Marshall M, Gray A, Lockwood A et al 1997 Case management for severe mental disorders **(Cochrane Review)**. In: The Cochrane Library, Issue 2. Update Software, Oxford; MacPherson R, Cornelius F, Kilpatrick D et al 2002 Outcome of clinical risk management in the Gloucester rehabilitation service. Psychiatric Bulletin 26: 449–452

- There is no evidence that methods aimed at risk reduction such as the care programme approach and clinical risk assessment/management prevent homicides and suicides.
- Failures in processes then may also not affect serious outcomes.

Szmukler G 2000 Homicide inquiries: what sense do they make? Psychiatric Bulletin 24: 6–10

- Homicide inquiries were viewed as loathsome, pointless and punitive by healthcare professionals.
- The RCA process may be more acceptable with its systematic and consistent non-legal approach.

Conclusions

- The evidence base on the benefits of RCA is yet to emerge.
- The process does appear to be more efficient and consistent, and less threatening and demoralising to clinical staff.

Routine use of mental health outcome assessments

Salvi G, Leese M, Slade M 2005 Routine use of mental health outcome assessments: choosing the measure. British Journal of Psychiatry 186: 146–152

This study compares the results from four staff-rated measures recommended for routine clinical use. The two goals were:

1. to identify the extent to which there is overlap in the information provided by these outcome measures
2. to make recommendations about the measure providing the most clinically relevant information for adult mental health services.

Department of Health and Aged Care 1999 Mental Health Information Development. Commonwealth Department of Health and Family Services, Canberra

- There is increasing pressure to use outcome measures in routine clinical practice.

Gilbody SM, House AO, Sheldon TA 2002 Psychiatrists in the UK do not use outcome measures: national survey. British Journal of Psychiatry 180: 101–103

- Found that the majority of psychiatrists in the UK do not routinely measure patients' care needs and outcomes in a standardised way.

Slade M, Cahill S, Kelsey W et al 2002 Threshold assessment grid (TAG): the development of a valid and brief scale to assess the severity of mental illness. Social Psychiatry and Psychiatric Epidemiology 35: 78–85

- 10 mental health teams throughout London participated in the study between 1999 and 2000.

Measures

All staff-rated and recommended for routine clinical use by the references authors.

The HoNOS, CANSAS and GAF have been translated into many languages and are used world-wide.

1. *Health of the Nation Outcomes Scales (HoNOS)*: Wing JK, Beevor AS, Curtis RH et al 1998 Health of the Nation Outcome Scales: research and development. British Journal of Psychiatry 172: 11–18.
   - Assesses social disability in 12 domains, each being scored from 0 (no problem) to 4 (severe problem), with the total score being the sum of all 12 domains.
2. *Camberwell Assessment of Need Short Appraisal Schedule (CANSAS)*: Phelan M, Slade M, Thornicroft G et al 1995 The Camberwell Assessment of Need (CAN): the validity and reliability of an instrument to assess the needs of people with severe mental illness. British Journal of Psychiatry 167: 589–595.
   - Assesses health and social needs across 22 domains, scored 0 (no need), 1 (met need), 2 (unmet need) and 9 (not known).
   Produces to subtotals:
   Total unmet needs and total met needs (Andreasen R, Caputi P, Oades IG 2001 Interrater reliability of the

Camberwell Assessment of Need Short Appraisal Schedule. Australian and New Zealand Journal of Psychiatry 35: 856-861). The sum is total needs = maximum of 22.

3. *Global Assessment of Functioning (GAF)*: Jones SH, Thornicroft G, Coffey M et al 1995 A brief mental health outcome scale: reliability and validity of the Global Assessment of Functioning (GAF). British Journal of Psychiatry 166: 654–659.
   - Rates symptoms and social functioning on a scale from 10 to 100.
4. *Threshold Assessment Grid (TAG)*: Slade et al 2002 (see above).
   - Assesses the severity of a person's mental health issues across seven domains.
   - Scores range from 0 to 4, 4 being very severe when immediate action is required.

Correlation analysis of total scores and factor analysis using combined data for the scales were performed.

Results

- Relationship between the total scores of the four measures was examined.
- CANSAS 'total needs met' score showed low association with the other measures.
- There was a degree of correlation between GAF, TAG, HoNOS and CANSAS 'total unmet needs' score.

Conclusions

- A global severity factor accounts for only a small percentage (16%) of the variance and is best measured with TAG or GAF.
- CANSAS and HoNOS both provide detailed characterisation of the patient, covering clinical and social needs.
- CANSAS is superior at looking at met needs (not covered by HoNOS).

See also Assessment tools and rating scales, below.

Treatment – Psychopharmacology

Rapid tranquillisation of violent or agitated patients in a psychiatric emergency setting

Alexander J, Tharyan P, Adams C et al 2004 Rapid tranquillisation of violent or agitated patients in a psychiatric emergency setting. Pragmatic randomised trial of intramuscular lorazepam versus haloperidol plus promethazine. British Journal of Psychiatry 185: 63–69

Method

- 200 patients were included.
- Half of the patients received treatment with a mixture of haloperidol (10 mg) and promethazine (25–50 mg).
- The remaining patients received lorazepam 4 mg IM.

Results

- At blind assessment 99.5% of patients were asleep or tranquil.
- Being asleep was more likely in patients who received the combined haloperidol–promethazine treatment.
- The combination treatment produced faster onset of tranquillisation or sedation and resulted in more clinical improvement over the first 2 hours.
- Neither intervention differed in the number then requiring physical restraint, numbers absconding or adverse effects.
- Both treatments proved effective in controlling violence and aggression.
- Combination therapy may be desirable if a faster rate of sedation is required.

Tardiff K, Sweillam A 1982 Assaultive behaviour among chronic patients. American Journal of Psychiatry 139: 212–215; Tardiff K, Koenigsberg HW 1985 Assaultive behaviour among psychiatric outpatients. American Journal of Psychiatry 142: 960–963

- Found that violence or aggression is a common reason for emergency psychiatric presentations, with 3–10% demonstrating assaultative behaviour.

Huf G, Coutinho ESF, Fagundes HM Jr et al 2002a Current practices in managing acutely disturbed patients at three hospitals in Rio De Janeiro–Brazil: a prevalence study. BMC Psychiatry 2:4.

- Haloperidol and promethazine, an antihistamine with sedative effects and effects which guard against dystonic reactions, is used in combination in India and Brazil.
- Intramuscular lorazepam is increasingly used in India and costs the same as the haloperidol–promethazine mix and limits the extrapyramidal or dystonic effects; however, its efficacy in comparison is unclear.

Treatment – Others

Complementary medicines in psychiatry

Werneke U, Turner T, Proebe S 2006 Complementary medicines in psychiatry. British Journal of Psychiatry 188: 109–121

- A review of the effectiveness and safety of complementary medicines in psychiatry.
- It found that there is some evidence for the use of:
  - ginkgo and hydergine in dementia
  - passion flower and valerian for sedation
  - St John's wort and S-adenosylmethionine in depression
  - selenium and folate as adjunctive therapy in depression.
- The evidence was not significant for:
  - omega 3 fatty acids in schizophrenia
  - melatonin for tardive dyskinesia
  - 18-methoxycoronaridine in cocaine and opiate addiction.
- Other studies with inconclusive results are not included here.

Birks J, Grimley Evans J, Van Dongen M 2002 Ginkgo biloba for cognitive impairment and dementia (**Cochrane Review**). In: The Cochrane Library, Issue 2. Update Software, Oxford; Kanowski S, Hoerr R 2003 Ginkgo biloba extract EGb 761 in dementia: intent-to-treat analyses of a 24-week, multi-center, double-blind, placebo-controlled, randomized trial. Pharmacopsychiatry 36(6): 297–303

- Found some improvement in cognitive performance in patients with Alzheimer's disease given ginkgo biloba.

van Dongen M, van Rossum E, Kessels A et al 2003 Gingko for elderly people with dementia and age-associated memory impairment: a randomized clinical trial. Clinical Epidemiology 56: 367–376

- This trial did not find that ginkgo biloba was effective in elderly people with Alzheimer's disease or age-related cognitive impairment.

Olin J, Schneider L, Novit A et al 2001 Hydergine for dementia (**Cochrane Review**). In: The Cochrane Library, Issue 4. Update Software, Oxford

- Hydergine was found to have beneficial effects on cognitive impairment in patients with dementia.
- The diagnostic criteria for dementia was not formalised.

Stevinson C, Ernst E 2000 Valerian for insomnia: a systematic review of randomised clinical trials. Sleep Medicine 1: 91–99

- Previous studies have found that valerian has useful sedative properties.
- This systematic review did not find a significant benefit.

Akhondzadeh S, Naghavi HR, Vazirian M et al 2001 Passion flower in the treatment of generalized anxiety: a pilot double-blind randomized controlled trial with oxazepam. Journal of Clinical Pharmacy and Therapeutics 26: 369–373

- Passion flower contains chrysin which acts as a partial agonist at benzodiazepine receptors.
- This study compared passion flower with oxazepam and found no difference between their effects.

MacMahon KMA, Broomfield NM, Espie CA 2005 A systematic review of the effectiveness of oral melatonin for adults (18 to 65 years) with delayed sleep phase syndrome and adults (18 to 65 years) with primary insomnia. Current Psychology Reviews 1: 103–113

- This study concluded that melatonin shows beneficial effects in the treatment of delayed sleep phase disorder.
- It is not helpful for primary sleep disorder.

Szegedi A, Kohnen R, Dienel A et al 2005 Acute treatment of moderate to severe depression with hypericum extract WS5570 (St John's wort): randomised controlled double blind non-inferiority trial against paroxetine. British Medical Journal 330: 503–506

- This study compared St John's wort in high dose with paroxetine in the treatment of moderate and severe depression.
- St John's wort and paroxetine were found to have equivalent effects.
- This is at odds with recent systematic reviews which suggest a role for St John's wort in mild depression.

Taylor MJ, Carney S, Geddes J et al 2004 Folate for depressive disorders (Cochrane Review). In: The Cochrane Library, Issue 1. Update Software, Oxford

- Concluded that folate has beneficial effects in the treatment of depression when used as an adjunct to antidepressant therapy.

Bressa GM 1994 S-adenosyl-1-methionine (SAMe) as antidepressant: meta-analysis of clinical studies. Acta Neurologica Scandinavica 154 (Suppl): 7–14

- S-adenosylmethionine is required in the methylation of a number of neurotransmitters.
- Folate is involved in the endogenous production of S-adenosylmethionine.
- This study found that S-adenosylmethionine, when given parenterally, is more effective than placebo in the treatment of depression.

Delle Chiaie R, Pancheri P, Scapicchio P 2002 Efficacy and tolerability of oral and intramuscular S-adenosyl-L-methionine 1,4-butanedisulfonate (SAMe) in the treatment of major depression: comparison with imipramine in 2 multicenter studies. American Journal of Clinical Nutrition 76 (Suppl): 1172S–1176S

- Parenteral S-adenosylmethionine was found to be as effective as imipramine in the treatment of depression and needed to be given as approximately one quarter of the oral dose.

Neurosurgery for mental disorder

Christmas D, Morrison C, Eljamel MS, Matthews K 2004 Neurosurgery for mental disorder. Advances in Psychiatric Treatment 10: 189–199

There has been a shift in the conceptualisation of the purpose of neurosurgery. It is no longer performed with a view to suppressing undesirable or unwanted behaviours but to engender a release of adaptive behaviour. There has been a dramatic reduction in rates of neurosurgery for mental disorder, a major change in both the selection of target sites and the techniques employed, and a reduction of the recognised indications for treatment.

The UK centre with the greatest clinical experience of neurosurgery for mental disorder (the Geoffrey Knight Unit, London) closed a number of years ago and since then stereotactic subcaudate tractotomy, previously the most commonly performed procedure, is no longer available. This leaves two UK centres for neurosurgery for mental disorder. The centre at Ninewells in Dundee performed 33 procedures between 1990 and 2001. The centre at the University Hospital of Wales in Cardiff performed 39 procedures between January 1994 and June 2000.

Three broad categories of psychiatric disorder may benefit from modern neurosurgery: obsessive–compulsive disorder, anxiety disorders and depressive disorders. It is generally accepted that only those disorders of substantial chronicity and treatment refractoriness should be considered. In the past, neurosurgery was crudely performed, with a lack of rigorous investigation regarding effectiveness and a lack of detailed assessment of adverse effects on personality and cognition. Procedures performed previously (bilateral amygdalotomy, thalamotomy and hypothalamotomy) for the treatment of aggression and hypersexuality are no longer thought appropriate.

Anterior capsulotomy interrupts frontothalamic fibres of connection and is used in the UK for depression and obsessive–compulsive disorder. Anterior cingulotomy was originally developed for the treatment of intractable pain, but its uses now also include anxiety disorders, depressive disorders and obsessive–compulsive disorder. Stereotactic subcaudate tractotomy and limbic leucotomy are no longer performed in the UK.

No systematic review or meta-analysis has been done. There are a number of methodological difficulties hindering research in this area, including:

- low numbers treated at any single site
- small populations in many studies
- the ethical considerations for the control group
- the logistical challenges that tertiary referral centres experience when following up patients over many years.

Those to be referred for neurosurgery must have had continuous, vigorous treatment of their illness, using a combination of pharmacological, psychological and socially based treatment strategies (including ECT for depression).

Recent advancements in neurosurgery for mental disorder (NMD) include vagus nerve stimulation and deep brain stimulation. Both procedures are potentially reversible and do not involve destruction of brain tissue. As the stimulation can be turned on or off it may be possible to conduct relatively pure double-blind controlled studies of efficacy. Recent studies suggest that vagus nerve stimulation may be most effective in patients with less chronic and treatment-refractory forms of depression.

Barraclough BM, Mitchell-Heggs NA 1978 Use of neurosurgery for psychological disorder in British Isles during 1974–6. British Medical Journal 2: 1591–1593

- The rate of leucotomy in the UK was 3.4 million operations per million population per annum.
- This included patients over 15 between 1974 and 1976.
- There were 431 patients in total.
- Depression was the most common indication, followed by anxiety, with 'violence' coming last.

CRAG Working Group on Mental Illness 1996 Neurosurgery for mental disorder. CRAG, Edinburgh

- Neurosurgery for mental disorder retains an important role in treating a small number of carefully selected patients.

Spangler WJ, Cosgrove GR, Ballantine HT Jr et al 1996 Magnetic resonance imaging-guided stereotactic cingulotomy for intractable psychiatric disease. Neurosurgery 38: 1071–1076; discussion 1076–1078

- Seizures occur in 1–6% of cases in the postoperative period.
- This rarely progressed to epilepsy.
- Anterior capsulotomy is associated with an all-condition success rate of 67% (55% for affective disorder and 45% for OCD).
- Anterior congulotomy is associated with a 67% success rate (65% for affective disorder and 56% for OCD).
- Subcaudate tractotomy is associated with a 37% success rate.
- Limbic leucotomy is associated with success rates of 78% for affective disorder and 61% for OCD.

Royal College of Psychiatrists 2000 Neurosurgery for mental disorder: report from the Neurosurgery Working Group of the Royal College of Psychiatrists. Royal College of Psychiatrists, London

- Examined the outcomes of 727 people with depression, 478 people with OCD and 290 people with affective disorder treated with neurosurgery.
- Marked improvement was found in 63% of people with depression, 58% of people with OCD and 52% of people with affective disorder.
- Between 1 and 2% of people were worse following treatment.
- No response to treatment was found in 14% of people with depression, 14% of people with OCD and 21% of people with affective disorder.

Montoya A, Weiss AP, Price BH et al 2002 Magnetic resonance imaging-guided stereotactic limbic leucotomy for treatment of intractable psychiatric disease. Neurosurgery 50: 1043–1049; discussion 1049–1052

- Reviewed six patients with major depressive disorder who underwent limbic leucotomy.
- 33% met the criteria for response when measured as a 50% reduction in BDI score.
- Reviewed 15 patients who underwent limbic leucotomy for obsessive–compulsive disorder.
- 42% were responded on the basis of improvement on the CGI.
- 33% achieved a 35% reduction in their Y-BOCS score.
- Apathy and anergia were reported in the postoperative period in up to 24% of cases.
- The suicide rate for limbic leucotomy was 10% on follow-up.

Lovett LM, Shaw DM 1987 Outcome in bipolar affective disorder after stereotactic tractotomy. British Journal of Psychiatry 151: 113–116

- Followed nine patients for 5 years after stereotactic subcaudate tractotomy.
- A reduction in the frequency of mood cycling was found.
- A greater response to medication was also reported after surgery.

Poynton A, Bridges PK, Bartlett JR 1988 Resistant bipolar affective disorder treated by stereotactic subcaudate tractotomy. British Journal of Psychiatry 152: 354–358

- Reported positive improvements in mood cycling in nine female patients after stereotactic subcaudate tractotomy.
- 33% had mild to moderate impairment of cognitive function.

Dougherty DD, Baer L, Cosgrove GR et al 2002 Prospective long-term follow up of 44 patients who received cingulotomy for treatment of refractory obsessive compulsive disorder. American Journal of Psychiatry 159: 269–275

- A study of 44 patients with obsessive–compulsive disorder who underwent stereotactic cingulotomy.
- 44% demonstrated a response or partial response.
- There was an average reduction of 28.7% on the Y-BOCS.
- Memory and concentration problems occurred and persisted for between 6 and 12 months in 5%.
- The suicide rate after anterior cingulotomy was 2%.

Kim C-H, Chang JW, Koo MS et al 2003 Anterior cingulotomy for refractory obsessive compulsive disorder. Acta Psychiatrica Scandinavica 107: 283–290

- A study of anterior cingulotomy for obsessive–compulsive disorder revealed an average improvement of 36% on the Y-BOCS after 12 months.

Rück C, Andreewitch S, Flyckt K et al 2003 Capsulotomy for refractory anxiety disorders: long term follow-up of 26 patients. American Journal of Psychiatry 160: 513–521

- A study of thermocapsulotomy in 26 patients with generalised anxiety disorder, social phobia or panic disorder.
- 92% of patients showed a response after 12 months.
- 67% of patients showed a response long term.
- The mean length of follow-up was 13 years.
- 28% of patients had clinical symptoms indicating frontal lobe dysfunction, suggesting that procedure- and disorder-related factors may be features in these cases.
- The suicide rate after anterior capsulotomy was 4%.

Bridges PK, Bartlett JR, Hale AS et al 1994 Psychosurgery: stereotactic subcaudate tractotomy. An indispensable treatment. British Journal of Psychiatry 165: 599–611; discussion 612–613

- A series of more than 1300 patients who underwent subcaudate tractotomy.
- There was no report of significant personality change (significant not defined).

Goktepe EO, Young LB, Bridges PK 1975 A further review of the results of stereotactic subcaudate tractotomy. British Journal of Psychiatry 126: 270–280

- Reported rates of personality change of 6.7% as reported by relatives.
- Noted the difficulties in differentiating between irreversible personality damage and unmasking of premorbid personality traits.

Rush AJ, George MS, Sackheim HA 2000 Vagus nerve stimulation (VNS) for treatment resistant depression: a multicentre study. Biological Psychiatry 47: 276–286; Sackheim HA, Rush AJ, George MS et al 2001 Vagus nerve stimulation (VNS) for treatment resistant depression: efficacy, side effects and predictors of outcome. Neuropsychopharmacology 25: 713–728

- The combined results of two multicentre open pilot studies found that 31% (18 of 59) of the subjects were deemed to have a clinical response within 12 weeks.
- Clinical response was designated as a reduction of 50% or more on the Hamilton Rating Scale for Depression.
- 15% (9) met criteria for complete response
- 5% (3) worsened during the treatment period.

Marangell LB, Rush AJ, George MS et al 2002 Vagus nerve stimulation (VNS) for major depressive disorder: one year outcomes. Biological Psychiatry 51: 280–287

- A follow-up study.
- 46% ($n = 28$) met the criteria for clinical response after 12 months of vagus nerve stimulation; 10 were also 'responders' at 12 weeks.
- Adverse effects include hoarseness, throat or neck pain, cough, dyspnoea and headache.
- Adverse effects significantly reduced over the course of 12 months of stimulation.
- No patient discontinued the stimulation because of adverse effects
- The only reports of cardiac effects are six instances of asystole lasting 10–20 seconds during implantation and first stimulation, none of which resulted in long-term sequelae.
- There have been isolated reports of hypomanic episodes occurring during vagus nerve stimulation

Gabriëls LA, Cosyns PR, Meyerson BA et al 2003 Long-term electrical capsular stimulation in patients with obsessive–compulsive disorder. Neurosurgery 52: 1263–1274

- A study of 12 patients with Parkinson's disease who received deep brain stimulation of the subthalamic nucleus.
- There were improvements in self-reported mood, HRSD scores and emotional memory during stimulation, with no change in cognitive performance.

Berney A, Vingerhoets F, Perrin A et al 2002 Effect on mood of subthalamic deep brain stimulation for Parkinson's disease: a consecutive series of 24 patients. Neurology 59: 1427–1429

- Reported a significant worsening of mood state in 6 of 24 patients who received subthalamic nucleus deep brain stimulation for Parkinson's disease.

Definitions

Psychosurgery – the selective surgical removal or destruction of nerve pathways for the purposes of influencing behaviour. (*Source:* WHO 1977, www.who. int.)

Neurosurgery for mental disorder – a surgical procedure for the destruction of brain tissue for the purposes of alleviating specific mental disorders carried out by a stereotactic or other method capable of making an accurate placement of the lesion. (*Source:* Royal College of Psychiatrists 2000 Neurosurgery for mental disorder. Report from the Neurosurgery Working Group of the Royal College of Psychiatrists. Royal College of Psychiatrists, London.)

See also the 'Treatment – Others' sections in Chapter 2 (Affective disorders), page 39, and Chapter 16 (Obsessive–compulsive disorder), page 245.

Assessment Tools and Rating Scales

BASIS-32

- Self-report for psychiatric inpatients.
- Measure of symptom and problem difficulty.
- Used predominantly to measure treatment outcomes.
- Administered by a healthcare professional prior to treatment.
- Re-administration to monitor treatment progress.
- Treatment benefit associated with reduced scores on self-reported symptoms and problem difficulties.

Weblink BASIS*plus*™ – www.basissurvey.org.

Clinical Global Impression Scale (CGI)

Guy W 1976 ECDEU Assessment Manual for Psychopharmacology – Revised (DHEW Pupl No ADM 76-338). National Institute of Mental Health, Bethesda, MD

- Assesses global severity of illness and the clinical condition over time.
- Performed by a trained assessor.
- Normally completed after clinical interview in a couple of minutes.
- 4-point scale from none to outweighs therapeutic effect.
- Has subscales for specific disorders.
- Standardised assessment tool. Three global subscales include:
  - severity of illness: 7-point scale from normal (1) to extremely ill (7)
  - global improvement: 7-point scale from very much improved (1) to very much worse (7)
  - efficacy index.
- Used widely in research.

General Health Questionnaire (GHQ)

Goldberg D 1972 The detection of psychiatric illness by questionnaire: a technique for the identification and assessment of non-psychotic psychiatric illness. Maudsley Monographs No. 21. Oxford University Press, London; Goldberg D, Hilier VP 1979 A scaled version of the General Health Questionnaire (GHQ-28). Psychological Medicine 9: 139–145. Online. Available: www.nfer-nelson.co.uk

- Self-administered questionnaire.
- Measure of ability to carry out normal functions and presence of novel experiences.
- Identifies non-psychotic psychiatric illness.
- Provides scaled scores over the past month.
- Four versions:
  - GHQ-60   Complete version
  - GHQ-30   Measure of physical illness
  - GHQ-28   Measure of somatic, neurotic and affective symptoms and their impact on social function
  - GHQ-12   Short research version.

Global Assessment of Functioning (GAF)

Luborsky L 1962 Clinicians' judgements of mental health. Archives of General Psychiatry 7: 407–417; American Psychiatric Association 2000 Diagnostic and statistical manual of mental disorders, 4th edn, Text Revision. American Psychiatric Association, Washington DC, p 34

- Global judgement following semi-structured interview.
- Rates overall psychological, social and occupational functioning, excluding impairment due to physical or environmental factors.
- Performed by a trained health professional.
- Score given after a clinical interview by clinician.
- Included in the DSM-IV as the Axis V assessment.
- Rates from 1 to 100 (Table 12.2).
- Children's and parent–infant relationship versions available.

HoNOS

Royal College of Psychiatrists 2006 Health of the Nation Outcome Scales (HoNOS). Royal College of Psychiatrists London. Online. Available: www.rcpsych.ac.uk

Table 12.2 Global Assessment of Functioning (GAF) rating score

GAF score	Clinical situation
90+	None
80	Now asymptomatic
70	Mild symptoms
60	Moderate symptoms
50	Serious symptoms
40	Severe symptoms
30 and over	Very severe. Should be hospitalised

There are six versions of the HoNOS:
- HoNOS for working age adults
- HoNOS65+for people > 65 years
- HoNOSCA for children and adolescents
- HoNOS-Secure
- HoNOS-LD for learning disabled people
- HoNOS-ABI for people with acquired brain injuries.

HoNOS

- Measure of health and social function in people with severe mental illness.
- Initially developed as a tool to monitor progress for the Health of the Nation targets.
- 12-item clinician rating instrument which measures behaviour, impairment, symptoms and social functioning.
- Completed after routine clinical assessment.
- Can monitor change.

HoNOS65+

12 scales which measure:
- behavioural disturbance
- non-accidental self-injury
- problem drinking or drug use
- cognitive problems
- problems related to physical illness or disability
- problems associated with hallucinations and/or delusions or false beliefs
- problems associated with depressive symptoms
- other mental and behavioural problems
- problems with social or supportive relationships
- problems with activities of daily living
- overall problems with living conditions
- problems with work and leisure activities.

4-point scoring from no problem (0) to severe problem (4) on each of the above scales.

HoNOS-Secure

- Need for clinical risk management procedures.
- Seven scales which measure:
  - risk of harm to adults or children
  - risk of self-harm (deliberate or accidental)
  - need for building security to prevent physical escape
  - need for a safely staffed living environment
  - need for escort on leave (beyond the secure perimeter)
  - risk to individual from others
  - need for risk management procedures.

See also the 'Assessment tools and rating scales' sections in Chapter 10 (Forensic psychiatry), page 168, Chapter 17 (Old age psychiatry), page 269.

Illness Behaviour Questionnaire (IBQ)

Pilowsky I, Spence N 1994 Manual for the illness behaviour questionnaire (IBQ), 3rd edn. University of Sydney, Adelaide

- 62 item self-report.
- Investigates patients' beliefs regarding their illness, in particular unhelpful or inappropriate responses to ill-health.

Millon Clinical Multiaxial Inventory (MCMI)

Millon T 1969 Modern psychopathology. WB Saunders, Philadelphia.

- Structured interview to assess presence of DSM-IV personality disorders.
- Rates the patient using 175 true/false questionnaires, by 20 categories.
- They relate to:
  - basic personality styles (8)
  - pathological personality styles (3)
  - disorder scales of moderate severity (6)
  - disorder scales of extreme severity (3).
- Enables the diagnosis of the 14 subtypes of personality disorder within DSM.

Modified Overt Aggression Scale (MOAS)

Kay SR, Wolkenfeld F, Murril LM 1988 Profiles of aggression among psychiatric patients. I. Nature and prevalence. Journal of Nervous and Mental Disease 176: 539–546

Measures four categories of aggression:

1. Verbal aggression
2. Physical aggression against self
3. Physical aggression against objects
4. Physical aggression against others.

Patients were considered to be violent if they expressed overt and intentional violence against others or a verbal threat with an accompanying weapon = score over 3.

Minnesota Multiphasic Personality Inventory (MMPI)

Minnesota Multiphasic Personality Inventory. Online. Available: www1.umn.edu/mmpi

* Most frequently used personality test in mental health.
* 567 true/false items for adults > 18
* Short 370 items for an adolescent version
* 10 clinical scales (Box 12.2) and three validity scales, which should be interpreted by a skilled and competent psychologist.

Premorbid Adjustment Scale (PAS)

Cannon-Spoor HE, Potkin SG, Wyatt RJ 1982 Measurement of premorbid adjustment on chronic schizophrenia. Schizophrenia Bulletin 8: 470–484

* The PAS defines the premorbid phase from birth to 6 months before the onset of illness.
* A widely used premorbid scale for psychosis.
* 36 items which examine the level of functioning before the onset of psychosis.

Box 12.2

MMPI clinical scales

Scale 0	Social introversion
Scale 1	Hypochondriasis
Scale 2	Depression
Scale 3	Hysteria
Scale 4	Psychoapathic deviate
Scale 5	Masculinity/femininity
Scale 6	Paranoia
Scale 7	Psychasthenia
Scale 8	Schizophrenia
Scale 9	Hypomania

---

* Examines:
  - sociability and withdrawal
  - peer relationships
  - scholastic performance
  - adaptation to school
  - capacity to develop sociosexual relationships.
* Assesses this at four stages of life:
  - childhood (up to 11 years)
  - early adolescence (12–15 years)
  - late adolescence (16–18 years)
  - adulthood (19 years and beyond).
* Rating is based on interviews with patient and/or family.
* Scores from 0 (best level of functioning) to 6 (worst level of functioning).

Guidelines

A growing evidence base for management guidelines

A growing evidence base for management guidelines. Revisiting... Guidelines for the management of acutely disturbed patients. MacPherson R, Dix R, Morgan S. Advances in Psychiatric Treatment 2005; 11: 404–415

There is a growing evidence base regarding the use of rapid tranquillisation derived from specialist care units and intensive psychiatric care units in particular. The majority of psychiatric hospitals have policies for rapid tranquillisation and emergency treatment. Formal guidelines have also been developed.

This article discusses patient assessment, risk assessment and the place of the Mental Health Act. It also discusses the serious adverse effects associated with rapid tranquillisation including, for example, respiratory depression and hypotension.

Caution is advised when prescribing for patients who are elderly, debilitated or have learning disabilities.

The National Audit Office 2003 A safer place to work – protecting hospital and ambulance staff from violence and aggression. The Stationery Office, London

* There was a 40% increase in self-reported violence on NHS staff between 1999 and 2002.
* The rate of violence is 2.5 times higher in mental health and learning disability trusts when compared with other specialties.
* Underreporting is high.
* Violent incidents are estimated to cost the NHS £69 million a year, not including human costs.

- There were widespread variations in staff training in risk assessment and aggression management.
- Doctors were particularly poorly trained.
- There were also variations in how staff were supported after an incident.
- Successful prosecution by assaulted staff was rare.

Lader M 1992 Expert evidence. Committee of Inquiry into Complaints about Ashworth Hospital (Cm 2028). HMSO, London

- Patients are at risk of sudden cardiopulmonary collapse.
- This is associated with the use of antipsychotics and physical arousal.

Banerjee S, Bingley W, Murphy E 1995 Deaths of detained patients. Mental Health Foundation, London

- The deaths of 206 detained patients were examined.
- 15 deaths were thought to be due to iatrogenic causes.
- The use of high dose medication and polypharmacy by inexperienced and junior staff were of particular concern.

Agid O, Kapur S, Arenovich T et al 2003 Delayed-onset hypothesis of antipsychotic action. A hypothesis tested and rejected. Archives of General Psychiatry 60: 1228–1235

- Antipsychotic medication can be beneficial in the rapid improvement of symptoms of psychosis and mania.
- These effects can be greater than those produced by benzodiazepines.

Crowner M, Dougon R, Convit A et al 1990 Akathisia and violence. Psychopharmacology Bulletin 26: 115–118

- Side effects of antipsychotic medication, akathisia in particular, are associated with suicidality and physical assault.

Fenton M, Coutinho EFS, Campbell C 2001 Zuclopenthixol acetate in the treatment of acute schizophrenia and similar serious mental illnesses (**Cochrane Review**). In: The Cochrane Library, Issue 4. Update Software, Oxford

- Whilst zuclopenthixol acetate was as effective as oral haloperidol, it may show more rapid and greater sedation.

Chouinard G 1985 Antimanic effects of clonazepam. Psychosomatics 26 (Suppl): 7–12

- Benzodiazepines are of benefit in the treatment of mania.

Dubin WR 1988 Rapid tranquillisation: antipsychotics or benzodiazepines. Journal of Clinical Psychiatry 49: 5–11

- Benzodiazepines are beneficial in the treatment of mild behaviour disturbance associated with substance misuse.

Stimmel GL 1996 Benzodiazepines in schizophrenia. Pharmacotherapy 16: 1485–1515

- Benzodiazepines are helpful in the treatment of schizophrenia-associated behavioural disturbance.

Broadstock M 2001 The effectiveness and safety of drug treatment for urgent sedation in psychiatric emergencies. New Zealand Health Technology Assessment 4: 1–38

- Respiratory depression is a recognised effect of benzodiazepine use.

Fava M 1997 Psychopharmacological treatment of pathologic aggression. Psychiatric Clinics of North America 20: 427–451

- Behavioural disinhibition can result from benzodiazepine use in some individuals.

McAllister-Williams RH, Ferrier IN 2002 Rapid tranquillisation: time for a reappraisal of options for parenteral therapy. British Journal of Psychiatry 180: 485–489

- Haloperidol, when used for rapid tranquillisation, has been associated with sudden death.
- It is likely that this is due to further prolongation of a QTc already lengthened by acute behavioural disturbance.

Royal College of Psychiatrists 1997 The association between antipsychotic drugs and sudden death (Council Report 57). Royal College of Psychiatrists, London

- Zuclopenthixol acetate should not be used for rapid tranquillisation as there are reports of sudden deaths and fatal cardiac events with its use.

Lindberg SR, Beasley CM, Alaka K et al 2003 Effects of intramuscular olanzapine vs haloperidol and placebo on QTc intervals in acutely agitated patients. Psychiatry Research 119: 113–123

- Intramuscular preparations of olanzapine do not appear to be associated with the high risks of QT prolongation.
- The bradycardia, syncope and vasovagal collapse that occur appear to be benign and self-limiting.

Kumar A 1997 Sudden unexplained death in a psychiatric patient – a case report: the role of phenothiazines and physical restraint. Medicine, Science and the Law 37: 170–175

- The situation where a struggling patient is physically restrained and given intramuscular medication must be viewed as a dangerous situation.
- Restraint is traumatic and humiliating to staff and its use impacts on the relationships between patients and staff.
- Issues of dignity, privacy, gender and location must not be forgotten.

Standard Nursing and Midwifery Advisory Committee 1999 Mental health nursing: addressing acute concerns. Department of Health, London. Online. Available: www.advisorybodies.doh.gov.uk/snmac/snmacmh.pdf

- Both patients and nursing staff can find the prolonged observation of patients difficult, counterproductive and distressing.

Definition

Rapid tranquillisation – the administration of medication to calm or sedate an agitated, aggressive patient. It aims to reduce patient suffering, allow improved communication, reduce risks to the patient and others, and to do no harm.

Violence: the short term management of disturbed/violent behaviour in psychiatric inpatient settings and emergency departments. NICE Clinical Guideline 25*
(see pages 203-205)

Observation

Policy

- Each service should have a policy on observation and engagement, adhering to the terminology and definitions used in this guideline (see 'Levels of observation', below) that includes:
  - who can instigate observation above the general level and who can change the level of observation
  - who should review the level of observation and when reviews should take place (at least every shift)
  - how the service user's perspectives will be taken into account
  - a process through which a review by a full clinical team will take place if observation above the general level continues for more than 1 week.ⓓ

Levels of observation

- The terminology adopted in this guideline should be adopted across England and Wales.ⓓ

General observation ⓓ

- This is the minimum acceptable level for all service users
- The location of the service user should be known to staff at all times but they are not necessarily within sight
- Positive engagement with the service user should take place at least once a shift
- Evaluate the service user's moods and behaviours associated with disturbed/violent behaviour, and record these in the notes

Intermittent observation ⓓ

- This level is appropriate for service users potentially at risk of disturbed/violent behaviour, including those who have previously been at risk but are in the process of recovery
- The service user's location should be checked every 15–30 minutes (specify exact times in the notes)
- Intrusion should be minimised and positive engagement with the service user should take place

Within eyesight observation ⓓ

- Service users who could, at any time, make an attempt to harm themselves or others should be observed at this level
- The service user should be within eyesight and accessible at all times, day and night
- Any possible tools or instruments that could be used should be removed, if deemed necessary
- Searching of the service user and their belongings may be necessary, which should be conducted sensitively and with due regard to legal rights
- Positive engagement with the service user is essential

Within arms length observation ⓓ

- Service users at the highest levels of risk of harming themselves or others may need to be observed at this level
- The service user should be supervised in close proximity
- More than one staff member may be necessary on specific occasions
- Issues of privacy and dignity, consideration of gender issues, and environmental dangers should be discussed and incorporated into the care plan
- Positive engagement with the service user is essential

B, C and **D** indicate grades of recommendation; **GPP** indicates a good practice point (see Appendix II for full details). * Reproduced with permission from the National Institute for Health and Clinical Excellence, London.

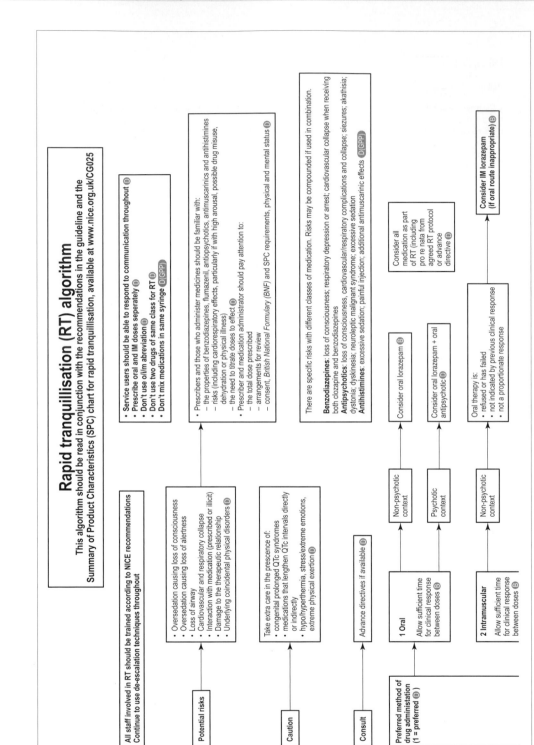

Rapid tranquillisation (RT) algorithm

This algorithm should be read in conjunction with the recommendations in the guideline and the Summary of Product Characteristics (SPC) chart for rapid tranquillisation, available at www.nice.org.uk/CG025

All staff involved in RT should be trained according to NICE recommendations. Continue to use de-escalation techniques throughout

- Service users should be able to respond to communication throughout (D)
- Prescribe oral and IM doses seperately (D)
- Don't use oil/im abreviation (D)
- Don't use two drugs of same class for RT (D)
- Don't mix medications in same syringe (D)(GPP)

Potential risks

- Oversedation causing loss of consciousness
- Oversedation causing loss of alertness
- Loss of airway
- Cardiovascular and respiratory collapse
- Interaction with medication (prescribed or illicit)
- Damage to the therapeutic relationship
- Underlying coincidental physical disorders (D)

- Prescribers and those who administer medicines should be familiar with:
  - the properties of benzodiazepines, flumazenil, antipsychotics, antimuscarinics and antihistimines
  - risks (including cardiorespiratory effects, particularly if with high arousal, possible drug misuse, dehydration or physical illness)
  - the need to titrate doses to effect (D)
- Prescriber and medication administrator should pay attention to:
  - the total dose prescribed
  - arrangements for review
  - consent, *British National Formulary (BNF)* and SPC requirements, physical and mental status (D)

Caution

Take extra care in the prescence of:
- congenital prolonged QTc syndromes
- medications that lengthen QTc intervals directly or indirectly
- hypo/hyperthermia, stress/extreme emotions, extreme physical exertion (D)

There are specific risks with different classes of medication. Risks may be compounded if used in combination.

Benzodiazepines: loss of consciousness; respiratory depression or arrest; cardiovascular collapse when receiving both clozapine and benzodiazepines
Antipsychotics: loss of consciousness, cardiovascular/respiratory complications and collapse; siezures; akathisia; dystonia; dyskinesia; neuroleptic malignant syndrome; excessive sedation
Antihistimines: excessive sedation; painful injection; additional antimuscarinic effects (D)(GPP)

Consult

Advance directives if available (D)

Consider all medication as part of RT (including pro re nata from agreed RT protocol or advance directive) (D)

Preferred method of drug administration
(1 = preferred (D))

1 Oral

Allow sufficient time for clinical response between doses (B)

Non-psychotic context → Consider oral lorazepam (B)

Psychotic context → Consider oral lorazepam + oral antipsychotic (D)

2 Intramuscular

Allow sufficient time for clinical response between doses (B)

Non-psychotic context → Oral therapy is:
- refused or has failed
- not indicated by previous clinical response
- not a proportionate response

→ Consider IM lorazepam (if oral route inappropriate) (B)

B, C and D indicate grades of recommendation; GPP indicates a good practice point (see Appendix II for full details). * Reproduced with permission from the National Institute for Health and Clinical Excellence, London.

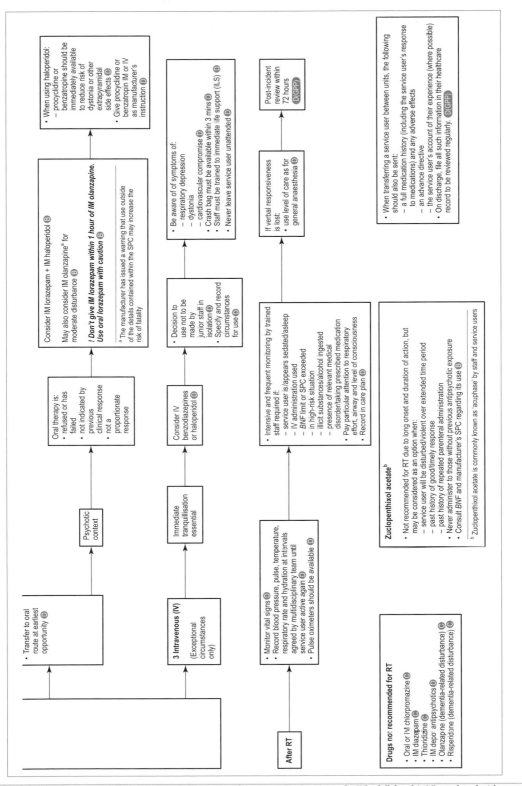

B, **C** and **D** indicate grades of recommendation; **GPP** indicates a good practice point (see Appendix II for full details). * Reproduced with permission from the National Institute for Health and Clinical Excellence, London.

Zaleplon, zolpidem and zopiclone for the short-term management of insomnia. NICE Technology Appraisal Guidance 77*

Guidance

When, after due consideration of the use of non-pharmacological measures, hypnotic drug therapy is considered appropriate for the management of severe insomnia interfering with normal life, it is recommended that hypnotics should be prescribed for short periods of time only, in strict accordance with their licensed indications.

It is recommended that, because of the lack of compelling evidence to distinguish between zaleplon, zolpidem, zopiclone and the shorter-acting benzodiazepine hypnotics, the drug with the lowest purchase cost (taking into account daily required dose and product price per dose) should be prescribed.

It is recommended that switching from one of these hypnotics to another should occur only if a patient experiences adverse effects considered to be directly related to a specific agent. These are the only circumstances in which drugs with higher acquisition costs are recommended.

Patients who have not responded to one of these hypnotic drugs should not be prescribed any of the others.

---

* Reproduced with permission from the National Institute for Health and Clinical Excellence, London.

Hyperkinetic disorders 13

Chapter contents

General topics

ADHD in adults

Zwi M, York A 2004 Attention deficit hyperactivity disorder in adults: validity unknown. Advances in Psychiatric Treatment 10: 248–259

It is argued that DSM-IV diagnostic criteria are too stringent when applied to adults. There is limited evidence regarding the pharmacological treatment of adult ADHD.

DSM-III was the first classification system to suggest that symptoms might continue into adulthood as 'attention-deficit disorder (hyperactivity), residual state'. The trend towards extension into adulthood continued in DSM-III-R for whom 'impairment in the workplace' is specifically mentioned. However, field trials for DSM-IV did not include adults.

Still GF 1902 Some abnormal physical conditions in children: the Goulstonian Lectures. Lancet 1: 1008–1012, 1077–1082

- Described children with hyperactivity and poor attention skills as having a 'defect of moral control'.

Bradley C 1937 The behaviour of children receiving benzedrine. American Journal of Psychiatry 94: 577–585

- Wrote about the use of amfetamines in children to reduce hyperactivity.

Zwi M, Ramchandani P, Joughin C 2000 Evidence and belief in ADHD. British Medical Journal 321: 975–976

- Notes the heterogeneity of clinical signs, symptoms, comorbidities and presentations.
- The progression of evolving diagnostic systems is also discussed.
- Concludes that ADHD is possibly best conceptualised as a heterogeneous, complex neurodevelopmental constellation of problems rather than a single disorder.

Timimi S 2001 Evidence and belief in attention-deficit hyperactivity disorder. British Medical Journal 322: 555

- The cut-off between normal behaviour and ADHD is arbitrary.
- There are a variety of definitions which exist for different reasons.
- Poses the question that ADHD is a research-generated concept with little relation to the complexity found in clinical practice.

Barkley RA 2002 International consensus statement on ADHD. Journal of the American Academy of Child and Adolescent Psychiatry 41: 1389

- The consensus statement from a consortium of 74 internationally acclaimed ADHD researchers.
- Argued in favour of the validity of the diagnosis, in response to the 'periodic inaccurate portrayal' of ADHD in the media.
- The statement describes ADHD as a syndrome characterised by deficiencies in a set of psychological

abilities that pose serious harm to most of those who have it.

- At the core of the disorder are deficits in behavioural inhibition and sustained attention.
- These lead to impaired social, educational and occupational functioning.
- There are difficulties with social rules, norms and laws, and increased physical injury and accidental poisoning.
- The document is a statement of opinion rather than a scientific argument.

Three cohort studies of children with diagnoses of ADHD have followed individuals from childhood into adulthood. They all report relatively low rates of ADHD in the adult years compared with childhood and adolescence. They also report that people with childhood ADHD showed higher rates of impairments when compared with controls. These include impaired educational and occupational outcomes, antisocial personality disorder, substance misuse and persistent social impairment.

Weiss G, Hechtman L, Milroy T et al 1985 Psychiatric status of hyperactives as adults. A controlled prospective 15-year follow-up of 63 hyperactive children. Journal of the American Academy of Child Psychiatry 24: 211–220

- Followed 63 hyperactive children and 41 controls for 15 years.
- Diagnostic interviews were not blinded and the loss to follow-up over 15 years was 33.6%.
- All children had a diagnosis of ADD(H).
- The majority had an associated conduct disorder.
- 66% of hyperactive individuals (compared with 7% of the control group) complained of at least one disabling symptom.
- The rates of ADHD (DSM-III) were not reported for the period of the study.
- The only DSM-III diagnosis that differed between the two groups was antisocial personality disorder.
- 23% of the hyperactive individuals and 2.4% of the controls had antisocial personality disorder.
- Of the hyperactive individuals, 90% had received 10–20 therapeutic interviews and 10% family therapy during childhood and adolescence.

Mannuzza S, Klein RG, Bessler A et al 1998 Adult psychiatric status of hyperactive boys grown up. American Journal of Psychiatry 155: 493–498

- A New York cohort study.
- 207 boys referred to a child psychiatry clinic were followed from their childhood to their early twenties.
- The boys were predominantly middle class, white and of average intelligence.

- Conduct disorder was virtually absent as those with aggression or antisocial behaviour were excluded.
- Assessors were blind.
- There was loss to follow-up of 12–18% over a period of 15–21 years.
- 85–90% of those with hyperactivity had been prescribed stimulant drugs in childhood, in some continuing on for many years.
- In late adolescence ADHD was present in 40% of the index cases and 3% of the controls.
- 27% of the index group and 8% of the controls had antisocial personality disorder.
- By mean age 25 'clinically impairing ADHD symptoms and syndromes' were present in 11% of the index group and in only 1% of the controls.
- In a second cohort only 4% of the index group and none of the controls had the disorder.

Rasmussen P, Gillberg C 2000 Natural outcome of ADHD with developmental coordination disorder at age 22 years. A controlled, longitudinal, community-based study. Journal of the American Academy of Child and Adolescent Psychiatry 39: 1424–1431

- A Swedish study.
- A longitudinal study of a community sample of 61 children with ADHD and comorbid developmental coordination disorder and 46 controls from childhood to adulthood.
- Using DSM-IV criteria the group consisted of 39 individuals with ADHD and developmental coordination disorder, 11 with ADHD only and five with developmental coordination disorder only.
- None of the index cases ever received stimulants.
- Follow-up extended over 15 years and loss to follow-up in both groups was 10%.
- Assessments of psychiatric status in adulthood were blind.
- At age 22, 49% of the index cases and 9% of the controls had 'marked symptoms of ADHD'.
- 60% of the children in the index group and 13% in the control group had a 'poor outcome'.
- Poor outcomes included drug or alcohol misuse, receiving a disability pension or welfare benefits, major personality disorder, chronic severe psychiatric disorder, autistic-spectrum disorder, and conviction for a criminal offence.

Mannuzza S, Klein RG, Klein DF et al 2002 Accuracy of adult recall of childhood attention deficit hyperactivity disorder. American Journal of Psychiatry 159: 1882–1888

- Adults reporting symptoms of ADHD in childhood were able to provide sufficient information to confirm a retrospective ADHD diagnosis.

- The blinded interviews achieved high sensitivity (0.78) and specificity (0.89) for adult recall of childhood ADHD symptoms.
- This study was performed in adults with a diagnosis of childhood ADHD resulting in a higher prevalence of true positive cases of ADHD.
- When the figures were recalculated assuming a 5% prevalence of ADHD in the general population, the false-positive rate rose substantially to 75%.
- Contemporaneous data are vital to substantiate retrospective diagnoses.

Loeber R, Green S, Lahey BB et al 1992 Developmental sequences in the age of onset of disruptive child behaviors. Journal of Child and Family Studies 1: 21–41

- Hyperactive–impulsive symptoms emerge initially in childhood before declining with age.

Applegate B, Lahey BB, Hart EL et al 1997 Validity of the age-of-onset criterion for ADHD. A report from the DSM-IV field trials. Journal of the American Academy of Child and Adolescent Psychiatry 36: 1211–1221

- Symptoms of inattention may emerge later and predominate with age.

Weiss M, Murray C, Weiss G 2002 Adults with attention-deficit/hyperactivity disorder. Current concepts. Journal of Psychiatric Practice 8: 99–111

- In longitudinal studies as many as 66% continue to report the presence of at least one ADHD symptom severe enough to cause impairment.
- If diagnostic criteria are overly restrictive, this will lead to underreporting in adults.

Murphy KR, Barkley RA, Bush T 2002 Young adults with attention deficit hyperactivity disorder: subtype differences in comorbidity, educational and clinical history. Journal of Nervous and Mental Disease 190: 147–157

- Note that DSM-IV diagnostic criteria include the presence of symptoms before the age of 7 years.
- If used, it may be difficult to confirm a diagnosis in the absence of a clearly documented history of childhood ADHD.

Murphy K, Barkley RA 1996 Attention deficit hyperactivity disorder in adults. Comorbidities and adaptive impairments. Comprehensive Psychiatry 37: 393–401

- Adults attending clinics are usually self-referred, compared with children who are usually taken by their parents.

- Factors associated with self-referral, such as educational and socioeconomic status, may influence the composition of this population.
- Patterns of comorbidity also varied.
- Clinic-referred adults were more likely to have comorbid anxiety disorders (50% affected).
- Hyperactive children were more commonly found to have conduct, substance misuse and antisocial personality disorders.

Studies investigating the pharmacological treatment of adult ADHD are listed in Table 13.1.

Weblink Attention Deficit Disorder Information and Support Service in the UK – www.addiss.co.uk.

ADHD is best understood as a cultural construct

Timimi S, Taylor E 2004 ADHD is best understood as a cultural construct. British Journal of Psychiatry 184: 8–9

There is some debate regarding the issues of diagnosis, and what exactly psychiatrists are and should treat. Increasing rates of ADHD may reflect the actual increase in incidence. It may reflect society's intolerance of behaviour that does not conform.

The argument for ADHD as a cultural construct might include the following considerations:

- No markers or tests exist for ADHD.
- There are uncertainties regarding definition, leading to wide variation in quoted prevalence rates (0.5–26%).
- Criteria may vary between different cultures.
- Researchers have not compared unmedicated children diagnosed with ADHD with age-matched controls, despite large numbers of neuroimaging studies.
- Sample studies have been small and have produced varied and inconsistent results.
- Genetic studies have shown that being male is a risk factor – boys are 4–10 times more likely to get this diagnosis in practice.
- Comorbidity is extremely high, which might suggest the diagnosis is not specific.
- There is no specific treatment and methylphenidate shows similar effects in normal children.
- There is no established prognosis.
- Association and cause are often confused in the literature.
- The medicalisation of behaviours can foster dependence on doctors and discourage children and families from problem solving themselves.

Prout A, James A 1997 Constructing and reconstructing childhood: contemporary issues in the sociological study of childhood. Falmer Press, London

Table 13.1 Pharmacological treatment of adult ADHD

Study	Treatment: may be beneficial
Spencer T, Wilsen T, Biederman J et al 1995 A double blind crossover comparison of methylphenidate and placebo in adults with childhood onset attention deficit hyperactivity disorder. Archives of General Psychiatry 52: 434–443	Methylphenidate
Dorrego MF, Canevaro L, Kuzis G et al 2002 A randomised double blind crossover study of methylphenidate and lithium in adults with attention deficit/hyperactivity disorder. Preliminary findings. Journal of Neuropsychiatry and Clinical Neurosciences 14: 289–295	Methylphenidate and lithium
Spencer T, Biederman J, Wilens T et al 2001 Efficacy of a mixed amphetamine salts compound in adults with attention deficit/hyperactivity disorder. Archives of General Psychiatry 58: 775–782	Mixed amfetamine salts
Wilens TE, Spencer TJ, Biederman J et al 2001 A controlled trial of bupropion for attention deficit hyperactivity disorder in adults. American Journal of Psychiatry 158: 282–288	Desipramine
Tylor FB, Russo J 2000 Efficacy of modafinil compared to dextroamphetamine for the treatment of attention deficit hyperactivity disorder in adults. Journal of Child and Adolescent Psychopharmacology 10: 311–320	Modafinil
Wilens TE, Biederman J, Spencer TJ et al 1999 Controlled trial of high doses of pemoline for adults with attention deficit/hyperactivity disorder. Journal of Clinical Psychopharmacology 19: 257–264	Pemoline
Michelson D, Adler L, Spencer T et al 2003 Atomoxetine in adult with ADHD: two randomised, placebo-controlled studies. Biological Psychiatry 53: 112–120	Atomoxetine (noradrenaline transporter)

- In modern western culture there are many factors that can adversely affect the mental state of children and their families.
- These include:
  - loss of extended family support
  - mother blame
  - pressure on schools
  - breakdown in the moral authority of adults
  - parents being in a double bind on discipline issues
  - busy family life
  - market economy value system emphasising individuality
  - competitiveness
  - independence.

Timimi S 2002 Pathological child psychiatry and the medicalization of childhood. Brunner-Routledge, Hove

- Children are being victimised and placed on highly addictive drugs with no proven long-term benefits.

The argument against ADHD as a cultural construct

- Suggests that hyperactivity is derived from an interaction of genetic and social influences.
- Genetic studies showing some molecular genetic variations (especially of genes affecting dopamine systems) have been robustly replicated.
- Consistent associations with changes in brain structure have been found, even in unmedicated children, with neuroimaging.
- Suggests evidence is lacking for the hypothesis that the institutions of society can cause the problem.
- Twin studies suggest that individual differences are barely influenced by the shared environment.
- One thing social factors can do is determine the degree of hyperactivity that is seen as a problem.
- Tolerance varies and it is others who determine their caseness.

- In the US, there is suspicion of overtreatment with stimulants, with a high rate of preschool children on stimulants. In the UK, however, there seems to be evidence of undertreatment and lack of identification.

Schachar R, Tannock R 2002 Syndromes of hyperactivity and attention deficit. In: Rutter M, Taylor E (eds) Child and adolescent psychiatry, 4th edn. Blackwell, Oxford, pp 399–418

- Brain structure and function and DNA composition are the physical counterparts of individual difference in hyperactivity.

Taylor E, Chadwick O, Heptinstall E et al 1996 Hyperactivity and conduct problems as risk factors for adolescent development. Journal of the American Academy of Child and Adolescent Psychiatry 35: 1213–1226

- Severe hyperactivity is a strong predictor of poor psychosocial adjustment.
- People with this disorder are more prone to accidents, conduct disorder, adolescent psychiatric disorders, educational and occupational failure, and lack of satisfactory relationships.

Sayal K, Taylor E, Beecham J et al 2002 Pathways to care in children at risk of attention-deficit hyperactivity disorder. British Journal of Psychiatry 181: 43–48

- Suggests the obstacle most probably lies in medical attitudes rather than public ones.
- Broad social influences contribute to the recognition of the disorder rather than its presence.
- These do not amount to a social construction of disorder – rather, in the UK at least, they work against recognition of a treatable risk.

Treatment – Psychopharmacology

Stimulant medication for the treatment of ADHD

Bailey L 2005 Stimulant medication for the treatment of attention-deficit hyperactivity disorder: evidence-b(i)ased practice. Psychiatric Bulletin 29: 284–287

Opinion and debate

There is ongoing debate on the status of ADHD as an illness and whether the prescription of stimulant medication is warranted. ADHD is an operationally defined concept built on a series of non-specific behaviours. Hyperkinetic behaviour can result from a range of biopsychosocial factors including sensory impairment, sleep disturbance, bereavement, mania, child abuse and inadequate parenting.

Much of the information required for the diagnosis is provided by informant history which has implications with regard to neutrality, especially in the case of a child with difficult behaviours. The name ADHD suggests impairment of attention but in clinical practice attention is rarely formally assessed in children with ADHD.

Considerations

- The mode of action of stimulant medication is unknown in ADHD.
- Little is known of the long-term effectiveness of stimulant treatment of ADHD.
- Stimulant medication is not a specific treatment for ADHD.
- Medication can lead to addiction and misuse.
- Pharmaceutical companies use aggressive marketing techniques to promote their drugs.
- ADHD is a commonly diagnosed behavioural disorder of childhood for which studies, including randomised trials, have established the efficacy of stimulants in alleviating ADHD symptoms.
- ADHD is an operationally defined disorder built on a series of non-specific behaviours of which specific aetiology is unknown and for which there is no single diagnostic test.

Koschack J, Kunert H, Derichs G et al 2003 Impaired and enhanced attentional function in children with attentional deficit/hyperactivity disorder. Psychological Medicine 33: 481–489

- Children with the disorder functioned within the normal range on attentional testing.
- They responded faster on all attentional tests and performed with significantly fewer errors on the Divided Attention test compared with controls.

Treatment – Psychological Therapies

Family therapy for attention deficit/ hyperactivity disorder

Bjornstad G, Montgomery P 2005 Family therapy for attention deficit disorder or attention deficit/hyperactivity disorder in children and adolescents **(Cochrane Review)**. In: The Cochrane Library, Issue 2. CD005042. Update Software, Oxford

- Two studies were found:
  - one showed no difference between behavioural family therapy and treatment as usual in the community
  - the other slightly favoured treatment over medication or placebo.

Assessment Tools and Rating Scales

Conners' Parent and Teacher Rating Scale

Gladman M, Lancaster S 2003 A review of the behaviour assessment system for children. School Psychology International 24: 276–291

- Diagnostic scale for ADHD using DSM criteria.
- Includes measures of behaviour described by parents and teachers.
- Behaviour scales include:
  - oppositional behaviour
  - anxiety
  - cognitive problems
  - social problems
  - perfectionism
  - ADHD symptoms.

Guidelines

Guidance on the use of methylphenidate (ritalin, equasym) for attention deficit/hyperactivity disorder (ADHD) in childhood. NICE Technology Appraisal 13*

Guidance

Methylphenidate is recommended for use as part of a comprehensive treatment programme for children with a diagnosis of severe attention deficit/hyperactivity disorder (ADHD). 'Severe ADHD' is broadly similar to a diagnosis of hyperkinetic disorder (HKD), although in some cases treatment may be appropriate for children and adolescents who do not fit the diagnostic criteria for HKD but are experiencing severe problems due to inattention or hyperactivity/impulsiveness.

Methylphenidate is not currently licensed for children under the age of 6 or for children with marked anxiety, agitation or tension symptoms or a family history of tics or Tourette's syndrome, hyperthyroidism, severe angina or cardiac arrhythmia, glaucoma or thyrotoxicosis. Caution is required in the prescribing of methylphenidate for children and young people with epilepsy, psychotic disorders, or a history of drug or alcohol dependence.

Diagnosis should be based on a timely, comprehensive assessment conducted by a child/adolescent psychiatrist or a paediatrician with expertise in ADHD. It should also involve children, parents and carers and the child's school, and take into account cultural factors in the child's environment. Multidisciplinary assessment, which may include educational or clinical psychologists and social workers, is advisable for children who present with indications of significant comorbidity.

Treatment with methylphenidate should only be initiated by child and adolescent psychiatrists or paediatricians with expertise in ADHD, but continued prescribing and monitoring may be performed by general practitioners, under shared care arrangements with specialists.

Careful titration is required to determine the optimal dose level and timing. The drug should be discontinued if improvement of symptoms is not observed after appropriate dose adjustment.

A comprehensive treatment programme should involve advice and support to parents and teachers, and could, but does not need to, include specific psychological treatment (e.g. behavioural therapy). While this wider service is desirable, any shortfall in its provision should not be used as a reason for delaying the appropriate use of medication.

Children on methylphenidate therapy should receive regular monitoring. When improvement has occurred and the child's condition is stable, treatment can be discontinued at intervals, under careful specialist supervision, in order to assess both the child's progress and the need for continuation of therapy.

This guidance relates only to children and adolescents with ADHD.

Evidence

A large number of randomised controlled trials (RCTs) of methylphenidate have been conducted. However, this evidence is predominantly from the US and does not necessarily generalise to a UK context.

There is evidence from placebo-controlled RCTs that methylphenidate is effective at reducing hyperactivity, inattention and impulsiveness in the short term while children continue to take medication.

There is insufficient evidence to judge the relative effectiveness of methylphenidate, dexamphetamine and antidepressants.

Direct randomised comparisons suggest that medication is more effective than behavioural intervention. However, this evidence is of mixed quality.

There is RCT evidence, some of relatively good quality, which suggests that the addition of medication to behavioural treatment programmes is beneficial. Improvements in short- and medium-term outcomes were observed across a number of dimensions.

Evidence from placebo-controlled clinical trials ($n = 1257$) shows that common side effects of methylphenidate are relatively mild and short lived, and that more severe side effects are very rare. However, these data are based on treatment and follow-up of less than 1 year. None of the studies included assessment of longer-term side effects or the risk of addiction or abuse with methylphenidate.

UK estimates suggest that the additional cost of methylphenidate therapy compared to no treatment would be in the region of £10,000–15,000 per quality adjusted life year (QALY) gained. These estimates are based on the assumption that quality of life would be improved by about 6–7 percentage points over 1 year of treatment. Changes to this and other assumptions suggest that the incremental cost-effectiveness ratio could be as low as £5000 or as high as £28,000 per QALY gained. There is no reliable estimate of the incremental cost per QALY gained of adding methylphenidate to behavioural therapy, although this would be expected to be somewhat higher than the above estimates.

---

* Reproduced with permission from the National Institute for Health and Clinical Excellence, London.

Attention deficit and hyperkinetic disorders in children and young people. SIGN Publication Number 52**

Websites

ADDnet UK
www.web-tv.co.uk
Children and Adults with ADHD
www.chadd.org
Training and publications for health and education professionals
www.devdis.com/index.html
Information for parents and professionals
www.attention.com
ADD Warehouse (books, videos, etc.)
www.addwarehouse.com
School Psychology Resources Online
www.bcpl.lib.md.us/~sandyste/school_psych.html

Diagnostic criteria

The core symptoms of ADHD and HKD comprise developmentally inappropriate levels of:
* inattention
  (difficulty in concentrating)
* hyperactivity
  (disorganised, excessive levels of activity)
* impulsive behaviour

In order to meet diagnostic criteria it is essential that symptoms:
* have their onset before the age of 7 years (ADHD) or 6 years (HKD)
* have persisted for at least 6 months
* must be pervasive
  (present in more than one setting, e.g. at home, at school, socially)
* have caused significant functional impairment
* are not better accounted for by other mental disorders
  (e.g. pervasive developmental disorder, schizophrenia, other psychotic disorders, depression or anxiety).

Assessment

The important components of assessment include:
* parent/care giver interview
* child/young person interview
* questionnaires
* psychological educational assessment
* clinical examination
* ancillary assessment including physical, psychiatric and psychological assessments.

Certain complications including preterm delivery, maternal smoking, drug and alcohol abuse may be associated with ADHD/HKD.

✓   If ADHD/HKD associated with significant impairment is suspected following preliminary assessment, refer for assessment by a child and adolescent psychiatrist or paediatrician.

B   Parental report of their children's symptoms is an essential component of the diagnostic assessment.
A history should be obtained of obstetric and perinatal complications.
A developmental history should be obtained to show a chronological development of difficulties.

C   An assessment of the child's presentation in their educational placement is important for confirming diagnosis and identifying educational underachievement.

B   Laboratory assessments should not be used routinely.

Management

ADHD/HKD may be chronic and persistent and in many cases long-term, multimodal, multidisciplinary management is required, drawing upon different treatment methods at different times. Intervention must be individualised with treatment packages and programmes of intervention developed depending on the specific needs of the child or young person and their family.

Non-pharmacological management

There is limited evidence for the effectiveness of psychosocial interventions in the management of the core symptoms of ADHD/HKD. Nevertheless, all symptoms presented by a child/young person must be assessed. Co-morbid conditions can be treated with psychosocial intervention.

A   Family-based psychosocial interventions of a behavioural type are recommended for the treatment of comorbid behavioural problems.

B   Individual psychosocial interventions are not routinely recommended.

A   Children with ADHD/HKD require an individualised school intervention programme including behavioural and academic interventions.

Pharmacological management

The initiation of pharmacological treatment for children with ADHD should only be undertaken by a specialist in child and adolescent psychiatry or paediatrics who has training in the use and monitoring of psychotropic medication in children and adolescents.

A   **Psychostimulants** (methylphenidate and dexamphetamine) should be considered as the first line of drug treatment for the core symptoms of ADHD/HKD.

A   **Tricyclic antidepressants** (TCAs) should be considered in the treatment of behavioural symptoms of ADHD/HKD.

☑   When prescribing psychostimulants, commence with the smallest possible dose and titrate to a 2–3 times daily schedule of increasing dosage at weekly intervals until a satisfactory response is obtained or side effects intrude.

☑   Blood testing should be carried out at the discretion of the supervising clinician and only when clinically indicated.

Combined drug therapy

C   Combined drug treatment may be indicated in certain cases, especially where comorbidity is a feature, but should be supervised by a specialist with expertise in the field.

Other drug therapy

☑   The use of alternative pharmacological agents should be supervised by clinicians with specialist knowledge

Alternative therapies

There is insufficient evidence at present to support the routine use of dietary, complementary and alternative interventions.

A, B and **C** indicate grades of recommendation; ☑ indicates a good practice point (see Appendix II for full details). ** Reproduced with permission from the Scottish Intercollegiate Guidelines Network, Edinburgh.

Possible drug side effects and management options

Anorexia, nausea, weight loss	Monitor carefully, give medication with meals, give calorie supplements
Growth concerns	If significant (rare in long term) or causing parental anxiety, attempt weekend or vacation medication breaks
Sleep difficulties	Monitor carefully, reduce or omit late afternoon or evening medication (but note that some patients improve with added evening medication)
Dizziness and headache	Monitor carefully (check blood pressure), ensure medication is taken with meals and encourage fluid intake
Involuntary movements, tics and Tourette's syndrome	Reduce or if persistent discontinue medication. Consider alternative (e.g. TCA) if symptoms are severe
Loss of spontaneity, dysphoria, agitation	Reduce or discontinue medication (discontinue if thought disorder or psychosis suspected – this is rare)
Irritability, behavioural rebound	Monitor carefully, reduce or overlap afternoon dose, evaluate for comorbidity (ODD/CD)

Learning disabilities psychiatry

14

Chapter contents

Ethical issues

Seeking consent: working with people with learning disabilities

> Department of Health 2001 Seeking consent: working with people with learning disabilities. DH, London

For a person's consent to be valid, the person must be:
- capable of taking that particular decision ('competent')
- acting voluntarily (not under pressure or duress from anyone)
- provided with enough information to enable them to make the decision.

Seeking consent is described as a process. To aid the process you should ensure when seeking consent that sufficient time and support is given. It is acceptable for someone to change their mind and accept a treatment previously refused (or vice versa). Patients should be made aware of this. If a patient changes their mind during a procedure then the procedure should be stopped at a safe juncture. It may be that an objection signifies pain or distress rather than a wish to withdraw consent.

Adults with the capacity to make a decision can refuse treatment, even if that might have detrimental effects. This may not be true for those being treated under mental health legislation for mental disorder. Detention under mental health legislation does not give the power to treat unrelated physical disorders without consent.

Consent forms act as a method of recording consent. Legally it makes no difference whether consent is verbal or written. For complex procedures or those incurring significant risk it is good practice to seek written consent.

If it is not possible for a patient who has capacity to give written consent, it should be noted that oral or non-verbal consent has been given.

Capacity

Capacity to make healthcare decisions is assumed until the opposite has been shown. This is true for all adults, regardless of any learning disability. A multidisciplinary assessment involving learning disability teams and speech and language therapists may be required if there is doubt regarding a patient's capacity to make the decision in question.

For people to have the capacity to take a particular decision, they must be able to:
- comprehend and retain information material to the decision, especially as to the consequences of having or not having the intervention in question
- use and weigh this information in the decision-making process.

For adults with learning disability it is essential that the information is provided in an accessible and appropriate way.

Methods of assessing comprehension and ability to use information to make a choice include:
- exploring the patient's ability to paraphrase what has been said (repeating and rewording as necessary)
- exploring whether the patient is able to compare alternatives, or to express any thoughts on possible consequences other than those which you have disclosed
- exploring whether the patient applies the information to their own case.

Adults with learning disability may receive support from family, carers, friends or advocates in understanding issues and coming to a decision. Members of the learning disability community teams can act in the role of health facilitator on behalf of the patient.

Some people may have the capacity to consent to some interventions but not to others. It should not be assumed that an adult is unable to make a decision because they have been unable to take a particular decision in the past. Nor should it be assumed that a person lacks capacity because their decision seems irrational or unreasonable. It may be that further information and discussion are required, but it is not appropriate to coerce a person into changing their decision and it should be remembered that different people will make different decisions.

To make a decision about consent to treatment, people need information about:

• the benefits and the risks of the proposed treatment
• what the treatment will involve
• what the implications of not having the treatment are
• what alternatives may be available
• what the practical effects on their lives of having, or not having, the treatment will be.

It may be necessary to use interpreters or communication aids to facilitate communication with an adult with learning disability. This might include the use of pictures, of short sentences and plain English. Communication boards where people can indicate 'yes' or 'no' may be helpful. Interpreters may be required where the first language is not English or if a sign language such as Makaton is used. Picture booklets can be helpful. Involvement of people close to the patient and members of the learning disability team may also be required.

When adults lack capacity Some people will not be capable of taking some decisions. If a person is not capable of giving or refusing consent it is still possible to lawfully provide treatment and care. Any treatment or care should be in the person's 'best interests'. No-one can give consent on behalf of an adult who is not able to give consent. It is good practice to include those close to a patient in decisions regarding treatment, unless it is clear that the patient does not wish a particular individual involved.

Advance directives

An advance refusal of certain treatments is legally binding if the person made the decision at a time when they were legally competent, having understood the implications of their decision and that the refusal is applicable to their situation. An advance directive setting out desired care is not legally binding, although they should be considered.

Best interests

Best interests are not limited to medical benefits. Lawfully other factors such as general well-being, relationships, spiritual and religious welfare are included in the meaning. An adult who does not have the capacity to make a decision may well still express a preference on the question in hand. Such preferences should also be taken into account. Best interests are limited to the person's best interests. It is not lawful to include the interests of family members or of health professionals.

If those close to the patient and the healthcare team are unable to come to a decision, then the courts can be asked to determine what is in the person's best interests. Certain procedures (including sterilisation and tissue donation) should always be referred to the court.

It is unlawful and discriminatory to assume that a treatment is not appropriate merely because a patient has learning disability.

Health professionals are not required to perform a procedure desired by family members. It is good practice to explain to family members why a treatment is thought inappropriate and a second opinion should be offered.

When a decision is made to provide treatment on the grounds of best interests, a written record of the reasons behind the decision and the involvement of others in that decision should be recorded. Any disagreements between the clinical team and those close to the patient should also be recorded.

Research

The same principles apply when seeking consent for research as for consent to treatment. The law is unclear when people are unable to give consent. It is generally not appropriate to carry out research on adults who are unable to give consent unless it is in that person's best interests.

Therapeutic research Where the available treatment for a condition is non-existent or of limited effectiveness, it may be in a patient's best interests to be entered into a clinical trial of a new treatment.

Non-therapeutic research It has been suggested that it can be lawful to carry out research in an incapacitated adult which is not beneficial to that adult as long as it is not against the interests of that individual. This has not been tested in the courts. In principle, such research should not be carried out in an incapacitated adult if it is possible to carry it out in an adult with capacity.

Withdrawing and withholding life-prolonging treatment

The same broad principles apply to providing, or withholding, life-prolonging treatment as apply to any other kind of treatment:

• If people with capacity refuse treatment, the refusal must be accepted.
• If people do not have capacity, the decision to provide or withhold life-prolonging treatment must be based on an assessment of their best interests.
• If a person has refused the treatment in advance in a valid advance directive, this refusal must be honoured.

Ideally decisions about whether or not cardiopulmonary resuscitation is appropriate should be made in advance and should involve the competent adult unless they make it very clear that they do not wish to discuss the subject.

When considering what will be in the person's best interests you should never make assumptions about the quality of life of someone with severe learning disabilities, or how that person values their life. Their ordinary life with their disability should be used as a baseline when considering any extra burden treatment might impose on them.

For those in a persistent vegetative state the courts have stated that it is good practice for court approval to be sought before artificial nutrition and hydration are withdrawn.

Definition

Seeking consent – helping the person make their own, informed choice.

See also the 'Ethical issues' section in Chapter 9 (Ethical issues), page 125.

General Topics

Aerobic exercise training programmes

Andriolo RB, El Dib RP, Ramos LR 2005 Aerobic exercise training programmes for improving physical health and psychosocial health in adults with Down syndrome **(Cochrane Review)**. In: The Cochrane Library, Issue 3. CD005176. Update Software, Oxford

- Two studies were included.
- One used walking/jogging and the other rowing training.
- The results showed an improvement in maximal treadmill grade in the intervention group.
- No other significant differences were found.
- There was insufficient evidence to support the use of aerobic exercise training programmes for physical or physiological outcomes.

Anxiety disorders in people with learning disabilities

Cooray SE, Bakala A 2005 Anxiety disorders in people with learning disabilities. Advances in Psychiatric Treatment 11: 355–361

Current psychiatric classification systems are based on studies that excluded people with learning disabilities. Deficits in language and/or abstract thinking make emotional symptoms difficult to identify. Limited social experience can influence the content of psychiatric symptoms. There is a tendency for clinicians to overlook psychiatric symptoms, attributing them to learning disability.

The evidence base relating to anxiety disorders in people with learning disabilities is poor. Most studies use some form of modified criteria, with a resultant lack of consistency. People with learning disabilities frequently contend with a lifetime of adversity, inadequate social support and poor coping skills. These contribute to increased vulnerability to stressful life events and trigger anxiety disorders. Types of fear reported in this population demonstrate similarities with children of equivalent mental age.

The treatment for anxiety disorders in people with learning disabilities broadly parallels that in the rest of the population, with the aim of targeting the maximum gains from the lowest effective dose and with minimum adverse effects.

Anxiety disorders are at least as common, and probably more common, among people with learning disabilities as among the general population. All the criteria for anxiety disorders in ICD-10 and DSM-IV can be applied validly and reliably in people with learning disability, but behavioural equivalents may be more appropriate in severe learning disability.

Reiss S, Levitan GW, Szyszko J 1982 Emotional disturbance and mental retardation: diagnostic overshadowing. American Journal of Mental Deficiency 86: 567–574

- Anxiety disorders may be underreported in learning disability.

Veerhoven WMA, Tuinier S 1997 Neuropsychiatric consultation in mentally retarded patients. European Psychiatry 12: 242–248

- Anxiety disorders are underdiagnosed in learning disability.

Cooper B 1972 Clinical and social aspects of chronic neurosis. Proceedings of the Royal Society of Medicine 65: 509–512

- In a sample of learning disabled people, higher rates of anxiety disorders were found in the elderly individuals than in the younger age groups.

Deb S, Thomas M, Bright C 2001 Mental disorder in adults with intellectual disability. 1: Prevalence of functional psychiatric illness among a community-based population aged between 16 and 64 years. Journal of Intellectual Disability Research 45: 495–505

- A study cohort comparing people with learning disabilities with the general population.
- There were significantly higher rates of phobic disorders in the group with learning disabilities.

Raghavan R 1997 Anxiety disorders in people with learning disabilities: a review of the literature. Journal of Learning Disabilities for Nursing, Health and Social Care 2: 3–9

- A literature review revealed a similar if not higher prevalence of generalised anxiety disorder in people with learning disabilities.

Moss S, Emerson E, Kiernan C et al 2000 Psychiatric symptoms in adults with learning disability and challenging behaviour. British Journal of Psychiatry 17: 452–456

- Anxiety disorders were identified as more prevalent in individuals with self-injurious behaviour than in those without such behaviour.

Masi G, Brovedani P, Mucci M et al 2002 Assessment of anxiety and depression in adolescents with mental retardation. Child Psychiatry and Human Development 32: 227–237

- In general, all criteria for anxiety disorders in ICD-10 or DSM-IV-TR can be applied validly and reliably in people with mild to moderate learning disabilities.

Matson JL, Smiroldo BB, Hamilton M et al 1997 Do anxiety disorders exist in persons with severe and profound retardation? Research in Developmental Disabilities 18: 39–44

- Concluded that when anxiety cannot be expressed, especially in people with more severe degrees of learning disability, it might manifest as a behavioural disorder.

Khreim I, Mikkelson E 1997 Anxiety disorders in adults with mental retardation. Psychiatric Annals 27: 271–281

- Greater emphasis should be placed on phenomena such as agitation, screaming, crying, withdrawal, regressive/clingy behaviour or freezing.
- These symptoms could be interpreted as manifestations of fear.

Kessler RC, McGonagle KA, Zhao S et al 1994 Lifetime and 12 month prevalence of DSM-III-R psychiatric disorders in the United States. Report from the National Comorbidity Survey. Archives of General Psychiatry 51: 8–19

- Reported that all types of mental disorder, including anxiety, decline with increasing educational level.

Levitas AS, Reid CS 1998 Rubinstein–Taybi syndrome and psychiatric disorders. Journal of Intellectual Disability Research 42: 284–292

- Fragile X syndrome is associated with social anxiety disorder.
- Rubinstein–Taybi and Prader–Willi syndromes are associated with obsessive–compulsive disorder.

Einfield SL, Tonge BJ, Rees VW 2001 Longitudinal course of behavioural and emotional problems in Williams syndrome. American Journal of Mental Retardation 106: 73–81

- Williams syndrome is associated with anxiety.

Dykens EM 2003 Anxiety, fears and phobias in persons with Williams syndrome. Developmental Neuropsychology 23: 291–316

- Williams syndrome is associated with phobias.

Hyman P, Oliver C, Hall S 2002 Self-injurious behaviour, self-restraint, and compulsive behaviours in Cornelia de Lange syndrome. American Journal on Mental Retardation 107: 146–154

- Noted significantly high compulsive behaviour in Cornelia de Lange syndrome.

Lindsay W, Neilson C, Lawrenson H 1997 Cognitive behaviour therapy for anxiety in people with learning disabilities. In: Stenfert Kroese B, Dagnan D, Loumides K (eds) Cognitive–behaviour therapy for people with learning disabilities. Routledge, London, pp 124–140; Lindsay WR 1999 Cognitive therapy. The Psychologist 12: 238–241

- Evidence from case studies of adults with mild or borderline learning disability and anxiety disorders demonstrates the effectiveness of cognitive–behavioural therapy.
- The principles may require modification to meet the abilities of the individual.

Martin NT, Gaffan EA, Williams T 1998 Behavioural effects of long-term multi-sensory stimulation. British Journal of Clinical Psychology 37: 69–82

- Reported a successful outcome with relation to achieving relaxation in individuals with severe-to-profound learning disability using multisensory stimulation (Snoezelen environment).

Comprehensive health care services

Lindsey M 2002 Comprehensive health care services. Advances in Psychiatric Treatment 8(2): 138–147

There are a number of factors that should be considered when planning effective health services for people with learning disability. People with learning disabilities should have equal access to all health services. They should not be excluded. They may require support to enable them to access services and staff may require disability awareness training to facilitate this. People with more complex and special needs require specialist services. The community learning disability teams should be involved in the development of individualised healthcare planning (e.g. Health Action Plans) and the facilitation of appropriate health service contact. Agencies, service users and carers should work in collaboration to ensure that social, educational and healthcare needs are met.

People with learning disability have the ordinary healthcare needs of the rest of the population. This includes health promotion, health screening and access to primary care, community and specialist health services. However, barriers to access exist. These can arise from:

* learning and communication difficulties (e.g. lack of understanding of healthy lifestyles)
* the importance of health screening
* failure to recognise symptoms of illness or their significance
* an inability to express pain, illness or unhappiness
* the knowledge, attitudes and beliefs of carers, clinicians and managers of services (e.g. misinterpretation of changes that indicate health problems)
* beliefs that changed or unusual behaviours that are due to learning disability rather than discomfort or mental health issues.

Carers and professionals may undervalue people with learning disabilities and consider their health needs to be unimportant, leading in extreme cases to neglect, ill treatment or discrimination. These issues can be combated with accessible information for patients (picture books, specialist well-woman and well-man clinics, etc.) and training and education for carers and staff. Regular health (including dental and sensory) checks to detect problems by symptom screening and physical examination are important. Screening for mental health problems should include standardised screening tools such as the Psychiatric Assessment Schedule for Adults with Developmental Disabilities.

There are also physical barriers to health care, including unsuitable buildings, signs, support, information about appointments, timing of appointments and information about treatment.

The special healthcare needs of people with learning disabilities should be remembered. They are at a rate much higher than in the general population, with high rates of general health problems, problems particular to genetic and syndromal causes, mental health problems, epilepsy, sensory impairment, cerebral palsy and other physical disabilities. Families are also at risk of mental health problems as they come to terms with the diagnosis.

Multidisciplinary working should aim to develop skills and approaches to overcome disabilities. Physiotherapy can aid the development of gross motor skills, occupational therapy the fine motor skills, and speech and language therapy better communication skills. Mental health professionals can advise on the promotion of good mental health through the development of emotional security, self-confidence and self-esteem, and through bonding to care givers.

The cause of the disability should be established where possible to anticipate the particular physical or mental health needs associated with that condition.

Psychiatric morbidity

* There are higher rates of mental health problems in this population.
* Between 10 and 39% of people with learning disabilities have additionally diagnosed psychiatric and behavioural disorders.
* It is important to consider the developmental disorders which frequently coexist and the need for specialist assessment and treatment in children and adolescents with learning disability.
* Schizophrenia and other disorders have been shown to be more common in this group, and there is some evidence that the rate of some psychiatric disorders, such as anxiety and depression, is higher in community settings than it was in the institutions.
* Up to 50% of children and adolescents with learning disability will require special services at some point in their childhood.
* There is a high prevalence of dementia in the elderly population with learning disability. Challenging behaviour estimates vary and often are long-term behavioural patterns rather than time-limited illnesses. There are associations with mental illness and communication problems.

Specific health needs

* Access to specialist services for epilepsy is required as 13–24% of people with learning disability are affected by epilepsy, often with more complex and refractory seizure disorders.
* Sensory impairments must be detected and remedied to minimise consequent disability, as about 30% of people with learning disability have significant sight problems and 40% significant hearing problems. There is a high rate of underdetection of treatable impairments.
* Up to 30% also have physical disabilities, most often owing to cerebral palsy, with a large number of related serious health problems (reflux disease, aspiration pneumonia, risk of choking, joint pains and muscle spasm). The chronic discomfort may present as a behavioural disorder. Pain management is particularly important for those who cannot easily communicate their discomfort.

Future care and service provision

The provision of health care for people with learning disabilities has shifted from institutional care to personalised community care. This should lead to increased use of community health services and a reduction in the barriers to care. Service users and carers are increasingly involved in planning service provision. People with learning disability are living longer and services will have to provide for the health needs of individuals with complex disabilities who now live into adulthood. Most people with learning disabilities live into old age.

Specialist mental health services are required to meet the needs of people with learning disabilities with complex needs. This includes children, adolescents and older people with learning disabilities. Services will need to provide for people with developmental disorders and people with complex seizure disorders.

See also the 'General topics' section in Chapter 27 (Service provision), pages 405-406.

Down's syndrome and dementia

Stanton LR, Coetzee RH 2004 Down's syndrome and dementia. Advances in Psychiatric Treatment 10: 50–58

Although baseline cognitive testing in early adulthood would be useful in people with Down's syndrome, there needs to be some consensus on which test batteries are used. More research is required, particularly in the treatment of Alzheimer's disease in Down's syndrome.

Tyrell J, Cosgrave M, McCarron M et al 2001 Dementia in people with Down's syndrome: the relevance of cognitive ability. International Journal of Geriatric Psychiatry 16: 1168–1174

- Study of 285 people with Down's syndrome.
- Found a 13% prevalence of Alzheimer's disease.

Holland AJ, Hon J, Huppert FA et al 2000 Incidence and course of dementia in people with Down's syndrome: findings from a population-based study. Journal of Intellectual Disability Research 44: 138–146

- Age-related cognitive decline and frontal lobe dementia appear to be more prevalent in the younger age groups (30–49 years of age).
- Frontal lobe dementia appears to be more prevalent in those with severe learning disability.
- These findings need to be confirmed with further studies.
- Personality change is often associated with early involvement of the frontal lobes.

Holland AJ, Hon J, Huppert FA et al 1998 Population-based study of the prevalence and presentation of dementia in adults with Down's syndrome. British Journal of Psychiatry 172: 493–498

- There appears to be no relationship between the level of learning disability and the risk of dementia or age at onset of dementia.

Oliver C, Crayton L, Holland A et al 1998 A four year prospective study of age-related cognitive change in adults with Down's syndrome. Psychological Medicine 28: 1365–1377

- The deterioration in cognitive decline appears to increase with age.
- In general, symptom acquisition mimics that seen in Alzheimer's disease.

Temple V, Jozsvai E, Konstantareas MM 2001 Alzheimer dementia in Down's syndrome: the relevance of cognitive ability. Journal of Intellectual Disability Research 45: 47–55

- The level of pre-existing cognitive function is closely associated with the rate of decline.
- Environmental factors have the greatest impact on cognitive function.

Cosgrave MP, Tyrell J, McCarron M et al 2000 A five year follow-up study of dementia in persons with Down's syndrome: early symptoms and patterns of deterioration. Irish Journal of Psychological Medicine 17: 5–11

- Deterioration in memory, learning and orientation tend to be the first signs of a developing dementia.
- Early symptoms are often accompanied by increased dependence.

Cooper SA, Prasher VP 1998 Maladaptive behaviours and symptoms of dementia in adults with Down's syndrome compared with adults with intellectual disabilities of other aetiologies. Journal of Intellectual Disability Research 42: 293–300

- Alzheimer's disease in Down's syndrome presents with a greater prevalence of:
  - low mood
  - excessive overactivity/restlessness
  - disturbed sleep
  - excessive uncooperativeness
  - auditory hallucinations.

Aylward EH, Burt DB, Thorpe LU et al 1997 Diagnosis of dementia in individuals with intellectual disability. Journal of Intellectual Disability Research 41: 152–164

- This working group suggested consensus criteria for the diagnosis of dementia in Down's syndrome.
- The group suggested the use of ICD-10 as a framework, because of its emphasis on non-cognitive changes.

Simard M, Van Reekum R 2001 Dementia with Lewy bodies in Down's syndrome. International Journal of Geriatric Psychiatry 16: 311–320

- Depression, motivational syndromes and psychotic symptoms may be more common in dementia with Lewy bodies.
- Those with dementia with Lewy bodies are particularly prone to adverse side effects of psychotropic medication, especially typical antipsychotics.
- Atypical antipsychotics may be better tolerated.

Bouman WP, Pinner G 2002 Use of atypical antipsychotic drugs in old age psychiatry. Advances in Psychiatric Treatment 8: 49–58

- The behavioural and psychological symptoms of dementia, although preferably handled by non-pharmacological means, can be treated as recommended for the general adult population.

Prasher VP, Huxley A, Haque MS 2002 A 24 week, double blind, placebo-controlled trial of donepezil in patients with Down syndrome and Alzheimer's disease. Pilot study. International Journal of Geriatric Psychiatry 17: 270–278

- There is some evidence that cognitive enhancers may be useful in this group of patients.

Hemingway-Eltomey JM, Lerner AJ 1999 Adverse effects of donepezil in treating Alzheimer's disease associated with Down's syndrome. American Journal of Psychiatry 156: 1470

- There have been concerns that cognitive enhancers in this group may be poorly tolerated.

Weblinks Alzheimer's Society – www.alzheimers.org.uk. Down's Syndrome Association – www.downs-syndrome. org.uk.

See also the 'General topics' section in Chapter 17 (Old age psychiatry), page 257.

Improving the general health of adults with learning disability

Kerr M 2004 Improving the general health of adults with learning disability. Advances in Psychiatric Treatment 10: 200–206

Individuals with learning disabilities are a heterogeneous group with varying needs. They receive a complex array of healthcare provision. The impact of societal and environmental factors on health status is greater in this group.

This article focuses on how health improvements can be made in terms of the disparity in health between the general and learning disabled populations, the health needs of adults with learning disability, existing barriers to health care and the provision of health care by primary care.

There are disparities between the health of people with learning disability and the rest of the population. People with learning disability have a lower expectancy of life, high levels of morbidity (in particular epilepsy, sensory impairment and behavioural disorder) and decreased involvement in health promotion and screening. Other factors include an increased risk of being overweight and underweight, low levels of employment and poorer social networks. Antipsychotic prescribing is high in this population – including people who do not have a psychotic illness. Adults with learning disability have high rates of undiagnosed illness.

There are barriers to health care for people with learning disability. Physical barriers exist and include factors such as poor mobility and disabled access. Adults may have a lack of understanding of the role of health services and may not be able to communicate their wishes. Communication with health professionals may be impaired with subsequent effects on assessment and treatment of illness. Fear, lack of support and education and consequent problem behaviours can prevent the necessary examination and investigations from being performed. The knowledge of care teams, health professionals, etc. and attitudes about illness in this population may act as barriers to appropriate care.

Welsh Office 1996 The Welsh Health Survey 1995. Summary of findings. Welsh Office, Cardiff

The following results are specific to people with learning disabilities:

- They had a higher rate of psychiatric illness (32.2%) than the general population (11.2%).
- They had more illness than the general population.
- Only 6% reported no illness compared with 37% of the general population.
- The prevalence of epilepsy was 22.1%.
- Eyesight was poor in 19.1%, compared with 8% of the general population.
- The family doctor was the most frequently contacted professional in the previous year (79.5%).
- Only one in 10 individuals had a healthy diet, and one in three had an unhealthy diet.
- 28.8% were overweight.
- 23.6% were obese.

McCulloch DL, Sludden PA, McKeon K et al 1996 Vision care requirements among intellectually disabled adults. Journal of Intellectual Disability Research 40: 140–150

- An institutional survey of vision.
- Poor visual acuity was found in:

- 12% of mildly disabled
- over 40% of severely disabled
- 100% of profoundly disabled patients.

Evenhuis HM, Mul M, Lemaire EKG et al 1997 Diagnosis of sensory impairment in people with intellectual disability in general practice. Journal of Intellectual Disability Research 41: 422–429

- Identified hearing loss in 25–42% of people with learning disabilities living in the community.

Mariani E, Ferini-Strambi L, Sala M et al 1993 Epilepsy in institutionalised patients with encephalopathy. Clinical aspects and nosological considerations. American Journal on Mental Retardation 98: 27–33

- Found a 32% prevalence of epilepsy in an institutional study.

Morgan CL, Scheepers MIA, Kerr MP 2003 Prevalence of epilepsy and associated health service utilisation and mortality among patients with intellectual disability. American Journal on Mental Retardation 108: 293–300

- A community study of epilepsy in learning disabled people.
- Epilepsy had a prevalence of 16.1%.

Morgan CL, Scheepers MIA, Kerr MP 2001 Mortality in patients with intellectual disability and epilepsy. Current Opinion in Psychiatry 14: 471–475

- Mortality rates (standardised mortality ratios and reduced life expectancy) are higher in people with learning disabilities, compared with the general population.

Richards BW, Siddiqui AQ 1980 Age and mortality trends in residents of an institution for the mentally handicapped. Journal of Mental Deficiency Research 24: 99–105

- There is a trend towards longer life expectancy in the learning disabled population.

Strauss D, Anderson TW, Shavelle R et al 1998 Causes of death of persons with developmental disabilities. Comparison of institutional and community residents. Mental Retardation 36: 386–391

- Predictors of mortality include the severity of the learning disability, reduced mobility, feeding difficulties and the presence of Down's syndrome.

Forssman H, Aksesson HO 1970 Mortality of the mentally deficient. A study of 12903 institutionalised subjects. Journal of Mental Deficiency Research 14: 276–294; Leestma JE, Walczak T, Hughes JR et al 1989 A prospective study of sudden unexpected death in epilepsy. Annals of Neurology 26: 195–203

- People with learning disability with epilepsy have increased mortality.
- They are at greater risk of sudden unexplained death in epilepsy.

Minihan PM, Dean DH 1990 Meeting the needs for health services of persons with mental retardation living in the community. American Journal of Public Health 80: 1043–1048

- A US study.
- 20% of learning disabled patients could be examined or treated only after measures such as premedication or pre-visits for desensitisation had been arranged.

Minihan PM, Dean DH, Lyons CM 1993 Managing the care of patients with mental retardation: a survey of physicians. Mental Retardation 31: 239–246

- Only one in five primary care physicians reported that they felt well prepared to handle a patient who refused to cooperate with an examination or with treatment.

Wilson DN, Haire A 1990 Health care screening for people with mental handicap living in the community. British Medical Journal 301: 1379–1381

- Carers failed to predict sensory impairment in 50% of patients who had difficulties in hearing or seeing.

Wilson DN, Haire A 1990 Health care screening for people with mental handicap living in the community. British Medical Journal 301: 1379–1381

Examination of any community-based population of people with learning disabilities receiving primary care will consistently uncover three serious problems:

- untreated, yet treatable, medical conditions
- untreated specific health issues related to the individual's disability
- a lack of uptake of generic health promotion, such as blood pressure screening.

Beange H, McElduff A, Baker W 1995 Medical disorders of adults with mental retardation. A population study. American Journal of Mental Retardation 99: 595–604

- There were significantly greater levels of obesity, vision and hearing impairment, hypersomnia, endocrine disease, skin disease and psychiatric disorders in adults with learning disabilities.
- Non-Down's syndrome women had increased hypertension and showed a lack of sufficient exercise.

- People with learning disability appear to visit their general practitioner at least as often as the general population.
- People with learning disability have been shown to use specialist services and to be hospitalised more frequently than the general population.
- 74% of 202 individuals with learning disabilities had conditions for which specialist care was needed.
- This care had not always been received and half of the identified conditions were found to be inadequately managed.

Whitefield ML, Lagan J, Russell O 1996 Assessing general practitioners' care of adult patients with learning disability: case control study. Quality in Health Care 5: 31–35

- This study compared a random sample of learning disabled people taken from the patient register of a primary health care team in an English city with age- and gender-matched controls from the same register.
- They found a significant increase in the use of antipsychotic and anticonvulsant medication in people with learning disabilities.
- There are higher rates of consultations for neurological and skin conditions in people with learning disability.
- The control population was significantly more likely to receive regular blood pressure monitoring.

Jones RG, Kerr MP 1997 A randomised control trial of an opportunistic health screening tool in primary care for people with intellectual disability. Journal of Intellectual Disability Research 41: 409–415

- Attempts in the UK to carry out a more structured assessment in normal primary care were unsuccessful.

See also the 'General topics' section in Chapter 21 (Physical health), pages 306 and 309

Long term affective disorder in people with mild learning disability

Richards M, Maughan B, Hardy R et al 2001 Long term affective disorder in people with mild learning disability. British Journal of Psychiatry 179: 523–527

- A study of the risk of affective disorder in those classified as having mild learning disabilities in the British 1946 birth cohort.
- Investigated the risks associated with affective disorder in childhood and adulthood.
- The Present State Examination was used at age 36 years.
- The Psychiatric Symptom Frequency Scale was used at age 43 years.

- People with learning disabilities had a four-fold increase in the risk of affective disorder, not accounted for by social and material disadvantage or by medical disorder.
- In young life, factors associated with affective disorder included paternal occupational social class, maternal education, family size, overcrowding, parental divorce or death and prolonged hospitalisation.
- At age 36, factors associated with affective disorder included socioeconomic status, educational attainment, family circumstances, employment, financial hardship, poor material home conditions, recent medical complaints and adverse life events.

Management of people with challenging behaviour

Xeniditis K, Russell A, Murphy D 2001 Management of people with challenging behaviour. Advances in Psychiatric Treatment 7(2): 109–116

Previous studies report a prevalence of challenging behaviour between 5.7 and 14%. Challenging behaviour occurs more commonly in males. It increases in prevalence from childhood, with a peak between 15 and 34 years and a subsequent decline. Aggression and self-injurious behaviour are greater at the more severe end of the spectrum.

Aetiology is believed to be multifactorial. Associated factors include:
- genetic influences
- brain structure and function
- psychosocial factors.

Assessment and treatment in the learning disability population are important as challenging behaviour can pose a significant obstacle to resettlement.

The general principles of management are:
- a patient-centred focus
- needs tailored to the individual person
- multiagency and multidisciplinary involvement
- the use of a number of treatment modalities (pharmacotherapy and psychosocial interventions)
- consideration of the safety of the patient and others
- treatment in a safe and secure environment (if necessary under the Mental Health Act in a specialised unit).

A systematic approach to assessment and treatment would include:
- identification of target behaviour(s)
- quantitative measurement of said behaviour:
  - direct naturalistic observations of the behaviour and related events, systematically recorded on ABC charts, or

- idiosyncratic observational schemes, with real time observation of behaviour at set intervals
- generation of hypotheses (medical, psychological and social) about the initiating and maintaining factors
- delivery of an appropriate therapeutic intervention
- evaluation of this intervention
- consideration of the use of standardised assessment tools.

Specific therapeutic interventions suggested include the following:

- Pharmacotherapy: treatment of an underlying mental disorder, epilepsy or other physical condition.
- Self-injury: trial of an antidepressant (e.g. naloxone or naltrexone).
- Sexually inappropriate behaviour: cyproterone acetate for recidivist sex offenders or those repeatedly exhibiting unacceptable or dangerous sexual behaviour.
- Aggression:
  - neuroleptics
  - benzodiazepines (beware paradoxical excitement)
  - mood stabilisers
  - antidepressants have all been used.
- Psychological treatments:
  - behaviour modification (using reinforcement programmes)
  - cognitive behavioural therapy (mild end of spectrum, some early research)
  - psychodynamic and systematic therapies (data are limited, especially in learning disability).

Definition

Challenging behaviour – culturally abnormal behaviour of such an intensity, frequency or duration that the physical safety of the person or others is likely to be placed in serious jeopardy, or behaviour which is likely to seriously limit the use of, or result in the person being denied access to, ordinary facilities. (*Source:* Emerson E 1995 Challenging behaviour. Analysis and intervention in people with learning difficulties. Cambridge University Press, Cambridge.)

Mental health services for adults with learning disabilities

Bouras N, Holt G 2004 Mental health services for adults with learning disabilities. British Journal of Psychiatry 184: 291–292

Services for people with learning disabilities have undergone major changes since deinstitutionalisation occurred. There has been a shift towards integration, participation, inclusion and choice. Normalisation and the provision of care by mainstream services have support. Others have argued for specialist expertise in the diagnosis and treatment of psychiatric disorders in this population.

When people with learning disabilities are admitted to mainstream units they often require longer admissions and additional support. The complex needs of this heterogeneous group can leave staff feeling ill-equipped.

Service responses vary both nationally and internationally. The most common form of care in England has been provided by community learning disability teams. These are often led by social services, with multiprofessional staff who provide a range of inputs, including physical and mental health care, resettlement and social care.

The authors suggest that specialisation of mental health services for people with learning disabilities, provided by mainstream mental health services at a tertiary level, offers a way forward.

Deb S, Thomas M, Bright C 2001 Mental disorder in adults with intellectual disability: prevalence of functional psychiatric illness among a community based population between 16 and 64 years. Journal of Intellectual Disability Research 45: 495–505

- Psychiatric disorders are more prevalent in adults with learning disability than in the general population.

Royal College of Psychiatrists 2003 Meeting the mental health needs of adults with a mild learning disability (Council Report CR115). Royal College of Psychiatrists, London

- Demands on mental health services for people with learning disabilities have increased since the move away from institutions.
- Additional services and resources have not been forthcoming.

Department of Health 2001 From words into action: London Learning Disability Strategic Framework. The Stationery Office, London

- The closure of institutions and the lack of local resources and funding have led to several thousand people with learning disabilities and psychiatric disorders being placed in residential facilities outwith their place of origin.
- Government policy states that care should be undertaken by mainstream mental health services.
- In practice, however, services struggle to meet the needs with both diagnoses.

Day K 1988 Services for psychiatrically disordered mentally handicapped adults. Australia and New Zealand Journal of Developmental Disabilities 14: 19–25

- Mainstream services do not see a role in the care of people with learning disabilities.
- It is believed that services are already struggling to meet the demands of the general population.

Department of Health 2001 Valuing people: a new strategy for learning disability for the 21st century. The Stationery Office, London

- Reviewing the role of the community learning disability team.
- Proposes that these teams enable access to mainstream services as much as possible.

Van Minnen A, Hoogduin CAL, Broekman TG 1997 Hospital versus outreach treatment of patients with mental retardation and psychiatric disorders: a controlled study. Acta Psychiatrica Scandinavica 95: 515–522

- Showed a reduction in hospitalisation when a service is provided by a community learning disability team.

Coelho RJ, Kelley PS, Deatsman-Kelly C 1993 An experimental investigation of an innovative community treatment model for persons with dual diagnosis (DD/MI). Journal of Rehabilitation 54: 37–42

- Examined intensive case management provided in a specialist programme by a mainstream community health team in the US.
- ICM led to improved adaptive functioning in a group with learning disabilities and psychiatric disorders.

Tyrer P, Hassiotis A, Ukoumunne O et al 1999 Intensive case management for psychotic patients with borderline intelligence: UK 700 Group. Lancet 354: 999–1000

- Found that a subgroup with borderline cognitive impairment from the UK 700 study spent significantly less time in hospital if they had received intensive community care.

Moss S, Bouras N, Holt G 2000 Mental health services for people with intellectual disability: a conceptual framework. Journal of Intellectual Disability Research 46: 340–355

- Postulated a matrix model for the development and evaluation of services for people with mental illness and learning disability.

Campbell M, Fitzpatrick R, Haines A et al 2000 Framework for design and evaluation of complex interventions to improve health. British Medical Journal 321: 694–696

- Systematic evaluation and exploratory clinical trials might be more appropriate at present for research into mental health services for people with learning disabilities.

- This would consider services in place and look at ways of improving practice.

See also the 'General topics' section in Chapter 27 (Service provision), pages 405-406.

Out of borough placements for people with learning disability

Jaydeokar S, Piachaud J 2004 Out of borough placements for people with learning disability. Advances in Psychiatric Treatment 10: 116–123

Out of borough placements are not usually the satisfactory choice for individuals, families or professionals. Local authorities continue to place a significant number of people with learning disabilities in residential care distant from their own community due to a lack of appropriate local facilities. The amount of out of borough services purchased appears to be related to the volume of local accommodation and the competence of local services in managing complex needs. Exporting boroughs tend to include city areas where house prices are high. The importing boroughs are mainly the shires – rural areas where large properties are less expensive and there is less likelihood of local opposition being organised. Many of the long-stay hospitals were situated away from population centres, and skilled staff were concentrated in these areas. With the closure of these hospitals, many staff left to run residential homes and services in the same area. The problem is also linked to the shortage of beds for short-term admissions and the difficulty of moving people through these beds into appropriate long-term accommodation. Rural quietness is a valid argument for some people. The measure of quality of life is complex and highly personal. An individual placed out of borough can have a good quality of life and may choose to live there. Out of borough placements will increase parental concerns due to less control and less involvement.

Local authorities have a responsibility to provide full time education to all children up to the age of 19. Those with very complex needs, particularly difficult behaviours, and those with pervasive developmental disorders may be placed in residential schools outside the borough. Their returning to the borough at the age of 19 requires good planning based on needs and service provision. Failure of such planning may lead to a person remaining out of borough against the wishes of the individual and the family. Out of borough placements may be the only discharge option for clinicians with the pressure for acute admission beds and if there is no suitable local care package. Service planning is important.

Psychiatrists should know what is planned and what is possible in the system, so that they can advise patients and carers appropriately. Membership of joint commissioning boards is an important role for a senior clinician. Good working relationships with senior managers in the health and social services, as well as with those in the voluntary and private sectors, allow clinicians to use their influence to avoid unnecessary conflict, thus encouraging service development. Community learning disability services should be tracking learning disabled people who show challenging behaviour, as well as those about to leave school and in out of borough placements.

Bailey NM, Cooper SA 1998 The current provision of specialist health services to people with learning disabilities in England and Wales. Journal of Intellectual Disability Research 41: 52–59

- Found that, on average, NHS trusts managed 10.3 long-stay beds per 100,000 population.
- 20% of trusts had no long-stay NHS provision at all for people with learning disabilities.
- 40% had completed their resettlement process, but retained some NHS long-stay beds, having reprovided these within small community units directly managed by NHS trusts.
- The majority of NHS trusts provided assessment and treatment beds.
- All trusts provided community teams for learning disabilities, although they varied greatly in their professional composition.

Ryan T 1998 Lost opportunities: purchasing strategies in housing and support for people with learning difficulties. Mental Health Care 1: 296–299

- For those with complex needs, out of borough placements are often seen as the only option on grounds of both cost and suitability.
- Reasons cited include:
  - lack of adequate local accommodation and support services
  - fears about potential risks to the community
  - costs
  - cost–benefit analyses.

Richardson A, Ritchie J 1989 Letting go: dilemmas for parents whose son or daughter has a mental handicap. Open University Press, Buckingham

The characteristics sought by parents for their child's living arrangements are:
- a 'home'
- caring, secure and permanent environment
- highly personalised approach
- small in size
- atmosphere should give a sense of being accepted
- adequate staffing and supervision
- needs of the residents should come before those of the staff and of the organisation.

Richardson A, Ritchie J 1986 Making the break: parents' views about adults with a mental handicap leaving home. King's Fund, London

- Parents' views on making the break from their disabled child vary considerably.
- Some actively seek residential placements, believing it is in everyone's interests for them to gain independence from the family.
- Some cannot contemplate a move at all and believe that paid carers could never replace parental love and concern.
- Some are deeply ambivalent, with resulting anxiety.

Department of Health 2003 Community care statistics 2003. Supported residents (adults), England. DH, London

- There are 40,335 people with learning disabilities supported by local authorities.
- 37,985 are in residential placements.
- 2350 are in nursing care placements.
- 24.6% of residential placements are outside the local borough.
- 29.2% of nursing placements are outside the local borough.

Definition

Nimbyism (acronym) – not in my back yard. (*Source:* Foster A, Roberts VZ (eds) 1998 'Not in my backyard': the psychosocial reality of community care. In: Managing mental health in the community: chaos and containment. Routledge, London, pp 27–37.)

Service innovations: risk assessment in learning disability

Bhaumik S, Nadkarni SS, Biswas AB at al 2005 Service innovations: risk assessment in learning disability. Psychiatric Bulletin 29: 28–31

Aims

To establish the effectiveness of the care programme approach (CPA) in adults with learning disabilities in a specialist treatment unit for adults with learning disability.

Method

- Case records were audited over a 6-month period and staff on the unit completed questionnaires about the patients, including CPA screening and risk assessment/management.

- Carers also completed questionnaires on their views regarding risk and information sharing.
- A 12-bed, low secure locked door unit was the location of the audit.

Results

- Over the 6-month period there were 15 admissions to the unit.
- Three patients were admitted with purely mental health needs and seven were judged to be a risk to others.
- The risks mainly presented by patients were aggression, dependency and mental health problems.
- Admission appeared to reduce dependency in general.
- Only 60% of patients had a CPA discharge planning meeting.
- 27% of patients had an evident risk management plan prior to discharge.
- A lack of sharing information regarding risk was elicited.

Discussion

- The audit revealed that there were major deficiencies in risk identification, management and information sharing.

McGrother CW, Bhaumik S, Thorp CF et al 2002 Prevalence, morbidity and service needs among South Asian and white adults with intellectual disability in Leicestershire, UK. Journal of Intellectual Disability Research 46: 299–309

- Patients with learning disabilities are at increased risk, given their increased incidence of mental health and behavioural disorders.

Bhaumik S, Collacott RA, Gandhi D et al 1995 A naturalistic study in the use of antidepressants in adults with learning disabilities and affective disorders. Human Psychopharmacology 10: 283–288

- Linguistic and communication problems can mean that mental health difficulties go unrecognised.

Roy A 2000 The care programme approach in learning disability psychiatry. Advances in Psychiatric Treatment 6: 280–387

- The use of CPA in learning disabilities has been variable across the country and introduced later than in mainstream services.

Saunders M 1998 Risk management. In: Thompson T, Mathias P (eds) Standards and learning disability. Baillière Tindall, London, pp 249–259

- Defined good risk assessment and management as an explicit, logical process benefiting patients, carers and service managers.
- It is an essential part of CPA that aids placement and allows people to be consistent with the information shared.
- In people with learning difficulties the risks may be lifelong despite treating the underlying condition and training and support.
- Risk assessment should cover:
  - inherent and mental health risks
  - risks related to environmental hazards
  - social and family circumstances
  - communication difficulties
  - inadequate coping skills
  - being easily influenced by others.

Policy and Legislation

Health needs assessment

Public Health Institute of Scotland 2004 People with learning disabilities in Scotland. Health needs assessment. PHIS, Glasgow. Online. Available: www.phis.org.uk/pdf. pl?file=publications/LDSummary.pdf

Contains recommendations aimed at reducing health inequalities, to encourage social inclusion.

Compared with the rest of the population, people with learning disability in Scotland have:

- a lower life expectancy
- higher levels of general health needs
- higher levels of specific health needs
- higher levels of unmet health needs
- different and more complex health needs
- different main causes of death.

The current health inequalities are partly due to the differences noted above. They also reflect the barriers to health care that people with learning disabilities experience.

Current health policies in Scotland are likely to lead to greater health inequalities. Specific interventions and policies for people with learning disabilities are required to address these issues.

The current closure programme for long-stay hospitals means that community services and supports must continue to be developed. Both generic and specific services for people with learning disabilities need to have the capacity and expertise to meet the needs of people with learning disabilities.

The needs of family carers are also not adequately addressed.

The 25 recommendations aim to improve health for people with learning disabilities and to reduce inequality. They address five main areas of concern:

1. Leadership and accountability
2. Infrastructure: development, planning and monitoring
3. Specific intervention:
   - health screening programme
   - national governance development, including an audit of all deaths of people with learning disabilities
   - improved primary care services
   - improved advocacy
   - specialist community-based services for children, adults and older persons with learning disabilities
4. Information
   - including a better understanding of the needs of persons with learning disabilities from ethnic minority communities
5. Education
   - including the involvement of paid and family carers.

See also the 'General topics' section in Chapter 21 (Physical health), page 303.

Home at last?

> Scottish Executive 2004 Home at last? The same as you? National Implementation Group. Report of the short-life working group on hospital closure and service reprovision. Scottish Executive, Edinburgh. Online. Available: www.scotland.gov.uk/Publications/2004/01/18742/31614

A key recommendation of *The same as you?* was that all long-stay learning disability hospitals should close by 2005. People should not have a hospital as their home. In 1980 there were over 7000 people in learning disability hospitals, compared with 900 in 2003. A further 652 should be discharged by 2005. Of these, 220 were still awaiting assessment and 275 did not have services commissioned.

Resettlement placements

Over 60% of adults with learning disabilities will be resettled in to a single tenancy.

Of those discharged in 2002 (574 in total), 31% moved to single tenancy, 33% to a house where between two and four share, 15% to group homes and 21% to nursing homes.

The report identified that there were barriers to meeting the closure deadlines. These were due to:

- delays in agreeing resettlement plans and their funding
- patients with complex needs being left until last
- difficulties with commissioning services, with accessing housing and with recruiting staff.

In December 2002 there were still 899 beds in learning disability hospitals in Scotland: 73% were long-stay beds,

18% assessment and treatment beds, and 9% specialist forensic beds. There is some variance in the definition of bed use and some people are in 'Assessment and Treatment' beds which have no throughput.

Of the 30 dedicated specialist forensic beds in the State Hospital at Carstairs, 11 were occupied by people ready to move on. Discharge had been delayed as there were no services available to meet their needs.

89 people remained in out of area NHS hospitals or other NHS funded resources. These and those awaiting resettlement from assessment and treatment beds should be included in resettlement plans.

> **Definition**
>
> **Commissioning** – deciding what services are needed and then getting someone to provide these by signing a contract.
>
> *See also The same as you? (p. 230) and Valuing people (p. 231), this chapter.*
>
> *See also the 'Policy and legislation' section in Chapter 27 (Service provision), page 406.*

Joint future directive

A Scottish Executive policy on joint working between local authorities, NHS Scotland and other organisations to provide better community care services.

The aims are to:

- support people to remain in their own homes
- provide a better quality of life for people with learning disabilities and others
- promote early assessment and intervention
- remove barriers within the care journey
- promote integrated services locally
- develop 'whole person' approaches to care.

A single shared assessment should be developed to:

- create a single point of entry for assessment of need and community care services for users
- ensure that agencies adopt a holistic approach
- reduce bureaucracy and duplication in assessment and planning care.

Weblink Scottish Executive – www.scotland.gov.uk
See also the 'Policy and legislation' section in Chapter 27 (Service provision), page 406.

Partnership for care

> Scottish Executive 2003 Partnership for care. Scotland's Health White Paper. The Stationery Office, Edinburgh. Online. Available: www.scotland.gov.uk/Publications/2003/02/16476/18730

Aims to promote a culture of continuous improvement in NHS Scotland, to devolve power to those best placed to make a difference and to better involve people in promoting the right changes for our health care.

Proposals build on *Our Healthier Nation: A Plan for Action, A Plan for Change*. Patients and national standards are seen as the key drivers of change. Partnership at national and local level with local authorities, the voluntary sector and local communities is also crucial.

Aims are:

* to improve Scotland's health (physical and mental)
* to reduce the health inequalities within our society
* to focus on the social groups most at risk
* to encourage the participation, empowerment and partnership of patients
* to consider clinical and local targets (to be monitored by NHS Quality Improvement Scotland).

Chapter 5 focuses on 'Partnership, Integration and Redesign'. There is legislation to create new community health partnerships in line with social work services and with stronger roots in the community. Integrated health care should be developed through managed clinical networks.

In Chapter 7 – 'Organising for Reform' – the move from NHS Trusts to NHS Boards as the key operational units is discussed. The purpose of this is to remove unnecessary organisational and legal barriers. This will support the development of integrated, decentralised healthcare services that meet the needs of individual patients and local communities. The existence of a number of separate statutory organisations reinforces institutional, professional and service delivery barriers.

See also the 'Policy and legislation' section in Chapter 27 (Service provision), page 406.

Promoting health, supporting inclusion

Scottish Executive 2002 Promoting health, supporting inclusion. The national review of the contribution of all nurses and midwives to the care and support of people with learning disabilities. Scottish Executive, Edinburgh. Online. Available: www.scotland.gov.uk/Publications/2002/07/15072/8572

This was undertaken to reflect the important changes and developments that are impacting significantly upon the lives of people with learning disabilities and their families. The central aim is to ensure that all nurses and midwives, wherever they practise, recognise the particular needs of people with learning disabilities, and work towards promoting and improving their lives.

The national review considered the health needs of all children and adults with learning disabilities in the context of the tiered model of care, as well as examining the key messages from this review (Box 14.1).

Social inclusion strategy

The Scottish Office 1999 Social inclusion – opening the door to a better Scotland: Strategy. The Scottish Office, Edinburgh. Online. Available: www.scotland.gov.uk/library/documents-w7/sima-00.htm

The health of children

The strategy aims to focus on children and young people. It focuses on the following:

* Education
* Expansion of childcare provision
* Family centres
* Children's services plans
* Starting Well (a new health demonstration project which will develop and disseminate best practice in supporting children's health from preconception through to school entry and will have particular regard to maternal health and postnatal depression)
* Alternatives to exclusion from school
* Study support
* New community schools, which will bring together in a single team of professionals from a range of services, including school education, social work, family support and health education and promotion services.

Learning disability

* The inclusiveness of the education system is particularly important to children who have special educational needs.
* The aim is to ensure that the vast majority of children with special educational needs are fully integrated into mainstream education, with the appropriate support.
* Children with disabilities and those affected by disability in the family have a right to an assessment of their needs and an action plan to ensure that those needs are met.

The Beattie Committee has been set up to consider what more can be done for young people who need additional support to participate in further education and training, or employment. It will question whether the need for support stems from physical or learning difficulties or mental health problems, or from lack of skills or motivation.

Weblink Scottish Executive – www.scotland.gov.uk

Box 14.1

National review of the health needs of children and adults with learning disabilities – tiered model and key messages

Tiered model

Tier 0: Community, public health and strategic approaches to care

- Community resources and supports, housing and support packages, education and learning, employment, public health initiatives and policy development.

Tier 1: Primary care and directly accessed health services

- Primary healthcare services, directly accessed services and their supporting services, and paid and family carers.

Tier 2: Health services accessed via primary care

- Generic secondary (outpatient, inpatient and tertiary) health services accessed via primary healthcare services and their supporting services, and paid and family carers.

Tier 3: Specialist locality health services

- Specialist learning disabilities services provided by local authorities, NHS Scotland and the independent sector, and paid and family carers in support of these.

Tier 4: Specialist area health services

- Supra-specialist (tertiary) learning disabilities services provided by local authorities, NHS Scotland and the independent sector, and paid and family carers in support of these.

Key messages

Tier 0

- Many people with learning disabilities have unrecognised and unmet health needs.
- Services must be organised and delivered locally in response to sound evidence and assessed need.
- The promotion of good health and well-being must be given greater priority at a strategic and local level.

Tier 1

- All people with learning disabilities should be enabled and supported appropriately to access primary care-based health services.
- Improving the health of people with learning disabilities by health assessment, health education and health promotion must be a priority.
- Planning and practice must be needs based.
- Good health enables social inclusion.

Tier 2

- Many people with learning disabilities have greater health needs than the general population.
- The assessment and treatment of health needs can be complex, requiring access to specialist skills.
- Partnership working needs to be developed with primary and secondary care and specialists in learning disabilities to support assessments of health needs, provide advice and coordinate care.

Tier 3

- Specialist services, including health, must be in place for people with complex needs.
- Specialist health services have a vital role to play in working with those who have the most complex needs.
- Nurses should be core members of specialist teams.
- People with learning disabilities, their families and carers need practical care, advice and support when caring for those with complex needs.

Tier 4

- Specialist services need to be in place on an area or region-wide basis for a small, but significant, number of people with learning disabilities.
- Nurses have skills that should be utilised in different settings to support people with learning disabilities in the least restrictive way.

The same as you?

Scottish Executive 2000 The same as you? A review of services for people with learning disabilities. Scottish Executive, Edinburgh. Online. Available: www.scotland.gov.uk/ldsr/docs/tsay-00.asp

Disabled people, whatever the origin, nature and seriousness of their handicaps and disabilities, have the same fundamental rights as their fellow citizens of the same age, which implies first and foremost the right to enjoy a decent life, as normal and full as possible.

United Nations (1975) The Declaration on the Rights of Disabled Persons.

People with learning disabilities should have a range of support and services to meet their needs. These include everyday needs, extra needs because of their learning disability and complex needs.

People with learning disabilities are mostly supported by their family. Families often have to provide social and nursing care: 25% of people with learning disabilities are looked after by a carer of over 65 years; 20% have two carers over 70 years. Older carers may well be worried about who will take over this care after they die.

Seven principles emerged during the consultation process:

- People with learning disabilities should be valued. They should be asked and encouraged to contribute to the community they live in. They should not be picked on or treated differently from others.
- People with learning disabilities are individual people.
- People with learning disabilities should be asked about the services they need and be involved in making choices about what they want.
- People with learning disabilities should be helped and supported to do everything they are able to do.
- People with learning disabilities should be able to use the same local services as everyone else, wherever possible.
- People with learning disabilities should benefit from specialist social, health and educational services.
- People with learning disabilities should have services which take account of their age, abilities and other needs.

The review lists some 29 recommendations regarding services for people with learning disabilities, including:

- the creation and training of local area coordinators to manage care and coordinate services
- a personal life plan for those who wish one
- direct payments for all those who require them by 2003
- the creation of the Scottish Centre for Learning Disability to offer advice, training and support; it should be responsible for a long-term public awareness programme
- the creation of a national network for people with an autistic spectrum disorder
- all health boards to have plans for closing all remaining long-stay hospitals for people with learning disabilities by 2005
- a reduction in specialist assessment and treatment places to four for every 100,000 population; there should be appropriate community services to avoid inpatient assessments and treatment
- modern, flexible and responsive community services to support people in the community through employment, lifelong learning and social activities
- greater employment opportunities (health boards should set an example)
- accessible public transport
- health board funding and resources to develop community-based short breaks for people with learning disabilities

- multiagency policies and guidelines on protecting vulnerable adults
- training and assessment services for dementia
- the provision of additional support teams for those with challenging behaviour and/or complex needs
- research into adults with learning disabilities in prison and forensic services; there should be an appropriate adult scheme for those coming into contact with the police.

Definitions

Challenging behaviour – A term used to describe when someone is acting in a way that might do themselves or others harm. People who care for these people are 'challenged' to stop the harm.

Learning disabilities – people with learning disabilities have a significant, lifelong condition that started before adulthood. It affected their development and means they need help to understand information, learn skills and cope independently.

Social inclusion – helping people to feel and be part of the society in which they live, i.e. they are 'socially included'.

Valuing people

Department of Health 2001 Valuing people: a new strategy for the 21st century. White Paper. DH, London

Valuing People sets out how the government will provide new opportunities for children and adults with learning disabilities and their families to live full and independent lives as part of their local communities.

It recognises major problems with current services, which include:

- poorly coordinated services for families with disabled children, especially for those with severely disabled children
- poor planning for young disabled people at the point of transition into adulthood
- insufficient support for carers, particularly for those caring for people with complex needs
- the limited choice or control that people with learning disabilities have over many aspects of their lives
- the often unmet substantial health care needs of people with learning disabilities
- limited housing choice
- day services that are often not tailored to the needs and abilities of the individual
- limited opportunities for employment
- the needs of people from minority ethnic communities, which are frequently overlooked

- inconsistency in expenditure and service delivery
- few examples of real partnership between health and social care or involving people with learning disabilities and carers.

Only 6% of people with learning disabilities have control over who they live with and only 1% over the choice of carer. Advocacy services are patchy and inconsistent. Less than 10% of people with learning disabilities are in employment and remain, therefore, heavily dependent on social security benefits. Social isolation remains a problem.

> Hester Adrian Research Centre 1999 The quality and costs of residential supports for people with learning disabilities: summary and implications. University of Manchester, Manchester

- This study found that only 30% of people with learning disabilities had a friend who was not either learning disabled, or part of their family or paid to care for them.

> Centre for Research in Primary Care 2004 The needs of people with learning disabilities from minority ethnic communities. University of Leeds, Leeds

- The prevalence of learning disability in some South Asian communities can be up to three times greater than in the general population.
- Diagnosis is often made at a later age than for the population as a whole and parents receive less information about their child's condition and the support available.
- Social exclusion is made more severe by language barriers and racism; negative stereotypes and attitudes contribute to disadvantage.
- Carers who do not speak English receive less information about their support role and experience high levels of stress.
- Agencies often underestimate people's attachments to cultural traditions and religious beliefs.

The four key principles which address the needs of people with learning disabilities are:
- rights
- independence
- choice
- inclusion.

Improving health

- People with learning disabilities have the same right of access to mainstream health services as the rest of the population.
- Health facilitators will be appointed from each local community learning disability team to support people with learning disabilities in getting the health care they need.

- All people with learning disabilities will be registered with a GP and have their own health action plan.
- Local specialist services will be developed as a priority for people with severe challenging behaviour.

Definition

Social exclusion – occurs when individuals or areas suffer as a consequence of socioeconomic factors such as unemployment, poor skills, low incomes, poor housing, high crime environments, bad health and family breakdown.

Weblink Valuing People Support Team – www.valuingpeople.gov.uk

Treatment – Psychopharmacology

Anti-psychotic medication versus placebo for people with both schizophrenia and learning disability

> Duggan L, Brylewski J 2006 Anti-psychotic medication versus placebo for people with both schizophrenia and learning disability **(Cochrane Review)**. In: The Cochrane Library, Issue 2. Update Software, Oxford

- No useable randomised controlled trial evidence was found.
- Will have to continue to extrapolate from trials of people with schizophrenia (without learning disability) and from non-randomised trials.

See also the 'Treatment – Psychopharmacology' section in Chapter 26 (Schizophrenia), page 379.

Antipsychotic medication for challenging behaviour in people with learning disabilities

> Brylewski J, Duggan L 2004 Antipsychotic medication for challenging behaviour in people with learning disabilities **(Cochrane Review)**. In: The Cochrane Library, Issue 3. CD000377. Update Software, Oxford

- Nine randomised controlled trials were included in the data.
- No evidence was obtained regarding the use of antipsychotic medication for this purpose.

Behavioural and cognitive–behavioural interventions for outwardly directed aggressive behaviour

Hassiotis A, Hall I 2004 Behavioural and cognitive–behavioural interventions for outwardly-directed aggressive behaviour in people with learning disabilities **(Cochrane Review)**. In: The Cochrane Library, Issue 1. CD003406. Update Software, Oxford

- Of three studies identified it was only possible to use the data from two.
- Modified relaxation, assertiveness training with problem solving, and anger management appear to have some impact on reduction of aggressive behaviour.
- This was not maintained at follow-up.

See also the 'Treatment – Psychological therapies' section in Chapter 25 (Psychological therapies), page 395.

Behavioural symptoms among people with severe and profound intellectual disabilities

Thompson CL, Reid A 2002 Behavioural symptoms among people with severe and profound intellectual disabilities: a 26 year follow up. British Journal of Psychiatry 181(1): 67–71

- A long-term prospective cohort study.
- Aimed to clarify the natural history of challenging behaviour and psychiatric disorder in people with severe and profound degrees of intellectual disability.
- In 1975, 100 individuals were randomly selected and their behaviour recorded via informant interviews, psychiatric assessment and using the Modified Manifest Abnormality Scale of the Clinical Interview Schedule.
- Repeat studies were performed in 1981/82 and 1992/93.
- Presence and severity of psychiatric disorder were also recorded.
- The study was repeated again in 2001, when the Checklist of Challenging Behaviour was also used.
- Results showed that behavioural symptomatology is remarkably persistent, in particular symptoms of stereotypy, emotional abnormalities, eye avoidance and overactivity.
- The severity of overall psychiatric disorder does show some abatement over time.
- It is important to consider these issues particularly with regard to the efficacy of treatment and management and with regard to placement.

Discontinuation of thioridazine in patients with learning disabilities

Davies SJ Cooke LB, Moore AG, Poto J 2002 Discontinuation of thioridazine in patients with learning disabilities: balancing cardiovascular toxicity with adverse consequences of changing drugs. British Medical Journal 324: 1519–1521

Patients with learning disabilities and psychiatric illness have been placed at higher risk when an antipsychotic drug is stopped or another is substituted than if the drug had been continued.

18 patients had their thioridazine discontinued. This led to:
- moderate to severe difficulties in 7
- behavioural disturbance in 5
- psychotic symptoms in 4
- detention with prolonged admission in 3
- neuroleptic malignant syndrome in one patient after a new antipsychotic medication was commenced.

Many people with learning disabilities lack the capacity to give their own consent to medical interventions, and psychiatrists may be reluctant to override guidelines when responsibility for making decisions cannot be shared with the patient.

See also the 'Treatment – Psychopharmacology' section in Chapter 26 (Schizophrenia), page 379.

Assessment Tools and Rating Scales

Diagnostic Criteria for Learning Disability (DC-LD)

Royal College of Psychiatrists 2001 Diagnostic criteria for use with adults with learning disabilities/mental retardation. Occasional Paper OP 48. Gaskell, London

This paper described an operationalised classification system for psychiatric disorders for use with adults with moderate to profound learning disabilities.

In adults with mild learning disability it can be used in conjunction with other classification systems (e.g. ICD-10 and DSM-IV).

It contains:
1. Axis I – Severity of learning disabilities
2. Axis II – Causes of learning disabilities
3. Axis III – Psychiatric disorders

- Level A Developmental disorders
- Level B Psychiatric issues:
  - Dementia
  - Delirium
  - Non-affective psychosis
  - Affective disorders
  - Neurotic and stress-related disorders
  - Eating disorders
  - Hyperkinetic disorder
- Level C Personality disorders
- Level D Problem behaviours
- Level E Other disorders.

Glasgow Depression Scale (GDS-LD)

Cuthill M, Espie CA, Cooper S-A 2003 Development and psychometric properties of the Glasgow Depression Scale for people with a learning disability: individual and carer versions. British Journal of Psychiatry 182: 347–353

- Derived from the Diagnostic Criteria for Learning Disability (DC-LD).
- 20-item individual version.
- Three-item response:
  - Never/No
  - Sometimes
  - Always.
- Primary questions have suggested supplementary questions.
- Could be used for population screening, symptom monitoring and evaluation of change.
- Takes 10–15 minutes to complete, depending on the ability of the informants.
- Carer scale contains objective observable components of depression.

Psychiatric Assessment Schedule for Adults with Developmental Disability (PAS-ADD)

Moss S, Ibbotson B, Prosser H et al 1997 Validity of the PAS-ADD for detecting psychiatric symptoms in adults with learning disability. Social Psychiatry and Psychiatric Epidemiology 32(6): 344–354

- A semi-structured interview.
- Completed by respondents with learning disability and key informants.
- Screening instrument designed to help carers recognise the presence of mental health problems in people with intellectual disabilities.

- Quick and easy to use.
- PAS-ADD 10 contains items selected from PSE-10.1.
- Interview sections are:
  - Physical illness
  - Eating and weight change
  - Sleep
  - Tension
  - Worries and fears
  - Depression
  - Substance abuse (including alcohol)
  - Auditory hallucinations
  - Hallucinations of other senses
  - Thought interference, replacement of will, delusions
  - Observational items
  - Retrospective ratings.
- The following diagnoses are covered:
  - F20.1-9   Schizophrenia
  - F29   Unspecified non-organic psychosis
  - F30.0   Hypomania
  - F32.0-3   Depressive episode
  - F40.0-2   Phobic anxiety disorders
  - F41.0-1   Panic and generalised anxiety disorders
  - F51.1   Non-organic hypersomnia.

Moss S, Prosser H, Costello H et al 1998 Reliability and validity of the PAS-ADD Checklist for detecting psychiatric disorders in adults with intellectual disability. Journal of Intellectual Disability Research, 42: 173–183

- Short version for use: PAS-ADD Checklist – screening tool for use by non-trained people.
- Five scales combine to produce scores for:
  - affective/neurotic disorder
  - possible organic disorder
  - psychotic disorder.

Vineland Adaptive Behaviour Scales

Sparrow SS, Balla DA, Cicchetti DV 1984 Vineland Adaptive Behavior Scales (Interview Edition). American Guidance Service, Circle Pines, MD

- Structured interview.
- Revised form of the Vineland Social Maturity Scale by E.A. Doll.
- Original scale was created for children (subjects) and mothers (informants).
- Completed with subject and informant or informant alone.
- Four domains:
  - Communication (67 items)
  - Daily living scales (92 items)
  - Socialisation (66 items)
  - Motor skills domain (36 items).

- Provides subscores on
  - Communication: receptive, expressive, written
  - Daily living scales: personal, domestic, community
  - Socialisation: interpersonal relationships, play and leisure, coping skills
  - Motor skills: gross, fine
- Creates age-equivalent scores.

Liaison psychiatry

15

General Topics

Is liaison psychiatry a separate speciality?

> Molodynski A, Bolton J, Guest L 2005 Is liaison psychiatry a separate speciality? Comparison of referrals to liaison psychiatry service and a community mental health team. Psychiatric Bulletin 29: 342–345

In the UK and Ireland, liaison psychiatry is a separate entity from general adult psychiatry, but there is debate as to whether it should have full specialty status. There are limited published data on the problems encountered and managed by liaison-specific teams.

Method

- This study compares the referrals to an established liaison service and a CMHT within the same catchment area.

Results

- The mean rate of referral was higher for the liaison service.
- The liaison service had a smaller ongoing case load than the CMHT.
- The liaison service received a larger number of urgent referrals.
- There were different proportions of certain primary diagnoses in patients referred to the two services.
- Nearly 25% of those referred to the liaison service had a primary organic disorder – largely delirium or dementia in older adults.

- Another skill required was the management of mental illness in the context of physical illness, including the appropriate use of psychotropics and psychological therapy.
- Self-harm referral numbers were high.

Discussion

- Liaison and general psychiatry services provide treatment to different patients with different problems.
- Different skills are required.
- Despite the fact that delirium and dementia in older adults form a large part of the clinical work, liaison psychiatry does not have specific old age psychiatry training.
- Management of people who self-harm also requires specific expertise.
- Separate services are valid and require different skills and specialist training.

See also the 'General topics' section in Chapter 17 (Old age psychiatry), page 263.

Value of measuring suicidal intent in the assessment of people attending hospital following self-poisoning/injury

> Harriss L, Hawtom K, Zahl D 2005 Value of measuring suicidal intent in the assessment of people attending hospital following self-poisoning or self-injury. British Journal of Psychiatry 186: 60–66

Studies have shown associations between the risk of dying by suicide and acts of self-harm in the preceding

12 months. The degree to which a person wants to die has been investigated as a potential risk factor. Follow-up studies have produced inconsistent results concerning the relationship between suicidal intent and future suicidal behaviour. Suicidal intent is nonetheless routinely assessed by psychiatric teams.

Methods

* Patients were identified through the Oxford Monitoring System for Attempted Suicide between 1993 and 2000.
* Self-harm was defined as intentional self-injury or self-poisoning irrespective of the motivation.
* The Suicide Intent Scale was completed.

Results

* 2727 males and 3767 females were included.
* There were 10,690 episodes of self-harm in total.
* Analysis was available for 4415 persons.
* 2719 were involved in the follow-up analysis.
* Suicide Intent Scale results:
  – males tended to score higher on the SIS than females
  – the SIS scores were lowest for those engaging in cutting behaviour
  – the SIS scores were highest amongst those engaging in other methods of self-injuring.
* High suicidal intent was associated with increasing age in both genders.
* After univariate analysis, male patients with the following variables were associated with having high suicidal intent scores:
  – age > 55
  – widowed
  – divorced or separated
  – having a single previous episode of self-harm
  – absence of alcohol misuse.
* 12.4% of high score males went on to have further episodes of self-harm in the subsequent 12 months compared with 22.3% of low score males.
* The differences were maintained after 3 years.
* In females high suicidal intent was associated with:
  – age > 55
  – widowed
  – divorced or separated
  – having a single previous episode of self-harm
  – living in a lonely household.
* 17.4% of high score females engaged in self-harm in the following year – this did not differ significantly from low score females.
* After 3 years the differences between high and low score females became significant.
* 30 (2.9%) males and 24 (1.7%) females died by suicide.
* Of those who committed suicide, significant numbers had had high SIS scores at the index episode – 63% of males and 79% of females.

* 42.1% of patients died within 12 months of the index episode.
* 12.5% who died from suicide had recorded a low SIS score.
* Suicidal intent at the time of self-harm is associated with a risk of subsequent suicide, particularly within the first year after an episode.

See also the 'General topics' section in Chapter 29 (Suicide and self-harm), page 413.

Treatment – Psychopharmacology

Anticonvulsant drugs for acute and chronic pain

Wiffen P, Collins S, McQuay H et al 2006 Anticonvulsant drugs for acute and chronic pain **(Cochrane Review)**. In: The Cochrane Library, Issue 1. Update Software, Oxford

* 23 trials were included (*n* = 1074).
* One trial compared sodium valproate and placebo in the treatment of acute pain.
* Sodium valproate did not have any beneficial effects on pain.
* Three placebo-controlled trials of carbamazepine for trigeminal neuralgia were included.
* Carbamazepine led to significant improvements in levels of pain (pooled NNT 2.5).
* Treatment with gabapentin was associated with reductions in postherpetic pain in one small placebo-controlled trial (NNT 3.2).
* Treatment with anticonvulsant medication was related to improvements in pain associated with diabetic neuropathy.
* The NNTs (from one RCT each) are:
  – carbamazepine 2.3
  – gabapentin 3.8
  – phenytoin 2.1.
* Phenytoin was not found to lead to beneficial effects on symptoms of irritable bowel syndrome.

Antidepressants for neuropathic pain

Saarto T, Wiffen PJ 2006 Antidepressants for neuropathic pain **(Cochrane Review)**. In: The Cochrane Library, Issue 1. Update Software, Oxford

* 50 trials were included (*n* = 2515).

- 19 different antidepressant medications were studied.
- Tricyclic antidepressants are of benefit in the treatment of neuropathic pain.
- Treatment with amitriptyline was associated with a reduction in pain levels (NNT 2; moderate pain relief).
- For diabetic neuropathy the NNT was 1.3.
- For postherpetic neuralgia the NNT was 2.2.
- TCAs were not found to have beneficial effects on neuropathies relating to HIV infection.
- The data regarding the effects of SSRIs on pain were limited.
- There was insufficient data available regarding the use of other antidepressant medications, including St John's wort, venlafaxine and L-tryptophan.

Carbamazepine for acute and chronic pain

Wiffen PJ, McQuay HJ, Moore RA 2006 Carbamazepine for acute and chronic pain **(Cochrane Review)**. In: The Cochrane Library, Issue 1. Update Software, Oxford

- 12 small trials were included ($n = 404$).
- Treatment with carbamazepine was associated with improvements in pain levels in patients with:
  - trigeminal neuralgia (NNT 1.8)
  - diabetic neuropathy (numbers too small for NNT).
- Carbamazepine was found to be as likely as placebo to cause major harm and has a NNH (minor harm) of 3.7.
- Carbamazepine was not found to be effective in the treatment of acute pain.

Treatment of anxiety and depressive disorders in patients with cardiovascular disease

Davies SJC, Jackson PR, Potokar J et al 2004 Treatment of anxiety and depressive disorders in patients with cardiovascular disease: a clinical review. British Medical Journal 328: 939–943

A review of the safety and efficacy of a range of antidepressants in the treatment of patients with cardiovascular disease. It specifically examines whether there is any potential for improving outcomes from a cardiovascular perspective. There is an association between anxiety, depression and cardiovascular disorders. This association is examined.

Prospective studies have shown an excess of poorer cardiovascular outcomes in those with depression or anxiety, suggesting that it cannot be attributed to them being psychologically undermined by the diagnosis.

Anxiety disorders and depression go undetected in hospital settings. It can be difficult to discriminate between psychological and cardiac symptoms.

Frasure-Smith N, Lesperance F, Talajic M 1995 Depression and 18-month prognosis after myocardial infarction. Circulation 91: 999–1005

- There is strong evidence linking depression with coronary artery disease and hypertension.
- 16% of MI patients fulfilled the criteria for major depressive disorder.
- There is a 3.5-fold increase in mortality in patients with depression within 6 months of myocardial infarction.

Davies SJ, Ghahramani P, Jackson PR et al 1999 Association of panic disorder and panic attacks with hypertension. American Journal of Medicine 107: 310–316

- There is evidence of an association between anxiety and hypertension.

Kawachi I, Sparrow D, Vokonas PS et al 1994 Symptoms of anxiety and risk of coronary heart disease. The normative aging study. Circulation 90: 2225–2229

- Cardiovascular disease subsequent to anxiety or sudden death has also been found in several prospective studies.

Sauer WH, Berlin JA, Kimmel SE 2003 Effect of antidepressants and their relative affinity for the serotonin transporter on the risk of myocardial infarction. Circulation 108: 32–36

- Serotonin increases the risk of hypertension and cardiovascular risk.

Serebruany VL, Glassman AH, Malinin AI et al 2003 Platelet/endothelial biomarkers I depressed patients treated with the selective serotonin reuptake inhibitor sertraline after acute coronary events: the Sertraline AntiDepressant Heart Attack Randomized Trial (SADHART) Platelet substudy. Circulation 108: 939–944

- Serotonin decreases the risk of an event by reducing platelet activation and restoring heart rate variability.

Esler M, Rumantir M, Kaye D et al 2001 The sympathetic neurobiology of essential hypertension: disparate influences of obesity, stress and noradrenaline transporter dysfunction? American Journal of Hypertension 14(6 Pt 2): S139–146

- Increased levels of noradrenaline and adrenaline have also been reported in those with hypertension and panic disorder.
- Treatment with tricyclic antidepressants causes concern in patients with cardiovascular disease. This relates to :
  - adverse effects on contractility
  - dysrhythmias and severe hypotension observed after overdose
  - ECG studies implying the theoretical risk of proarrhythmic action similar to type 1 antiarrhythmic drugs.

Davies SJ, Jackson PR, Ramsay LE et al 2003 Drug intolerance due to non-specific adverse effects related to psychiatric morbidity in hypertensive patients. Archives of Internal Medicine 163: 592–600

- Anxiety and depressive disorders are associated with intolerance to antihypertensive medication.
- The link is strongest when the person describes atypical side effects from the medication.

Roose SP, Laghrissi-Thode F, Kennedy JS et al 1998 Comparison of paroxetine and nortriptyline in depressed patients with ischaemic heart disease. Journal of the American Medical Association 279: 287–291

- Concluded that treatment with tricyclic antidepressant medication does not lead to a worsening of heart failure.
- There is no increased risk of sudden death with normal doses.
- The studies are small but may suggest that treatment can lead to a lower mortality from MI.
- Paroxetine when compared to nortriptyline was found to cause fewer problems from a cardiovascular perspective.

Glassman AH, O'Connor CM, Califf RM et al 2002 Sertraline treatment of major depression in patients with acute MI or unstable angina. Journal of the American Medical Association 288: 701–709

- Nortriptyline is less likely than other tricyclics to cause a significant drop in blood pressure.

Strik JJ, Honig A, Lousberg R et al 2000 Efficacy and safety of fluoxetine in the treatment of patients with major depression after first myocardial infarction: findings from a double-blind, placebo-controlled trial. Psychosomatic Medicine 62: 783–789

- Venlafaxine may be used in patients with coronary heart disease.
- Caution is required at doses of more than 300mg as there is a dose-dependent escalation in blood pressure.

Strik JJ, Honig A, Lousberg R et al 1998 Cardiac side effects of two selective serotonin reuptake inhibitors in middle-aged and elderly depressed patients. International Clinical Psychopharmacology 13: 263–267

- Fluoxetine improved symptoms of depression in patients who had suffered a MI.

Glassman AH, O'Connor CM, Califf RM et al 2002 Sertraline treatment of major depression in patients with acute MI or unstable angina. Journal of the American Medical Association 288(6): 701–709

- A double-blind, placebo-controlled trial.
- 369 patients with depression were included.
- Patients were assessed within 30 days of admission with either acute MI or unstable angina.
- Treatment was with either sertraline or placebo for 24 weeks.
- Sertraline was shown to be significantly more effective than placebo for those with severe depression.
- Sertraline produced significantly more improvement on a global scale for all of the subjects.
- There was no difference with regard to safety within cardiac parameters between the two drugs.

See also the 'Treatment – Psychopharmacology' sections in Chapter 2 (Affective disorders), page 31, and Chapter 3 (Anxiety disorders), page 53.

Treatment – Psychological Therapies

Can CBT reduce hypochondriasis?

Gottlieb S 2004 Can cognitive behaviour therapy reduce hypochondriasis? British Medical Journal News 328: 725

Reports a study that assessed treatment with individualised cognitive behaviour therapy for patients with hypochondriasis. It had previously been believed that this disorder was refractory to psychological or drug treatment.

Hypochondriasis was defined as a persistent fear of or belief in having a serious undiagnosed illness.

Barsky A, Ahern D 2004 Cognitive behavior therapy for hypochondriasis: a randomized controlled trial. Journal of the American Medical Association 291: 1464–1470

- An American randomised trial between 1997 and 2001 comparing cognitive behavioural therapy and treatment as usual.

- 102 people were treated with CBT – one 90-minute session a week for 6 weeks.
- There were 82 patients in the control group.
- CBT can have long-term benefits in the reduction of symptoms of hypochondriasis in patients who are willing to try a psychological approach.
- At 12-month follow-up, patients in the CBT group had greater reductions in hypochondriasis scores than the patients in the control group.

See also the 'Treatment – Psychological therapies' section in Chapter 25 (Psychological therapies), page 362.

Effectiveness of opportunistic brief interventions for problem drinking in a general hospital setting

Emmen M, Schippers GM, Bleijenberg G et al 2004 Effectiveness of opportunistic brief interventions for problem drinking in a general hospital setting: systematic review. British Medical Journal 328: 318–320

A systematic review which aimed to determine the effectiveness of opportunistic brief interventions for problem drinking in a hospital setting.

Results

- Eight studies were found – there were a number of methodological weaknesses.
- One short-term study of a relatively intensive intervention was associated with a significant reduction in alcohol consumption in the intervention group.
- The review concluded that the effectiveness of opportunistic brief interventions in a general hospital setting for problem drinkers is still inconclusive.

Heather N 1995 Brief intervention strategies. In: Hester RK, Miller WR (eds) Handbook on alcoholism treatment approaches: effective alternatives. Allyn and Bacon, Needham Heights, MA, pp 105–122

- Brief interventions aimed at problem drinkers are not a type of treatment but a category of intervention.
- They share general characteristics that offer them conceptual coherence.
- They aim to increase harm-free drinking as opposed to total abstinence.
- Most comprise:
  - assessment
  - advice
  - counselling
  - educational elements
  - possibly self-help information.
- The interventions in general hospital settings are generally opportunistic.

Babor TF, Grant M 1992 Programme on substance abuse. Project on identification and management of alcohol related problems. Report on phase II: a randomised clinical trial of brief interventions in primary health care. World Health Organization, Geneva

- A RCT performed by the World Health Organization.
- The most influential study of the effectiveness of brief interventions for problem drinking.
- Simple advice and brief counselling led to reductions in hazardous and harmful alcohol consumption by both sexes in various healthcare settings.

Maheswaren R, Beevers M, Beevers DG 1992 Effectiveness of advice to reduce alcohol consumption in hypertensive patients. Hypertension 19: 79–84

- Only one study reviewed found significant reductions in weekly alcohol consumption in the intervention group.
- The other studies showed no significant differences.
- This review does not agree with the mostly positive results reported elsewhere for brief alcohol interventions in general health care.
- This study reviewed general hospital settings only and not primary care.

Poikolainen K 1999 Effectiveness of brief interventions to reduce alcohol intake in primary health care populations: a meta-analysis. Preventive Medicine 28: 503–509

- A review of brief interventions in primary care only did not show strong evidence of an effect.

See also the 'Treatment – Psychological therapies' sections in Chapter 1 (Addictions psychiatry), page 19.

Psychological interventions for multiple sclerosis

Thomas PW, Thomas S, Hillier C et al 2006 Psychological interventions for multiple sclerosis **(Cochrane Review)**. In: The Cochrane Library, Issue 1. Update Software, Oxford

- 16 trials were included and studied in four subgroups which involved people with:
  - cognitive impairments
  - moderate to severe disability
  - multiple sclerosis (no other variables defined)
  - depression.
- There was evidence that cognitive rehabilitation led to some improvement in cognitive outcomes.
- Treatment with psychotherapy in patients with moderate to severe disability was associated with some improvement in symptoms of depression.

* The results from three trials suggested that cognitive behavioural therapy may be associated with adjusting to and coping with a diagnosis of MS.
* Two studies of people with MS and depression found a significant improvement in patients who were treated with cognitive behavioural therapy.

Psychological interventions for symptomatic management of non-specific chest pain in patients with normal coronary anatomy

Kisely S, Campbell LA, Skerritt P 2006 Psychological interventions for symptomatic management of non-specific chest pain in patients with normal coronary anatomy **(Cochrane Review)**. In: The Cochrane Library, Issue 1. Update Software, Oxford

* Eight studies were included $(n = 403)$.
* All types of psychotherapy were included in the literature search.
* Treatment with psychotherapy was associated with:
  - significant improvements in chest pain in the first 12 weeks
  - significant decrease in the number of chest pain days.
* Improvements continued in the following 3–9 months.
* Cognitive behavioural therapy was noted to be particularly effective.

Psychosocial treatments for multiple unexplained physical symptoms

Allen LA, Escobar JI, Lehrer PM et al 2002 Psychosocial treatments for multiple unexplained physical symptoms: a review of the literature. Psychosomatic Medicine 64: 939–950

Patients with multiple symptoms which are medically unexplained ('polysymptomatic somatisers') may use a number of health services and may not respond to standard treatment.

Method

* A literature search was performed which focused on functional somatic syndromes and somatisation disorder.
* Studies that included single symptom disorders were excluded.
* 34 RCTs were identified.

* Effect sizes were calculated from each study where possible.

Results

* The results of treatment of people with multiple medically unexplained symptoms with psychosocial treatment show only modest effect sizes.
* 67% of the studies reported significant improvements in the primary outcome measure – change in physical symptoms.
* Almost half of the studies which examined the impact of treatment on psychological distress reported greater improvements in the treatment groups.
* Less than one in four adults showed long-term improvement, where the mean follow-up was 6.4 months.

Kasher TM, Rost K, Cohen B et al 1995 Enhancing the health of somatization disorder patients: effectiveness of short-term group therapy. Psychosomatics 36: 462–470

* Patients with somatisation disorder treated with group psychotherapy showed improvements in physical function and reduced mental health complaints in comparison to patients who received standard care.
* The group treatment focused on emotional expression, support and improved coping skills.

Sumathipala A, Hewege R, Hanwella R et al 2000 Randomised controlled trial of cognitive behaviour therapy for repeated consultations for medically unexplained symptoms: a feasibility study in Sri Lanka. Psychological Medicine 30: 747–57

* Patients with five or more unexplained physical symptoms had greater improvements in somatic complaints when treated with individual CBT than patients who received standard care.

Svedlund J, Sjodin I, Ottosson JO et al 1983 Controlled study of psychotherapy in irritable bowel syndrome. Lancet 2: 589–592

* Dynamic therapy was associated with benefit in patients with symptoms of irritable bowel syndrome.

Whorell PJ, Prior A, Farragher EB 1994 Controlled trial of hypnotherapy in the treatment of severe refractory irritable bowel syndrome. Journal of Consulting and Clinical Psychology 62: 576–582

* Hypnotherapy was associated with benefit in patients with symptoms of irritable bowel syndrome.

Blanchard EB, Greene B, Scharff L et al 1993 Relaxation training as a treatment for irritable bowel syndrome. Biofeedback and Self-Regulation 18: 125–132

- Progressive muscle relaxation was associated with benefit in patients with symptoms of irritable bowel syndrome.

Greene B, Blanchard EB 1994 Cognitive therapy for irritable bowel syndrome. Journal of Consulting and Clinical Psychology 62: 576–582

- Individual cognitive therapy was associated with an improvement in symptoms of irritable bowel syndrome.
- This has not been consistently replicated by other studies.

Vollmer A, Blanchard EB 1998 Controlled comparison of individual versus group cognitive therapy for irritable bowel syndrome. Behavior Therapy 29: 19–33

- Group cognitive therapy was associated with an improvement in symptoms of irritable bowel syndrome.

Corney RH, Stanton R, Newell R et al 1991 Behavioural psychotherapy in the treatment of irritable bowel syndrome. Journal of Psychosomatic Research 35: 461–469

- A programme of bowel retraining, operant pain management techniques and increased activity levels did not show benefits over standard medical treatment at the end of treatment.

Fulcher KY, White PD 1997 Randomised controlled trial of graded exercise in patients with the chronic fatigue syndrome. British Medical Journal 341: 1647–1652

- Patients with chronic fatigue syndrome treated with a graded exercise programme showed greater improvements in levels of fatigue, level of functioning and general health compared with a group treated with relaxation/flexibility interventions.

Wearden AJ, Morris RK, Mullis R et al 1998 Randomised, double-blind, placebo-controlled treatment trial of fluoxetine and graded exercise for chronic fatigue syndrome. British Journal of Psychiatry 172: 485–490

- A study which compared fluoxetine treatment alone with fluoxetine treatment combined with graded exercise and a no treatment control group.
- Neither graded exercise nor fluoxetine treatment was associated with improvement in levels of fatigue.

McCain GA, Bell DA, Mai FM et al 1988 A controlled study of the effects of a supervised cardiovascular fitness training program on the manifestations of primary fibromyalgia. Arthritis and Rheumatism 31: 1135–1141

- A three-times-a-week exercise programme led to greater reductions in objectively measured levels of tenderness than a three-times-a-week flexibility training programme.

Martin L, Nutting A, Macintosh BR et al 1996 An exercise program in the treatment of fibromyalgia. Journal of Rheumatology 23: 1050–1053

- A three-times-a-week exercise programme led to greater reductions in objectively measured levels of tenderness than a relaxation programme.

Buckelew SP, Conway R, Parker J et al 1998 Biofeedback/relaxation training and exercise interventions for fibromyalgia: a prospective trial. Arthritis Care and Research 11: 196–209

- Compared an exercise group, a relaxation group, a combined exercise/relaxation group and an education/control group.
- Treatments that included exercise led to better physical function than control group treatment.
- There were no differences between the groups in terms of myalgia scores or self-reported pain.
- Receiving any of the three treatments was associated with reduced tenderness levels compared with the control group.

Keel PJ, Bodoky C, Gerhard U et al 1998 Comparison of integrated group therapy and group relaxation training for fibromyalgia. Clinical Journal of Pain 14: 232–238

- Treatment with group CBT in patients with fibromyalgia was not associated with benefits at the end of treatment greater than those for the control group.
- This finding is in agreement with other studies.
- Treatment with group CBT was associated with improvements in pain intensity 4 months after treatment.

See also the 'Treatment – Psychological therapies' section in Chapter 25 (Psychological therapies), page 350.

Obsessive–compulsive disorder

16

Chapter contents

Treatment – Others

Transcranial magnetic stimulation for the treatment of obsessive–compulsive disorder

Martin JLR, Barbanoj MJ, Perez V, Sacristan M 2003 Transcranial magnetic stimulation for the treatment of obsessive–compulsive disorder **(Cochrane Review)**. In: The Cochrane Library, Issue 2. CD003387. Update Software, Oxford

- Three trials were included, with two providing data suitable for quantitative analysis.
- A meta-analysis was not possible.
- No differences were noted between rTMS and sham TMS using the Yale–Brown Obsessive Compulsive Scale or the Hamilton Depression Rating Scale for all time periods analysed.

Assessment tools and Rating Scales

Yale–Brown Obsessive Compulsive Scale (Y-BOCS)

Goodman WK, Price LH, Rasmussen SA et al 1989 The Yale–Brown Obsessive Compulsive Scale, I: development, use, and reliability. Archives of General Psychiatry 46: 1006–1011

- Clinician-rated semi-structured interview.
- Rates the severity and type of symptoms in OCD.
- Covers the week prior to interview
- Takes about 30 minutes to complete.
- Gold standard for OCD symptoms.
- Well suited for assessing the severity of symptoms and monitoring change.
- Divided into obsession and compulsion subsets.
- Starts with a symptom checklist and then the patient is asked to focus on the three most upsetting obsessions and compulsions.

Guidelines

Obsessive–compulsive disorder: core interventions in the treatment of obsessive–compulsive disorder and body dysmorphic disorder. NICE Clinical Guideline 31*
see pages 246 & 247

The stepped-care model

Who is responsible for care?	What is the focus?	What do they do?
Step 6 Inpatient care or intensive treatment programmes CAMHS Tier 4	OCD or BDD with risk to life, severe self-neglect or severe distress or disability	Reassess, discuss options, care coordination SSRI or clomipramine, CBT (including ERP), or combination of SSRI or clomipramine and CBT (including ERP), augmentation strategies; consider admission or special living arrangements
Step 5 Multidisciplinary care with expertise in OCD/BDD CAMHS Tiers 3 and 4	OCD or BDD with significant comorbidity, or more severely impaired functioning and/or treatment resistance, partial response or relapse	Reassess, discuss options **For adults:** SSRI or clomipramine, CBT (including ERP), or combination of SSRI or clomipramine and CBT (including ERP); consider care coordination, augmentation strategies, admission, social care **For children and young people:** CBT (including ERP), then consider combined treatments of CBT (including ERP) with SSRI, alternative SSRI or clomopramine. For young people consider referral to specialist services outside CAMHS if appropriate
Step 4 Multidisciplinary care in primary or secondary care CAMHS Tiers 2 and 3	OCD or BDD with comorbidity or poor response to initial treatment	Assess and review, discuss options **For adults:** CBT (including ERP), SSRI, alternative SSRI or clomipramine, combined treatments **For children and young people:** CBT (including ERP), then consider combined treatments of CBT (including ERP) with SSRI, alternative SSRI or clomipramine
Step 3 GPs, primary care team, primary care mental health workers, family support team CAMHS Tiers 1 and 2	Management and initial treatment of OCD or BDD	Assess and review, discuss options **For adults according to impairment:** Brief individual CBT (including ERP) with self-help materials (for OCD), individual or group CBT (including ERP), SSRI, or consider combined treatments; consider involving the family/carers in ERP **For children and young people:** Guided self-help (for OCD), CBT (including ERP), involve family/carers and consider involving school
Step 2 GPs, practice nurses, school heath advisors, health visitors, general health settings (including hospitals) CAMHS Tier 1	Recognition and assessment	Detect, educate, discuss treatment options, signpost voluntary support organisations, provide support to individuals/families/carers/work/schools, or refer to any of the appropriate levels
Step 1 Individuals, public organisations, NHS	Awareness and recognition	Provide, seek and share information about OCD or BDD and its impact on individuals and families/carers

Reproduced with permission from the National Institute for Health and Clinical Excellence, London.

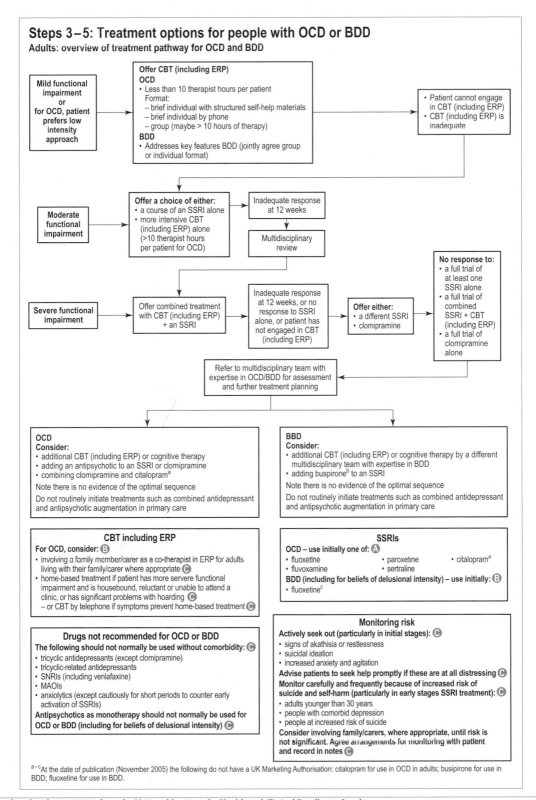

Steps 3–5: Treatment options for people with OCD or BDD
Adults: overview of treatment pathway for OCD and BDD

Mild functional impairment or for OCD, patient prefers low intensity approach

Offer CBT (including ERP)
OCD
- Less than 10 therapist hours per patient
  Format:
  – brief individual with structured self-help materials
  – brief individual by phone
  – group (maybe > 10 hours of therapy)
BDD
- Addresses key features BDD (jointly agree group or individual format)

- Patient cannot engage in CBT (including ERP)
- CBT (including ERP) is inadequate

Moderate functional impairment

Offer a choice of either:
- a course of an SSRI alone
- more intensive CBT (including ERP) alone (>10 therapist hours per patient for OCD)

Inadequate response at 12 weeks

Multidisciplinary review

Severe functional impairment

Offer combined treatment with CBT (including ERP) + an SSRI

Inadequate response at 12 weeks, or no response to SSRI alone, or patient has not engaged in CBT (including ERP)

Offer either:
- a different SSRI
- clomipramine

No response to:
- a full trial of at least one SSRI alone
- a full trial of combined SSRI + CBT (including ERP)
- a full trial of clomipramine alone

Refer to multidisciplinary team with expertise in OCD/BDD for assessment and further treatment planning

OCD
Consider:
- additional CBT (including ERP) or cognitive therapy
- adding an antipsychotic to an SSRI or clomipramine
- combining clomipramine and citalopram[a]

Note there is no evidence of the optimal sequence

Do not routinely initiate treatments such as combined antidepressant and antipsychotic augmentation in primary care

BBD
Consider:
- additional CBT (including ERP) or cognitive therapy by a different multidisciplinary team with expertise in BDD
- adding buspirone[b] to an SSRI

Note there is no evidence of the optimal sequence

Do not routinely initiate treatments such as combined antidepressant and antipsychotic augmentation in primary care

CBT including ERP
For OCD, consider: **B**
- involving a family member/carer as a co-therapist in ERP for adults living with their family/carer where appropriate **C**
- home-based treatment if patient has more severe functional impairment and is housebound, reluctant or unable to attend a clinic, or has significant problems with hoarding **C**
  – or CBT by telephone if symptoms prevent home-based treatment **C**

SSRIs
OCD – use initially one of: **A**
- fluoxetine
- fluvoxamine
- paroxetine
- sertraline
- citalopram[a]

BDD (including for beliefs of delusional intensity) – use initially: **B**
- fluoxetine[c]

Drugs not recommended for OCD or BDD
The following should not normally be used without comorbidity: **C**
- tricyclic antidepressants (except clomipramine)
- tricyclic-related antidepressants
- SNRIs (including venlafaxine)
- MAOIs
- anxiolytics (except cautiously for short periods to counter early activation of SSRIs)

Antipsychotics as monotherapy should not normally be used for OCD or BDD (including for beliefs of delusional intensity) **C**

Monitoring risk
Actively seek out (particularly in initial stages): **C**
- signs of akathisia or restlessness
- suicidal ideation
- increased anxiety and agitation

Advise patients to seek help promptly if these are at all distressing **C**

Monitor carefully and frequently because of increased risk of suicide and self-harm (particularly in early stages SSRI treatment): **C**
- adults younger than 30 years
- people with comorbid depression
- people at increased risk of suicide

Consider involving family/carers, where appropriate, until risk is not significant. Agree arrangements for monitoring with patient and record in notes **C**

[a–c] At the date of publication (November 2005) the following do not have a UK Marketing Authorisation: citalopram for use in OCD in adults; buspirone for use in BDD; fluoxetine for use in BDD.

Psychological interventions

All healthcare professionals offering psychological treatments for OCD or BDD to people of any age should advise patients who request other forms of psychological therapy, such as psychoanalysis, transactional analysis, hypnosis or marital/couple therapy, that there is no convincing evidence to support their use. [C]

Using psychological interventions in adults

Obsessive thoughts without covert compulsions
* Consider CBT (including exposure of the obsessive thoughts and response prevention of mental rituals and neutralising strategies). [B]

OCD
* Consider cognitive therapy adapted for OCD: [C]
    - as an addition to ERP to enhance long-term symptom reduction
    - for people who refuse or cannot engage with treatments that include ERP.

Using psychological interventions in children and young people

* Consider including rewards to enhance motivation and reinforce desired behaviour changes. [C]

Pharmacological interventions

Using SSRIs in adults

* Advise patients verbally and in writing that:
    - craving and tolerance do not occur [C]
    - discontinuation/withdrawal symptoms may occur on stopping the drug, or missing or reducing doses [C]
    - there is a range of potential side effects (including worsening anxiety, suicidal thoughts and self-harm) that need to be carefully monitored, especially in the first few weeks of treatment [C]
    - onset of effect is commonly delayed for up to 12 weeks (although depressive symptoms improve more quickly). [C]

Monitoring
* For people at high risk of suicide: [C]
    - prescribe a limited amount of medication
    - consider, particularly in patients with comorbid depression, additional support such as more frequent direct contacts with primary care staff, or telephone contacts, particularly in first few weeks of treatment.
* Around the time of dose change, monitor for any new symptoms or worsening of the condition. [C]
* If marked and/or prolonged akathisia, restlessness or agitation develops, review the use of the drug. Change to a different SSRI if the patient prefers. [C]
* Monitor more intensively adults with BDD not receiving appropriate treatment or not responding to treatment, because of the high risk of suicide in people with BDD. [GPP]

Continuing treatment
* If effective, continue treatment for at least 12 months to prevent relapse and allow for further improvement. [C]

Discontinuing treatment
* When reducing or stopping SSRI treatment, taper the dose gradually over several weeks, according to the patient's need. Take account of the starting dose, drug half-life and particular profile of adverse effects when determining the rate of reduction. [C]
* Encourage the patient to seek advice if they experience significant discontinuation/withdrawal symptoms. [C]

Using clomipramine in adults

* Consider clomipramine when: [C]
    - an adequate trial of at least one SSRI was ineffective, or
    - an SSRI was poorly tolerated, or
    - the patient prefers clomipramine, or
    - there has been a previous good response to clomipramine.
* For people at significant risk of cardiovascular disease, carry out an ECG and a blood pressure measurement before prescribing clomipramine. [C]

C indicates the grade of recommendation; **GPP** indicates a good practice point (see Appendix II for full details).

Old age psychiatry

Chapter contents

Ethical issues

Advance statements in old age psychiatry

Williams L, Rigby J 2004 Advance statements in old age psychiatry. Advances in Psychiatric Treatment 10: 260–266

An advance statement details the wishes of an individual in the event of the loss of capacity to make decisions in the future. Advance statements were developed in the 1960s in the United States. They were later introduced in the UK. The House of Lords concluded that they could represent legally binding treatment refusals if certain criteria were met.

The Draft Mental Incapacity Bill in England and Wales states that advance refusals should be respected if they are valid and applicable. The Adults with Incapacity Act in Scotland makes it possible to confer a welfare power of attorney to protect the wishes of an individual.

- An *advance statement* requests that a person's wishes be considered. However, the person cannot demand treatment and the advance statement is not legally binding.
- An *advance directive* (or advance treatment refusal or living will) is a particular form of advance statement which is a more explicit declaration regarding the refusal of specific treatments.

Any competent adult has the right to refuse medical treatment based on the legal principle of self-determination. Advance statements could potentially promote patient autonomy, enhance communication and relieve the burden felt by relatives.

Advance statements can be oral. Written statements provide the clearest record of the wishes of the patient. The patient must be capable at the time of writing. If prepared in collaboration with the medical team, this can provide an opportunity to discuss diagnosis, prognosis and treatment options. A solicitor is not required to witness the statement. Capacity can be suggested if the statement is witnessed by both the doctor and the solicitor. Advance statements apply to the present situation. They only become active when capacity is lost.

Examples include the following:

- For a patient with dementia, early discussion might involve the provision of physical treatments such as PEG feeding and the treatment of infections.
- In patients with functional illness, the choice of medication or accommodation placements may be discussed.
- Consent to involvement in research can also be considered.

Where advance statements or refusals cannot be followed, careful discussion and documentation are essential.

Advance refusals can be overridden by the Mental Health Act if it is thought that an individual is at risk or for the protection of others. It is good practice to respect advance statements where possible.

Treatment refusals are not applicable where the control of infectious diseases and issues of public health are involved.

Treatment refusals do not include refusal of basic care and hygiene measures (e.g. the changing of soiled bed linen).

It is not possible to refuse analgesia in an advance directive as this could cause distress to carers.

Advance statements cannot cover all scenarios. They should be reviewed regularly in view of medical advances. Once capacity is lost, the statement is considered permanent and irreversible.

Fazel S, Hope T, Jacoby R 1999 Dementia, intelligence, and the capacity to complete advance directives. Lancet 354: 48

- A study of the capacity of patients with dementia to make decisions at first presentation to an old age clinic.
- 20% of these patients had the capacity to make an advance directive at first presentation.

Weblinks

Age Concern – www.ageconcern.org.uk

Alzheimer's Society – www.alzheimers.org.uk

Mind (National Association for Mental Health) – www.mind.org.uk

See also the 'Ethical issues' section in Chapter 9 (Ethical issues), page 119.

Elder abuse

Lachs MS, Pillemer K 2004 Elder abuse. Lancet 364(9441): 1236–1271

Elder abuse is recognised internationally as a growing problem. In 1997 the International Network for the Prevention of Elder Abuse was established due to increasing concern regarding the mistreatment of older people.

Bonnie R, Wallace R (eds) 2002 Elder mistreatment: abuse, neglect, and exploitation in an aging America. National Academy Press, Washington, DC.

The US National Academy of Sciences suggested a set of statements to define elder abuse. These are:
- intentional actions that cause harm or create a serious risk of harm (whether or not harm is intended) to a vulnerable elder by a caregiver or other person who stands in a trust relationship to the elder, or
- failure by a caregiver to satisfy the elder's basic needs or protect the elder from harm.

Types of abuse include physical, psychological, sexual, financial and neglect. The frequency is difficult to determine with accuracy.

Thomas C 2002 First National Study of Elder Abuse and Neglect: contrast with results from other studies. Journal of Elder Abuse and Neglect 12: 1–14

- Elder abuse is thought to be between 2 and 10%.

Pillemer K, Finkelhor D 1988 The prevalence of elder abuse: a random sample survey. Gerontologist 28: 51–57

- A non-institutional sample of elderly people in urban Boston.
- The overall rate of elder abuse was 3.2%.

Comijs HC, Penninx BW, Knipscheer KP et al 1999 Psychological distress in victims of elder abuse: the effects of social support and coping. Journal of Gerontology: Psychological Sciences and Social Sciences 54: 240–245

- A Dutch study of four types of abuse.
- Found a 1-year rate of elder abuse of 5.8%.

Lachs MS, Williams C, O'Brien S et al 1997 Risk factors for reported elder abuse and neglect: a nine-year observational cohort study. Gerontologist 37: 469–474

- Abuse occurs in a multitude of settings from the person's own home to hospitals and care homes.
- Shared living is a risk factor.

Choi NG, Kulick VN, Murphy KP et al 1999 Financial exploitation of elders: analysis of risk factors based on county adult protective services data. Journal of Elder Abuse and Neglect 10: 39–61

- Higher rates of financial abuse occur amongst those living alone.

Paveza GJ, Cohen D, Eisdorfer C et al 1992 Severe family violence and Alzheimer's disease: prevalence and risk factors. Gerontologist 32: 493–497

- Higher rates of physical abuse are described in people with dementia.
- Carers could also be victim to assault by a confused elderly person and this may lead to stress, distress and retaliation.
- Elderly carers can also be the victims of abuse by relatives with dementia.

Compton SA, Flanagan P, Gregg W 1997 Elder abuse in people with dementia in Northern Ireland: prevalence and predictors in cases referred to a psychiatry of old age service. International Journal Geriatric Psychiatry 12: 632–635

- Social isolation is a risk factor for stress and elder abuse.

Reay AM, Browne KD 2001 Risk factor characteristics in carers who physically abuse or neglect their elderly dependants. Aging and Mental Health 5: 56–62

- A history of mental illness in the perpetrator is associated with elder abuse.
- Depression is a common characteristic of elder abusers.
- This has been verified by a number of other studies.

Anetzberger GJ, Korbin JE, Austin C 1994 Alcoholism and elder abuse. Journal of Interpersonal Violence 9: 184–193

- Perpetrators of elder abuse are more likely to abuse alcohol.

Greenberg JR, McKibben M, Raymond JA 1990 Dependent adult children and elder abuse. Journal of Elder Abuse and Neglect 2: 73–86

- It is generally the case that people who commit elder abuse are themselves dependent on the person that they abuse.
- Abuse may be a way of obtaining money or other resources.

The evidence is not clear regarding the association between the victim's health and functional ability and levels of abuse. Physical impairment could make an elderly patient more vulnerable to abuse. Studies have not found any relationship between the level of an elder's dependency resulting in stress on carers and elder abuse.

There are arguments for and against screening for elder abuse. At present there are no valid and reliable screening tools.

Physical signs can also be misleading:
- injuries can be sustained by falling or by being mistreated
- weight loss could reflect physical ill-health or neglect
- medication errors may be entirely innocent or intentional attempts to cause harm.

The older person may wish to conceal being a victim of abuse and is not always able to freely describe the problem. Increased awareness amongst professionals and education are of great importance.

Lachs MS, Williams CS, O'Brien S et al 1998 The mortality of elder abuse. Journal of the American Medical Association 280: 428–443

- A longitudinal study of old people.
- People who were mistreated were over three times more likely to die during the 3-year study period than those who were not abused.
- After 13 years, only 9% of old people who were mistreated were still alive, compared with 41% of those who had not been mistreated.

Lachs MS, Williams CS, O'Brien S et al 2002 Adult protective service home use and nursing home placement. Gerontologist 42: 734–739

- Being the victim of elder abuse is associated with increased rates of adverse life events (e.g. placement in a nursing home).

- It is also associated with higher levels of morbidity (e.g. increased rates of depression).
- The article goes on to discuss what action might be taken in the event of suspected or actual elder abuse.

General Topics

Alcohol use disorders

O'Connell H, Chin A, Cunningham C et al 2003 Alcohol use disorders in elderly people: redefining an age-old problem in old age. British Medical Journal 327: 664–667

Media attention and public health initiatives toward alcohol misuse tend to focus on younger age groups. Alcohol use disorders are common amongst the elderly and are associated with significant health problems. Alcohol misuse is often not detected or is misdiagnosed in older people.

The prevalence of alcohol problems in older adults is thought to be less than in younger adults but this may be an underestimate. Most prevalence studies have been conducted in North America. These may not generalise to UK culture.

UK National Digital Archive of Datasets 1994 General household survey, UK, 1994. Online. Available: www.ndad.nationalarchives.gov.uk

- An estimate for the prevalence of alcohol misuse/dependence in the community is 2–4%.
- The rates are higher when excessive consumption is included:
  - 17% for men
  - 7% for women.
- Even higher rates are seen in hospitals:
  - 14% in the emergency department
  - 18% in medical inpatients
  - 23–44% in psychiatric inpatients.

Saunders PA, Copeland JR, Dewey ME et al 1991 Heavy drinking as a risk factor for depression and dementia in elderly men. Findings from the Liverpool longitudinal community study. British Journal of Psychiatry 159: 213–216

- Alcohol abuse is associated with being male.

Bristow MF, Clare AW 1992 Prevalence and characteristics of at-risk drinkers among elderly acute medical inpatients. British Journal of Addiction 87: 291–294

- Alcohol abuse is associated with being socially isolated and single.

Ekerdt DJ, deLabry LO, Glynn RJ et al 1989 Change in drinking behaviours with retirement: findings from the normative ageing study. Journal of Studies in Alcohol 50: 347–353

- Alcohol abuse is associated with being separated or divorced.

Disorders of alcohol use are frequently undetected and misdiagnosed by health professionals. This may occur because:
- the patient may be reluctant to reveal the history
- health workers have a lower suspicion in the elderly
- health workers are less likely to refer patients to specialist services
- health professionals may consider the person's alcohol problem as 'understandable' in the context of changing social and health status related to age.

Callahan CM, Tierney WM 1995 Health services use and mortality among older primary care patients with alcoholism. Journal of the American Geriatrics Society 43: 1378–1383

- A primary care study.
- 10% of the population had evidence of alcohol-related problems.
- Less than half of patients identified with alcohol-related problems had this documented in their medical records.

The presentation of alcohol problems is not always obvious but they may come to light following a history of falls, confusion or depression. A psychiatric diagnosis or physical health problems may mask symptoms.

Safe limits for alcohol consumption are not defined for the elderly but are likely to be lower than for younger adults in view of the changes in body composition with ageing.

Screening questionnaires and diagnostic criteria may not be relevant in this population.

Reid MC, Anderson PA 1997 Geriatric substance use disorders. Medical Clinics of North America 81: 999–1016

- DSM-IV criteria may not apply in the ageing population.
- Elderly people have changes in their roles and in their social circumstances as well as varying health needs.
- Elderly people are more likely to experience the physical health consequences than the social, legal and occupational complications that the younger population with alcohol use problems undergo.

Hurt RD, Finlayson RE, Morse RM et al 1988 Alcoholism in elderly persons: medical aspects and prognosis of 216 inpatients. Mayo Clinic Proceedings 63: 753–760

- Elderly people who misuse alcohol are much more likely than their peers to have serious medical disorders.

Colsher PL, Wallace RB 1990 Elderly men with histories of heavy drinking: correlates and consequences. Journal of Studies in Alcohol 51: 528–535

- Factors associated with ever having been a heavy drinker are long lasting.
- People who have ever been a heavy drinker are more likely to have:
  - major illnesses
  - a lower self-reported health status
  - more visits from the doctor
  - greater numbers of depressive symptoms
  - less satisfaction with life
  - smaller social networks.

Ruitenberg A, van Sweiten JC, Witteman JCM et al 2002 Alcohol consumption and risk of dementia: the Rotterdam study. Lancet 359: 281–286

- A study of the potential health benefits of consuming alcohol.
- Light to moderate alcohol intake was associated with reductions in the risk of:
  - coronary heart disease
  - stroke
  - dementia.

Curtis JR, Geller G, Stokes EJ et al 1989 Characteristics, diagnosis and treatment of alcoholism in elderly patients. Journal of the American Geriatrics Society 37: 310–316

- Elderly people are as likely as the younger population to benefit from treatment.

Liskow BI, Rinck C, Campbell J et al 1989 Alcohol withdrawal in the elderly. Journal of Studies in Alcohol 50: 414

- Elderly people with alcohol use disorders have:
  - high levels of medical comorbidity
  - increased severity of alcohol withdrawals
  - increased duration of alcohol withdrawals.

Hurt RD, Finlayson RE, Morse RM et al 1988 Alcoholism in elderly persons: medical aspects and prognosis of 216 inpatients. Mayo Clinic Proceedings 63: 753–760

- Elderly people have:
  - increased sensitivity to the adverse effects of medication
  - altered pharmacokinetics.
- This is particularly true for inpatients who are older and have serious illness.

Dunne FJ 1994 Misuse of alcohol or drugs by elderly people. British Medical Journal 308: 608–609

- Disulfiram can lead to an acute confusional state in elderly people.

- It should be used with caution and only in the short term.

Oslin DW, Mellow AM 1998 Neurotransmitter-based therapeutic strategies in late-life alcoholism and other addictions. In: Gomberg E, Hegedus AM, Zucker RA (eds) Alcohol problems and aging. NIAA Research Monograph No 33. NIH Publication No 98-4163. National Institute on Alcohol Abuse and Alcoholism, Bethesda, MD

- Naltrexone is associated with a reduction in relapse rate in people with alcohol use disorders aged between 50 and 74 years.

Kofoed LL, Tolon RL, Atkinson RM et al 1987 Treatment compliance of older alcoholics: an elder-specific approach is superior to 'mainstreaming'. Journal of Studies in Alcohol 48: 47

- Older people with alcohol use disorders who receive psychological treatments (psychoeducation, counselling and motivational interviewing) may respond better when the treatments are provided in same age settings.

Brennan PL, Moos RH 1991 Functioning, life context, and help-seeking among late-onset problem drinkers: Comparisons with non problem and early-onset drinkers on skid row. British Journal of Addiction 86: 1139

- Alcohol use disorders arising late in life may relate to life events such as bereavement, a change in role or onset of illness.

Adams SL, Waskel SA 1991 Late onset of alcoholism among older Midwestern men in treatment. Psychological Reports 68: 432

- Between 11 and 33% of elderly people develop alcohol use disorders later in life.

Ewing JA 1984 Detecting alcoholism: the CAGE questionnaire. Journal of the American Medical Association 252: 1905–1907

- The CAGE questionnaire has been found to have reasonable sensitivity and specificity in older people.
- Further questions should be asked, such as, 'Why do you think you should cut down?'

Weblinks

International Psychogeriatric Association – www.ipa-online.org

National Institute on Alcohol Abuse and Alcoholism – www.niaaa.nih.gov.

See also the 'General topics' section in Chapter 1 (Addictions psychiatry), pages 12-15.

Carers as partners in mental health services for older people

Oyebode JR 2005 Carers as partners in mental health services for older people. Advances in Psychiatric Treatment 2005 11: 297–304

A systematic planned approach that engages carers as an integral part of the system of care has potential benefits for patients, carers and services. The input of carers can range from the provision of a collaborative history, involvement in review meetings and outpatient appointments to being taught specific skills for the care of the patient. Such skills can include communication skills and behavioural management techniques. At present, carers may only be offered help when they are struggling with day-to-day care. Difficulties in evaluating the effectiveness of carer-provided interventions are discussed. Carer interventions can be provided in a group setting and examples of this are given.

Office for National Statistics 2001 Census 2001. ONS, London

- 10% of the population provides unpaid care.

Department of Health 1999 The National Strategy for Carers. The Stationery Office. London, p 13

- Discusses the provision of information for carers so that they become real partners in the provision of care to the person they are looking after.

Wolff JL, Agree EM 2004 Depression among recipients of informal care: the effects of reciprocity, respect, and adequacy of support. Journal of Gerontology: Psychological Sciences and Social Sciences 59: S173–S180

- This study found that in terms of health the perceived quality of care and the relationship with the carer are more important than actual health.

Schulz R, O'Brien A, Czaja S et al 2002 Dementia caregiver intervention research: in search of clinical significance. Gerontologist 42: 589–602

- A review of studies comparing carer interventions, environmental interventions and pharmacological interventions in patients with dementia.
- Measured outcomes of carer health, social significance, carer quality of life and acceptability of treatments.
- Psychosocial interventions for carers led to significant beneficial effects in all outcomes except carer quality of life.

Brodaty H, Green A, Koshera A 2003 Meta-analysis of psychosocial interventions for caregivers of people with dementia. Journal of the American Geriatrics Society 51: 657–664

- This meta-analysis found that dementia carer interventions (not respite care) led to significant beneficial effects in terms of improved psychological distress levels, carer knowledge and the patient's mood.
- The results were equivocal with regard to the time to institutionalisation.
- No effects on carer burden were found.

Challis D, von-Abendorff R, Brown P et al 2002 Care management, dementia care and specialist mental health services: an evaluation. International Journal of Geriatric Psychiatry 17: 315–325

- Intensive case management in dementia, where the needs of the patient and carer are closely attended to, shows greater benefits than usual care.
- Benefits include reduced need, lower risk of coming to harm, improvements in activities of daily living and improved social contacts.
- Carers reported lower stress levels when involved in intensive case management.
- Patients receiving intensive management were more likely to remain at home at the end of 2 years than those receiving usual care (51 and 33%, respectively).

Marriot A, Donaldson C, Tarrier N et al 2000 Effectiveness of cognitive-behavioural family intervention in reducing the burden of care in carers of patients with Alzheimer's disease. British Journal of Psychiatry 176: 557–562

- This intervention involved an in-depth assessment of the needs of the patient and main carer.
- This was followed by 14 fortnightly therapy sessions with the carer.
- Sessions involved the sharing of information and education regarding stress management and coping skills.
- RCT evidence shows that the intervention was beneficial in reducing psychiatric morbidity and depression in carers at 3-month follow-up.
- Patients also had improvements in activities of daily living.

Clare L, Woods R 2001 Cognitive rehabilitation in dementia. Psychology Press, Hove

- In cognitive rehabilitation the carer can be co-therapist and address issues such as the retention or the enhancement of skills in patients with dementia.

Quayhagen MP, Quayhagen M 1996 Discovering life quality in coping with dementia. Western Journal of Nursing 18: 120–135

- Two studies found that cognitive rehabilitation, where the patient's spouse is involved as therapist, has beneficial effects on cognitive function.

The future of memory clinics

Passmore AP, Craig DA 2004 The future of memory clinics. Psychiatric Bulletin 28: 375–377

Memory clinics were first developed in the US and later in the UK. They were created in the UK in the 1980s as a service for people with dementia. The principle was to provide a specialist clinic for the diagnosis, education and management of people with dementia in a multidisciplinary setting. Research was also a feature.

The introduction of anticholinesterase medication for people with dementia has led to the need for consensus on their use. The National Institute for Clinical Excellence (NICE) and the National Service Framework for Older People (Department of Health 2001) concur that memory clinics should be further developed.

The function of a memory clinic can include:
- acting as a referral point for other professionals
- aiming for early diagnosis by a specialist
- initiating and monitoring therapy where appropriate
- referring to other agencies
- education and support for patients and carers.

Patients seen at a memory clinic are likely to differ from those seen at standard old age psychiatry clinics in that they:
- are more likely to be younger
- are generally less impaired
- are living at home
- have first contact with services 2 years earlier in the course of their disease.

A benefit of early diagnosis may be that there is a delay until inception into care facilities.

The ideal structure of a memory clinic is not clear. It will likely involve a psychiatrist supported by nursing staff, with input from psychology and voluntary agencies. Clinics will require adequate funding to maintain the service and prevent delays to first appointment due to waiting lists.

Hypersexuality in dementia

Series H, Degano P 2005 Hypersexuality in dementia. Advances in Psychiatric Treatment 11: 424–431

Sexually disinhibited behaviours are quite common in people with dementia (2–17%). This article discusses the prevalence, nature, ethical issues, assessment and management of this problem. There are no published studies of specific behavioural treatments for sexually disinhibited behaviour in this group. Staff training is recommended regarding education, support and agreement of how behaviours should be managed. No medications are licensed for this population and there is little available evidence. The majority of evidence is drawn from the treatment of sexual offenders.

Burns A, Jacoby R, Levy R 1990 Psychiatric phenomena in Alzheimer's disease. IV: Disorders of behaviour. British Journal of Psychiatry 157: 86–94

- Studied sexually disinhibited behaviour in people with Alzheimer's disease living at home, in residential care and in hospital.
- Sexually disinhibited behaviour occurred in:
  - 6.9% of 178 people
  - 8% of the men
  - 7% of the women.
- Behaviours included:
  - exposure
  - obscene sexual language
  - masturbation
  - propositioning others.
- Sexually disinhibited behaviour was associated with increasing severity of dementia.

Rabins RV, Mace NL, Lucas MJ 1982 The impact of dementia on the family. Journal of the American Medical Association 248: 333–335

- Inappropriate sexual behaviour was reported by 2% of caregivers (one family).

Kumar A, Koss E, Metzler D et al 1988 Behavioural symptomatology in dementia of the Alzheimer type. Alzheimer Disease and Associated Disorders 2: 363–365

- A comparison between 28 people with Alzheimer's disease and a control group.
- There were no significant differences between the groups with regard to assaultative or sexually inappropriate behaviour.
- These behaviours occurred in both groups at a rate of 7%.

Zeiss AM, Davies HD, Tinklenberg JR 1996 An observational study of sexual behaviour in demented male patients. Journal of Gerontology 51: M325–329

- An observational study of the types of sexual behaviour displayed by 40 people with dementia resident in a care home.
- There were 94 episodes of sexually inappropriate or ambiguous behaviour.
- Staff did not respond to any of these behaviours.

- Staff also ignored more than half of appropriate sexual behaviours.

Management of depression in later life

Baldwin R, Wild R 2004 Management of depression in later life. Advances in Psychiatric Treatment 10: 131–139

Depression is the most common psychiatric diagnosis in the elderly population. Although antidepressants and psychological treatment are effective, prognosis could be improved. Depression in old age is associated with chronicity and a high risk of relapse after recovery. It is the leading cause of suicide in older people. There is little evidence regarding the effectiveness of treatments for minor and major depression in older people. Consensus opinion regarding the initiation, type, dosage and side effects of medications are given.

Penninx BW, Deeg DJ, van Eijk JT et al 2000 Changes in depression and physical decline in older adults: a longitudinal perspective. Journal of Affective Disorders 61: 1–12

- Depressive disorder in older people is associated with:
  - a poorer quality of life
  - increased disability secondary to physical disorder.

Cuijpers P, Smit F 2002 Excess mortality in depression: a meta-analysis of community studies. Journal of Affective Disorders 72: 227–236

- Depression in older people is an independent predictor of mortality.
- Minor and major depression in this group share similar risk factors.
- The adverse outcomes associated with having minor depression lie halfway between the adverse outcomes for major depression and having no depression at all.

Beekman AT, Copeland JR, Prince MJ 1999 Review of community prevalence of depression in later life. British Journal of Psychiatry 174: 307–311

- A meta-analysis of the prevalence of depressive disorder in older people living in the community.
- Depression is the most frequent psychiatric illness amongst older adults.
- 13.5% had significant depression.
- 2% had major depression.
- Rates are much higher in hospital and care homes.

Yesavage JA, Brink TL, Rose TL et al 1983 Development and validation of a geriatric depression screening scale:

preliminary report. Journal of Psychiatric Research 17: 37–49.

- The Geriatric Depression Scale (www.stanford. edu/~yesavage/GDS.html) is the screening test with the most validation.
- There are a number of forms (4-, 5- and 15-item versions) with yes/no answer formats.
- The 15-item version includes questions on satisfaction with life, boredom, happiness, helplessness, etc. for the preceding 7 days.

Williams JW, Barrett J, Oxman T et al 2000 Treatment of dysthymia and minor depression in primary care: a randomized controlled trial in older adults. Journal of the American Medical Association 284: 1519–1526

- Paroxetine was associated with moderate benefits in older people with persistent minor depression and dysthymia.
- Problem-solving therapy was not effective in this group.

Baldwin RC, O'Brien J 2002 Vascular basis of late-onset depressive disorder. British Journal of Psychiatry 180: 157–160

- Described a syndrome of vascular depression with underlying ischaemic white matter changes.
- This has features of:
  - apathy
  - psychomotor retardation
  - poor executive function
  - lower rates of depressive thinking
  - late age of onset.

Cole MG, Bellavance F 1997 The prognosis of depression in old age. American Journal of Geriatric Psychiatry 5: 4–14

- 60% of patients in secondary care responded to treatment or had subsequent episodes which also responded to treatment.
- 20% of patients went on to have chronic symptoms.
- Patients who lived in the community had poorer outcomes.

Tuma TA 2000 Outcome of hospital-treated depression at 4.5 years. An elderly and a younger adult cohort compared. British Journal of Psychiatry 176: 224–228

- The high mortality of depression in older patients is largely due to physical illness.

Unutzer J, Katon W, Callachan C et al 2002 Collaborative care management of late-life depression in the primary care setting. Journal of the American Medical Association 288: 2836–2845

- A primary care study.
- 50% of patients expressed a preference for psychological treatment over medication when given a choice.
- Problem-solving treatment was associated with some benefits.

Pinquart M, Sorensen S 2001 How effective are psychotherapeutic and other psychosocial interventions with older adults? A meta-analysis. Journal of Mental Health and Aging 7: 207–243

- In adults with mild to moderate depression, psychological treatment and treatment with medication are equally effective.

Thompson LW, Coon DW, Gallagher-Thompson D et al 2001 Comparison of desipramine and cognitive/ behavioural therapy in the treatment of elderly outpatients with mild to moderate depression. American Journal of Geriatric Psychiatry 9: 225–240

- Cognitive behavioural therapy is efficacious in the treatment of depression in older adults.
- Antidepressant medication in combination with psychological treatment is more effective than treatment with either alone.
- Benefits are particularly noted in relapse prevention.

Tew JD, Mulsant BH, Haskett RF et al 1999 Acute efficacy of ECT in the treatment of major depression in the Old-Old. American Journal of Psychiatry 156: 1865–1870

- ECT is the most effective treatment for older people with severe depression.
- It is associated with recovery in four out of five patients.
- It is well tolerated.

McCusker J, Cole M, Keller E et al 1998 Effectiveness of treatments of depression in older ambulatory patients. Archives of General Medicine 158: 705–712

- Approximately one-third of patients do not respond to first-line antidepressant treatment.

See also the 'General topics' section in Chapter 2 (Affective disorders), pages 25, 30-31.

Older people with longstanding mental health illness: the graduates

Jolley D, Kosky N, Holloway F 2004 Older people with longstanding mental health illness: the graduates. Advances in Psychiatric Treatment 10: 27–36

Ageing and elderly adults with chronic psychiatric illness of long duration have specific needs. The care of these adults has moved from the old asylum hospitals to the community. The ongoing care of this population needs to be appropriately planned with consideration of the roles for general, rehabilitation and old age psychiatry.

Much of the available evidence relates to older long-stay inpatients resettled as community patients. There is less evidence for the 'new' generation of graduate patients although they may share many of the social and psychological problems.

There is a growing elderly population due to the rise in life expectancy in the developed world. The needs of this population are considered in the National Service Framework for Older People. The creation of a framework specifically for this population can be problematic. It can assume that the older population does not have any of the needs of the younger 'working age' population. It has also meant that illnesses such as stroke and dementia are raised in the framework for older people whilst not being exclusive to this age group.

Campbell P, Ananth H 2002 Graduates. In: Jacoby R, Oppenheimer C (eds) Psychiatry in the elderly, 3rd edn. Oxford Medical Publications, Oxford, pp 762–798

- Mental hospital graduates include people with:
  - chronic schizophrenia (50–70%)
  - unstable mood disorder (10–15%)
  - dementia, often of early onset (5–20%)
  - miscellaneous conditions, including personality disorder, alcohol dependence, brain damage and multiple pathology.
- Patients with chronic schizophrenia continued to have active delusional beliefs (36% compared with 60% on admission), hallucinations (40%, similar to the rate on admission) and negative symptoms (70% versus 60%).
- The graduates had had long contact with psychiatric services, little contact with their family or community, poor employment records, few marriages, marriages that failed and no home to speak of other than their hospital.
- The graduates had ongoing problems with impulsivity, risk of self-harm, risk of violence, lack of insight and the impact their behaviours might have on other people.
- The graduated often lacked initiative, had poor motivation and needed support in activities of daily living.
- The graduated were more likely to have problems with physical illness than the general population.

Trieman N, Wills W, Leff J 1996 TAPS Project 28. Does reprovision benefit elderly long-stay mental patients? Schizophrenia Research 21: 199–208

Team for the Assessment of Psychiatric Services (TAPS):
- 130 elderly long-stay patients were discharged from the Friern Barnet hospital.

- 71 patients were still alive 3 years later.
- Half of the remaining patients had returned to the hospital.
- The patients who continued to live in the community were functioning at a higher level than those in hospital.
- There were no differences in mortality rates for those remaining in hospital and those living in the community.
- One person living in the community committed suicide and one person was imprisoned.

Dayson D 1993 TAPS Project 12. Crime, vagrancy, death and readmission of the long-term mentally ill during their first year of local reprovision. British Journal of Psychiatry 162: 40–44

- Six of 278 patients discharged to community living were living on the streets within 12 months.

Anderson J, Dayson D, Wills W et al 1993 TAPS Project 13. Clinical and social outcomes of long stay psychiatric patients after one year in the community. British Journal of Psychiatry 162: 45–56

- Resettlement into the community was associated with:
  - being able to name more friends
  - improved social contacts
  - increased satisfaction with treatment and accommodation.

Royal College of Psychiatrists 2005 Caring for people who enter old age with enduring or relapsing mental illness ('graduates'). Council Report CR110. Royal College of Psychiatrists, London. Online. Available: www.rcpsych.ac.uk/files/pdfversion/cr110.pdf

- Agencies responsible for commissioning and providing mental health services for graduate populations should actively identify such groups of patients.
- Each individual should have their physical, mental and social needs reviewed and catered for.
- The Care Programme Approach can be used in the ongoing monitoring of the needs of these patients.

Preventing dementia

Purandare N, Ballard C, Burns A 2005 Preventing dementia. Advances in Psychiatric Treatment 11: 176–183

- Large epidemiological studies have shown that diabetes increases the risk of Alzheimer's and vascular dementia. It is not known if treatment of diabetes reduces the risk of dementia.

- There are associations between carotid atherosclerosis and dementia. There is no evidence regarding the treatment of atheromatous emboli and the effects on cognitive decline.
- It has been established that myocardial infarction and atrial fibrillation are risk factors for both Alzheimer's dementia and vascular dementia.
- Low folate and vitamin B12 measured by increased total homocysteine levels have been associated with dementia and cognitive impairment. It is not clear what impact homocysteine level reduction has on cognitive function.
- It is suggested that prevention strategies be targeted at those in middle life when some of the risk factors for dementia may already be having an impact. It is important then to identify target groups to make this economically viable.
- An alternative approach would be to target an older population with mild cognitive impairment. Studies tend to focus on primary outcomes of stroke and heart disease, not dementia and cognitive impairment.

Jorn AF, Korten AE, Henderson AS 1987 The prevalence of dementia: a quantitative integration of the literature. Acta Psychiatrica Scandinavica 76: 465–479

- The prevalence of dementia would fall by 50% if risk reduction strategies (Box 17.1) were successful in delaying its onset by 5 years.

Box 17.1

Strategies for the prevention of dementia

Treatment of vascular risk factors
- Hypertension
- Hypercholesterolaemia
- Diabetes
- Carotid atherosclerosis
- Heart disease
- Smoking

Neuroprotection
- Folate and vitamin B12
- Antioxidants (vitamins C and E, alcohol)
- Anti-inflammatory agents

Building up neuronal reserves
- Cognitive activity
- Physical activity
- Social and leisure activity

Launer LJ, Ross GW, Petrovitch H et al 2000 Midlife blood pressure and dementia: the Honolulu–Asia aging study. Neurobiology of Aging 21: 49–55

- An ageing study of 3500 Japanese–American men aged over 25.
- Untreated hypertension increases the risk of dementia four- to five-fold.

Murray MD, Lane KA, Gao S et al 2002 Preservation of cognitive function with antihypertensive medications: a longitudinal analysis of a community-based sample of African Americans. Archives of Internal Medicine 162: 2090–2096

- Treatment of hypertension was associated with a 38% reduction in Alzheimer's and vascular dementia.

Forette F, Seux ML, Staessen JA et al 2003 The prevention of dementia with antihypertensive treatment: new evidence from the Systolic Hypertension in Europe (Syst-Eur) study. Archives of Internal Medicine 162: 2046–2052

- Use of a calcium channel blocker reduced the risk of Alzheimer's disease by half over a 2- year period.

Tzourio C, Anderson C, Chapman N et al (PROGRESS Collaborative Group) 2003 Effects of blood pressure lowering with perindopril and indapamide therapy on dementia and cognitive decline in patients with cerebrovascular disease (PROGRESS trial). Archives of Internal Medicine 163: 1069–1075

- There was a significant reduction in incidence of dementia in stroke patients treated with an angiotensin-converting enzyme (ACE).
- It is not clear if improvements in cognitive function result from the reduction of blood pressure or from another neuroprotective effect.

Moroney JT, Tang MX, Berglund L et al 1999 Low density lipoprotein cholesterol and the risk of dementia with stroke. Journal of the American Medical Association 282: 254–260

- A 2-year follow-up study of 2000 older people in New York.
- Those with the highest levels of cholesterol were at increased risk of dementia, in particular vascular dementia.

Kivipelto M, Helkala EL, Laakso MP et al 2002 Apolipoprotein E epsilon4 allele, elevated midlife total cholesterol level, and high midlife systolic blood pressure are independent risk factors for late-life Alzheimer disease. Annals of Internal Medicine 137: 149–155

- A 21-year follow-up study.
- Raised cholesterol (≥ 6.5 mmol/l) in middle age was independently associated with double the risk of dementia. This included Alzheimer's dementia.

Etminan M, Gill S, Samii A 2003 The role of lipid-lowering drugs in cognitive function: a meta-analysis of observational studies. Pharmacotherapy 23: 726–730

- A meta-analysis
- Statins were associated with a significant reduction in risk of cognitive impairment. Other lipid lowering agents were not.

Ott A, Slooter AJC, Hofman A et al 1998 Smoking and the risk of dementia and Alzheimer's disease in a population-based cohort study: the Rotterdam study. Lancet 351: 1840–1843

- Smoking is a risk factor for Alzheimer's disease.
- Those currently smoking have double the incidence of dementia and Alzheimer's disease.

Nordberg A, Hellstrom-Lindahl E, Lee M et al 2002 Chronic nicotine treatment reduces beta-amyloidosis in the brain of a mouse model of Alzheimer's disease (APPsw). Journal of Neurochemistry 81: 655–658

- Previous studies suggested that smoking is thought to double the risk of Alzheimer's disease.
- This study suggested that smoking may have neuroprotective effects.
- The mechanism of action may be via reduction in amyloid burden.

Sano M, Ernesto C, Thomas RG et al 1997 A controlled trial of selegiline, alpha-tocopherol, or both as treatment for Alzheimer's disease. The Alzheimer's Cooperative Study. New England Journal of Medicine 336: 1216–1222

- In this RCT people with moderate to severe Alzheimer's disease (n = 341) were randomised to receive selegiline and/or vitamin E or placebo.
- All active treatments had a beneficial effect in reducing disease progression over a 2-year period.
- Outcomes measured were time to death, time to institutionalisation, performance of daily living skills and vascular dementia.

Ruitenberg A, van Sweiten JC, Witteman JC et al 2002 Alcohol consumption and risk of dementia: The Rotterdam study. Lancet 359: 281–286

- This large study (n = > 5000) of 6 years' duration found that moderate alcohol consumption (1–3 drinks per day) reduced the risk of dementia (Alzheimer's disease and vascular dementia).

In't Veld BA, Ruitenberg A, Hofman A et al 2001 Non-steroidal anti-inflammatory drugs and the risk of Alzheimer's disease. New England Journal of Medicine 345: 1515–1521

- This study suggested that the conflicting evidence regarding the impact of NSAIDs on risk of Alzheimer's disease may be due to inaccurate and retrospective recording of data.
- Following review of computerised pharmacy records (n = 7000) from a 7-year period, it was found that NSAIDs are associated with a reduced risk of Alzheimer's disease.
- Duration of NSAID use is important.

Wilson RS, Mendes De Leon CF, Barnes LL et al 2002 Participation in cognitively stimulating activities and risk of incident Alzheimer disease. Journal of the American Medical Association 287: 742–748

- There are no randomised trials of the impact of cognitive activity on the risk of dementia.
- This study records the frequency of seven common activities of 801 older members of the clergy over a 4-year period.
- Activities included reading, watching television and doing crosswords.
- After controlling for age, education and gender it was found that an increase in cognitive activity by one point was associated with a 33% reduction in the risk of Alzheimer's disease.
- Physical activity was also associated with a risk reduction but this was thought to be via cognitively stimulating activities rather than physical activity alone.

Wang H-X, Karp A, Winblad B et al 2002 Late-life engagement in social and leisure activities is associated with a decreased risk of dementia: a longitudinal study from the Kungsholmen project. American Journal of Epidemiology 155: 1081–1087

- Participation in stimulating mental, social or productive activities reduced the risk of developing dementia by half over a 6-year period.

Burns A, Zaudig M 2002 Mild cognitive impairment in older people. Lancet 360: 1963–1965

- Mild cognitive impairment has a community prevalence of 17–34%.
- There is an annual conversion to dementia in 10–15%.

Treatment of psychosis

Karim S, Byrne EJ 2005 Treatment of psychosis in elderly people. Advances in Psychiatric Treatment 11: 286–296

Psychotic symptoms in the elderly may arise from a wide range of conditions, including delirium, drug-induced psychosis, schizophrenia and related disorders, affective disorder and neurodegenerative conditions. Antipsychotic medication has traditionally been used and there is an established evidence base for their general use. The evidence regarding neuroleptic medication in the elderly population specifically is sparse. There have been recent concerns regarding the safety of antipsychotic medication in dementia.

Targum SD, Abbott JL 1999 Psychosis in the elderly: a spectrum of disorders. Journal of Clinical Psychiatry 60 (Suppl 8): 4–10

- The prevalence of psychotic symptoms in the elderly population is estimated at between 0.2 and 4.7%.

Zayas EM, Grossberg GT 1998 The treatment of psychosis in late life. Journal of Clinical Psychiatry 59 (Suppl 1): 5–12

- Symptoms of psychosis in nursing homes are higher and range from 10 to 63%.

Östling S, Skoog I 2002 Psychotic symptoms and paranoid ideation in a non-demented population-based sample of the very old. Archives of General Psychiatry 59: 53–59

- A 3-year follow-up study of psychotic symptoms in a population-based sample of people over 85 years without dementia.
- Between 7.1 and 13.7% experienced psychotic symptoms.
- Hallucinations and paranoid ideations were associated with an increased risk of dementia and death in the subsequent 3 years.

Jeste DV 2004 Tardive dyskinesia rates with atypical antipsychotics in older adults. Journal of Clinical Psychiatry 65 (Suppl 9): 21–24

- Tardive dyskinesia can be the cause of a number of physical and psychological complications.
- These include:
  - problems with eating
  - problems with swallowing
  - loss of weight
  - falls
  - problems with balance
  - depression.

- Atypical medication is associated with lower rates of tardive dyskinesia than for typical antipsychotic medication.

Kane JM 1999 Prospective study of tardive dyskinesia in the elderly. In: Syllabus and Proceedings of the 1999 American Psychiatric Association Annual Meeting (Abstract NO32C: 79). APA, Washington, DC

- Typical antipsychotic medication is associated with a five to six times greater increase in risk of tardive dyskinesia in older people.

Holmes C, Fortenza O, Powell J et al 1997 Do neuroleptic drugs hasten cognitive decline in dementia? Carriers of apolipoprotein E epsilon 4 allele seem particularly susceptible to their effects. British Medical Journal 10: 1411

- Antipsychotics can increase the rate of cognitive decline.

Duff G 2004 Atypical antipsychotic drugs and stroke: message from Professor Gordon Duff, Chairman, Committee on Safety of Medicines (CEM/CMO/2004/1). Online. Available: www.mhra.gov.uk

- Risperidone and olanzapine are associated with twice the risk of stroke in people treated for BPSD.
- The Committee on Safety of Medicines concluded that these two drugs should not be used in dementia.

Herrmann N, Mamdani M, Lanctot KL 2004 Atypical antipsychotics and risk of cerebrovascular accidents. American Journal of Psychiatry 161: 1113–1115

- Found no difference between risperidone, olanzapine and typical antipsychotic medications in the treatment of dementia.

Royal College of Psychiatrists, Royal College of General Practitioners, British Geriatrics Society et al 2004 Guidance for the management of behavioural and psychiatric symptoms in dementia and the treatment of psychosis in people with a history of stroke/TIA following CSM restriction on risperidone and olanzapine. Faculty of the Psychiatry of Old Age, Royal College of Psychiatrists, London. Online. Available: www.rcpsych.ac.uk

- Concluded that there was a small but significant risk of cerebrovascular adverse events in elderly people treated with risperidone and olanzapine.
- The risks were more marked in those over the age of 80 years.
- The group advised that the prescription of these medications requires adequate consideration and that their use may still be considered necessary when other treatments are not suitable or have potentially harmful effects of their own.

- The decision to withdraw or continue medication requires adequate consideration of the patient's past history and the risks of recurrence.
- The rationale for treatment should be clearly documented and the general practitioner should be involved in discussions.

Cohen CI, Cohen GD, Blank K et al 2000 Schizophrenia and older adults: an overview. Directions for research and policy. American Journal of Geriatric Psychiatry 8: 19–28

- The prevalence of schizophrenia (onset at any age) in adults aged over 65 years is approximately 1%.

Jeste DV, Twamley EW 2003 Understanding and managing psychosis in late life. Psychiatric Times XX (3)

- One in four patients with schizophrenia aged over 65 years will have a late onset illness.

Barak Y, Wittenberg N, Naor S et al 1999 Clozapine in elderly psychiatric patients: tolerability, safety and efficacy. Comprehensive Psychiatry 40: 320–325

- A review of the few small studies of clozapine in the elderly population.
- Sedation, lethargy and postural hypotension are commonly occurring adverse effects.
- Treatment of psychotic illness with clozapine was associated with moderate/marked improvements in symptoms.
- The mean dose of medication was relatively low (134 mg/day).
- Agranulocytosis may be more common in the older age group.

Katz IR, Jeste DV, Mintzer JE et al 1999 Comparison of risperidone and placebo for psychosis and behavioural disturbances associated with dementia: a randomized, double blind trial. Risperidone Study Group. Journal of Clinical Psychiatry 60: 107–115

- Treatment with risperidone is associated with significant improvements in clinical symptoms.
- Low doses of risperidone (1.5–6 mg) were tolerated well.

Madhusoodanan S, Suresh P, Brenner R 1999 Experience with the atypical anti-psychotics risperidone and olanzapine in the elderly. Annals of Clinical Psychiatry 11: 113–118

- A study of 151 hospital inpatients with a mean age of 71 years.
- Patients received either risperidone or olanzapine.
- Both treatments led to significant improvements in symptoms of schizophrenia.

- 17% of patients receiving olanzapine reported adverse effects.

Zayas EM, Grossberg GT 2002 Treatment of late-onset psychotic disorders. In: Copeland JRM, Abou-Saleh MT, Blazer D (eds) Principles and practice of general psychiatry, 2nd edn. Wiley, Chichester, pp 511–525

- A literature review.
- Concluded that quetiapine is safe when used in the elderly population.
- There is no associated weight gain.
- Slow titration from a low starting dose can reduce initial adverse effects of postural hypotension, dizziness and agitation.

Madhusoodanan S, Brenner R, Gupta S et al 2004 Clinical experience with aripiprazole treatment in ten elderly patients with schizophrenia or schizoaffective disorder: retrospective case studies. CNS Spectrum 9: 862–867

- 10 patients were treated with aripiprazole.
- Aripiprazole was found to be safe, with improvements in positive and negative symptoms.

Jeste DV, Finkel SI 2000 Psychosis of Alzheimer's disease and related dementias. Diagnostic criteria for a distinct syndrome. American Journal of Geriatric Psychiatry 8: 29–34

- Concluded that between 30 and 50% of people with Alzheimer's disease have psychotic symptoms.

Bassiony MM, Steinberg MS, Warren A et al 2000 Delusions and hallucinations in Alzheimer's disease: prevalence and clinical correlates. International Journal of Geriatric Psychiatry 15: 99–107

- A community study of Alzheimer's disease.
- One in three patients had symptoms of psychotic illness, with delusions occurring more often than hallucinations.

Katz IR, Jeste DV, Mintzer JE et al 1999 Comparison of risperidone and placebo for psychosis and behavioural disturbances associated with dementia: a randomized, double blind trial. Risperidone Study Group. Journal of Clinical Psychiatry 60: 107–115

- A randomised double-blind trial of risperidone versus placebo in patients resident in nursing homes.
- Risperidone was found to be more effective than placebo.
- The recommended dose of risperidone was 1 mg per day.

Street JS, Clark WS, Gannon KS et al 2000 Olanzapine treatment of psychotic and behavioural symptoms in patients with Alzheimer disease in nursing care facilities:

a double-blind, randomized, placebo-controlled trial. The HGEU Study Group. Archives of General Psychiatry 57: 968–976

- A double-blind, placebo-controlled comparison of olanzapine and placebo.
- Treatment with olanzapine was associated with a significant reduction in psychotic symptoms when a dose of 5 mg was used.

McKeith IG, Del Ser T, Spano P et al 2000 Efficacy of rivastigmine in dementia with Lewy bodies: a randomized, double-blind, placebo-controlled international study. Lancet 356: 2031–2036

- A large multicentre double blind trial comparing rivastigmine with placebo in patients with Lewy body dementia.
- Treatment with rivastigmine was associated with significant reductions in delusions and hallucinations.

Hoeh N, Gyalai L, Weistraub D et al 2003 Pharmacological management of psychosis in the elderly. A critical review. Journal of Geriatric Psychiatry and Neurology 16: 213–218

- Clozapine is effective in reducing symptoms of psychosis in Parkinson's disease.
- A low dose is required to reduce symptoms with minimal adverse effects.
- The optimal dose is between 6.25 and 50 mg per day.

See also the 'General topics' section in Chapter 26 (Schizophrenia), page 367.

The value of cranial CT in old age psychiatry

Fielding S 2005 The value of cranial computed tomography in old age psychiatry: a review of the results of 178 consecutive scans. Psychiatric Bulletin 29: 21–23

Effective evaluation and early diagnosis may allow prevention of dementia and clarify if cholinesterase inhibitors or antiplatelet medications are required.

Aims

To assess the value of computed tomography (CT) in patients presenting to old age psychiatry services over a 2-year period.

Method

- A retrospective review of consecutive CT referrals.

Results

- 178 patients were included.

- 10 patients with dementia of potentially reversible cause (PRC) were correctly identified.
- Prevalence of infarcts was 11.9%.
- Prevalence of small vessel disease was 32.8%.
- The prevalence of PRCs of dementia was low at 2.3%.
- The apparent decrease in dementia with PRC may be due to a lower threshold in requesting cranial CT.
- No patient had a fully reversible cause for cognitive impairment identified by CT.
- There was a high prevalence of evidence of small and large vessel cerebrovascular disease in the study population.
- A real benefit of scanning may be to raise the discovery rates of vascular dementia.

Jobst KA, Barnetson LPD, Shepstone BJ (on behalf of the Oxford project to investigate memory and aging) 1998 Accurate prediction of histologically confirmed Alzheimer's disease and the differential diagnosis of dementia: the use of the NINCDS-ADRDA and DSM-III-R criteria, SPECT, X-Ray CT, and Apo E4 in medial temporal lobe dementias. International Psychogeriatrics 10: 271–310

- Evidence that SPECT scanning is useful in determining the subtype of dementia.

The Royal College of Psychiatrists 1995 Consensus statement on the assessment of an elderly person with suspected cognitive impairment by a Specialist Old Age Psychiatry Service (Council Report CR49). Royal College of Psychiatrists, London

- All patients should be scanned unless the history is typical or the history is greater than 1 year in duration.

Cummings JL 2000 Neuroimaging in the dementia assessment: is it necessary? Journal of the American Geriatrics Society 48: 1345–1346

- Suggests that everyone with dementia requires a scan.

Branton T 1999 Use of computerized tomography by old age psychiatrists: an examination of criteria for investigation of cognitive impairment. International Journal of Geriatric Medicine 14: 567–571

- The prevalence of PRCs was 7.8%.

What exactly do we mean by 'mild cognitive impairment'?

Coen R 2005 What exactly do we mean by 'mild cognitive impairment'? Old Age Psychiatrist 37: 10–11

Mild cognitive impairment (MCI) is a term used to describe objective cognitive impairment that does not fulfil diagnostic criteria for dementia. The impairments are not limited to memory.

It can be difficult to separate cognitive decline due to normal ageing from the mild cognitive impairment that represents the early stages of a pathological dementia process.

The International Working Group on Mild Cognitive Impairment recommends emphasis on impaired cognition rather than just memory impairment.

There are clinical and research interests in this field. The identification of patients with MCI can be a challenge. It requires a clinical judgement that the patient is suffering from MCI as opposed to the very early stages of dementia.

Criteria to consider in the diagnosis of MCI are:
* subjective memory complaints (preferably corroborated by an informant)
* objective memory impairment
* memory deficits out of proportion to normal changes in cognitive functioning should be essentially intact
* informant history may be required regarding activities of daily living
* the patient does not meet the criteria for dementia.

Who cares wins: old age psychiatry in general hospitals

Royal College of Psychiatrists 2005 Who cares wins. Report of a working group for the Faculty of Old Age Psychiatry. Royal College of Psychiatrists, London

A Royal College report which draws attention to the care of older people with mental disorder in general hospitals. This is felt to be an area of clinical practice and service provision that has been neglected. It suggests that specialist liaison mental health services for the elderly are developed. The liaison service for working-age adults is a relatively well-developed specialty and failure to deliver a similar service for older adults may represent an ageist policy.
* Older people occupy two-thirds of NHS beds at any given time.
* 60% of older people admitted to a general hospital have or will develop a mental disorder during their admission.
* Three disorders account for 80% of these cases:
  – depression
  – dementia
  – delirium.
* These three disorders are more common in the general hospital setting than in the wider community.

Having a mental disorder is associated with worse outcomes for an individual. Individuals with mental disorder who are admitted to hospital with a hip fracture have longer admission lengths and reduced survival. There are associated cost implications.

Intervention can improve outcome by reducing the length of inpatient stay and utilising appropriate resources. Interventions to improve outcomes should include:
* training and education of general staff about the issues relevant to mental health
* care plans with integrated information about mental state
* identification of patients at high risk of developing psychiatric disorders
* appropriate treatment.

Service models vary. The liaison model may be preferable to the more traditional consultation model of psychiatric care in general medical and surgical wards. It is likely that the general care team could manage simple mental health problems but a specialist mental health service would respond quickly to more difficult cases. There may be some advantages to being based on the general hospital site. A multidisciplinary team could be the single point of access. Nursing liaison with consultant supervision could be considered.

See also the 'General topics' section in Chapter 15 (Liaison psychiatry), page 237.

Policy and Legislation

The National Service Framework for Older People

Department of Health 2001 The National Service Framework for Older People. DH, London

This Department of Health publication describes the 10-year action plan for the promotion of good health and the development of services for older adults. It recognises that older people are major users of health and social care services but do not always have their needs adequately addressed.

The focus for improving services will be achieved by working toward eight specific standards in different domains of health and social care. The standards will be set by the National Institute for Clinical Excellence (NICE) and National Service Frameworks. Progress will be monitored by the Commission for Health Improvement and a programme of patient and service user surveys.

Standard One: Rooting out age discrimination
* Aim: to ensure that older people are never discriminated against in accessing NHS or social care services as a result of their age.
* Standard: NHS services will be provided on the basis of clinical need alone, regardless of age. Social care

services will not use age to restrict access to available services.

Standard Two: Person-centred care

- Aim: to ensure that older people are treated as individuals and that they receive appropriate and timely care which meets their needs, regardless of health or social service boundaries.
- Standard: NHS and social care services treat older people as individuals and enable them to make choices about their own care. This will be achieved through the single assessment process and integrated provision of services.

Standard Three: Intermediate care

- Aim: to provide integrated services to promote faster recovery from illness, prevent unnecessary hospital admissions, support timely discharge and maximise independent living.
- Standard: older people will have access to a range of intermediate care services at home or designated care settings. This will prevent unnecessary hospital admission, prevent premature or unnecessary inception into long-term care and enable early discharge from hospital.

Standard Four: General hospital care

- Aim: to ensure that older people receive the specialist help they need and gain maximum benefit from having been in hospital.
- Standard: older people's care in hospital to be delivered by staff who have the right set of skills to meet their needs.

Standard Five: Stroke

- Aim: to reduce the incidence of stroke in the population and to ensure that those who have had a stroke have prompt access to integrated stroke care services.
- Standard: the NHS will work with other agencies where appropriate to prevent strokes. People who are thought to have had a stroke will have access to diagnostic services, will be treated by a specialist stroke service and participate in a multidisciplinary programme of secondary prevention and rehabilitation.

Stroke is the single biggest cause of severe disability and the third most common cause of death in the UK.

Standard Six: Falls

- Aim: to reduce the number of falls which result in serious injury and to ensure effective treatment and rehabilitation for those who have fallen.
- Standard: the NHS will work in partnership with councils to prevent falls and reduce injuries in the elderly. Older people who have fallen will receive effective treatment and, along with their carers, advice on prevention through a specialist falls service.

Falls are a major cause of disability and the leading cause of mortality due to injury in people aged over 75 years in the UK. Up to 14,000 people a year die in the UK as a result of an osteoporotic hip fracture. A fall can precipitate admission into long-term care and the fear of falling has an impact on confidence for daily activities.

Standard Seven: Mental health in older people

- Aim: to promote good mental health and to treat and support those with depression and dementia.
- Standard: older people with mental health problems will have access to mental health services to ensure effective diagnosis, treatment and support for them and their carers.

Mental health problems among the elderly exact a large social and economic toll on the individual, their families, carers and the statutory agencies. Underdetection of mental illness in the elderly is widespread, partly because many older adults live alone. Depression in the elderly is especially underdiagnosed, particularly amongst care home residents. Mental health services for older people should be community orientated and provide seamless care.

Standard Eight: The promotion of health and active life in older age

- Aim: to extend the healthy life expectancy of older people.
- Standard: promote the health of older people by action from the NHS with support of councils.

The NHS Plan commits an extra £1.4 billion for older people to be provided annually by 2004. It also provides for increases in staffing, including an extra 85 old age psychiatrists. From April 2002 the National Care Standards Commission will register and inspect all private and voluntary care homes. *See also the 'Policy and legislation' section in Chapter 22 (Policy and legislation), page 329.*

Treatment – Psychopharmacology

Antidepressants versus placebo for the depressed elderly

Wilson K, Mottram P, Sivanranthan A, Nightingale A 2001 Antidepressants versus placebo for the depressed elderly **(Cochrane Review)**. In: The Cochrane Library, Issue 1. CD000561. Update Software, Oxford

- 17 trials were included where 245 patients were treated with TCAs, 365 patients with SSRIs and 58 patients with MAOIs.
- Using a fixed effects model, odds ratios of 0.32 for TCAs, 0.51 for SSRIs and 0.17 for MAOIs were calculated.
- They were all effective in both institutionalised and community patients, including those likely to have severe physical illness.

See also the 'Treatment – Psychopharmacology' section in Chapter 2 (Affective disorders), page 31.

Do neuroleptic drugs hasten cognitive decline in dementia?

McShane R, Keene J, Gedling K et al 1997 Do neuroleptic drugs hasten cognitive decline in dementia? Prospective study with necropsy follow up. British Medical Journal 314: 266–271

Method

- A 2-year prospective, longitudinal study.
- Patients were interviewed every 4 months.
- Necropsy was performed.

Results

- 71 adults with dementia were included and 42 later underwent postmortem examination.
- All subjects lived at home, initially with an informant.
- Information was collected regarding cognitive function, behavioural problems and postmortem examination.
- Treatment with neuroleptic medication was mainly with thioridazine, promazine, haloperidol and chlorpromazine.
- The mean MMSE score at inception was 15.5 with a mean duration of dementia at that time of 5.7 years.
- Treatment with neuroleptic medication was associated with a two-fold increase in decline on cognitive score.
- Increase in decline on cognitive score was associated in turn with aggression, disturbed diurnal rhythm and the presence of persecutory ideation.
- Treatment with neuroleptic medication and the severity of persecutory ideation were the only variables independently associated with an increased rate in cognitive decline.
- Initiation of neuroleptic medication coincided with the onset of a more rapid decline.
- Prior to neuroleptic treatment the median rate of cognitive decline was 5 points per year.
- After commencing neuroleptic medication the rate of cognitive decline was 11 points per year.

- Seven of the 42 patients who underwent necropsy had Lewy body pathology.
- The presence of Lewy body pathology at necropsy was not associated with neuroleptic use and faster cognitive decline.

Pharmaceutical interventions for emotionalism

House HO, Hackett ML, Anderson CS et al 2006 Pharmaceutical interventions for emotionalism after stroke **(Cochrane Review)**. In: The Cochrane Library, Issue 1. Update Software, Oxford

- Five trials ($n = 103$) comparing psychotropic medication with placebo in patients with post-stroke emotionalism were included.
- Four trials showed that psychotropic medication was associated with beneficial effects:
  - a decrease in emotionalism by 50%
  - a decrease in frequency of compulsive laughter
  - a decrease in pathological laughing and crying.
- Confidence intervals were wide.
- One study found that psychotropic medication was associated with a worse outcome in people treated for post-stroke emotionalism.
- Treatment with psychotropic medication was associated with a greater dropout rate.
- The trials did not find in favour of any specific drug or class of drug.

Therapies for depression in Parkinson's disease

Shabnam Ghazi-Noori S, Chung TH, Deane KHO et al 2003 Therapies for depression in Parkinson's disease **(Cochrane Review)**. In: The Cochrane Library, Issue 2. CD003465. Update Software, Oxford

- No eligible trials of ECT or behavioural therapy were found.
- Insufficient data were available on the effectiveness and safety of any antidepressants in Parkinson's disease.
- One crossover trial of nortriptyline versus placebo showed a greater improvement in the treatment group but it was not statistically significant.
- Another RCT of citalopram versus placebo did not show any statistical significance after 52 weeks with the Hamilton Depression Scale.
- A third randomised controlled trial of fluvoxamine versus amitriptyline showed similar numbers with a

50% reduction in Hamilton score, but the complete trial data were not available.

• Visual hallucinations and confusion were reported in patients with fluvoxamine and amitriptyline.

See also the 'Treatment – Psychopharmacology' section in Chapter 2 (Affective disorders), page 31.

Treatment – Psychological Therapies

Non-pharmacological interventions in dementia

Douglas S, James I, Ballard C 2004 Non-pharmacological interventions in dementia. Advances in Psychiatric Treatment 10: 171–179

It is the preferred choice that non-pharmacological interventions are used before treatment with medication is initiated. This is not always the case. Cognitive approaches have been the main focus. It is increasingly understood that a number of non-cognitive symptoms are problematic for patients and carers. These are termed challenging behaviours or the 'behavioural and psychiatric symptoms of dementia' (BPSD) and include agitation, aggression, mood disorders and psychosis. Others are sexual disinhibition, eating problems and abnormal vocalisations. A number of therapies are discussed.

Schultz R, Williamson GH 1991 A 2-year longitudinal study of depression among Alzheimer's caregivers. Psychology and Aging 6: 569–578

• BPSD are often the reason for institutionalisation.
• These symptoms increase the burden on carers and therefore carers' levels of stress.

Margallo-Lana M, Swann A, O'Brien J et al 2001 Prevalence and pharmacological management of behavioural and psychological symptoms amongst dementia sufferers living in care environments. International Journal of Geriatric Psychiatry 16: 39–44

• Estimated that 40% of people with dementia cared for in residential and nursing homes receive neuroleptic medication.
• This is of concern when the considerable side effect profiles are considered.

Ballard CG, O'Brien J, James I et al 2001 Dementia: management of behavioural and psychological symptoms. Oxford University Press, Oxford

• Concluded that neuroleptic medication is associated with lower levels of well-being and poorer quality of life.

McShane R, Keene J, Gedling K et al 1997 Do neuroleptic drugs hasten cognitive decline in dementia? Prospective study with necropsy follow-up. British Medical Journal 314: 211–212

• Neuroleptic medication may accelerate cognitive decline in patients with dementia.

Cohen-Mansfield J 2000 Use of patient characteristics to determine non-pharmacological interventions for behavioural and psychological symptoms of dementia. International Psychogeriatrics 12(1): 373–380

• Produced an 'unmet needs model for agitation'.
• There are three main functions of behaviours:
    – to obtain or meet a need (e.g. pacing for stimulation)
    – to communicate a need (e.g. repetitively asking a question)
    – the result of an unmet need (e.g. aggression triggered by pain or discomfort).

Psychotherapies with older people

Hepple J 2004 Psychotherapies with older people: an overview. Advances in Psychiatric Treatment 10: 371–377

Psychological therapies traditionally have not been a priority in old age psychiatry. This may be due in part to prejudice regarding the older population and a lack of development of expertise in the area. Negative stereotypes about the treatability of older people may have a negative effect on the expectations of clinicians regarding the effectiveness of treatment in this age group.

Psychotherapy theories have tended to focus on early life and child development with the exception of Erikson and his theory of the 'eight ages of man'. He described dichotomies to explore developmental changes up to late life when the final stage – 'ego integrity versus despair' – may be reached.

The biological model has dominated in old age psychiatry with less of a focus on psychological explanations for illness and distress in the elderly. Many professionals feel that psychological therapies are not being well delivered to older people. This, coupled with low expectation of a successful outcome, is reflected in a disproportionately low referral rate.

Cognitive behavioural therapy

This therapy focuses on negative thoughts with their reinforcing behaviours and challenges dysfunctional cycles by identifying unhelpful thinking. A graded exposure model is used to address avoidant behaviours. In older adults the emphasis may need to be on maintaining focus on the work, exploring feelings of guilt and helplessness at the onset of life events and awareness of the interaction with physical disease.

Wilkinson P 2002 Cognitive behaviour therapy. In: Hepple JN, Pearce J, Wilkinson PW (eds) Psychological therapies with older people. Developing treatments for effective practice. Brunner-Routledge, Hove

- Cognitive behavioural therapy (CBT) has been shown to be efficacious in the treatment of depression, anxiety disorders and problem behaviours in dementia.

Teri L, Curtis J, Gallagher-Thompson D et al 1994 Cognitive/ behaviour therapy with depressed older adults. In: Schneider LS, Reynolds CF, Lebowitz B et al (eds) Diagnosis and treatment of depression in the elderly. Proceedings of the NIH Consensus Development Conference. American Psychiatric Press, Washington, DC

- Reported a series of studies by Gallagher and Thompson with older people in the US.
- CBT was effective in the depressed elderly, in both hospital and community settings.
- This was true when CBT was given as group or individual therapy.

Barraclough C, King P, Colville J et al 2001 A randomised controlled trial of effectiveness of cognitive behavioural therapy and supportive counselling for anxiety symptoms in older adults. Journal of Consulting and Clinical Psychology 69: 756–762

- Compared CBT and supportive counselling for anxiety symptoms.
- CBT is more effective than supportive counselling in the treatment of anxiety disorders.

Cognitive analytical therapy

CAT provides a brief, structured and collaborative therapy. It connects current experiences with past trauma using dialogue and meaning. The evidence base is yet to be established. In later life, coping skills are challenged by changes in social role, disability and loss events. This can lead to resurfacing of pre-existing traumas that could give rise to depression, anxiety and self-destructive behaviours. CAT acts to link past and present with an emphasis on the need to find meaning.

Psychodynamic therapy

This aims to develop insight into repressed material from earlier life and to address relevant issues within the therapeutic relationship. Therapists may be reluctant to acknowledge the infantile needs of the elderly person if there is a subconscious fear of it reflecting their own potential dependence and helplessness in old age. The psychodynamic model may be useful for working with material derived from the patient's struggles to adjust to old age. This can include feelings of abandonment, despair, isolation and loss of creativity.

Psychotherapies are not usually considered for patients with dementia because of the presence of memory impairment.

Thompson L, Gallagher D, Breckenridge JS 1987 Comparative effectiveness of psychotherapies for depressed elders. Journal of Consultant and Clinical Psychology 55: 385–390

- Psychodynamic therapy in older people with depression was as effective as treatment with CBT.

Interpersonal therapy

IPT is a practical, focused, brief therapy that requires basic training but is used by a variety of professionals.

The therapy focuses on disturbances in current relationships and aims to improve communication to renegotiate role relationships, thus reducing symptoms and improving function.

Reynolds CF, Frank E, Peral JM 1999 Nortriptyline and interpersonal psychotherapy on maintenance therapies for recurrent major depression: a randomised controlled trial in patients older than 59 years. Journal of the American Medical Association 281: 39–44

- IPT was associated with improvements in the acute phase of treatment for acute depression in older adults.
- It is also effective for relapse prevention.

Systemic therapy

There is minimal evidence regarding the use of systemic or family therapy approaches in the elderly population.

Qualls SH 2000 Therapy with ageing families: rationale, opportunities and challenges. Ageing and Mental Health 4: 191–199

- Found that a systematic approach can be helpful to communicate and come to terms with a diagnosis of dementia.
- It can be beneficial in reducing symptoms of somatisation.

Thornton S, Brotchie J 1987 Reminiscence: a critical review of the literature. British Journal of Clinical Psychology 26: 93–111

- Reminiscence therapy can be used to improve communication and enhance self-esteem.

- There is the risk that a group reminiscence therapy approach will assume that all individuals in an age bracket will share the same life experiences.

Reality orientation

Reality orientation attempts to correct a person's misinterpretation of their environment by reorientation.

Sutton L 2004 Cultures of care in severe depression and dementia. In: Hepple JN, Pearce J, Wilkinson PW (eds) Psychological therapies with older people. Developing treatments for effective practice. Brunner-Routledge, Hove

- Concluded that reality orientation acts as a constant and repeated reminder of the decline in cognitive function in the care setting.

Validation therapy

This therapy explores interpersonal interaction with attempts by the carer to validate and share its content.

Feil N 1982 Validation. The Feil Method. Edward Feil Productions, Cleveland, OH

- Validation therapy can be cathartic and allow patients with dementia to reconnect to their environment.
- A highly active therapist is required.
- The method of development of a psychological therapies network for older people is described, as are suggested therapies for specific disorders.

See also the 'Treatment – Psychological therapies' section in Chapter 25 (Psychological therapies), page 349.

Treatment – Others

Aromatherapy in dementia

Holmes C, Ballard C 2004 Aromatherapy in dementia. Advances in Psychiatric Treatment 10: 296–300

Aromatherapy uses pure essential oils obtained from plants. Highly fragrant oils are produced by distillation.

There has been recent interest in the use of lavender and lemon balm essential oils in people with dementia with regard to potential calming and cognitive enhancing effects.

Psychological responses to odour are possible and depend on a person's perception of whether the scent is pleasant or not. High concentrations may be perceived as unpleasant whereas lower concentrations of the same smell are described as pleasant. Scents are linked with emotional responses, partly because of the afferent links from the olfactory bulb to the amygdala. The pharmacological mechanism of action is not thought to be because of a perceived odour; it is thought that compounds within the essential oils can enter the body and have a direct effect on the brain. There are methodological difficulties in the creation of a double-blind trial.

Vance D 1999 Considering olfactory stimulation for adults with age-related dementia. Perceptual and Motor Skills 88: 398–400

- Concluded that people with dementia are anosmic due to early loss of olfactory neurones.

Henry J, Rusius CW, Davies M et al 1994 Lavender for night sedation of people with dementia. International Journal of Aromatherapy 5(2): 28–30

- A crossover study of nine patients.
- Lavender oil was associated with an increased duration of sleep.

Brooker DJR, Snale M, Johnson E et al 1997 Single case evaluation of the effects of aromatherapy and massage on disturbed behaviour in severe dementia. British Journal of Clinical Psychology 36: 287–296

- Single case study design of four patients with senile dementia.
- Patients received treatment with ambient lavender, massage with lavender oil, massage without oil and no treatment.
- Massage with lavender oil is associated with improvements in behaviour in the hour after treatment.

Holmes C, Hopkins V, Hensford C et al 2001 Lavender oil as a treatment for agitated behaviour in severe dementia. International Journal of Psychogeriatric Psychiatry 17: 305–308

- A small, placebo-controlled trial.
- Masked observer ratings of 15 patients with severe dementia during lavender stream aromatherapy and placebo were made.
- 60% of patients showed improvements during the aromatherapy treatment.
- One person became more agitated during treatment.

Ballard CG, O'Brien JT, Reichelt K et al 2002 Aromatherapy as a safe and effective treatment for the management of agitation in severe dementia: the results of a double blind placebo controlled trial with Melissa. Journal of Clinical Psychiatry 63: 553–558

- The largest placebo-controlled study comparing lemon balm with placebo (sunflower oil).
- 72 patients were involved.

- This showed that lemon balm was associated with improvements in behavioural symptoms at rates akin to the benefits seen with neuroleptic treatment in less severe dementia.
- There were also improvements in activity and quality of life.

Electroconvulsive therapy for the depressed elderly

Van der Wurff FB, Stek ML, Hoogendijk WL, Beekman ATF 2003 Electroconvulsive therapy for the depressed elderly **(Cochrane Review)**. In: The Cochrane Library, Issue 2. CD003593. Update Software, Oxford

- There is little randomised evidence.
- Three trials were included: one trial of efficacy of ECT versus sham ECT (O'Leary 1994), one trial of unilateral versus bilateral ECT (Fraser 1980) and the other comparing the efficacy of once a week and thrice a week ECT (Kellner 1992).
- All studies had methodological problems and only the results of the second trial could be analysed.
- ECT was superior to sham ECT, but caution was advised in interpretation of the results.
- There was no clear difference between unilateral and bilateral ECT with regard to efficacy.
- It was not possible to analyse data regarding side effects.
- There were no data regarding patients with comorbid dementia, cerebrovascular disorders or Parkinson's disease.

See also the 'Treatment – Others' section in Chapter 2 (Affective disorders), page 39.

Assessment Tools and Rating Scales

Cambridge Cognitive Capacity Scale (CAMCOG)

Grevett C, O'Brian J 2002 A new database for CAMCOG. Old Age Psychiatrist 28: 9

- Structured interview.
- Assesses cognition in the elderly, including those with dementia.
- A trained interviewer conducts the interview.
- Takes approximately 20 minutes to complete.
- Component of the Cambridge Examination for Mental Disorders in the Elderly (CAMDEX.)

- Generates scores in eight domains:
  - orientation
  - language
  - memory
  - attention
  - praxis
  - calculation
  - abstract thinking
  - perception.
- A total score is also generated.
- The CAMCOG database is available to interpret results.
- Scores are more normally distributed than with the MMSE – the ceiling effect is less of a problem.

Clinical dementia rating (CDR)

Morris JC 1993 The clinical dementia rating (CDR): current version and scoring rules. Neurology 43: 2412–2414

- Semi-structured interview with patient and informant.
- Designed to rate the severity of dementia.
- Conducted by a trained health professional.
- Examines the previous week.
- Separate structured interviews with patients and carer.
- Scores are determined for six independent categories:
  - memory
  - orientation
  - judgement and problem solving
  - community affairs
  - home and hobbies
  - personal care.
- Scores are allocated by comparing the patient's characteristics with a descriptive guideline for each score. Algorithms then compute the global rating score.

Clock drawing test

Sunderland T, Hill JL, Mellow AM et al 1989 Clock drawing in Alzheimer's disease. A novel measure of dementia severity. Journal of the American Geriatrics Society 37: 725–729

- Clinician-rated patient activity which screens for cognitive impairment in dementia. Measures spatial dysfunction and neglect.
- Performed by a trained health professional.
- Takes approximately 5 minutes to complete, but no time limit for patients.
- Simple and quick.
- Poorly standardised.
- In the presence of an abnormal MMSE it is a fairly sensitive and specific adjunct for detecting executive cognitive dysfunction.

Disability assessment for dementia (DAD)

Gelinas I, Gauthier L, McIntyre M, Gauthier S 1999 Development of a functional measure for persons with Alzheimer's disease: the disability assessment for dementia. American Journal of Occupational Therapy 53: 471–481

- Structured interview or questionnaire for the patient's carer.
- Quantifies functional abilities in ADLs in patients with dementia and other cognitive impairments.
- A clinician conducts the interview in approximately 20 minutes.
- Originally for patients with Alzheimer's disease living in care settings.
- 40 items relating to basic self-care and instrumental aspects of ADL.
- Scored from 0 (most impairment) to 100 (least impairment.)

GBS (Gottfries–Brane–Steen) scale

Gottfries CG, Brane G, Gullberg B, Steen G 1982 A new rating scale for dementia syndromes. Archives of Gerontology and Geriatrics 1: 311–330

- Clinician-rated scale.
- Designed to give a quantitative measure of dementia, independent of aetiology.
- Based on observation or liaison with carer.
- Based on the recent time period.
- Takes 30 minutes to complete.
- Four subscales estimate motor, intellectual and emotional impairments; the fourth covers six common symptoms in dementia.
- Not a diagnostic scale but can monitor change and can be used in clinical trials.

Geriatric depression scale

Yesavage JA, Brink TL, Rose TL et al 1982–83 Development and validation of a geriatric depression screening scale: a preliminary report. Journal of Psychiatric Research 17: 37–49

- Observer rated.
- Scored out of 15 (0 = no depression).
- Used in research.

See also the 'Assessment tools and rating scales' section in Chapter 2 (Affective disorders), page 43.

Mini-Mental State Examination (MMSE)

Folstein M, Folstein S, McHugh PR 1975 'Mini-Mental State.' A practical method for grading the cognitive state of patients for the clinician. Journal of Psychiatric Research 12: 189–198

- Structured clinician-rated interview scale featuring pencil and paper tasks.
- Screens for presence of cognitive impairment caused by dementia.
- Performed by trained health professionals.
- Takes 5–10 minutes to complete and covers the present time.
- Most widely used tool for assessing cognitive impairment in the elderly.
- Easy to perform.
- Tests nine items:
  - memory
  - orientation
  - attention
  - verbal fluency
  - nominal aphasia
  - receptive aphasia plus receptive apraxia
  - alexia
  - agraphia
  - constructional apraxia.
- Limitations:
  - ceiling effect
  - floor effect
  - fails to detect changes in subtle impairment or in established severe dementia.

Neuropsychiatric inventory (NPI)

Cummings JL, Mega M, Gray K et al 1994 The neuropsychiatric inventory: comprehensive assessment of psychopathology in dementia. Neurology 44: 2308–2314

- Clinician-rated scale.
- Assesses behavioural and neuropsychological disturbances in patients with dementia. Includes affective abnormalities and psychosis.
- Performed by a trained health professional in consultation with the carer.
- Considers the previous week.
- Takes 30 minutes to complete.
- 12 behavioural disturbances are assessed:
  - delusions
  - hallucinations
  - agitation
  - dysphoria
  - euphoria

- anxiety
- apathy
- irritability
- disinhibition
- aberrant motor activity
- night-time behavioural disturbances
- eating disturbances.

• Assesses both severity and frequency. Only positive responses are examined and scored.

Pseudodementia checklist

Wells CE 1979 Checklist differentiating pseudodementia from dementia. American Journal of Psychiatry 136: 895–900

• Semi-structured interview to differentiate pseudodementia from dementia.
• Performed by an experienced rater.
• Takes 15 minutes to complete.
• Measures the present time state.
• 22-item checklist focusing on clinical course and history, complaints, clinical behaviour and mental capacity.
• Has been well validated using psychometric test battery, CT and EEG.
• For clinical use.

Guidelines

Committee on Safety of Medicines: atypical antipsychotics and stroke

Committee on Safety of Medicines (CSM) 2004 Atypical antipsychotics and stroke. MHRA, London

No atypical antipsychotics are licensed for the treatment of behavioural disturbance in dementia but they are often used for this purpose. The CSM has reviewed the evidence and determined that there is a three-fold increase in the risk of stroke when patients are treated with risperidone as compared to treatment with placebo. Analysis of data for olanzapine shows a similar increase in the risk of stroke and a two-fold increase in all-cause mortality.

The mechanism for the increased risk of stroke is neither clear nor confined to patients with dementia and cerebrovascular disease. The risk should be considered relevant to any patient with a history of cerebrovascular disease.

The CSM advises that the magnitude of risk is sufficient to outweigh the likely benefits of treatment for behavioural symptoms in dementia and it is a cause for concern in any patient with a high baseline risk of stroke.

The CSM advises risperidone and olanzapine should not be used for the treatment of behavioural symptoms of dementia. Treatment with risperidone for acute psychosis in patients with dementia should be short term and only under specialist advice. Prescribers should consider the risk of cerebrovascular events and vascular risk factors before treating any patient with a history of stroke or transient ischaemic attack. Patients with dementia who are currently being treated with an atypical antipsychotic drug should have their treatment reviewed.

Weblink Medicines and Healthcare Products Regulatory Agency – www.mhra.gov.uk

See also the 'Guidelines' section in Chapter 21 (Physical health), pages 313-314.

Atypical antipsychotics and psychiatric symptoms of dementia

Royal College of Psychiatrists Faculty for the Psychiatry of Old Age 2004 Atypical antipsychotics and psychiatric symptoms of dementia – prescribing update for old age psychiatrists. Royal College of Psychiatrists, London

This document was developed following collaboration by the Royal College of Psychiatrists (Old Age Faculty), the British Geriatrics Society, the Royal College of General Practitioners and the Alzheimer's Society in response to the safety message by the CSM in 2004. It raises concerns that the CSM guidance has been inappropriately interpreted – for example, situations where patients have had their medication withdrawn or changed to others with potentially more harmful side effects without consideration of individual circumstances. There are also longstanding concerns about inappropriate prescribing, polypharmacy, excessive doses and insufficient review.

The CSM alert showed there was an increased risk of adverse cerebrovascular events with risperidone and olanzapine. The greatest risk appears to be amongst those aged over 80 years. People with risk factors for cerebrovascular disease could be considered at increased risk but there is no trial evidence to support this assumption. The increased risk may also apply to quetiapine.

Medication, environmental approaches and behavioural techniques can be used concurrently in the treatment of behavioural and psychiatric symptoms of dementia (BPSD). Drug treatments are not licensed for the treatment of BPSD. Medication can be considered first line where there is a specific indication such as concurrent depressive disorder. Medication may also be considered where symptoms are severe and prompt treatment is required. Medication should be started at low dose with slow titration and regular review, and discontinued as soon as is appropriate. In less pressing situations, environmental and behavioural techniques may be appropriate first line.

The patient's consent and capacity to give consent should be considered where medication is warranted. If the patient does not have the capacity to consent to medication, discussion should be sought with the patient's carer, family and GP. The relevant mental health legislation should be followed.

The use of atypical antipsychotics is associated with side effects including weight gain, impaired glycaemic control, sedation and (at higher doses) extrapyramidal effects. Typical antipsychotics are associated with higher levels of side effects including extrapyramidal effects, tardive dyskinesia, drowsiness and anticholinergic effects.

Long-term use of antipsychotic medication in dementia carries risks of cognitive decline, falls, etc. Some patients may have their medication successfully withdrawn if they have been symptom free for a sufficient period. Medication should be withdrawn gradually. It may be appropriate to continue atypical antipsychotic medication in patients who continue to display BPSD, particularly where alternatives are unsuitable and where problems are predicted if changes are made.

See also the 'Guidelines' section in Chapter 2 (Affective disorders), page 47.

College guidelines on electroconvulsive therapy: an update for prescribers

See the 'Guidelines' section in Chapter 2 (Affective disorders), page 44.

Donepezil, galantamine, rivastigmine and memantine for the treatment of Alzheimer's disease. NICE Appraisal Consultation*

- These recommendations review the guidance issued by NICE in 2001 on the use of acetylcholinesterase inhibitors for the treatment of Alzheimer's disease.
- The potential benefits in other types of dementia are not examined.
- Donepezil, galantamine and rivastigmine are recommended in Alzheimer's disease of moderate severity only.
- Moderate severity is inferred by a score between 10 and 20 on MMSE.

There are a number of requirements, which include the following:
- The diagnosis should be made in a specialist clinic.
- Standard diagnostic criteria should be used.

- There should be assessment of cognition, global and behavioural functioning, quality of life and activities of daily living prior to commencing medication.
- Where possible, compliance should be ensured by a carer.
- Treatment should be initiated by professionals who work with the elderly population only.
- The views of carers should be sought regarding the patient's condition and any change related to treatment.
- General practitioners and elderly care specialists should have agreed shared care protocols for the prescription of treatment once it has been initiated.
- Patients receiving treatment should be monitored every 6 months using the MMSE, global and behavioural assessment.
- The drug should be continued while the MMSE remains at or above 10, assuming that the treatment is considered to have a worthwhile effect on behaviour and global functioning.
- The lowest acquisition cost drug should be used.
- Memantine is not recommended for Alzheimer's disease treatment (except as part of a clinical study).
- People with mild Alzheimer's disease who are currently taking an acetylcholinesterase inhibitor may continue until they, their carer or the specialist decide to stop.

Many people with mild dementia cope well in the community but need more assistance as the disease progresses. The annual cost of care for people with dementia in England is £6billion (Audit Commission).

In 2003, donepezil accounted for more than three-quarters of prescriptions for acetylcholinesterase inhibitors. Randomised controlled trials have shown that treatment with donepezil was associated with improvements in MMSE scores when compared to placebo. Studies have found less deterioration in functional ability than in those on placebo but these findings were not statistically significant. Quality of life estimates remain unclear. Behavioural symptoms were found to improve or their deterioration to be delayed. Adverse events were higher in patients taking donepezil rather than placebo. The numbers of adverse events increased with increasing dose.

There are insufficient data regarding the comparative efficacy of the different acetylcholinesterase inhibitors. Studies were of poor quality and results were of limited significance.

Considerations regarding the cost-effectiveness of these treatments are complicated. The group advises treating the manufacturers' calculations with considerable caution. The acetylcholinesterase inhibitors may not be cost-effective for use in the NHS. Factors such as potential improvement in behavioural symptoms and potential benefit to carers are relevant here.

---

* Reproduced with permission from the National Institute for Health and Clinical Excellence, London.

Interventions in the management of behavioural and psychological aspects of dementia. SIGN Publication Number 22**

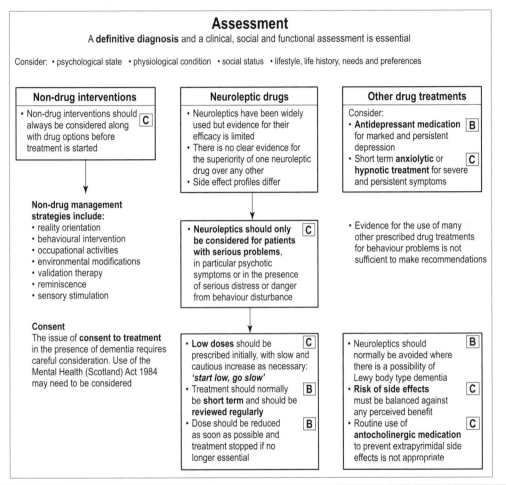

Assessment

A **definitive diagnosis** and a clinical, social and functional assessment is essential

Consider: • psychological state   • physiological condition   • social status   • lifestyle, life history, needs and preferences

Non-drug interventions

• Non-drug interventions should always be considered along with drug options before treatment is started [C]

Non-drug management strategies include:
• reality orientation
• behavioural intervention
• occupational activities
• environmental modifications
• validation therapy
• reminiscence
• sensory stimulation

Consent
The issue of **consent to treatment** in the presence of dementia requires careful consideration. Use of the Mental Health (Scotland) Act 1984 may need to be considered

Neuroleptic drugs

• Neuroleptics have been widely used but evidence for their efficacy is limited
• There is no clear evidence for the superiority of one neuroleptic drug over any other
• Side effect profiles differ

• **Neuroleptics should only be considered for patients with serious problems**, in particular psychotic symptoms or in the presence of serious distress or danger from behaviour disturbance [C]

• **Low doses** should be prescribed initially, with slow and cautious increase as necessary: *'start low, go slow'* [C]
• Treatment should normally be **short term** and should be **reviewed regularly** [B]
• Dose should be reduced as soon as possible and treatment stopped if no longer essential [B]

Other drug treatments

Consider:
• **Antidepressant medication** for marked and persistent depression [B]
• Short term **anxiolytic** or **hypnotic treatment** for severe and persistent symptoms [C]

• Evidence for the use of many other prescribed drug treatments for behaviour problems is not sufficient to make recommendations

• Neuroleptics should normally be avoided where there is a possibility of Lewy body type dementia [B]
• **Risk of side effects** must be balanced against any perceived benefit [C]
• Routine use of **antocholinergic medication** to prevent extrapyramidal side effects is not appropriate [C]

B and **C** indicate grades of recommendation (see Appendix II for full details). ** Derived from the National Clinical Guideline recommended for use in Scotland by the Scottish Intercollegiate Guidelines Network (SIGN), Edinburgh. Reproduced with permission.

Management of patients with dementia. SIGN Guideline 86**

Diagnosis

B   DSM-IV or NINCDS-ADRDA criteria should be used for the diagnosis of Alzheimer's disease.

B   The Hachinski Ischaemic Scale or NINDS-AIRENS criteria may be used to assist in the diagnosis of vascular dementia.

C   Diagnosis criteria for dementia with Lewy bodies and frontotemporal dementia should be considered in clinical assessment.

Initial cognitive testing

B   In individuals with suspected cognitive impairment, the MMSE should be used in the diagnosis of dementia.

✓   Initial cognitive testing can be improved by the use of Addenbrooke's Cognitive Examination.

Screening for comorbid conditions

☑ Physical investigations including laboratory tests should be selected on clinical grounds according to history and clinical circumstances.

B As part of the assessment for suspected dementia, the presence of comorbid depression should be considered.

The use of imaging

C Structural imaging should ideally form part of the diagnostic workup of patients with suspected dementia.

C SPECT may be used in combination with CT to aid the differential diagnosis of dementia when the diagnosis is in doubt.

Neuropsychological testing

B Neuropsychological testing should be used in the diagnosis of dementia, especially in patients where dementia is not clinically obvious.

Non-Pharmacological interventions

Behaviour management

B Behaviour management may be used to reduce depression in people with dementia.

Caregiver intervention programmes

B Caregivers should receive comprehensive training on interventions that are effective for people with dementia.

Cognitive stimulation

B Cognitive stimulation should be offered to individuals with dementia.

Multisensory stimulation and combined therapies

☑ For people with moderate dementia who can tolerate it, multisensory stimulation may be a clinically useful intervention.

☑ • Multisensory stimulation is not recommended for relief of neuropsychiatric symptoms in people with moderate to severe dementia.
• Bright light therapy is not recommended for the treatment of cognitive impairment, sleep disturbance or agitation in people with dementia.
• In people with dementia who show behavioural disturbance despite the use of psychotropic medication, aromatherapy may influence behaviour but cannot be recommended as a direct alternative to antipsychotic drugs, nor for the reduction of specific behavioural problems.

• The use of aromatherapy to reduce associated symptoms in people with dementia should be discussed with a qualified aromatherapist who can advise on contraindications.

Recreational and physical activities

B Recreational activities should be introduced to people with dementia to enhance quality of life and well-being.

☑ For people with dementia, a combination of structured exercise and conversation may help maintain mobility.

Reality orientation therapy

D Reality orientation therapy should be used by a skilled practitioner, on an individualised basis, with people who are disorientated in time, place and person.

Pharmacological interventions

Cholinesterase inhibitors

B Donepezil, at daily doses of 5 mg and above can be used:
• to treat cognitive decline in people with Alzheimer's disease
• for the management of associated symptoms in people with Alzheimer's disease

B Galantamine, at daily doses of 16 mg and above can be used:
• to treat cognitive decline in people with Alzheimer's disease and people with mixed dementias
• for the management of associated symptoms in people with Alzheimer's disease

B Rivastigmine, at daily doses of 6 mg and above can be used:
• to treat cognitive decline in people with Alzheimer's disease
• to treat cognitive decline in people with dementia with Lewy bodies
• for the management of associated symptoms in people with Alzheimer's disease and dementia with Lewy bodies.

Antipsychotics

B If necessary, conventional antipsychotics may be used with caution, given their side effect profile, to treat the associated symptoms of dementia.

☑ • An individualised approach to managing agitation in people with dementia is required.
• Atypical antipsychotics with reduced sedation and extrapyramidal side effects may be useful in practice, although the risk of serious adverse events such as stroke must be carefully evaluated.

- In patients who are stable, antipsychotic withdrawal should be considered.
- Where antipsychotics are inappropriate, cholinesterase inhibitors may be considered.

Antidepressants

D Antidepressants can be used for the treatment of comorbid depression in dementia providing their use is evaluated carefully.

✓ Trazodone may be considered for patients with depressive symptoms and dementia-associated agitation.

Herbal medicines

✓ - People with dementia who wish to use *Ginkgo biloba* should consult qualified herbalist for advice and should be made aware of possible interactions with other prescribed drugs.
- People with dementia who wish to use *Salvia officinalis* should consult a qualified herbalist for advice.

Information for patients and carers

C Patients and carers should be offered information tailored to the patient's perceived needs. Healthcare professionals should be aware that:

C - many people with dementia can understand this diagnosis, receive information and be involved in decision making

C - some people with dementia may not wish to know their diagnosis

D - in some situations disclosure of a diagnosis of dementia may be inappropriate.

✓ - The wishes of the person with dementia should be upheld at all times.
- The diagnosis of dementia should be given by a healthcare professional skilled in communication or counselling.
- Where diagnosis is not disclosed there should be a clear record of the reasons.
- Patients and carers should be provided with information about the services and interventions available to them at all stages of the patient's journey of care.
- Information should be offered to patients and carers in advance of the next stage of the illness.

Websites

Alzheimer Scotland - Action on Dementia
Website: www.alzscot.org.uk
Age Concern Scotland
Website: www.ageconcernscotland.org.uk
Help the Aged in Scotland
Email: infoscot@helptheaged.org.uk
Mental Health Foundation Scotland
Website: www.mentalhealth.org.uk

A, B, C and **D** indicate grades of recommendation; ✓ indicates a good practice point (see Appendix II for full details). ** Reproduced with permission from the Scottish Intercollegiate Guidelines Network, Edinburgh.

Perinatal psychiatry

Chapter contents

General Topics

Bipolar disorder and childbirth

> Jones I, Craddock, N 2005 Bipolar disorder and childbirth: the importance of recognising risk [editorial]. British Journal of Psychiatry 186: 453–454

Discusses the risk of suicide and infanticide during psychotic episodes in the postpartum period. Follows the report of the inquiry into the death of a psychiatric colleague published in October 2003, when Dr Daksha Emson took the life of herself and her 3-month-old daughter whilst psychotic. She had a history of BAD.

A confidential inquiry into maternal deaths in 2001 found that suicide had become the leading cause for maternal mortality in the UK, accounting for 28% of deaths, the majority of which were in the context of puerperal psychosis. 46% of these women had been in contact with psychiatric services – and half of these had been admitted previously with a severe episode of illness following childbirth.

In many, therefore, it is preventable. Most, however, did not have a detailed risk assessment, none had a detailed management plan, none was under close surveillance in the puerperium and none was under the care of the MBU/perinatal psychiatric service. The findings are sadly alike in the 2004 Confidential Enquiry into Maternal Deaths.

Puerperal psychosis occurs in 25–50% of those with a previous diagnosis of BAD (increasing to 60% in women with BAD and a personal or family history of puerperal psychosis).

It is clear that women with a history of BAD require careful management prior to conception, throughout pregnancy and during the postpartum period.

Strategies for minimising risk include the following:
- Be aware of high risk in the 2 weeks following delivery.
- Careful consideration of future pregnancies. All women should be screened in the antenatal period for known important risk factors and protocols should be in place to ensure formal treatment of women at risk.
- The risks of stopping medication prior to or during pregnancy should be the result of planning and risk analysis. (The same applies to starting medication in those who develop symptoms during pregnancy or breastfeeding.)
- Individualised risk factors should be available and close contact maintained during the period of risk.

> Stewart DE, Kompenhouwer J, Kendell RF et al 1991 Prophylactic lithium in puerperal psychosis. The experience of three centres. British Journal of Psychiatry 158: 393–397

- Some evidence exists for the use of prophylactic lithium in the immediate postpartum period.
- There is a need for well-conducted studies into use of antipsychotics in this context.
- Only anecdotal evidence is available to date.

Management of drug misuse in pregnancy

> Day E, George S 2005 Management of drug misuse in pregnancy. Advances in Psychiatric Treatment 11: 253–261

No figures are reported for the use of illicit drugs in pregnant women in the UK. The effects of drug use on the mother are the same as those for non-pregnant women. They include neglect of medical, nutritional and social well-being. Those who inject are at risk of blood-borne viruses and a number of medical complications. Illicit drug use can lead to involvement in crime: prostitution, robbery and burglary.

Parental drug misuse after birth can lead to physical and emotional abuse or neglect, inadequate parenting or supervision, separation, poverty, poor education, exposure to criminal behaviour and social isolation.

Screening for blood-borne viruses with subsequent immunisation and treatment to reduce long-term sequelae should be carried out. Steps should be taken to prevent mother-to-baby transmission where possible.

The evidence that exists regarding the long-term effects of drug misuse is contradictory.

This article goes on to discuss the specific treatments for neonatal abstinence syndromes and drug dependence. Evidence exists to support the use of both residential and outpatient treatment programmes in the treatment of drug-dependent pregnant women.

National Institute of Drug Abuse 1996 The National Pregnancy and Health Survey: drug use among women delivering livebirths 1992. National Institute of Drug Abuse, Rockville, MD

- 2613 American women completed a self-report.
- Women from urban and rural hospitals were included.
- Over 5% of those who gave birth during the study period had used illicit drugs.
- 2.9% had used cannabis and 1.1% had used cocaine during their pregnancy.
- 20% smoked tobacco and 18.5% drank alcohol.

US National Household Survey. Office of Applied Statistics. Online. Available: http://oas.samhsa.gov

Results from 1994 and 1995 were combined:
- 9.3% of women aged 15–44 years reported the use of illicit drugs.
- 2.3% used illicit drugs whilst pregnant.

Fischer G, Johnson RE, Eder H et al 2000 Treatment of opioid-dependent pregnant women with buprenorphine. Addiction 95: 239–244

- Neonates born to mothers who misuse drugs have a high incidence of preterm birth, low birth weight and poor nutritional status.
- Maternal infection, neglect and malnutrition are partly to blame.

Advisory Council on the Misuse of Drugs 2003 Hidden harm: responding to the needs of children of problem drug users. Home Office, London

- Estimated that, for 20,000–30,000 children in England and Wales, one or both parents have a serious drug misuse problem.

Drug use in a parent can impact on the child's welfare in a number of ways. Drug intoxication and withdrawal affect judgement, coordination and conscious levels, with subsequent effects on child rearing and supervision. Disinhibition can lead to aggression and physical abuse. Irritability and mood disturbance can result from drug withdrawal. Unemployment, poverty and criminality affect the function of the family and the purchase of drugs may be a higher priority than purchasing food and essentials for the home. Impaired supervision may leave children vulnerable to other people in the home as well as to the presence of drugs and injecting equipment in the house.

Osborn DA, Cole MJ, Jeffrey HE 2004 Opiate treatment for opiate withdrawal in newborn infants **(Cochrane Review)**. In: The Cochrane Library, Issue 3. Update Software, Oxford

- 48–94% of infants will show signs of opioid neonatal syndrome, including gastrointestinal disturbances, irritability, hyperactivity, feeding difficulties, sleeping difficulties and autonomic hyperactivity.
- This is particularly true for infants withdrawing from methadone rather than heroin.
- Seizures are rare and occur in less than 5%.
- The problems with sleep, feeding and weight loss can impact on the relationship between mother and baby.

Coghlan D, Milner M, Clarke T et al 1999 Neonatal abstinence syndrome. Irish Medical Journal 92: 232–236

- Withdrawal from methadone tends to be later in onset, longer in duration and of greater severity than withdrawal from heroin.

Bandstra ES, Burkett G 1991 Maternal–fetal and neonatal effects of in utero cocaine exposure. Seminars in Perinatology 15: 288–301

- Maternal cocaine use causes problems for the fetus, including placental abruption, intrauterine growth retardation, spontaneous abortion, pre-eclampsia, pulmonary oedema, seizures and cardiac arrhythmias.
- Congenital physical anomalies occur, most often affecting the ocular and urogenital systems.
- Heavy cocaine use in the immediate antenatal period can lead to neonatal intoxication with symptoms of irritability, hypertonia and sleep and appetite disturbances.

Sanchis A, Rosique D, Catala J 1991 Adverse effects of maternal lorazepam on neonates. DCIP: The Annals of Pharmacotherapy 25: 1137–1138

- Heavy benzodiazepine use is associated with cleft lip and palate.
- A neonatal abstinence syndrome is associated with a floppy baby who is lethargic and irritable with low muscle tone and respiratory depression.

Ornoy A, Michailevskaya V, Lukashov I et al 1996 The developmental outcome of children born to heroin-dependent mothers raised at home or adopted. Child Abuse and Neglect 20: 385–396

- Long-term effects of maternal heroin use, such as developmental disorders, may be as much to do with home environment as in utero heroin exposure.
- Maternal drug use continues to impact on child development in early life, with high levels of inattention, hyperactivity and aggression in preschool children.

Kandel D 1990 Parenting styles, drug use and children's adjustment in families of young adults. Journal of Marriage and the Family 52: 183–196

- A study of parents of primary school children.
- Past parental drug use was associated with more punitive parental discipline and less child supervision.

Kolar AF, Brown BS, Haertzen CA et al 1994 Children of substance abusers. The life experiences of children of opiate addicts in methadone maintenance. American Journal of Drug and Alcohol Abuse 20: 159–171

- Adolescents with drug-using parents are at higher risk of offending and bullying.
- They are also more likely to be absent from school, to have to repeat a year or to be suspended.

Johnson JL, Leff M 1999 Children of substance abusers: overview of research findings. Paediatrics 103: 1085–1099

- Adolescents who use drugs themselves are likely to have one or more parents who also use drugs.

Hepburn M 2002 Drug use and women's reproductive health. In: Peterson T, McBride A (eds) Working with substance misusers: a guide to theory and practice. Routledge, London

- It is important that drug-using women only become pregnant if they want to.
- Services should aim to help such women maximise their health and improve their lifestyle and diet before they conceive.
- Sudden withdrawal from benzodiazepines can cause maternal convulsions. This should be avoided.

Klee H, Jackson M, Lewis S 2002 Drug misuse and motherhood. Routledge, London

- Pregnant women who use drugs may not seek professional help; if they do, they may deny drug use.
- Early signs of pregnancy may be missed due to drug use and this can lead to women presenting late for treatment.
- Pregnant women who use drugs may fear others will view them as an irresponsible or inadequate parent.
- This may be worsened by poor self-esteem, guilt and depression.

Luty J 2003 What works in drug addiction? Advances in Psychiatric Treatment 9: 363–367

- The same basic principles for the good treatment of drug misuse apply to the treatment of drug misuse in pregnant women.
- Special attention should be paid to the health of the unborn child.

Finnegan LP 1991 Treatment issues for opioid-dependent women during the perinatal period. Journal of Psychoactive Drugs 23: 191–201

- Methadone maintenance programmes in pregnancy in combination with psychosocial treatment programmes are beneficial in reducing obstetric and fetal complications and neonatal morbidity and mortality.
- Opioid withdrawal in the first trimester is associated with miscarriage.
- Opioid withdrawal in the third trimester is associated with premature labour and fetal death.
- Some women may prefer to undergo detoxification than to have maintenance treatment.

Ward J, Mattick RP, Hall W (eds) 1998 Methadone maintenance during pregnancy. In: Methadone maintenance treatment and other opioid replacement therapies. Harwood Academic, Amsterdam

- Women on methadone maintenance programmes during pregnancy do consistently better than women who receive no treatment for their drug misuse.
- The use of street heroin leading to alternate intoxication and withdrawal is harmful to the fetus.
- Fetal death is associated with withdrawal.
- Maintenance treatment is preferable to complete detoxification.
- Complete detoxification can result in an abstinence syndrome, leading to fetal distress.
- Neonatal effects of heroin dependence are confounded by maternal lifestyle and other factors such as maternal smoking.

Fischer G 2000 Treatment of opioid dependence in pregnant women. Addiction 95: 1141–1144

- Methadone maintenance therapy for opioid dependent pregnant women was found to produce beneficial effects on physical and psychological health.
- Women receiving methadone maintenance were more stable and more likely to attend their prenatal care.

Householder J, Hatcher R, Burns W et al 1982 Infants born to narcotic-addicted mothers. Psychological Bulletin 92: 453–468

- The babies of women maintained on methadone during pregnancy are bigger and less likely to be born prematurely than the babies of women who receive no treatment for their drug misuse.

Dunlop AJ, Panjari M, O'Sullivan H et al 2003 Clinical guidelines for the use of buprenorphine in pregnancy. Turning Point Alcohol and Drug Centre, Fitzroy, Australia

- There is insufficient good evidence and insufficient follow-up regarding the safety of buprenorphine in pregnancy and breast feeding.

Kaltenbach K, Berghella V, Finnegan L 1998 Opioid dependence during pregnancy. Obstetrics and Gynecology Clinics of North America 25: 139–151

- There is no safe alternative to cocaine that can be prescribed in pregnancy for women who are dependent.

Mayo-Smith MF 1997 Pharmacological management of alcohol withdrawal: a meta-analysis and evidence-based practice guideline. Journal of the American Medical Association 160: 649–655

- Alcohol misuse occurs in many pregnant women who misuse drugs.

Camp JM, Finkelstein N 1995 Fostering effective parenting skills and healthy child development within residential substance abuse treatment settings. CAPP, Cambridge, MA

- Parenting training for people who misuse drugs can have beneficial effects on self-esteem, parenting attitudes and knowledge.

See also the 'General topics' section in Chapter 1 (Addictions psychiatry), pages 2, 3, 7-9.

Obstetric variables

Blackmore ER, Jones I, Doshi M et al 2006 Obstetric variables associated with bipolar affective puerperal psychosis. British Journal of Psychiatry 188: 32–36

Background

A number of factors have been associated with an increase in risk of postpartum puerperal psychosis, including:
- first pregnancy
- shorter pregnancy
- complications in pregnancy and delivery (including caesarean section)
- a female baby.

The findings have only been consistent for primiparity.

Method

- This study compared all of the deliveries of 129 women who had had an episode of bipolar affective puerperal psychosis.
- Patients were recruited from mental health teams, a national action group and through national and local publicity.

Results

- 84% of the women had bipolar I disorder.
- The remainder had a diagnosis of schizoaffective disorder.
- 287 pregnancies resulted in 242 live births. Only the latter were included.
- The women had a median number of two pregnancies and two deliveries.
- There were 167 episodes of puerperal psychosis in total for the 129 women, with 72% having one episode, 27% two episodes and one woman three episodes.

Conclusion

- This study concluded that there is an association between primiparity and puerperal psychosis.
- It also suggested that complications during delivery may be linked to having a severe postpartum episode.

Psychological impact of stillbirth on fathers in the subsequent pregnancy and puerperium

Turton P, Badenhorst W, Hughes P et al 2006 Psychological impact of stillbirth on fathers in the subsequent pregnancy and puerperium. British Journal of Psychiatry 188: 165–172

Method

- Psychological assessments were undertaken in 38 pregnant couples whose previous pregnancy had resulted in stillbirth and 38 pair-matched controls.
- Assessments were performed during the antenatal period and at 6, 26 and 52 weeks postnatally.
- The Beck Depression Inventory, the Spielberger State-Trait Inventory, the PTSD-1 Interview and the Golombok Rust Inventory of Marital Satisfaction were used.

Recruitment

- 105 mothers were initially identified.
- 16 had begun a new relationship since their stillbirth and 16 delivered their baby before an antenatal assessment could be performed.
- 32 couples declined to take part.
- Refusal by the father occurred more often than refusal by the mother.

Results

- Fathers who had previous experience of stillbirth had higher levels of psychiatric symptoms (anxiety and post-traumatic stress disorder) in the antenatal period. These symptoms remitted after the birth of a live baby.
- It was not possible to compare paternal PTSD between index and control groups due to the absence of a comparable trauma.
- Mothers who had had a previous stillbirth had higher levels of psychiatric symptoms at each psychological assessment when compared to fathers.
- Fathers in the index group had higher levels of anxiety symptoms compared to mothers when the subsequent pregnancy was delayed.
- Fathers' coping strategies included increased alcohol intake, prescription medication (18.4%), illegal drugs (7.9%) and professional support (47.4%). Professional support included hospital counsellors, religious ministers, other healthcare professionals and voluntary self-help groups.

Conclusion

- The vulnerability of fathers to psychological distress in the pregnancy subsequent to one ending in stillbirth needs to be recognised.

Policy and Legislation

Why mothers die: confidential enquiry into maternal deaths

> CEMACH 2003 Why mothers die 2000–2002: report on confidential enquiries into maternal deaths in the United Kingdom. Ch. 11A: Deaths from suicide and other psychiatric causes. Online. Available: www.cemach.org.uk/publications/WMD2000_2002/wmd-11a.htm

Background

- One in 10 new mothers develops depression; this will be severe in up to half of those cases.

- One in 50 women will be seen by a psychiatrist within 12 months of delivery.
- Four in 1000 women will be admitted to a psychiatric hospital.
- Two in 1000 women will suffer from puerperal psychosis.
- The risk of developing a severe mental illness is substantially elevated in the postpartum period, particularly in the first 3 months.
- For severe mental illness after childbirth the relative risks are:
  - developing a severe depressive illness   5
  - review by a psychiatrist   7
  - admission with psychosis   324
- Being pregnant is associated with a lower risk of developing a new psychiatric disorder than at any other time.
- Women who have had a previous episode of serious mental illness unrelated to pregnancy are at increased risk of postpartum illness, with a risk between 1 in 2 and 1 in 36.
- Women who have had a previous episode of mania at any time have a 1 in 2 chance of a postpartum episode.
- Suicide is the leading cause of maternal death.
- 50% of the women who died from suicide had a history of serious mental illness; in 25% this was related to pregnancy.

Results

- 54% of patients who committed suicide were severely depressed or psychotic.
- 65% used a violent method of suicide.
- 83% were over 25 years old.
- 55% had at least one previous childbirth.
- 57% had a history of serious mental illness.
- 76% of patients who committed suicide had no psychiatric management plan in place for the peripartum period. Information sharing generally was poor between involved professionals.
- Many women requiring inpatient care are not being admitted to specialist mother and baby units.

Substance abuse

- There is underidentification of substance misuse in pregnant women.
- Women who abuse substances are at substantially increased risk of maternal and perinatal morbidity and mortality.
- Close, multiagency supervision is required.
- Women using opioids should be prescribed substitution therapy.

Recommendations

- Every trust that provides maternity services must have guidelines regarding the care of women who are at risk of pregnancy-related serious mental illness.
- Every woman with serious postpartum mental illness must have access to a specialist perinatal mental health team.
- Specialist mother and baby units should be responsible for the care of women who require psychiatric admission following childbirth.
- There should be sufficient provision of regional mother and baby units.

Treatment – Psychopharmacology

Antidepressant prevention of postnatal depression

Howard LM, Hoffbrand S, Henshaw C, Boath L, Bradley E 2005 Antidepressant prevention of postnatal depression **(Cochrane Review)**. In: The Cochrane Library, Issue 2. CD004363. Update Software, Oxford

- Two trials were identified of women with a history of postpartum depression.
- Intention to treat analyses were not performed.
- Nortriptyline ($n = 26$) showed no benefit over placebo ($n = 25$).
- Sertraline ($n = 14$) reduced the recurrence of postnatal depression in comparison with placebo ($n = 8$).
- Sertraline also reduced the time to recurrence when compared with placebo.
- There was a lack of clear evidence to drive clinical practice.
- Larger trials are required.

See also the 'Treatment – Psychopharmacology' section in Chapter 2 (Affective disorders), page 31.

Antidepressant treatment for postnatal depression

Hoffbrand S, Howard L, Crawley H 2001 Antidepressant treatment for postnatal depression **(Cochrane Review)**. In: The Cochrane Library, Issue 2. CD002018. Update Software, Oxford

- Only one small trial could be included (Appleby 1997), limiting what conclusions are drawn.
- It reported that fluoxetine (given after an initial session of counselling) was as effective as a full course of

cognitive behavioural counselling in the treatment of postnatal depression.
- Further research in this area is required.

See also the 'Treatment – Psychopharmacology' section in Chapter 2 (Affective disorders), page 31.

Psychotropic medication in pregnancy

Kohen D 2004 Psychotropic medication in pregnancy. Advances in Psychiatric Treatment 10: 59–66

In the treatment of pregnant women, the current consensus is that no decision is risk-free but that mental health complications outweigh the risk of pharmacotherapy. To date there is no evidence of excessive placental passage of either antidepressant or psychotropic drugs, but increased maternal dosage typically increases umbilical cord passage, resulting in higher serum levels in the infant.

Although there is limited information about behavioural problems caused by psychotropic medication intake during pregnancy, long-term behavioural teratogenicity should be considered. It is also clear that untreated mothers may fail their children to the point of neglect and maternal separation, with the potential for adverse effects in adulthood.

- Clinical observation and data support the safety of both tricyclic and tetracyclic antidepressants.
- As yet there is no evidence regarding the impact of psychotropic medication on spontaneous abortion rates.
- There is limited published research regarding the use of trazodone, nefazodone and mirtazapine.
- There are few reliable reports on the safety of MAOIs in pregnancy and their use in pregnancy is therefore not advised.
- Lithium, carbamazepine and sodium valproate are known teratogens carrying an increased risk of malformation of the fetus. The lowest possible dose should be used and a high level of vigilance is advised.
- The teratogenic potential of lamotrigine, gabapentin and topiramate is not well documented.
- Early low dose use of conventional antipsychotics as antiemetics, followed by later animal studies and clinical observational studies, have shown that there is generally no increased teratogenic risk with high potency antipsychotics.
- No oral and depot conventional antipsychotic has been associated with teratology in the fetus, and it has therefore been concluded that these drugs are safe in pregnancy.
- Information about the use of atypical antipsychotics is based on single case studies and data collected by pharmaceutical companies but the lack of any reported sequelae needs to be replicated in larger and more rigorous studies.

Oates M 2001 Death from psychiatric causes. In: Lewis G, Drife L (eds) Why mothers die 1997–1999: confidential enquiries into maternal deaths in the United Kingdom. Royal College of Obstetricians and Gynaecologists Press, London, pp 165–187

- Suicide during the perinatal period is a serious risk in women with mental health problems.

Orr ST, Miller CA 1995 Maternal depressive symptoms and risk of poor pregnancy outcome: review of the literature and preliminary findings. Epidemiology Review 17: 165–171

- Antenatal depression and anxiety have been linked to low birth weight and smaller head circumference.
- Depression increases the risk of low birth weight.

Koren G, Pastuszak A, Ito S 1998 Drugs in pregnancy. New England Journal of Medicine 338: 1128–1137

- A useful treatment should not be stopped without a clear and plausible reason. Neonatal toxicity, prematurity and stillbirth, and morphological and behavioural teratology are potential risks and need to be considered.

Stowe ZN, Nemeroff CB 1998 Psychopharmacology during pregnancy and lactation. In: Schatzberg AF, Nemeroff CB (eds) Textbook of psycho-pharmacology. American Psychiatric Press, Washington, DC, pp 823–837

- The altered pharmacokinetic and pharmacodynamic changes in the body during pregnancy include delayed gastric emptying, delayed gastrointestinal motility, increased volume of distribution, decreased drug binding capacity, decreased albumin levels and enhanced hepatic metabolism with induced liver metabolic pathways.
- There is greater renal clearance and the glomerular filtration rate increases.
- Plasma volume increases by 5%.
- The fetus has lower plasma protein binding, lowered hepatic functioning, relatively increased cardiac output and greater permeability in the blood–brain barrier in comparison with adults.
- These changes highlight the need for cautious prescribing, lower doses of medication, monotherapy and regular review.

McElhatton PR, Bateman DN, Evans C et al 1998 Does prenatal exposure to ecstasy cause congenital malformation? A prospective follow-up of 92 pregnancies. British Journal of Clinical Pharmacology 45: 184

- In pregnant women comorbid severe mental illness and substance misuse leads to intrauterine death, increased risk of congenital defects, cardiovascular and musculoskeletal anomalies and fetal alcohol syndrome, all attributable to the misused substances.

Altshuler LL, Cohan L, Szuba MP et al 1996 Pharmacological management of psychiatric illness during pregnancy: dilemmas and guidelines. American Journal of Psychiatry 153: 592–606

- Animal studies with different tricyclics (imipramine, amitriptyline and dothiepin) and tetracyclics (maprotiline) using supramaximal doses have shown no increased risk of congenital malformations in first-trimester exposure.
- Benzodiazepines used in the first trimester have been linked to an increased risk of oral cleft lip (up to 0.6%) and congenital malformations of the central nervous system and the urinary tract.

Crombie DL, Pincent RJ, Fleming D 1972 Imipramine and pregnancy [letter]. British Medical Journal 2: 745

- Case studies of women who received imipramine and amitriptyline throughout pregnancy.
- Tricyclic antidepressants do not increase the risk of malformation.

McElhatton PR, Garbis HM, Elefant E et al 1996 The outcome of pregnancy in 689 women exposed to therapeutic doses of antidepressants. A collaborative of the European Network of Teratology Information Service (ENTIS). Reproductive Toxicology 10: 285–294

- A statistically rigorous study which investigated the outcome of pregnancy in 689 women exposed to therapeutic dosages of antidepressants.
- It included 283 women who were treated with tricyclic antidepressants from the first trimester onwards.
- There was no reported increase in malformations in the infants.

Nulman I, Rovet J, Stewart DE et al 2002 Child development following exposure to tricyclic antidepressants or fluoxetine throughout foetal life: a prospective controlled study. American Journal of Psychiatry 159: 1889–1895

- Found no increase in anatomical or behavioural teratology.
- There was no increase in later behavioural problems in children born to mothers taking tricyclics or fluoxetine during pregnancy.

Simon GE, Cunningham ML, Davis RL 2002 Outcomes of prenatal antidepressant exposure. American Journal of Psychiatry 159: 2055–2061

- Documented reversible perinatal complications in the form of withdrawal symptoms.

- Withdrawal symptoms commonly included irritability, eating and sleeping difficulties and convulsions.
- These symptoms particularly occur when tricyclics and fluoxetine have been used in high dosages and in the third trimester.

Einarsen A, Bumn F, Sarkar M et al 2001 Pregnancy outcome following gestational exposure to venlafaxine: a multicentre prospective controlled study. American Journal of Psychiatry 158: 1728–1730

- Venlafaxine has been used in 150 pregnant women without an increase in the rates of major malformations above the baseline rate of 1–3%.

Cohen LS, Friedman JM, Jefferson JW et al 1994 A re-evaluation of risk of in utero exposure to lithium. Journal of the American Medical Association 271: 146–150

- Lithium in pregnancy has a revised teratological risk based on meta-analysis of 0.05%.
- It has a relative risk 10–20 times that for the general population.

Viguera AC, Nonacs R, Cohen LS et al 2000 Risk of recurrence of bipolar disorder in pregnant and nonpregnant women after discontinuing lithium maintenance. American Journal of Psychiatry 157: 179–184

- Evidence based on prospective studies suggests that the risk to the fetus of lithium exposure might have been overestimated and the risk to the mother and child of lithium withdrawal underestimated.
- Found an average recurrence rate of up to 50% within 6 months of discontinuing lithium.
- Rapid discontinuation appears to increase the risk of relapse even further, regardless of whether the patients are pregnant or not.

Koch S, Jager-Roman E, Losche G et al 1996 Anti-epileptic drug treatment in pregnancy: drug side effects in neonates and neurological outcome. Acta Paediatrica 85: 739–746

- Examined the relationship between maternal antiepileptic therapy, neonatal behaviour and later neurological functions.
- Children exposed to valproate in utero showed neurological dysfunction and increased excitability in infancy and later life.
- Valproate concentration in the infant at birth was found to correlate with degree of neonatal hyperexcitability and neurological dysfunction at 6 years.

Slone D, Siskind V, Heinonen RP et al 1977 Antenatal exposure to the phenothiazines in relation to congenital malformations, perinatal mortality rate, birth weight and intelligence quotient score. American Journal of Obstetrics and Gynecology 128: 486–488

- The California Child Health Development Project (1959–1966).
- A study of 19,000 births.
- There was no significant increase in congenital abnormalities following prenatal exposure to oral or injectable antipsychotics.

Sacker A, Done DJ, Crow TJ 1996 Obstetric complications in children born to parents with schizophrenia: a meta-analysis of case control studies. Psychological Medicine 26: 279–287

- A meta-analysis of all studies examining the complications of offspring of women with schizophrenia.
- Although the effects were small, women with schizophrenia had an increased risk of pregnancy and birth complications.
- Low birth weight, preterm birth and perinatal infant death occurred more frequently.
- The incidence of poverty, smoking, substance misuse, violence and many other risk factors are increased in people with schizophrenia, suggesting that the higher frequency of some complications could be attributed to these environmental factors.

Tekell JL 2001 Managing pregnancy in the schizophrenic woman. In: Yonkers KA, Little BB (eds) Management of psychiatric disorders in pregnancy. Arnold, Oxford, pp 188–212

- Conventional antipsychotics do not seem to pose a risk in labour and the perinatal period.
- Complications in the infant are usually seen in the immediate postnatal period.

Wisner KL, Perel JM 1988 Psychopharmacological agents and electroconvulsive therapy during pregnancy and the puerperium. In: Cohen PL (ed.) Psychiatric consultation in childbirth settings. Plenum, New York, pp 165–206

- There are reports of possible teratogenicity associated with the use of anticholinergic drugs in combination with antipsychotics.
- Anticholinergic medication should be avoided where possible.
- If required, anticholinergic medication should be used in the lowest possible dosage.

Rubin PC 1981 Current concepts: beta blockers in pregnancy. New England Journal of Medicine 305: 1323–1326

- Beta-blockers for akathisia in pregnancy are not associated with any increase in congenital malformations.

Assessment Tools and Rating Scales

Edinburgh Postnatal Depression Scale (EPDS)

Cox JL, Holden JM, Sagovsky R 1987 Edinburgh Postnatal Depression Scale (EPDS). British Journal of Psychiatry 150: 782–786

- Self-rated scale which assists primary care health professionals to detect mothers suffering from postnatal depression.
- Covers the previous week and present.
- Takes less than 5 minutes to complete.
- 10 short statements followed by options of varying severity.
- Mother underlines response that comes closest to how she has been feeling in the previous 7 days.

See also the 'Assessment tools and rating scales' section in Chapter 2 (Affective disorders), page 43.

Guidelines

Postnatal depression and puerperal psychosis. SIGN Publication Number 60*

Definitions

Postnatal depression (PND) is regarded as any non-psychotic depressive illness of mild to moderate severity occurring during the first postnatal year. It is important to distinguish PND from 'baby blues', the brief episode of misery and tearfulness that affects at least half of all women following delivery, especially those having their first baby. Puerperal psychosis is a mood disorder accompanied by features such as loss of contact with reality, hallucinations, severe thought disturbance and abnormal behaviour.

Diagnosis, screening and prevention

A   Procedures should be in place to ensure that all women are routinely assessed during the antenatal period for a history of depression.

There is no evidence to support routine screening in the antenatal period to predict development of PND.

D   All women should be screened during pregnancy for previous puerperal psychosis, history of other psychopathology (especially affective psychosis) and family history of affective psychosis.

☑   When assessing women in the postnatal period it is important to remember that normal emotional changes may mask depressive symptoms or be misinterpreted as depression.

☑   Primary care teams should be aware that with decreasing duration of stay in postnatal wards, puerperal psychosis is more likely to present following a mother's discharge home.

C   The EPDS should be offered to women in the postnatal period *as part of* a screening programme for PND.

C   The EPDS is not a diagnostic tool. Diagnosis of PND requires clinical evaluation.

☑   A cut-off on the EPDS of 10 or above is suggested for whole population screening.

☑   The EPDS should be used at approximately 6 weeks and 3 months following delivery and should be administered by trained health visitors or other health professionals.

☑   In high risk women it may be effective to have postnatal visits, interpersonal therapy and/or antenatal preparation.

☑   Women identified at high risk of puerperal psychosis should receive specialist psychiatric review.

Management

B   PND and puerperal psychosis should be treated.

D   PND should be managed in the same way as depression at any other time, but with the additional considerations regarding the use of antidepressants when breastfeeding and in pregnancy.

☑   St John's wort and other alternative medicines should not be used during pregnancy and lactation until further evidence as to their safety in these situations is available.

☑   The use of hormonal therapies in the routine management of patients with PND is not advised.

B   Psychosocial interventions should be considered when deciding on treatment options for a mother diagnosed as suffering from PND.

C   The effects of a mother's PND on other family members and their subsequent needs should be considered and treatment offered to them as appropriate.

C   Interventions that work with more than one family member at a time should be considered when assessing the treatment options available.

☑   The psychosocial treatment option chosen should reflect both clinical judgement and the mother's and family's preferences where possible.

D   Puerperal psychosis should be managed in the same way as psychotic disorders at any other time, but with the additional considerations regarding the use of drug treatments when breastfeeding and in pregnancy.

Mother and baby units

D   The option to admit mother and baby together to a specialist unit should be available. Mother and babies should not be admitted to general psychiatric wards routinely.

☑   A multiprofessional assessment, including social work, and involving family members, should take place to review the decision to admit mother and baby to a specialist unit either before or shortly after admission.

☑   Clinical responsibility for the baby whilst the mother is an inpatient needs to be clearly determined.

Prescribing

The following general principles governing prescription of new medication or the continuation of established therapy during pregnancy and in breastfeeding apply to all recommendations in this guideline.

*   establish a clear indication for drug treatment (i.e the presence of significant illness in the absence of acceptable or effective alternatives)

*   use treatments in the lowest effective dose for the shortest period necessary

*   drugs with a better evidence base (generally more established drugs) are preferable

*   assess the benefit/risk ratio of the illness and treatment for both mother and baby/fetus.

B   The risks of stopping tricyclic or SSRI antidepressant medication should be carefully assessed in relation to the mother's mental state and previous history. There is no indication to stop tricyclic or SSRI antidepressant medication as a matter of routine in early pregnancy.

C   There is no clinical indication for women treated with TCAs (other than doxepin) paroxetine, sertraline or fluoxetine to stop breastfeeding, provided the infant is healthy and its progress monitored.

Websites

The National Childbirth Trust,
Website: www.nctpregnancyandbabycare.com
Action on Puerperal Psychosis,
Website: www.bham.ac.uk/app
The Scottish Association for Mental Health,
Website: www.samh.org.uk

This guideline was issued in June 2002 and will be updated as new evidence becomes available. **A, B, C** and **D** indicate grades of recommendation ☑ indicates a good practice point (see Appendix II for full details). * Reproduced with permission from the Scottish Intercollegiate Guidelines Network, Edinburgh.

Personality disorders

General Topics

Admission patterns of patients with personality disorder

Dasgupta P, Barber J 2004 Admission patterns of patients with personality disorder. Psychiatric Bulletin 28: 321–323

This study examines the prevalence and admission patterns of patients with personality disorder admitted to general psychiatric wards in Scotland.

Method

- A retrospective case note study in Ayrshire, Scotland.
- Investigated patients with personality disorder admitted to hospital in 2001.
- The diagnosis of personality disorder was taken from discharge diagnoses.
- Data were collected on:
  - diagnosis
  - associated alcohol and substance misuse in 2001
  - number and length of admissions over a 5-year period, if the patient had had an admission of over 5 weeks in 2001.

Results

- Over 800 patients were included.
- 7.35% of patients were given a diagnosis of personality disorder, 38 of whom were women.

- More admissions were seen in the younger age group.
- Of the 62 patients with personality disorder:
  - 63% had a primary diagnosis of personality disorder
  - 30% had an additional diagnosis of psychiatric disorder
  - 19.3% had a diagnosis of alcohol or substance misuse disorder
  - 4.8% had both a psychiatric disorder due to alcohol or substance misuse and a personality disorder.
- Personality subtypes were:
  - 51.6%   Emotionally unstable
  - 25.8%   Unspecified
  - 12.9%   Dissocial
  - 4.8%   Anxious avoidant
  - 1.6%   Dependent/histrionic and other.
- 25 of the patients with personality disorder remained as inpatients for over 5 weeks.
- 24% of patients with admissions of over 5 weeks' duration had a diagnosis of emotionally unstable personality disorder.
- The average inpatient stay was 13.24 weeks, compared with 8.02 for the whole group.

Discussion

- Personality disorder accounted for just over 7% of all admissions to general adult psychiatric beds in 2001.
- The majority of those admitted with personality disorders are female, under 40 and with emotionally unstable personality disorder.
- The admission rates for this hospital were slightly higher than the figures quoted for Scotland as a whole over the same time period.

Bender DS, Dolan RT, Skodol AE et al 2001 Treatment utilisation by patients with personality disorders. American Journal of Psychiatry 158: 295–302

- Personality disordered patients place a great demand on health and social services.
- Borderline and schizotypal personality disorders are associated with extensive use of mental health services.

Information and Statistics Division Scotland 2001 Mental illness discharges by type of admission, year ending 31 March 2001. ISD Scotland 'National Statistics' release. ISD Scotland, Edinburgh

- 5% of acute psychiatric admissions in those under 65 years can be accounted for by those with personality disorder.

Zimmerman M, Mattia JI 1999 Differences between clinical and research practices in diagnosing borderline personality disorder. American Journal of Psychiatry 156: 1570–1574

- Research-orientated diagnostic criteria tend to increase the likelihood of clinicians making a diagnosis of personality disorder.

Department of Health 1995 Mental illness hospitals and units in England. Results from a mental health enquiry. Statistical bulletin. HMSO, London; Olfsun M, Machanic D 1996 Mental disorders in public, private non-profit and proprietary general hospitals. American Journal of Psychiatry 160: 274–283

- Found the prevalence of personality disorder in psychiatric inpatients to be 50% or more using standardised assessment instruments.

Management of personality disorders in acute inpatient settings 1: Borderline personality disorders

Fagin L 2004 Management of personality disorders in acute inpatient settings. Part 1: Borderline personality disorders. Advances in Psychiatric Treatment 10: 93–99

Indicators for admission of patients with a personality disorder include:
- crisis intervention, particularly to reduce the risk of suicide or violence to others
- treatment of comorbid psychiatric disorders – depression or psychosis
- chaotic behaviour endangering the patient and the treatment alliance
- stabilisation of existing medication regimens

- reviewing the diagnosis and treatment plan
- full risk assessment.

Admission can have a deleterious effect on patients and others, and should be taken into account. There should also be an awareness that not everyone can work with people with personality disorders. Some researchers have reported considerable improvements in specialised units run on psychodynamic, cognitive behavioural or dialectical behavioural lines; however, these interventions are not readily available in all districts.

Treatment in an acute inpatient setting can allow careful assessment by experienced staff, focusing on the present crisis and the need for containment in an informal setting. Significant others, carers, relatives and other agencies can be involved in the assessment. It is helpful to agree a care plan early on. There should be specified goals that are shared with the patient and all staff. There should be a focus on immediate needs, mostly of a practical nature. Clear boundaries should be set regarding tolerable behaviour, including aggression, absconding, suicidal gestures and the use of illicit substances or alcohol. Inpatient groups can be included in the treatment plan alongside medication if necessary. There should be staff support groups and adequate supervision, particularly of junior staff. The treatment plan can include early discharge arrangements for when the crisis has been overcome and a readiness to discharge if goals are not met. On discharge there should be consideration of a referral to community or specialist services with close and careful handovers through the care programme approach. A short duration of admission can be helpful.

In people who do not respond as predicted to treatment for an Axis I disorder, the coexistence of a comorbid personality disorder should be considered.

Important features in the management of people with personality disorder include:
- a flexible approach
- ensuring the patient is safe
- containment of strong emotions such as anger, aggression and hate
- encouraging reflection
- setting appropriate boundaries
- a collaborative approach
- watchfulness for splitting between and within staff teams
- awareness of countertransference.

Symptoms of affective dysregulation (mood lability, rejection sensitivity, inappropriate intense anger, depressive mood crashes or outbursts of anger) can respond to high dose fluoxetine or venlafaxine or to MAOIs.

When impulse control becomes the predominant feature (aggression, self-mutilation, self-damaging behaviour), SSRIs can be helpful, aided by the addition of lithium, carbamazepine, sodium valproate or low dose neuroleptics.

Bateman A, Tyrer P 2002 Effective management of personality disorder. National Institute of Mental Health in

England (NIMHE), Leeds. Online. Available: www.nimhe.org. uk/downloads/Bateman_Tyrer.doc

- Management principles in the treatment of personality disorders.
- Staff should devote effort to achieving adherence to the treatment.
- Treatment should:
  - be well structured
  - have a clear focus
  - have a theoretical basis that is coherent to both staff and patients
  - be relatively long term
  - be well integrated with other services available to the patient, using the care programme approach as the principal means of networking, communicating and reviewing plans between different elements of the service
  - involve a clear treatment alliance between staff and patient.

Duggan M 2002 Developing services for people with personality disorder: The training needs of staff and services. National Institute of Mental Health in England (NIMHE), Leeds. Online. Available: www.nimhe.org.uk/ downloads/ReportJuly112002.doc

- Key competencies of staff that help them work effectively with such patients include emotional resilience, clarity about personal and interpersonal boundaries, and ability to tolerate the intense emotional impact that these patients can have on them.

Kullgren G 1988 Factors associated with completed suicide in borderline personality disorder. Journal of Nervous and Mental Diseases 176: 40–44

- Analysis of completed suicides by patients with borderline personality disorder has shown that perceived rejection by caregivers has often been the precipitating cause.

Webster JM 1991 Rethinking inpatient treatment of borderline patients. Perspectives in Psychiatric Care 27: 17–20

- The aim of emergency admission is to restore a sense of responsibility and rely on the patient's previously good internal resources.

Gallop R 1992 Self destructive and impulsive behaviour in the patient with a borderline personality disorder: rethinking hospital treatment and management. Archives of Psychiatric Nursing 6: 178–182

A clear understanding of the meaning of suicidal behaviour and the aims of the staff's response can help patients in a number of ways:

- It can enable patients to improve their interpersonal skills during conflicts.
- It can increase the internal regulation of unwanted emotions.
- It can allow patients to develop the skills to tolerate emotional distress until change occurs.
- It can aid the patient to learn self-management.

Definition

Coercive bondage – when staff feel that they carry more of the responsibility for keeping these suicidal patients alive than do the patients themselves. (*Source*: Hendin H 1981 Psychotherapy and suicide. American Journal of Psychotherapy 35: 469–480.)

See also the 'General topics' section in Chapter 30 (Treatment settings), page 432.

Management of personality disorders in acute inpatient settings 2: Less common personality disorders

Fagin L 2004 Management of personality disorders in acute in-patient settings. Part 2: Less common personality disorders. Advances in Psychiatric Treatment 10: 100–106

Admissions of patients with paranoid personality disorder are rare and may end up confirming the patient's paranoid suspicions about services. The outcome will largely depend on the ability of staff to contain their paranoid projections without counterattacking or responding in a defensive manner.

Schizoid and schizotypal personality disorders rarely present. They may be misdiagnosed as schizophrenia. Staff may need to be prepared to accept the unfathomableness of some patients and to function as a supportive alter ego in practical areas such as personal care, reality testing and basic interpersonal skills. The possibility of beginning to establish a modicum of relatedness will obviously depend on the degree and severity of withdrawal.

Staff should be prepared to accept silence as a powerful form of communication, to feel rejected and distanced, and to accept the patient's rhythm and pace of change. Validation by other patients often carries more weight than validation by staff

Inpatient interventions for patients with antisocial personality disorder are best carried out in residential or inpatient psychotherapy units that work within clearly defined boundaries. Patients admitted in crisis should be quickly assessed and the decision taken either not to treat but to take risk management actions or, if there is scope for intervention, to refer to the relevant service as soon as possible. Meanwhile, strict boundaries and conditions should be set regarding aggression, sexual acting out, theft and drug importation, with clear consequences if boundaries are crossed.

Gabbard GO, Coyne L 1987 Predictors of response of antisocial patients to hospital treatment. Hospital and Community Psychiatry 38: 1181–1185

Predictors of a positive or negative response to hospital treatment are outlined in Box 19.1.

Lion J 1990 Countertransference in the treatment of the antisocial patient. In: Gabbard GO (ed.) Countertransference issues in psychiatric treatment. American Psychiatric Press, Washington, DC

- A level of scepticism is important, particularly during assessments.
- It is important not to deny or normalise dangerousness.
- There should be an awareness of the possible polarities in feeling.
- The potential for sexual seduction by patients should be considered.
- Arrangements for the supervision of less experienced staff should be made.

In patients with hysterical and histrionic personality disorders, admission often follows a relationship crisis, with subsequent dramatic acts of self-harm. Difficulties exist in treating such patients in inpatient settings. These include the formation of rivalrous relationships with other patients and erotic transferences to staff. There is the potential for a negative cycle of increasingly dramatic behaviour in order to attract attention. This can provoke strong negative countertransference feelings in staff, who then ignore any demands and reinforce the cycle.

Obsessive–compulsive personality disorder is an ego-syntonic disorder. It does not generally cause distress to patients themselves, but can affect those with whom they work or live. Patients with this disorder are unlikely to end up in inpatient facilities. Should admission occur, patients may have the need to be perfect patients, with attempts to control anger, sadness or despair provoking rambling, circumstantial conversations. Focussing on the patient's feelings rather than facts or words can be helpful.

Patients with avoidant personality disorder are unlikely to be admitted to hospital unless they present with an Axis I diagnosis. Dynamic and cognitive behavioural approaches are the treatment of choice in outpatient environments.

In dependent personality disorder the intense submissiveness and clinginess, linked with difficulties in decision making and a tendency to relinquish responsibility to others, can impact on treatment of comorbid Axis I disorders. Clinical strategies should focus on the patient's responsibilities and independence. It should be borne in mind that improvement can be seen as a potential threat. The setting of time limits can be helpful.

See also the 'General topics' section in Chapter 30 (Treatment settings), page 432.

Personality disorder and depression

Newton-Holmes G, Tyrer P, Johnson T 2006 Personality disorder and the outcome of depression: meta-analysis of published studies. British Journal of Psychiatry 188: 13–20

- A meta-analysis of 34 studies of comorbid depressive and personality disorders.
- Personality disorder was defined on a categorical scale.
- It was carried out in response to the conflicting evidence regarding the outcome of treatment for depression in people with comorbid personality disorder.
- It was found that people treated for depression who had comorbid personality disorder were at twice the risk of a poor outcome compared to patients who did not have a comorbid personality disorder.
- This was true in all treatment groups except for the small ECT group.
- There was a trend for psychotherapy to be associated with poorer outcome in people with comorbid personality disorder.
- The results were not significantly affected by the instrument used to measure depression outcome.

Box 19.1

Predictors of a positive or negative response to hospital treatment

Positive response
- Presence of anxiety
- Concurrent depressive disorder
- Concurrent psychotic illness (non-affective and not organic)

Negative response
- History of arrest or conviction for felony
- History of repeated lying, use of alternative names and fraud
- Ongoing legal issues on admission
- Hospitalisation as an alternative to imprisonment
- Previous violence to others
- Diagnosis of organic brain impairment

Personality and comorbidity of common psychiatric disorders

Khan AA, Jacobson KC, Gardner CO, Prescott CA, Kendler KS 2005 Personality and comorbidity of common psychiatric disorders. British Journal of Psychiatry 186: 190–196

- Little is known about the degree to which comorbidity arises from variation in normal personality.
- This study aimed to examine the association between variations in normal personality and the comorbidity of eight common psychiatric and substance use disorders.
- 7588 participants were assessed from a population-based twin registry.
- Assessments were made of internalising (depression, anxiety, panic and phobias) and externalising disorders (drug and alcohol dependence, antisocial personality and conduct disorders).
- Personality dimensions of neuroticism, extraversion and novelty seeking were assessed.
- High neuroticism appears to be a broad vulnerability factor for comorbid psychiatric disorders.
- Novelty seeking is modestly important for comorbid externalising disorders.

See also the 'General topics' section in Chapter 12 (General psychiatry), page 184.

Predictors of antisocial personality

Simonoff E, Elander J, Holshaw J et al 2004 Predictors of antisocial personality. Continuities from childhood to adult life. British Journal of Psychiatry 184: 118–127

Aims

This study aimed to explore the independent and joint effects of childhood characteristics on the persistence of antisocial behaviour into adult life.

Method

- 107 twin pairs were recruited in childhood and followed up 10–25 years later.
- They were interviewed using a variety of measures regarding childhood and adult psychiatric disorder, psychosocial functioning, and psychosocial functioning and psychosocial and cognitive risk factors.

Results

- Using univariate analysis, childhood hyperactivity and conduct disorder showed equally strong prediction of ASPD and criminality in early and mid-adult life.

- Lower IQ and reading difficulties were most prominent in their relationships with childhood and adolescent antisocial behaviour.
- In multivariate modelling, childhood conduct disorder and hyperactivity predicted adult ASPD, even when intervening risk factors were accounted for.
- The number of hyperactive and conduct symptoms also predicted adult outcome.

Conclusions

- The study showed that childhood disruptive behaviour has powerful long-term effects on adult antisocial outcomes, which continue into middle adulthood.
- The importance of the number of symptoms, the presence of disruptive disorder and intermediate experiences highlight three areas where interventions might be targeted.

Robins LN 1978 Sturdy childhood predictors of adult antisocial behaviour: replications for longitudinal studies. Psychological Medicine 8: 611–622

- Found that around a third of those with conduct disorder in childhood go on to have antisocial personality disorder in adulthood.

Zoccolillo M, Pickles A, Quinton D et al 1992 The outcome of childhood conduct disorder: implications for defining adult personality and conduct disorder. Psychological Medicine 22: 971–986

- Found that one-third of children with conduct disorder go on to have other types of personality disorder, psychiatric and psychosocial difficulties.

Olweus D 1979 Stability in aggressive reaction patterns in males: a review. Psychological Bulletin 86: 852–875

- High levels of aggression in childhood predict later antisocial behaviour.

Farrington DP, Loeber R, Van Kammen WB 1990 Long term criminal outcomes of hyperactivity–impulsivity–attention deficit and conduct problems in childhood. In: Robins LN, Rutter M (eds) Straight and devious pathways from childhood to adulthood. Cambridge University Press, Cambridge, pp 62–81

- Hyperactivity in childhood is associated with later antisocial behaviour.

Kerr M, Tremblay RE, Pagani L et al 1997 Boys: behavioural inhibition and the risk of later delinquency. Archives of General Psychiatry 54: 809–816

- Aloofness or the absence of friendship in childhood predicts later antisocial behaviour.

Fergusson DM 1996 The role of adolescent peer affiliations in the continuity between childhood behavioural adjustment and juvenile offending. Journal of Abnormal Child Psychology 24: 205–221

- Having delinquent peer groups in childhood is associated with adult antisocial behaviour.

Caspi A, Elder JMH, Herbener ES 1990 Childhood personality and the prediction of life-course patterns. In: Robins LN, Rutter M (eds) Straight and devious pathways from childhood to adulthood. Cambridge University Press, Cambridge, pp 13–55

- Premature termination of education is associated with later antisocial behaviour.

Policy and Legislation

Personality disorder: no longer a diagnosis of exclusion

National Institute of Mental Health in England 2003 Personality disorder: no longer a diagnosis of exclusion. Policy implementation guidance for the development of services for people with personality disorder. NIMHE, Leeds[†] Online. Available: www.dh.gov.uk/assetRoot/04/05/42/30/04054230.pdf

Guidance produced to aid the implementation of the NSF for Mental Health as it applies to people with a personality disorder. The document provides information for trusts about the government's intentions for the delivery of personality disorder services within general mental health and forensic settings. All trusts delivering mental health services need to consider how to meet the needs of patients with a personality disorder who experience significant distress or difficulty as a result of their disorder. Funding will be available to enable trusts to develop personality disorder services over the 3-year period 2003–2006.

There is a perceived gap in services for people with a primary diagnosis of personality disorder in general adult and forensic settings. There is also a need for appropriate education and training for mental health practitioners in this area.

Key points

General adult mental health services
1. Good practice indicates that service provision for personality disorder can most appropriately be provided by means of:

- the development of a specialist multidisciplinary personality disorder team to target those with significant distress or difficulty who present with complex problems
- the development of specialist day patient services in areas with high concentrations of morbidity.

Forensic services
2. In future, forensic services will need to consider how to develop expertise in the identification and assessment of personality disordered offenders in order to provide effective liaison to MAPPPs.

3. The DH expects to prioritise the national development of a small number of personality disorder centres within regional forensic services to provide a dedicated infrastructure for the assessment, treatment and management of personality disordered offenders.

Staff selection, supervision, education and training
4. The DH will engage in dialogue with the Royal Colleges, regulatory bodies and curriculum setting bodies to:

- address the gap in training at pre-registration and pre-qualification for key disciplines
- influence the content of undergraduate syllabuses
- influence the mechanisms determining the selection of CPD educational opportunities.

5. The DH expects to develop new training opportunities, inviting tenders from recognised sites of good practice and from training providers to offer a range of inputs to trusts delivering personality disorder services, and to expand the pool and range of personality disorder courses available nationally. Training providers will need to consider how best to involve service users in training professionals.

See also the 'Policy and legislation' section in Chapter 27 (Service provision), page 406.

Treatment – Psychopharmacology

Drug treatment for personality disorders

Tyrer P, Bateman AW 2004 Drug treatment for personality disorders. Advances in Psychiatric Treatment 10: 389–398

Almost all drug trials for personality disorder have been for borderline personality disorder. It can be difficult to separate core components of personality disorder from secondary psychiatric components. A number of theories are discussed as to why drugs might be beneficial in personality disorder. With regard to the use of antipsychotic medications in personality disorder, although it is likely that they may be of benefit, their role has not been adequately defined. The risks of self-harm and overdose will likely outweigh the evidence that MAOIs have benefit in patients with borderline personality disorder. Newer reversible MAOIs have not been studied. Trials regarding the effects of carbamazepine have been limited in numbers, although there may be beneficial effects.

Zanarini MC, Frankenburg FR 2001 Olanzapine treatment of female borderline personality disorder patients: a double-blind, placebo-controlled pilot study. Journal of Clinical Psychiatry 62: 849–854

- Three out of four patients with borderline personality disorder had received polypharmacy.

Tyrer P, Mitchard S, Methuen C et al 2003 Treatment-rejecting and treatment-seeking personality disorders: Type R and Type S. Journal of Personality Disorders 17: 265–270

- Most people with personality disorder do not wish to be treated with drugs (treatment-resisting).
- It is suggested that the subgroup who are treatment-seeking should not be regarded as typical and that differences in patients regarding desire for treatment may have an impact on treatment outcomes.

Soloff PH, George A, Nathan RS et al 1986 Progress in pharmacotherapy of borderline disorders: a double blind study of amitriptyline, haloperidol and placebo. Archives of General Psychiatry 43: 691–697

- Amitriptyline was not helpful in the treatment of borderline personality disorder. Haloperidol was more effective than amitriptyline, even in treating symptoms of depression.
- This RCT found that low dose typical antipsychotic drugs (haloperidol) are beneficial in comparison with placebo and amitriptyline.
- These results were not replicated in a 4-month continuation study.

Cornelius JR, Soloff PH, Perel JM et al 1993 Continuation pharmacotherapy of borderline personality disorder with haloperidol and phenelzine. American Journal of Psychiatry 150: 1843–1848

- Haloperidol was beneficial when compared to placebo for the symptom of irritability.
- In general, phenelzine was of greater benefit than haloperidol.
- The treatment group had a dropout rate twice that of the placebo group.

Montgomery SA, Montgomery D 1982 Pharmacological prevention of suicidal behaviour. Journal of Affective Disorders 4: 291–298

- Flupenthixol was found to be beneficial in reducing the number of subsequent episodes of self-harm.

Tyrer P, Sievewright N, Ferguson B et al 1993 The Nottingham Study of Neurotic Disorder. Effect of personality status on response to drug treatment, cognitive therapy and self-help over two years. British Journal of Psychiatry 162: 219–226

- A RCT of the treatment of common anxiety and depressive disorders.
- Follow-up 2 years after the initial trial showed that patients treated with dothiepin had the same outcome regardless of whether they had a personality disorder or not.
- In comparison, patients with personality disorder who had psychological treatments (self-help and cognitive behavioural therapy) had worse outcomes than those who did not have a personality disorder.

Coccaro EF, Kavoussi RJ 1997 Fluoxetine and impulsive aggressive behaviour in personality-disordered subjects. Archives of General Psychiatry 54: 1081–1088

- These studies showed that SSRIs were of benefit in the reduction of aggressive, impulsive and angry behaviour in patients with borderline and aggressive personality disorders.

Healy D 2003 Lines of evidence on the risks of suicide with selective serotonin reuptake inhibitors. Psychotherapy and Psychosomatics 72: 71–79

- Suggested that suicidal behaviour may be provoked by SSRIs in a minority of patients.

Links PS, Steiner M, Boiago I et al 1990 Lithium therapy for borderline patients: preliminary findings. Journal of Personality Disorders 4: 173–181

- Lithium is found to have beneficial effects on aggression in patients with borderline personality disorder.

Hollander E, Tracy KA, Swann AC et al 2003 Divalproex in the treatment of impulsive aggression: efficacy in Cluster B personality disorders. Neuropsychopharmacology 28: 1186–1197

- A small RCT.
- Showed the efficacy of divalproex sodium in the treatment of borderline personality disorder.

Seivewright H, Tyrer P, Casey P et al 1991 A three year follow up of psychiatric morbidity in urban and rural primary care. Psychological Medicine 21: 495–503

- Benzodiazepines are widely used in patients with personality disorder despite fears regarding dependence.

- They are more likely to be used long term than in patients who do not have a personality disorder; this may relate to their efficacy rather than to dependence in this group.

Treatment – Psychological Therapies

Psychological treatment for personality disorders

Bateman AW, Tyrer P 2004 Psychological treatment for personality disorders. Advances in Psychiatric Treatment 10: 378–388

There is evidence that certain treatments have some efficacy in personality disorder. These, and the planning and management of treatment in patients with personality disorder, are considered here. The inherent difficulties of evaluating treatments in this group are discussed, including the choice of outcome measures. Results of a trial comparing a manualised dynamic therapy (transference focused psychotherapy), dialectical behaviour therapy and supportive psychotherapy are awaited.

Winston A, Pollack J, McCullough L et al 1991 Brief psychotherapy of personality disorders. Journal of Nervous and Mental Disease 179: 188–193

- Short-term dynamic psychotherapy and brief adaptational psychotherapy were equally effective and were beneficial in comparison with waiting list controls.
- Patients with borderline and narcissistic features were excluded.

Winston A, Laikin M, Pollack J et al 1994 Short-term dynamic psychotherapy of personality disorders. American Journal of Psychiatry 15: 190–194

- A further study which included patients with borderline and narcissistic personality disorders.
- It found similar results to the 1991 paper.

Bateman A, Fonaghy P 1999 The effectiveness of partial hospitalization in the treatment of borderline personality disorder: a randomised controlled trial. American Journal of Psychiatry 156: 1563–1569; Bateman A, Fonaghy P 2001 Treatment of borderline personality disorder with psychoanalytically oriented partial hospitalisation: an 18-month follow up. American Journal of Psychiatry 158: 36–42

- This randomised study found that a psychoanalytically orientated partial hospitalisation programme with standard psychiatric care for patients with borderline personality disorder had significant beneficial effects.

- This benefit was not apparent immediately.
- Benefit was greatest at 18 months and maintained after a further 18 months.
- This approach is fully manualised as a mentalisation-based treatment.
- It focuses on understanding, recognising and reflecting on the intentional mental state and actions of oneself and of others.
- Both group and individual therapy are used to allow patients to consider what feelings they evoke in others, and vice versa.

Clarkin JF, Foelsch P, Levy K et al 2001 The development of a psychodynamic treatment for patients with borderline personality disorder: a preliminary study of behavioural change. Journal of Personality Disorders 15: 487–495

- A cohort study of women with borderline personality disorder ($n = 23$).
- Patients who received transference focused psychotherapy had self-injurious behaviour of less severity, significantly fewer suicide attempts and reduced hospitalisation (numbers and lengths of admission) when compared with the previous year.
- Approximately one in five patients withdrew.

Chiesa M, Fonaghy P, Holmes J et al 2002 Health service use costs by personality disorder following specialist and non-specialist treatment: a comparative study. Journal of Personality Disorders 16: 160–173

- This study compared long-term residential treatment using a therapeutic community approach, a step-down programme (briefer inpatient therapeutic community treatment with subsequent community-based dynamic therapy) and general community psychiatric care.
- The step-down programme was better than the other two treatment approaches in terms of self-harm, suicide rates, readmission rates and cost.
- After 3 years, those in the step-down programme continued to show greater benefits than the inpatient group.

Ryle A, Golynkina K 2000 Effectiveness of time-limited cognitive analytic therapy of borderline personality disorder: factors associated with outcome. British Journal of Medical Psychology 73: 197–210

- Cognitive analytic therapy may be beneficial for patients with borderline personality disorder.
- It appears to be as beneficial as other psychological therapies.
- Cognitive analytic therapy may be preferred by patients but the figures in terms of dropout rates do not reach significance.

- A RCT comparing CAT with best available standard care is underway.

Tyrer P, Thompson S, Schmidt U et al 2003 Randomised controlled trial of brief cognitive behaviour therapy versus treatment as usual in recurrent deliberate self-harm: the POPMACT study. Psychological Medicine 33: 969–976

- This study compared manual-assisted cognitive behavioural therapy (which included some aspects of dialectical behaviour therapy) with treatment as usual.
- Treatment as usual included psychotherapy and problem-solving therapy.
- Up to seven sessions of therapy were offered to people displaying recurrent self-harm ($n = 480$).
- This large multicentre study used ordinary therapists who had been trained in the approach.
- Patients received no special care which meant that they were not seen at home if they did not attend.
- 60% of patients attended for the intervention therapy.
- 39% of the intervention group went on to repeat self-harm compared to 46% in the treatment-as-usual group ($p = 0.20$).
- There were seven suicides, with five of these in the treatment-as-usual group.

Tyrer P, van den Bosch LM, Koeter MW et al 2004 Dialectical behaviour therapy for women with borderline personality disorder: 12-month, randomised clinical trial in The Netherlands. British Journal of Psychiatry 182: 135–140

- The frequency of self-harm was reduced by half in the intervention group in comparison to the treatment-as-usual group; however, there were great variations in the episodes of self-harm.
- Manual assisted cognitive behavioural therapy for patients with borderline personality disorder cost more than for other personality disorders.
- The effects on self-harm were not as great as in other personality disorders.

Linehan MM, Armstrong H, Suarez A et al 1991 Cognitive-behavioural treatment of chronically parasuicidal patients. Archives of General Psychiatry 48: 1060–1064

- 44 female patients with repeated self-harm (two episodes in the last 5 years, with one within the last 8 weeks) and borderline personality disorder were randomised to treatment with dialectical behaviour therapy or to treatment as usual.
- Those who received DBT for 12 months had reduced suicide attempts (number and severity) and inpatient admission (frequency and length).
- There were no benefits on outcomes of depression, hopelessness or reasons for living.

Linehan MM, Heard HL, Armstrong HE 1993 Naturalistic follow-up of a behavioural treatment for chronically parasuicidal borderline patients. Archives of General Psychiatry 50: 971–974

- Follow-up of patients from the 1991 study found that the beneficial effects of DBT on parasuicidal behaviour at 6 months did not continue at 12 months.
- With regard to hospitalisation, DBT had beneficial effects at 12 months, but not at 6 months.

Verheul R, van den Bosch LM, Koeter MW et al 2003 Dialectical behaviour therapy for women with borderline personality disorder: 12-month, randomised clinical trial in The Netherlands. British Journal of Psychiatry 182: 135–140

- This is the only study that supports the original trial of DBT.
- This study randomly assigned 58 women with borderline personality disorder to either 12 months of DBT or treatment as usual.
- Patients were included from addictions and general psychiatry services.
- DBT had lower dropout rates and significant reductions in harm to self by self-mutilation or by impulsive acts.
- Patients with more severe self-harming behaviours appeared to be helped the most.

See also the 'Treatment – Psychological therapies' section in Chapter 25 (Psychological therapies), pages 356, 357, 361-363.

Pervasive developmental disorders

20

Chapter contents

- General topics 297
- Treatment – Psychopharmacology 301
- Treatment – Psychological therapies 301
- Treatment – Others 301

General Topics

Asperger syndrome: from childhood into adulthood

Berney T 2004 Asperger syndrome: from childhood into adulthood. Advances in Psychiatric Treatment 10: 341–351

A number of screening tools are discussed. Diagnosis should take into account function in childhood as well as current function. The needs of people with Asperger syndrome are not ideally met either by general psychiatry or by learning disability psychiatry services. This needs to be addressed by education of staff. Specialist support services can provide alternative or additional support, depending on the level of support required.

Tantam D 2003 The challenge of adolescents and adults with Asperger syndrome. Child and Adolescent Psychiatric Clinics of North America 12: 775–782

- Asperger syndrome is associated with a wide range of disorders including anxiety, depression, obsessive–compulsive disorder, attention deficit hyperactivity disorder and alcoholism.
- It is also associated with family and marital problems.
- It is doubtful that autistic spectrum disorder predisposes to schizophrenia.
- The inherent diagnostic difficulties occurring should not delay treatment.

- There may be an association between Asperger syndrome and violent aggression. This case series found that 'hitting people' occurred in 40% of the sample.

Fombonne E 2003 Epidemiological surveys of autism and other pervasive developmental disorders: an update. Journal of Autism and Developmental Disorders 33: 365–382

- Autism was originally considered a rare disorder which occurred mainly in individuals with significant learning disability.
- Population prevalence of autistic spectrum disorder (versus autism) is 0.6%.
- 70–90% of this group are of normal learning ability.
- This increase in prevalence reflects the changes in diagnostic concepts rather than a true increase in prevalence.

Tuchman R, Rapin I 2002 Epilepsy in autism. Lancet Neurology 1: 352–358

- More than a third of people with autistic spectrum disorder will develop epilepsy.
- The risk of epilepsy is associated with the degree of developmental delay and any receptive language deficit.
- Epilepsy in Asperger syndrome has not been studied specifically but is likely to be lower at around 5–10% and with later onset.

McDougle CJ, Naylor ST, Cohen DJ et al 1995 A double-blind, placebo-controlled study of fluvoxamine in adults with autistic disorder. Archives of General Psychiatry 53: 1001–1008

- Showed that SSRIs were of benefit in people with autism and depression.

Powell A 2002 Taking responsibility: good practice guidelines for services – adults with Asperger syndrome. National Autistic Society, London

- The function of a person with Asperger syndrome should be viewed in the context of structure and support to reduce stress.

Segar M 1997 A survival guide for people with Asperger syndrome. NoRSACA, Nottingham. Online. Available: www. autismandcomputing.org.uk/marc2.htm

- People with Asperger syndrome may need to be explicitly taught social skills that others may learn intuitively.
- These skills might include how to make social overtures, how to complain and how to avoid exploitation.

Attwood T 2004 Strategies for improving the social interaction of children with Asperger syndrome. Autism 4: 85–100

- Skills regarding self-care may have to be taught to people with Asperger syndrome.
- These include activities of daily living (shopping, laundry and cleanliness).
- Obsessionality in some areas may lead to reduced attention to self-care.
- Social skills need to be taught (conversation, dating, coping with authority and asking for help) in order that individuals develop a positive identity and competence in social situations.

Measures adapted by universities to help students with autistic spectrum disorders

- A disability support service that has the skills and status to liaise with departments to help them adapt to the needs of these students (e.g. by extending work deadlines or modifying arrangements to enable a student to complete placements, practicals or fieldwork).
- A public education programme and specific training for both staff and students to make them aware of autistic spectrum disorders and their difficulties, and of the support service.
- A keyworker, usually a postgraduate student or member of staff, to whom a student can go for immediate advice or pastoral support.

- Specialist tuition to develop suitable study skills (e.g. language skills, structuring their work and organising their approach to studying).
- The use of aids such as handouts and tape recordings of lectures.
- Help with managing allowances, budgeting and everyday skills such as laundry and shopping. Mentorship schemes, possibly through the students' union, can draw in other students.
- A support network for isolated students. Group seminars, tutorial and study groups can all contribute, as can paired or group assignments and recreational activities.
- An introductory programme that includes first contacts (e.g. with a tutor), good induction and orientation (e.g. with maps of the campus and lists of important contacts and their roles), positive family contacts when appropriate and, above all, a flexible approach that adapts to different students and their particular needs. Safe places on campus where students can withdraw, calm down and refocus when anxiety or anger threatens to get out of control. The involvement of all elements, including the campus police and the students' union, can allow fragile students to complete their course successfully as well as learn to manage their over-arousal.
- A clear and realistic plan for the student's exit from university/college when they have completed their course. There should be reviews in the final year and, if the student is under 25 years old, Connexions (the careers and employment advisory agency designed to help people throughout adolescence and into adulthood) can be contacted.

Weblink The National Autistic Society: Prospects is a programme run by the National Autistic Society which addresses issues pertaining to recruitment and retention of employment in people with autistic spectrum disorder – www.nas.org.uk

Autistic spectrum disorders: lessons from neuroimaging

Toal F, Murphy DGM, Murphy K 2005 Autistic spectrum disorders: lessons from neuroimaging. British Journal of Psychiatry 187: 395–397

The aetiology of autism remains unknown. Advances have been made in the understanding of the neurobiological basis of the condition. There is inequality between social and cognitive skills in autism, with this being particularly prominent in high functioning autism/Asperger syndrome. The biological associates of poor social functioning are little understood at present.

Some mental health services exclude people with autistic spectrum disorder, arguing that it is not a true psychiatric disorder. The hypothesised genetic neurodevelopmental nature of the disorder contradicts this, as does its inclusion in psychiatric classification systems. Although the cause is currently unknown, it is thought to be a complex combination of genetic and environmental factors. One of the earliest indicators that it was neurobiological in nature was the high rate of associated epilepsy. Epilepsy affects approximately one-third of autistic children.

The services that do exist are few in number for adults, and most child and adolescent services do not offer long-term follow-up into adulthood.

Charman T 2002 The prevalence of autism spectrum disorders. Recent evidence and future challenges. European Child and Adolescent Psychiatry 11: 249–256

- The prevalence of autism is approximately 60 per 10,000 for autistic spectrum disorder.

Bailey A, Le Couteur A, Gottesman I et al 1995 Autism as a strongly genetic disorder: evidence from a British twin study. Psychological Medicine 25: 63–72

- Have since shown it to be among the most heritable of neuropsychiatric disorders.

Kanner L 1943 Autistic disturbances of affective contact. Nervous Child 2: 217–250

- First reports of abnormal brain development with descriptions of 'large heads'.

Courchesne E 2004 Brain development in autism: early overgrowth followed by premature arrest of growth. Mental Retardation and Developmental Disabilities Research Reviews 10: 106–111

- Most consistent finding is of increased brain volume, with evidence that it may be age dependent.
- Proposed that there is a period of accelerated development followed by a period of slowed development.

McAlonan GM, Daly E, Kumari V et al 2002 Brain anatomy and sensorimotor gating in Asperger's syndrome. Brain 125: 1594–1606

- Found that adulthood brain ageing is significantly different in people with autistic spectrum disorder.
- The early biological differences most probably modify brain maturation across lifespan.
- People with Asperger syndrome had significantly less grey matter in frontostriatal and cerebellar regions than controls.
- People with Asperger syndrome had significant differences in ageing of the cerebral hemispheres and caudate nuclei.

Sokol DK, Edwards-Brown M 2004 Neuroimaging in autistic spectrum disorder (ASD). Journal of Neuroimaging 14: 8–15

- Some specific brain regions are particularly implicated:
  - frontal
  - limbic
  - basal ganglia
  - cerebellar regions.

McAlonan GM, Cheung V, Cheung C et al 2005 Mapping the brain in autism. A voxel-based MRI study of volumetric differences and intercorrelations in autism. Brain 128: 268–276

- A study of a group of Chinese children with high-functioning autism.
- In a different study, children with autistic spectrum disorder were found to have a significant difference in the grey matter volumes of the ventral and superior temporal lobes, and the white matter volumes of the cerebellum, internal capsule and fornices.

Critchley HD, Daly EM, Bullmore ET et al 2003 The functional neuroanatomy of social behaviour: changes in cerebral blood flow when people with autistic disorder process facial expressions. Brain 123: 2203–2212

- Hypoactivation of the 'face area' in the right fusiform gyrus has repeatedly been reported in adults with autistic spectrum disorder when subjects look at faces.

Pierce K, Haist F, Sedaghat F et al 2004 The brain response to personally familiar faces in autism: findings of fusiform activity and beyond. Brain 127: 2703–2716

- The hypoactivation can be modified if the face is familiar or if there are different levels of emotional content of the faces.

Castelli F, Frith C, Happe F et al 2002 Autism, Asperger syndrome and brain mechanics for the attribution of mental states to animated shapes. Brain 125: 1839–1849

- Found decreased activation in the medial prefrontal cortex and amygdala during so-called 'mentalising' tasks in autistic people.
- This suggests that these areas form a crucial component of the brain system that underlies normal understanding of other minds.

Murphy DG, Critchley HD, Schmitz N et al 2002 Asperger syndrome: a proton magnetic resonance spectroscopy study of brain. Archives of General Psychiatry 59: 885–891

- People with autistic spectrum disorder have significant abnormalities in prefrontal lobe neuronal integrity, which appears to be related to the severity of symptoms.

Horowitz B, Rumsey JM, Grady CL et al 1998 The cerebral metabolic landscape in autism. Intercorrelation of regional glucose utilisation. Archives of Neurology 45: 749–755

- Positron emission tomography (PET) has shown differences in the connectivity of cortical–cortical and cortical–basal ganglia circuits.

Chugani DC 2004 Serotonin in autism and paediatric epilepsies. Mental Retardation and Developmental Disabilities Research Reviews 10: 112–116

- Some studies reported significant differences in serotonin synthesis.
- 5HT acts as a trophic or differentiation factor during brain development and helps in the modulation of social and repetitive behaviour.
- There is also growing evidence that people with autistic spectrum disorder may benefit from SSRIs and atypical antipsychotics.

Boddaert N, Barthelemy C, Poline J-B et al 2005 Autism: functional brain mapping of exceptional calendar capacity. British Journal of Psychiatry 187: 83–86

- Postulated that savant capacities may be sustained by a memory-processing network involving the temporofrontal regions, including the hippocampus.
- Structures in the medial temporal lobe are essential for normal memory functions, including acquisition of new information.

Increase in autism is due to changes in diagnosis

Katikireddi V 2004 Increase in autism is due to changes in diagnosis, study claims. BMJ News 328: 364

- The study by Jick and Kaye (see below) concluded that the increase in the incidence of autism is due to changes in diagnostic practice.

Jick H, Kaye JA 2003 Epidemiology and possible cause of autism. Pharmacotherapy 12: 1524–1530

- The diagnosis of behavioural and developmental disorders has fallen by 20% per year from 1992 to 2000.
- The diagnosis of autism, however, has increased by similar amounts over the same time period.
- The increased prevalence of autism was believed to be an artefact.
- The increase relates to the changes in diagnostic practices such as:

- improved identification
- increased availability of services.
- A comparison was made between two groups of boys – a group with autism and a group without autism.
- The researchers sought to identify factors that could be associated with the condition.
- Both groups received the same frequency of vaccines (including MMR) and medications. There were no differences between the groups with regard to their mothers' medication or illnesses during pregnancy.

Study finds no connection between MMR vaccine and autism

Gottleib S 2004 Study finds no connection between MMR vaccine and autism. BMJ News 328: 421

This article reported on a study that found no relationship between the combined vaccination against measles, mumps and rubella (MMR) and the development of autism.

DeStefano F, Karapur B, Thompson WW et al 2004 Age at first measles-mumps-rubella vaccination in children with autism and school matched control subjects: a population-based study in metropolitan Atlanta. Pediatrics 113: 259–266

Some advocacy groups hold the belief that autism is due to the thimerosal (a preservative) in the MMR vaccine.

Scientists have hypothesised that if thimerosal crossed the blood–brain barrier it could cause brain damage.

Thimerosal is no longer used in the US, but is still used in some vaccines worldwide.

Method

- The study reported the vaccination histories of 624 children with autism.
- The vaccination history was compared with a control group of 1824 school-matched children without autism.

Results

- 70.5% of autistic children and 67.5% of controls were vaccinated by the recommended age of 12–15 months.
- The data showed no link between receipt of the MMR vaccine and the development of autism.
- There was no link in any of the subgroups of the children analysed – this included children who had an apparently normal development initially with later regression.

Treatment – Psychopharmacology

Combined vitamin B6–magnesium treatment in autistic spectrum disorder

Nye C, Brice A 2006 Combined vitamin B6–magnesium treatment in autistic spectrum disorder **(Cochrane Review)**. In: The Cochrane Library, Issue 2. Update Software, Oxford

- Three trials were reviewed.
- One crossover study had insufficient data to include in the analysis.
- A second crossover trial found no significant differences between treatment and control groups on any of the outcome measures of social interaction, communication, compulsivity, impulsivity or hyperactivity.
- The third study examined a group of children with pervasive developmental disorder presenting with symptoms which resemble pyridoxine-dependent epilepsy. The treatment group showed significant effects on IQ.

Treatment – Psychological Therapies

Parent-mediated early intervention for young children with autistic spectrum disorder

Diggle T, McConnachie HR, Randle VRL 2002 Parent-mediated early intervention for young children with autism spectrum disorder **(Cochrane Review)**. In: The Cochrane Library, Issue 2. CD003496. Update Software, Oxford

- Two studies were included.
- One study of parent training showed significant results on the outcomes of child language and maternal knowledge of autism.
- The clinician-delivered intervention in the second study had better child outcomes on direct measurement than the purely parent-mediated early intervention.
- There were no differences in parent and teacher measures.

See also the 'Treatment – Psychological therapies' section in *Chapter 25 (Psychological therapies), pages 360, 361.*

Treatment – Others

Gluten- and casein-free diets for autistic spectrum disorder

Millward C, Ferriter M, Calver S, Connell-Jones G 2004 Gluten and casein free diets for autistic spectrum disorder **(Cochrane Review)**. In: The Cochrane Library, Issue 2. CD003498. Update Software, Oxford

- One small trial was identified.
- A reduction in autistic traits was reported following a combined gluten- and casein-free diet.
- Results for cognitive skills, linguistic ability and motor ability were not significant.

Physical health

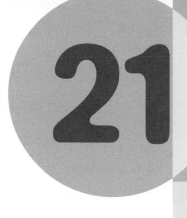

21

General topics

Causes of the excess mortality of schizophrenia

> Brown S, Barraclough B 2000 Causes of the excess mortality of schizophrenia. British Journal of Psychiatry 177: 212–217

Method

- A community cohort study of people with schizophrenia living in Southampton in the early 1980s.
- Aimed to calculate the standardised mortality ratio (ratio of deaths observed to deaths expected, expressed as a percentage).
- 370 patients with schizophrenia were followed over a 13-year period.
- The circumstances of death were examined.

Results

- Results were included for 96% of the original cohort.
- There were 79 deaths in the 13-year period.
- Standardised mortality ratios were significantly higher than for the general population, with rates of:
  - 298 for all causes of death
  - 232 for natural causes of death
  - 1273 for unnatural causes of death.

- There were higher levels of death due to:
  - circulatory, digestive, endocrine, nervous and respiratory disorders
  - smoking-related disease
  - suicide
  - undetermined causes.
- Deaths from cerebrovascular disease, diabetes and epilepsy were much higher than in the general population.

See also the 'General topics' section in Chapter 26 (Schizophrenia), pages 372-373.

A comparison of 10-year cardiac risk estimates in schizophrenia

> Goff DC, Sullivan LM, McEvoy JP et al 2005 A comparison of ten year cardiac risk estimates in schizophrenia patients from the CATIE study and matched cosntrols. Schizophrenia Research 80(1): 45–53

There is established evidence regarding the increased standardised mortality rates in schizophrenia.

Method

- 689 patients from the Clinical Trials of Antipsychotic Treatment Effectiveness (CATIE) Schizophrenia Trial were included.
- The 10-year risk of coronary heart disease was calculated at baseline and the result compared with matched controls.

Results

* There were significant increases in the 10-year CHD risk for male and female patients with schizophrenia when compared with the control group.
* The significant elevation in CHD was independent of BMI.
* In males the CHD was 9.4% compared with 7.0% in controls.
* In females the CHD was 6.3% compared with 4.2% in controls.
* People with schizophrenia were more likely to
  – smoke (68% versus 35%)
  – have diabetes (13% versus 3%)
  – have hypertension (27% versus 17%)
  – have lower HDL cholesterol levels (43.7 versus 49.3 mg/dl).
* There were no significant differences between the groups for total cholesterol levels.

Brown S, Brown J, Birtwistle L et al 1997 The unhealthy lifestyle of people with schizophrenia. British Journal of Psychiatry 171: 502–508

* A meta-analysis.
* Suicide and death by accident are:
  – generally increased in studies of people with schizophrenia
  – responsible for approximately 40% of the excess mortality.

See also the 'General topics' section in Chapter 26 (Schizophrenia), pages 372-373.

Diabetes mellitus and schizophrenia

Kohen D 2004 Diabetes mellitus and schizophrenia: historical perspective. British Journal of Psychiatry 184: S64–66

* A historical literature review.
* There is early evidence regarding an association between schizophrenia and diabetes mellitus, unrelated to the use of antipsychotic medication.
* More recent studies have found associations between the use of antipsychotic medication and the development of diabetes mellitus.

Results

* Historical literature described abnormal insulin and glucose levels and responses in people with severe mental illness, such as dementia praecox. These changes were found in patients prior to the introduction of antipsychotic medication.
* Early studies of people with schizophrenia proposed that a tendency towards diabetes could be uncovered by treatment with chlorpromazine.

Dietary improvement in people with schizophrenia

McCreadie RG, Kelly C, Connolly M et al 2005 Dietary improvement in people with schizophrenia. Randomised controlled trial. British Journal of Psychiatry 187: 346–351

Method

* The principal intervention in this RCT was the provision of free fruit and vegetables.
* Just over 100 people with schizophrenia were randomly allocated to receive free fruit and vegetables (along with dietary advice, instruction in meal planning and food preparation), free fruit and vegetables (alone) or treatment as usual.
* Bloods were taken to measure plasma folate, glucose, vitamins C and E and carotenoids, and serum total cholesterol and HDL cholesterol.
* Mental state was assessed using the PANSS.
* BMI was recorded as was the level of physical activity.
* At baseline and after 18 months, cardiovascular risk factors were measured including:
  – age
  – gender
  – smoking status
  – blood pressure
  – left ventricular hypertrophy
  – plasma glucose
  – serum total cholesterol and HDL cholesterol levels.

Results

* People with schizophrenia have a poorer diet than the general population.
* People with schizophrenia are less likely to eat fresh fruit and vegetables, low fat milk, potatoes, pasta or rice.
* This is more pronounced in men with schizophrenia.
* It was found that consumption of fruit and vegetables will increase if they are provided.
* The change in consumption of fruit and vegetables was not accompanied by a greater dietary change, with fruit and vegetables merely being added to the existing diet.
* There was no difference in mental state as assessed by PANSS in the groups receiving the fruit and vegetables.
* 12 months after the intervention there were no differences in fruit and vegetable consumption between the three groups.
* There were no differences at any time between the groups in micronutrients, BMI, physical activity or risk of CHD.
* The results showed that there is little value in providing additional information along with the fruit and vegetables as there were no differences in consumption between the two groups.

- The investigators concluded that although patients were willing to enter the study they were not motivated to change.
- Motivational interviewing may be required in addition to education.
- Patients with schizophrenia may benefit from being provided with foods that fulfil dietary requirements as they are not always able to make informed choices about dietary health.
- Primary and secondary care should probably be involved in the management of the physical health of people with schizophrenia.

Mortensen PD, Juel K1993 Mortality and causes of death in first admitted schizophrenic patients. British Journal of Psychiatry 163: 183–189

- Found that people with schizophrenia die early, especially from cardiovascular disease.

McCreadie R, Macdonald E, Blacklock C et al 1998 Dietary intake of schizophrenic patients in Nithsdale, Scotland: case-control study. British Medical Journal 317: 784–785

- People with schizophrenia make poor dietary choices.

Zino S, Skeaff M, Williams S et al 1997 Randomised controlled trial of effect of fruit and vegetable consumption on plasma concentration of lipid and antioxidants. British Medical Journal 314: 1787–1791

- Has shown that advice regarding fruit and vegetables has been successful in the general population.

McCreadie RG, Kelly C 2000 Patients with schizophrenia who smoke: private disaster, public resource. British Journal of Psychiatry 176: 109

- Found that two-thirds of their patients smoked, spending approximately a third of benefits on tobacco.

Department of Health 2005 School fruit and vegetable scheme. DH, London

- A free piece of fruit or vegetable has been provided for children in school in England as part of the National School Fruit and Vegetable Scheme.

Effects of antipsychotics on fat deposition and changes in leptin and insulin levels

Zhi-Jun Zhang, Zhi-Jan Yao, Wen Liu et al 2004 Effects of antipsychotics on fat deposition and changes in leptin and insulin levels. Magnetic resonance imaging study of previously untreated people with schizophrenia. British Journal of Psychiatry 184: 58–62

Weight gain is a common side effect of antipsychotic use and can lead to further morbidity and poor adherence to treatment. Mechanisms for antipsychotic-related weight gain are likely to be multifactorial.

This study looks specifically at effects of initial antipsychotic treatment on abdominal fat deposition and how this increase in body fat related to circulation of leptin, insulin and lipid levels in drug-naive patients with first episode psychosis.

Method

- This study was carried out in China.
- All subjects met DSM-IV criteria and were experiencing their first episode of psychosis.
- They had not had previous treatment with antipsychotic medication.
- 46 inpatients were recruited.
- Controls were age- and gender-matched members of hospital staff.
- The subjects had no concurrent medical conditions which would have an impact on their weight.
- Antipsychotic treatment (mainly risperidone and chlorpromazine) followed local practice.
- Clozapine and olanzapine were not studied.
- Diazepam or anticholinergic drugs were prescribed if required for side effects.
- Patients received an average of 2500 kcal (men) and 2200 kcal (women) and had the opportunity to have an hour's exercise per day.
- Measures of body fat indicators were weight, height, waist and hip circumference, BMI and WHR (waist: hip ratio) calculated on admission, weekly and at 10 weeks. Measurement of subcutaneous fat (SUB) and intra-abdominal fat (IAF) was performed by MRI scans performed on admission and at 10 weeks.

Results

- 30 patients were given risperidone (average of 4.77 mg for men and 4.26 mg for women). A further 15 were given chlorpromazine (average dose of 600 mg).
- There were significant increases in all weight and fat indicators after 10 weeks of treatment with antipsychotic medication in the patient group.
- Weight increase was most marked in men.
- There was substantial elevation in plasma leptin in the patient group after 10 weeks of treatment.
- A significant increase in non-fasting glucose was found after 10 weeks of treatment. Substantial and significant differences were also found in total and LDL cholesterol and triglycerides.

Thakore JH, Mann JN, Viahos L et al 2002 Increased visceral fat distribution in drug-naive and drug -free patients with schizophrenia. International Journal of Obesity 26: 137–141

- Reported that IAF but not SUB (determined by CT) was significantly increased in patients with schizophrenia – this was unrelated to antipsychotic medication.
- This occurred after treatment.

Cnop M, Landchild MJ, Vidal J et al 2002 The concurrent accumulation of intra-abdominal and subcutaneous fat explains the association between insulin resistance and plasma leptin concentrations: distinct metabolic effects of two fat compartments. Diabetes 51: 1005–1015

- Intra-abdominal fat is correlated with insulin resistance.

Newcomer JW, Haupt DW, Fucetola R et al 2002 Abnormalities in glucose regulation during antipsychotic treatment of schizophrenia. Archives of General Psychiatry 59: 337–345

- There is growing evidence that treatment with antipsychotics (particularly with clozapine and olanzapine) may impair glucose metabolism and increase the risk of diabetes.
- Showed these changes following chronic use of risperidone as well as more profound effects with olanzapine and clozapine.
- Drug-induced weight gain was not associated with symptom improvement.

Improving the physical health of long-stay psychiatric inpatients

Cormac I, Martin D, Ferriter M 2004 Improving the physical health of long-stay psychiatric in-patients. Advances in Psychiatric Treatment 10: 107–115

- Clinicians should give advice about smoking cessation and document it. They should consider the use of nicotine replacement therapy. Specialist smoking cessation clinics are successful. Induction of liver enzymes, by the ingested products of tobacco consumption, can affect drug metabolism.
- The Food Standards Agency recommends that five portions of fruit or vegetables should be consumed per day and at least two portions of oily fish per week.
- Thirst is a problem for many patients taking psychotropic medication. Patients may consume large quantities of carbonated and caffeine-containing drinks. Access to drinking water throughout the day should be provided.

- The Department of Health recommends 30 minutes of moderate intensity activity (e.g. brisk walking, heavy gardening and heavy housework) on at least 5 days per week. Opportunities for exercise may be limited for some long-stay patients and for others exercise may not be a realistic option.
- Psychiatrists must retain their basic medical skills. Nursing staff working in long-stay institutions must have competencies in physical health care.
- Psychiatric patients with physical disorders may not complain of symptoms or may have atypical symptoms. Psychiatric patients are not always referred to specialists, despite identified healthcare needs, and if referred may receive suboptimal treatment.
- Information about each patient's physical health should be stored in the same place in each medical record and should be readily accessible. Many long-stay patients receive an annual health check – the quality of information collected can be improved with the use of a semi-structured or structured interview. Long-stay patients should be given relevant information about health screening, be encouraged to take part and given the chance to attend.
- Dentists, opticians, hearing and speech and language therapists, chiropodists and dietitians should be involved in care.
- Monitoring of psychotropic medications and adverse effects should be undertaken.

Harris EC, Barraclough B 1998 Excess mortality of mental disorder. British Journal of Psychiatry 173: 11–53

- Over 27 forms of mental disorder were associated with an increased risk of premature death.
- 60% of deaths occurred due to natural causes.
- Increased mortality is related to the effects of the mental disorder and to the patient's altered lifestyle.

Brown S, Barraclough B, Inskip H 2000 Causes of the excess mortality of schizophrenia. British Journal of Psychiatry 177: 212–217

- In comparison with the general population, there is a three-fold increase in standardised mortality ratios for all causes, in particular for diseases of the circulatory, respiratory, digestive, endocrine and nervous systems.
- Excess mortality of schizophrenia could be lessened by reduction in smoking rates, reduced environmental risk factors and improved management of medical diseases.

Fisher WH, Barreira PJ, Geller JL 2001 Long stay psychiatric patients in state hospitals at the end of the 20th century. Psychiatric Services 52: 1051–1056

- 84% of long-stay psychiatric patients had an array of medical problems and nursing needs.

- The presence of significant medical problems is one of the barriers to discharge.

Department of Health 2000 National Service Framework for Coronary Heart Disease: Main Report. The Stationery Office, London

- The major causes of death in England and Wales are cardiovascular disease, cancer and respiratory disease.
- Modifiable lifestyle behaviours associated with these health risks are tobacco smoking, physical activity, poor diet and nutrition.

Meltzer H, Gill B, Petticrew M 1996 Economic activity and social functioning of residents with psychiatric disorders. OPCS Surveys of Psychiatric Morbidity in Great Britain, Report 6. HMSO, London

- Over 70% of long-stay patients smoke.
- The highest prevalence of smoking is in patients with psychotic disorders, with 52% smoking more than 20 cigarettes per day.

Allison DB, Mentore JL, Heo M 1999 Antipsychotic induced weight gain: a comprehensive research synthesis. American Journal of Psychiatry 156: 1686–1696

- Obesity is prevalent in many long-stay patients.
- It is exacerbated by physical inactivity and sometimes by medication, with the side effects of weight gain.

Fisher WH, Roberts R 1998 Primary health care service for long stay psychiatric inpatients. Psychiatric Bulletin 22: 610–612

- Primary care services delivering acute and chronic disease management according to NSF standards should be arranged for long-stay patients.
- The initial focus should be on those with the highest risk of coronary heart disease.

Definition

Long stay – in an institution for over 1 year.

Lifestyle and physical health in schizophrenia

Connolly M, Kelly C 2005 Lifestyle and physical health in schizophrenia. Advances in Psychiatric Treatment 11: 125–132

- Modifiable risk factors in patients with schizophrenia are discussed.

- It is noted that there have been no RCTs of the use of new anti-obesity drugs in the population of patients with schizophrenia and obesity.
- That atypical antipsychotics can affect lipid profiles is noted, although the precise mechanism is not clear.

Brown S 1997 Excess mortality of schizophrenia. A meta-analysis. British Journal of Psychiatry 171: 502–508

- People with schizophrenia are at increased risk of premature death when compared with their peers.
- Suicide accounts for over a quarter of this premature mortality.
- 12% of reported deaths were attributed to suicide.
- The majority of the remaining morbidity was due to natural causes, including cardiovascular disease, respiratory disease and diabetes.

Brown S, Birtwistle J, Roe L et al 1999 The unhealthy lifestyle of people with schizophrenia. Psychological Medicine 29: 697–701

- People with schizophrenia are significantly more likely to have a poor diet, take less exercise and smoke more heavily than matched groups in the general population.

McCreadie RG 2003 Diet, smoking and cardiovascular risk in people with schizophrenia. Descriptive study. British Journal of Psychiatry 183: 534–539

- Adults with schizophrenia in Scotland (n = 102) had diets which contained less than the recommended intake of fruit and vegetables, with consequent low carotenoid and vitamin C levels.
- There was a restricted range of intake from the major food groups.
- Two patients had folate deficiency.
- Female patients with schizophrenia were at significantly greater risk of being overweight or obese than the general female population.
- People with schizophrenia were also found to take little exercise. This may relate to features of schizophrenia and its treatment.

Kelly C, McCreadie R 2000 Cigarette smoking and schizophrenia. Advances in Psychiatric Treatment 6: 327–332

- People who have schizophrenia are much more likely to smoke compared to the general population (75–92% versus 30–40%).
- There appears to be an association between heavy smoking and more severe levels of illness.
- Smoking can induce hepatic enzymes with the subsequent metabolism of psychotropic medication. People who smoke often require higher doses of medication.

Meltzer HY, Fleischhacker WW 2001 Weight gain: a growing problem in schizophrenia management. Journal of Clinical Psychiatry 62 (Suppl 7): 1–43

- There is an association between higher body weight and higher levels of mortality.
- Weight gain can also lead to social stigmatisation.

Allison DB, Casey E 2001 Antipsychotic-induced weight gain. A review of the literature. Journal of Clinical Psychiatry 62 (Suppl 7): 22–31

- 1989 National Health Interview Survey.
- People with schizophrenia were more obese than people who did not have schizophrenia.
- This difference was significant in women with schizophrenia.

Tardieu S, Micallef J, Gentile S et al 2003 Weight gain profiles of new antipsychotics: public health consequences. Obesity Reviews 4: 129–138

- The effects of weight gain in people with schizophrenia include:
  - health risks – hypertension, atherosclerosis, type 2 diabetes, cardiovascular disease and stroke
  - stigmatisation
  - non-adherence to treatment
  - further impairment of quality of life
  - social withdrawal.
- Antipsychotic medication is associated with hyperglycaemia which can go undiagnosed.
- This may contribute to the excess morbidity and mortality found in patients with schizophrenia.

Fontaine KR, Moonseong H, Harrigan EP et al 2001 Estimating the consequences of antipsychotic induced weight gain on health and mortality rate. Psychiatric Research 101: 277–288

- This concluded that 492 deaths from suicide would be prevented per 100,000 patients with schizophrenia treated with clozapine.
- The consequences of the weight gained (which is presumed to be related to the use of antipsychotic medication) would lead to a further 416 deaths per 100,000 patients.

Kurtzthaler MD, Fleischhacker WW 2001 The clinical implications of weight gain in schizophrenia. Journal of Clinical Psychiatry 62 (Suppl 7): 32–37

- Patients with schizophrenia and obesity are 13 times more likely to request that their antipsychotic medication be stopped than those with schizophrenia who are not obese.

Dixon L, Welden P, Delahanty J et al 2000 Prevalence and correlates of diabetes in national schizophrenia samples. Schizophrenia Bulletin 26: 903–912

- This study compared the USA Schizophrenia Patient Outcomes Research Team (PORT) and National Health Interview Survey figures regarding schizophrenia and diabetes.
- The rate of diabetes in people with schizophrenia was greater than that in the general population between 1991 and 1996.
- This is relevant as it pre-dates the widespread use of atypical antipsychotics.

Ryan MCM, Collins P, Thakore JH 2003 Impaired fasting glucose tolerance in first episode, drug naive patients with schizophrenia. American Journal of Psychiatry 160: 284–289

- This study of untreated patients with first episode schizophrenia found that more than 15% had impaired fasting glucose compared with no cases in the healthy matched volunteers.

Henderson DC, Cagliero E, Gray C et al 2000 Clozapine, diabetes mellitus, weight gain, and lipid abnormalities. A five-year naturalistic study. American Journal of Psychiatry 157: 975–981

- A naturalistic uncontrolled follow-up study of 82 patients commenced on clozapine.
- There were 30 new cases of diabetes by the end of the fifth year.
- The patients had a mean age of 36.4 years and a mean BMI of 26.9.

Meyer JM 2001 Effects of atypical antipsychotics on weight and serum lipid levels. Journal of Clinical Psychiatry 62 (Suppl 7): 27–34

- Almost all the new cases of diabetes ($n = 30$) diagnosed in adults with schizophrenia were picked up at routine annual screening.
- Regular biochemical monitoring is required.

Ryan MCM, Thakore JH 2002 Physical consequences of schizophrenia and its treatment. The metabolic syndrome. Life Sciences 71: 239–257

- A metabolic syndrome in people with schizophrenia was described.
- Features of this syndrome are obesity (central or upper body), insulin resistance or hyperinsulinaemia, dyslipidaemia, impaired glucose tolerance or type 2 diabetes and hypertension.

Meaney AM, O'Keane V 2002 Prolactin and schizophrenia. Clinical consequences of hyperprolactinaemia. Life Sciences 71: 979–992

- Neuroleptic medication, in particular risperidone and conventional antipsychotics, can have negative effects on sexual and endocrine function.
- In women the negative effects include oligomenorrhoea, amenorrhoea and hypo-oestrogenism with associated cardiovascular effects.
- In men the negative effects include reduced steroidogenesis and spermatogenesis.

Naidoo U, Goff DC, Kilbanski A 2003 Hyperprolactinaemia and bone mineral density: the potential impact of antipsychotic agents. Psychoneuroendocrinology 28 (Suppl 2): 97–108

- There are a number of potential risk factors for osteoporosis in schizophrenia. These can be due to the schizophrenia itself, due to the treatment with medication or due to general factors.
- Factors due to schizophrenia include poor diet, limited weight-bearing exercise, smoking and polydipsia.
- Factors due to treatment with antipsychotic medication are hyperprolactinaemia and subsequent lowered oestrogen and testosterone.
- General factors associated with risks of fractures include sedation, postural hypotension with related dizziness and falls, and the use of anticonvulsant medication.

Hansen V, Jacobsen BK, Arnesen E 2001 Cause-specific mortality in psychotropic patients after deinstitutionalization. British Journal of Psychiatry 179: 438–443

- During the period of deinstitutionalisation there was a significant increase in the total mortality rate for patients with functional psychosis in Norway.

Salokangas RK, Honlonsen T, Stengard E et al 2002 Mortality in chronic schizophrenia during decreasing number of psychiatric beds in Finland. Schizophrenia Research 54: 265–275

- This study did not find an increase in mortality for patients with schizophrenia during the period of deinstitutionalisation.

Druss BG, Bradford WD, Rosenheck RA et al 2001 Quality of medical care and excess mortality in older patients with mental disorders. Archives of General Psychiatry 58: 565–572

- This study found that elderly patients with schizophrenia had significantly higher mortality rates after myocardial infarction.
- The excess mortality did not remain significant when factors regarding the provision and quality of care were included.
- It was not clear why patients with schizophrenia did not receive the same level of care as the general population or if this related to features of the patients or of the treatment providers.

See also the 'General topics' section in Chapter 26 (Schizophrenia), pages 372, 373.

Physical health and health risk factors in a population of long-stay psychiatric patients

Cormac I, Ferriter M, Benning R et al 2005 Physical health and health risk factors in a population of long-stay psychiatric patients. Psychiatric Bulletin 29: 18–20

The Department of Health has made improving the physical health of the population in the UK a priority. Chronic psychiatric disorders are associated with increased morbidity and premature mortality. The standardised mortality rate in people with schizophrenia is nearly three times that of the general population.

Aims

To evaluate the physical health and risk factors in a group of long-stay psychiatric patients in the Rampton High Secure Hospital.

Method

- Consenting patients were given a semi-structured interview to complete.
- Case notes were examined.
- Measurements of height, weight, waist circumference and blood pressure were taken and BMI calculated.

Results

- The mean age was 39 years
- Mean length of stay was nearly 9 years.
- The majority of patients had schizophrenia, with large numbers having disordered personalities or behaviours.
- 59 patients had learning disabilities, increasing the vulnerability to physical illness and with related communication barriers to obtaining health care.
- 71% smoked.

Obesity

- Rate of obesity was 36% in men and 75% in women compared with 17% and 22% in the general population, respectively.
- Three patients were underweight.
- Records showed there had been a substantial increase in weight during admission.
- With regard to waist size, 53% of men and 76% of women had waist sizes that required interventions to reduce health risk.

BMI and psychotropic medication

- There was no statistical difference between the mean waist size for female patients taking medication with a risk of weight gain and female patients on no medication with no risk of weight gain.
- Male patients taking medication with a risk of weight gain had a statistically significant greater mean waist size than male patients on no medication with no risk of weight gain.

Hypertension

- 48% of males and 9% of females were hypertensive compared with figures for the general population of 41% and 33%, respectively.

General morbidity

- 36% of the sample were breathless after climbing the stairs.
- 54% had one or more diagnosed health problems.

Discussion

- Aetiology of the physical health problems was not clear from this study.
- No invasive procedures took place.
- There are serious concerns about avoidable health risks in a population of long-stay psychiatric patients.
- Since completion of this study, Rampton has developed interventions for health promotion for long-stay patients.

Harris EC, Barraclough B 1998 Excess mortality of mental disorder. British Journal of Psychiatry 137: 11–53

- Attributed the poor physical health of psychiatric patients to:
  - poor health awareness
  - fewer opportunities for a healthy lifestyle
  - high rates of smoking
  - the risks associated with psychotropic medication.

Prevalence of diabetes and impaired glucose tolerance in patients with schizophrenia

Bushe C, Holt R 2004 Prevalence of diabetes and impaired glucose tolerance in patients with schizophrenia. British Journal of Psychiatry 184: S67–71

- A literature review.
- Difficulties in defining diagnostic criteria are noted for both type 2 diabetes and schizophrenia.
- The insidious onset of diabetes and the high rate of non-detection of diabetes in the community mean that it is a condition whose prevalence is difficult to establish.
- Prevalence also varies with age, ethnic origin and geographical location.
- Prevalence rates for diabetes range from 1.2 to 7.4%, depending on age.
- Prevalence rates for impaired glucose tolerance range from 6.3 to 16.7%.
- Studies of type 2 diabetes in people with schizophrenia have suggested that there may be a two- to four-fold increase in prevalence rates compared with the general population.

Results

- Evidence published prior to the introduction of antipsychotic medication noted an association between having a severe mental illness and the development of glycaemic abnormalities.
- Recent evidence suggests that people with schizophrenia are more likely to have diabetes and impaired glucose tolerance than the rest of the population.
- Impaired glucose tolerance in people with schizophrenia may pre-date treatment with antipsychotic medication.
- It was not possible to measure prevalence rates for diabetes or impaired glucose tolerance in this population.
- It was suggested that 15% of patients with schizophrenia may have diabetes, with similar numbers having impaired glucose tolerance.
- Screening for diabetes in patients with schizophrenia is recommended.

See also the 'General topics' section in Chapter 26 (Schizophrenia), pages 372, 373.

Risk for coronary heart disease in people with severe mental illness

Osborn DPJ, Nazareth I, King MB 2006 Risk for coronary heart disease in people with severe mental illness. Cross sectional comparative study in primary care. British Journal of Psychiatry 188: 271–277

People with severe mental illness have increasingly high rates of coronary heart disease. Deaths from CHD outnumber deaths from suicide.

Method

- A cross-sectional screening study in people with and without severe mental illness in primary care in North London.
- 182 patients with severe mental illness and 313 patients without severe mental illness were invited to attend for screening.
- The four most important risk factors for CHD were examined.
- Socioeconomic variables were recorded to examine the relationship between antipsychotic medication and the risk of coronary heart disease.

Results

- 225 patients were interviewed; of these, 75 had severe mental illness.
- Associations were found between severe mental illness and:
  - raised 10-year coronary heart disease risk scores
  - HDL cholesterol levels < 1.0 mmol/l
  - raised cholesterol/ HDL cholesterol ratios
  - diabetes mellitus
  - smoking.
- These associations were not fully explained by socioeconomic deprivation or by the effects of antipsychotic medication.
- There was a significant variation depending on age, with a more pronounced result as age approached 60 years.
- There were no differences between the groups for blood pressure levels or body mass indices.
- Over 60 years the CHD risk for people with SMI lowered; this may reflect a healthy survivor effect.

Patients with severe mental illness should be actively involved in CHD screening.

Policy and Legislation

The expert patient

Department of Health 2001 The expert patient: a new approach to chronic disease. Management for the 21st century. DH, London[†]

People are living longer. This increased longevity has brought with it an increased burden of morbidity (heart disease, stroke, cancer, arthritis, mental illness, etc.). The predominant disease pattern in most developed countries is of chronic or long-term illness rather than acute disease. The development of an Expert Patients Initiative was set out in *Saving Lives: Our Healthier Nation*.

Background

In Great Britain as many as 17.5 million adults may be living with a chronic disease. Older people suffer more.

For affected individuals and their families, living with long-term conditions can often mean physical and psychological difficulties, socioeconomic problems, reduced quality of life and, sometimes, social exclusion.

Although people have problems specific to their individual illness, there is a core of common needs:

- How to recognise and act upon symptoms
- Dealing with acute attacks or exacerbations of the disease
- Making the most effective use of medicines and treatments
- Accessing social and other services
- Dealing with fatigue
- Managing work
- Developing strategies to deal with the psychological consequences of the illness.

Research and practical experience in North America and Britain are showing that today's patients with chronic diseases need not be mere recipients of care – they can become key decision makers in the treatment process. By ensuring that knowledge of their condition is developed to a point where they are empowered to take some responsibility for its management and work in partnership with their health and social care providers, patients can be given greater control over their lives. Self-management programmes can be specifically designed to reduce the severity of symptoms and improve confidence, resourcefulness and self-efficacy.

The Expert Patients Programme, if successful, may lead to the following differences:

- More patients with chronic diseases improve, remain stable or deteriorate more slowly.
- More patients can effectively manage specific aspects of their condition (e.g. pain, complications, medication use).
- Patients with chronic diseases are less severely incapacitated by fatigue, sleep deprivation, low levels of energy and the emotional consequences of their illness.
- Patients with chronic diseases are effective in appropriately accessing health and social care services and gaining and retaining employment.
- More patients with chronic diseases are well informed about their condition and medication, feel empowered in their relationship with healthcare professionals and have higher self-esteem.

- People with chronic diseases contribute their skills and insight for the further improvement of services and as advocates of others.

The report recommends action over a 6-year period to introduce lay-led self-management training programmes for patients with chronic diseases within the NHS in England. The eight specific recommendations are as follows:

- Promote awareness and create an expectation that patient expertise is a central component in the delivery of care to people with chronic disease.
- Establish a programme for developing more user-led self-management courses to allow people with chronic illness to have access to opportunities to develop the confidence, knowledge and skills to manage their conditions better, and thereby gain a greater measure of control and independence to enhance their quality of life.
- Identify barriers to mainstreaming user-led self-management in the NHS and address these barriers, in the first instance through existing National Service Frameworks and others that are planned such as that on long-term health conditions.
- Integrate user-led self-management into existing NHS provision of health care – for example, into other National Service Frameworks, Healthy Living Centres and NHS Direct.
- Ensure that each primary care trust area has arrangements for user-led self-management programmes for key chronic conditions to be delivered or commissioned.
- Expand the practical support for user-led programmes provided by patients' organisations in partnership with health and social care professionals.
- Build, as part of continuing professional development programmes, a core course which would promote health professionals' knowledge and understanding about the benefits – for them as well as for patients – of user-led self-management programmes.
- Establish a national coordinating and training resource to enable health, social services and voluntary sector professionals to keep up to date with developments in the provision of self-management. Patients should be part of the process of developing professional education programmes.

Treatment – Psychopharmacology

Antipsychotic-induced weight gain

Allison DB, Mentore JL, Heo M et al 1999 Antipsychotic-induced weight gain: a comprehensive research synthesis. American Journal of Psychiatry 156: 1686–1696

Weight gain is associated with treatment with antipsychotic medication. It can impact on compliance with treatment and has implications for physical health.

Method

- A meta-analysis of studies of weight gain in patients treated with any antipsychotic medications.
- The analysis estimated the weight gain during the first 10 weeks of treatment.
- Qualitative information was also collected.

Results

- Treatment with placebo was associated with a mean weight reduction of 0.74 kg and may reflect preceding treatment with a neuroleptic medication.
- There was insufficient data regarding quetiapine.
- Treatment with:
  - clozapine was associated with a weight gain of 4.45 kg
  - olanzapine was associated with a weight gain of 4.15 kg
  - risperidone was associated with a weight gain of 2.10 kg.

Beasley CM Jr, Tollefson GD, Tran PV 1997 Safety of olanzapine. Journal of Clinical Psychiatry 58 (Suppl 10): 13–17, 19–21

- Antipsychotic-related weight gain appears to be greatest in individuals with a low initial body mass index.

Antipsychotics and diabetes

Haddad PM 2004 Antipsychotics and diabetes. British Journal of Psychiatry 184: S80–S86

Method

- A literature review.
- Non-prospective studies which examined the link between antipsychotic medication and diabetes mellitus.

Results

- Studies which are retrospective cannot estimate an association between antipsychotic medication and schizophrenia as they have not adequately considered other risk factors which may be at play.
- Retrospective studies do not sufficiently control for the variation in detection and diagnosis of diabetes.
- The majority of studies have found higher rates of diabetes in patients who are treated with antipsychotic

medication than people who do not receive antipsychotic medication.

- The rate of diabetes is higher in people with schizophrenia who receive atypical antipsychotic medication than people treated with conventional antipsychotic medication.
- People who are treated with atypical antipsychotic medication may be more actively screened for diabetes.

Further research should be performed using a prospective study design.

Antipsychotics and the risk of sudden cardiac death

Ray WA, Meredith S, Thapa PB et al 2001 Antipsychotics and the risk of sudden cardiac death. Archives of General Psychiatry 58(12): 1161–1167

There is evidence from case reports of a dose-related association between antipsychotic medication and sudden death. There are case reports regarding thioridazine, haloperidol and risperidone, amongst others. Antipsychotic medications have dose-related effects on cardiac electrophysiology.

Method

- A retrospective cohort study of 481,744 persons with a total follow up of 1,282,996 person-years.
- Computerised Medicaid pharmacy files provided data on the drug doses and days dispensed.
- Antipsychotics studied included haloperidol, fluphenazine, perphenazine, clozapine, chlorpromazine and thioridazine.
- Comparisons were made between low and moderate antipsychotic dosage (moderate dosage taken as greater than 100 mg of thioridazine equivalent).

Results

- There were 1487 confirmed sudden cardiac deaths (11.6 deaths per 10,000 person-years of follow-up).
- Patients receiving moderate doses of antipsychotic medication were more likely to be male, of younger age and have lower cardiovascular disease illness scores.
- Patients treated with antipsychotic medication at doses greater than 100 mg thioridazine equivalent had a 2.4-fold increase in the rate of sudden cardiac death.
- The risk of sudden death:
  - increased with age
  - is associated with being male
  - is higher in current users (multivariate rate ratio 2.39) than past users of antipsychotic medication
  - is associated with current treatment with antipsychotic medication

  - increased with increasing dose of antipsychotic medication.

Association between atypical antipsychotic agents and type 2 diabetes

Bushe C, Leonard B 2004 Association between atypical antipsychotic agents and type 2 diabetes: review of prospective clinical data. British Journal of Psychiatry 184: S87–S93

Background

- The majority of the evidence regarding the association between antipsychotic medication and diabetes mellitus in people with schizophrenia is retrospective.
- These studies have not adequately controlled for important confounding factors.

Method

- A systematic review of prospective studies of the association between schizophrenia, antipsychotic medication and diabetes.

Results

- There were no differences in glycaemic control between patients who were treated with antipsychotic medication and patients in the control group.
- There were no significant differences for any of the antipsychotic medication studies with regard to abnormalities in glycaemic control.
- There was no association between weight gain due to treatment and the risk of developing diabetes.
- The diabetogenic potential previously ascribed to atypical antipsychotic medication may be incorrect.
- Large prospective studies of sufficient length are required.
- There should be a consensus on the glucose measurement of choice.

Subramaniam M, Chong SA, Pek E 2003 Diabetes mellitus and impaired glucose tolerance in patients with schizophrenia. Canadian Journal of Psychiatry 48: 345–347

- A chart review of 607 patients with chronic schizophrenia treated with conventional antipsychotic medication.
- Patients found to have diabetes (4.9%) were excluded from further study.
- 194 patients gave informed consent and were investigated with fasting blood glucose and an oral glucose tolerance test.

- The prevalence of new cases of type 2 diabetes was 16%, leading to a total prevalence of 21%.
- An additional 31% of patients were found to have impaired glucose tolerance.

Conventional and atypical antipsychotics and the risk of hospitalisation for ventricular arrhythmias or cardiac arrest

Liperoti R, Gambassi G, Lapane KL et al 2005 Conventional and atypical antipsychotics and the risk of hospitalisation for ventricular arrhythmias or cardiac arrest. Archives of Internal Medicine 165(6): 696–701

Antipsychotic medication is linked with ventricular arrhythmias, cardiac arrest and sudden death. There is experimental evidence that atypical antipsychotics can prolong the QT interval; however, only clozapine has been associated with serious cardiac problems.

Method

- A case control study of American nursing home residents.
- Data were identified via Medicare claims.
- Patients admitted to hospital for ventricular arrhythmias or cardiac arrest in an 18-month period in 1998 and 1999 were included.
- Controls were identified (up to five per patient) from the same residential facilities.

Results

- 649 cases and 2962 controls were included.
- Treatment with typical antipsychotics was associated with almost twice the risk of admissions for ventricular arrhythmia or cardiac arrest.
- Admissions were particularly likely in people with cardiac disease.
- Atypical antipsychotic medication did not appear to increase the risk of arrhythmia or arrest.

Ray WA, Meredith S, Thapa PB et al 2001 Antipsychotics and the risk of sudden cardiac death. Archives of General Psychiatry 58: 1161–1167

- Investigated rates of sudden death in patients aged 15–84 years receiving treatment with typical antipsychotic medication.
- Patients receiving typical antipsychotic medication were twice as likely to die suddenly.
- The rate of sudden death in patients treated with thioridazine was associated with the dose of medication, with sudden death rate ratios of 1.3 in low

dose users (< 100 mg) and 2.39 in moderate dose users (> 100 mg).

Conley RR, Mahmoud R 2001 A randomised double-blind trial of risperidone and olanzapine in the treatment of schizophrenia or schizoaffective disorder. American Journal of Psychiatry 158: 765–774

- A double-blind trial comparing risperidone and olanzapine.
- Treatment with risperidone at high dose is associated with an increase in QT interval of 4.4 ms.
- Risperidone overdose was found to lead to severe QT prolongation in sporadic cases.

Dopamine antagonists and the development of breast cancer

Wang PS, Walker AM, Tsuang MT et al 2002 Dopamine antagonists and the development of breast cancer. Archives of General Psychiatry 59(12): 1147–1154

Method

- A retrospective cohort study comparing women who had been treated with dopamine antagonists ($n = 52,819$) and a control group ($n = 55,289$) in America.
- The women were over 20 years of age and did not have breast cancer at enrolment.
- Actual drug dispensing was used for an objective measure of medication use.
- Dopamine antagonists included were chlorpromazine, clozapine, haloperidol, perphenazine, pimozide and risperidone, amongst others.
- Prochlorperazine and metoclopramide were also reviewed.
- Cases of breast cancer were identified via a local cancer registry and breast cancer surgery statistics.

Results

- Treatment with dopamine antagonist antipsychotic medication was associated with a 16% increase in the risk of breast cancer.
- A dose–response relationship was noted.
- Treatment with dopamine antagonist antiemetic medication also increased the risk of breast cancer.
- There was no relationship between dopamine antagonists and the development of colon cancer – the control condition.

Schyve PM, Smithline F, Meltzer HY 1978 Neuroleptic-induced prolactin level elevation and breast cancer. Archives of General Psychiatry 35: 1291–1301

- Dopamine antagonist medication can increase serum prolactin levels.
- Elevations in serum prolactin levels are significantly higher in women when compared with men given equivalent doses.

Guidelines

Epilepsy and management of epilepsy in adults. SIGN Publication Number 70*
see pages 315-319

Introduction

In Scotland there are 20,000–30,000 people with active epilepsy and there will be between 2000 and 3500 new diagnoses each year. As it is a common condition, and the number of epilepsy specialists is very small, many people with epilepsy have been diagnosed and treated by non-specialists in both primary and secondary care.

MODELS OF CARE

D	A **structured management system** for epilepsy should be establised in primary care. As with other chronic diseases, an **annual review** is desirable.
D	The shared care management system adopted should seek to: • identify all patients with epilepsy, register/record basic demographic data, validate the classification of seizures and syndromes • make the provisional diagnosis in new patients, provide appropriate information and refer to a specialist centre • monitor seizures, aiming to improve control by adjustment of medication or re-referral to hospital services • minimise side effects of medications and their interactions. • facilitate structured withdrawal from medication where appropriate, and if agreed by the patient • introduce non-clinal interventions, and disseminate information to help improve quality of life for patients with epilepsy • address specific women's issues and needs of patients with learning disabilities
☑	• Services should be provided in acute hospitals to enable probable recent-onset seizures to be seen within 2 weeks of onset. • Hospitals should provide services to review people with drug-resistant epilepsy. • Subspeciality epilepsy clinics should also be available to meet the needs of specific groups of patients (epilepsy in learning disability, in pregnancy, in adolescence and in potential surgical candidates). • Each epilepsy tean should include epilepsy nurse specialists.

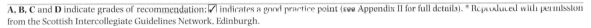

A, B, C and D indicate grades of recommendation; ☑ indicates a good practice point (see Appendix II for full details). * Reproduced with permission from the Scottish Intercollegiate Guidelines Network, Edinburgh.

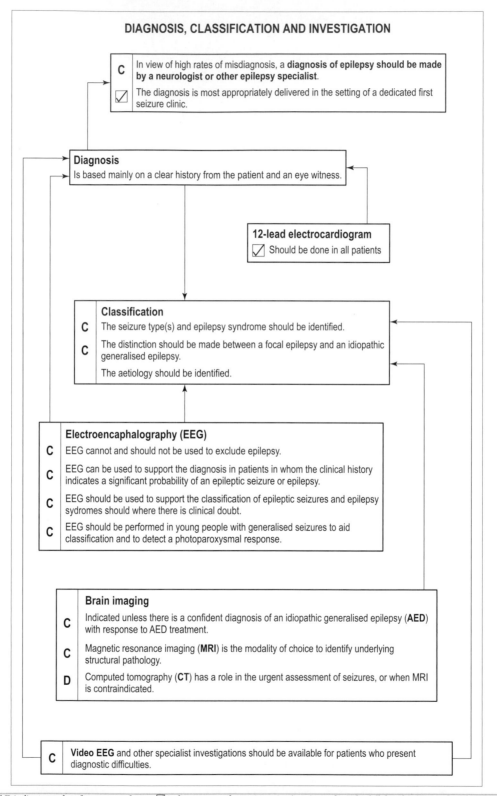

DIAGNOSIS, CLASSIFICATION AND INVESTIGATION

C — In view of high rates of misdiagnosis, a **diagnosis of epilepsy should be made by a neurologist or other epilepsy specialist**.

☑ The diagnosis is most appropriately delivered in the setting of a dedicated first seizure clinic.

Diagnosis
Is based mainly on a clear history from the patient and an eye witness.

12-lead electrocardiogram
☑ Should be done in all patients

Classification
C — The seizure type(s) and epilepsy syndrome should be identified.

C — The distinction should be made between a focal epilepsy and an idiopathic generalised epilepsy.

The aetiology should be identified.

Electroencaphalography (EEG)
C — EEG cannot and should not be used to exclude epilepsy.

C — EEG can be used to support the diagnosis in patients in whom the clinical history indicates a significant probability of an epileptic seizure or epilepsy.

C — EEG should be used to support the classification of epileptic seizures and epilepsy sydromes should where there is clinical doubt.

C — EEG should be performed in young people with generalised seizures to aid classification and to detect a photoparoxysmal response.

Brain imaging
C — Indicated unless there is a confident diagnosis of an idiopathic generalised epilepsy (**AED**) with response to AED treatment.

C — Magnetic resonance imaging (**MRI**) is the modality of choice to identify underlying structural pathology.

D — Computed tomography (**CT**) has a role in the urgent assessment of seizures, or when MRI is contraindicated.

C — **Video EEG** and other specialist investigations should be available for patients who present diagnostic difficulties.

A, B, C and **D** indicate grades of recommendation; ☑ indicates a good practice point (see Appendix II for full details). * Reproduced with permission from the Scottish Intercollegiate Guidelines Network, Edinburgh.

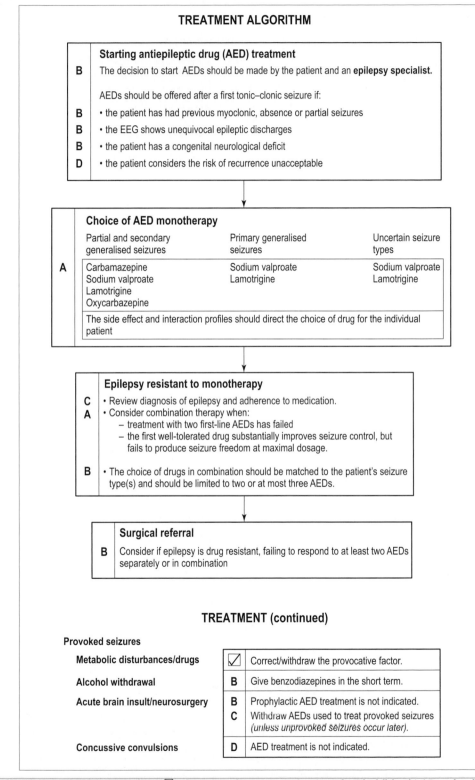

TREATMENT ALGORITHM

Starting antiepileptic drug (AED) treatment

B   The decision to start AEDs should be made by the patient and an **epilepsy specialist.**

AEDs should be offered after a first tonic–clonic seizure if:

B   • the patient has had previous myoclonic, absence or partial seizures
B   • the EEG shows unequivocal epileptic discharges
B   • the patient has a congenital neurological deficit
D   • the patient considers the risk of recurrence unacceptable

Choice of AED monotherapy

	Partial and secondary generalised seizures	Primary generalised seizures	Uncertain seizure types
A	Carbamazepine Sodium valproate Lamotrigine Oxycarbazepine	Sodium valproate Lamotrigine	Sodium valproate Lamotrigine

The side effect and interaction profiles should direct the choice of drug for the individual patient

Epilepsy resistant to monotherapy

C   • Review diagnosis of epilepsy and adherence to medication.
A   • Consider combination therapy when:
　　　– treatment with two first-line AEDs has failed
　　　– the first well-tolerated drug substantially improves seizure control, but fails to produce seizure freedom at maximal dosage.

B   • The choice of drugs in combination should be matched to the patient's seizure type(s) and should be limited to two or at most three AEDs.

Surgical referral

B   Consider if epilepsy is drug resistant, failing to respond to at least two AEDs separately or in combination

TREATMENT (continued)

Provoked seizures

Metabolic disturbances/drugs	☑	Correct/withdraw the provocative factor.
Alcohol withdrawal	B	Give benzodiazepines in the short term.
Acute brain insult/neurosurgery	B	Prophylactic AED treatment is not indicated.
	C	Withdraw AEDs used to treat provoked seizures (unless unprovoked seizures occur later).
Concussive convulsions	D	AED treatment is not indicated.

A, B, C and D indicate grades of recommendation; ☑ indicates a good practice point (see Appendix II for full details). * Reproduced with permission from the Scottish Intercollegiate Guidelines Network, Edinburgh.

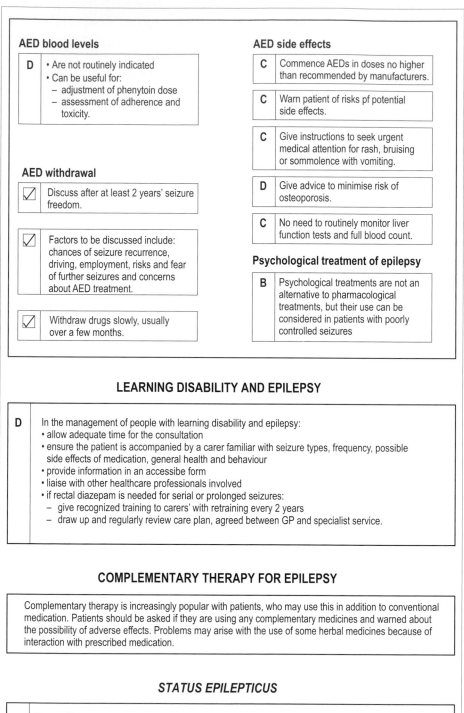

AED blood levels

D	• Are not routinely indicated • Can be useful for: – adjustment of phenytoin dose – assessment of adherence and toxicity.

AED withdrawal

☑	Discuss after at least 2 years' seizure freedom.
☑	Factors to be discussed include: chances of seizure recurrence, driving, employment, risks and fear of further seizures and concerns about AED treatment.
☑	Withdraw drugs slowly, usually over a few months.

AED side effects

C	Commence AEDs in doses no higher than recommended by manufacturers.
C	Warn patient of risks pf potential side effects.
C	Give instructions to seek urgent medical attention for rash, bruising or sommolence with vomiting.
D	Give advice to minimise risk of osteoporosis.
C	No need to routinely monitor liver function tests and full blood count.

Psychological treatment of epilepsy

B	Psychological treatments are not an alternative to pharmacological treatments, but their use can be considered in patients with poorly controlled seizures

LEARNING DISABILITY AND EPILEPSY

D	In the management of people with learning disability and epilepsy: • allow adequate time for the consultation • ensure the patient is accompanied by a carer familiar with seizure types, frequency, possible side effects of medication, general health and behaviour • provide information in an accessibe form • liaise with other healthcare professionals involved • if rectal diazepam is needed for serial or prolonged seizures: – give recognized training to carers' with retraining every 2 years – draw up and regularly review care plan, agreed between GP and specialist service.

COMPLEMENTARY THERAPY FOR EPILEPSY

Complementary therapy is increasingly popular with patients, who may use this in addition to conventional medication. Patients should be asked if they are using any complementary medicines and warned about the possibility of adverse effects. Problems may arise with the use of some herbal medicines because of interaction with prescribed medication.

STATUS EPILEPTICUS

A	**Prevention** Carers should treat serial or prolonged seizures in the community with rectal diazepam according to an agreed protocol (*protocol must include advice on when to transfer to hospital*).

A, B, C and D indicate grades of recommendation; ☑ indicates a good practice point (see Appendix II for full details). * Reproduced with permission from the Scottish Intercollegiate Guidelines Network, Edinburgh.

INFORMATION FOR PATIENTS AND CARERS

☑ Information should be given in an **appropriate manner** with sufficient time to answer questions. The type of information given should be recorded in the patient notes.

☑ Information should be **repeated** over time and reinforced to ensure understanding.

D The following checklist should be used to help healthcare professionsls to give patients and carers the information they need in an appropriate format:

☐ **General epilepsy information**
explanation of what epilepsy is*
probable cause
explanation of investigative procedures
classification of seizures*
syndrome
epidemiology
prognosis*
genetics
Sudden Unexpected Death in Epilepsy*

☐ **Antiepileptic drugs**
choice of drug*
efficacy*
side effects*
adherence*
drug interactions*
free prescriptions*

☐ **Seizure triggers**
lack of sleep*
alcohol and recreational drugs*
stress*
photosensitivity

☐ **First-aid**
general guidelines*
status epilepticus

☐ **Issues for women**
contraception*
pre-conception*
pregnancy and breastfeeding*
menopause

☐ **Lifestyle**
driving regulations*
employment
education (e.g. elementary school guidelines for teachers)
leisure
relationships
safety in the home*

☐ **Possible psychosocial consequences**
perceived stigma*
memory loss*
depression
anxiety
maintaining mental well-being
self-esteem*
sexual difficulties

☐ **Support organisations**
addresses and telephone numbers of national and local epilepsy organisations*

*essential information   Epilepsy Scotland helpline: 0808 800 2200 (**www.epilepsyscotland.org.uk**)

EPILEPSY IN WOMEN

Women with epilepsy, who are of childbearing age, need additional advice about issues such as contraception and pregnancy.

☑ Advice on contraception should be given before young women are sexually active.

D When the combined oral contraception is given with an enzyme-inducing AED, a minimum of 50 mcg of oestrogen should be used. Women should be warned that its efficacy is reduced. If breakthrough bleeding occurs the dose should be increased.

☑ Information about the risk of epilepsy and AEDs in pregnancy and the need for folate and vitamin K should be given to all women of childbearing age and repeated at review appointments.

☑ Pregnancy in women with epilepsy should be supervised in an obstetric clinic with access to a physician specialising in epilepsy.

A, B, C and **D** indicate grades of recommendation; ☑ indicates a good practice point (see Appendix II for full details). * Reproduced with permission from the Scottish Intercollegiate Guidelines Network, Edinburgh.

Policy and legislation

22

Policy and Legislation

The Adults with Incapacity Act

> Scottish Executive 2000 The Adults with Incapacity (Scotland) Act. Scottish Executive, Edinburgh. Online. Available: www.scotland.gov.uk/Topics/Justice/Civil/16360/4927

Decisions made for adults with incapacity must:
- be for the adult's benefit
- take into account the wishes of the adult, carer, relatives and guardian/attorney
- be the least restrictive option
- encourage the adult to develop new, or maximise existing, skills.

The Mental Welfare Commission has responsibilities to protect adults who lack capacity because of a mental disorder.

Local authorities are responsible for the welfare of adults who lack capacity.

The Public Guardian supervises and registers attorneys, guardians, intervention orders and anyone who can access a person's funds.

Individuals can arrange for a person to take over power of attorney for some or all of their property, finances, welfare and healthcare affairs, as long as it is registered with the Public Guardian.

Local authorities or anyone else claiming an interest in the person's affairs can apply to the Sheriff's Court for:
- an intervention order – a one-off order regarding a specific issue such as the disposal of property, or

- guardianship – for ongoing management of finances, welfare or health care.

The Act lays down safeguards for people who lack capacity who are to be involved in research.

See also the 'Policy and legislation' section in Chapter 14 (Learning disabilities psychiatry), page 227.

Care Programme Approach

> Department of Health 1990 The care programme approach for people with mental illness referred to the specialist psychiatric services: HC(90)23. DH, London

- Was introduced in 1991 to provide a framework for effective multidisciplinary mental health care.
- There are four stages:
  - systematic assessment of the individual's needs, both for health and socially
  - agreement of a package of care with the individual, carers and professionals involved
  - identification of a keyworker
  - regular review of the individual's needs and delivery of care
- CPA is now integrated with care management and has two levels: standard and enhanced.

Choosing Health

> Department of Health 2004 Choosing health. Making healthy choices easier. A White Paper. DH, London. Online. Available: www.dh.gov.uk/assetRoot/04/09/47/51/04094751.pdf

- Describes a new approach to public health issues in response to *Securing Good Health for the Whole Population*, produced in February 2004.
- The paper will tackle:
  - smoking
  - obesity
  - exercise
  - alcohol
  - sexual health
  - mental health.
- Credible, balanced information on health will be provided in combination with specific services and support. These will enable individuals to make healthier lifestyle choices.
- Adults have a responsibility to protect children who are too young or who do not have the capacity to make a healthy choice.
- Individuals will be protected from the effects of the unhealthy choices of others (e.g. passive smoking).
- The NHS and other agencies, including media, will work to develop a number of campaigns.
- Specific issues such as food labelling, salt content and portion sizes will be addressed in the food industry.
- There will be further restrictions on tobacco advertising.
- There will be a consultation on banning smoking in all enclosed public places.
- There will be investment in physical education in schools.
- Money will be provided to primary care trusts for health promotion.
- Health inequalities will be addressed. Specific target areas include social deprivation, young people and those with mental health problems.

The Community Care and Health (Scotland) Act 2002

Scottish Executive 2002 The Community Care and Health (Scotland) Act 2002. Scottish Executive, Edinburgh. Online. Available: www.opsi.gov.uk/legislation/scotland/acts2002/20020005.htm[†]

This Act aims to improve community care services with the provision of free nursing and personal care.
  It legislates with regard to:
- free personal and nursing care for everyone over the age of 65
- more expensive care than is usual, to be provided with additional payment from the client
- increased availability of direct payments from home care services which will allow people to have increased control over their care arrangements
- allowing 'deferred payments' where local authorities can contribute to care home fees so that a resident's

home need not be sold; payment is made to the local authority at a later date
- extending the right to assessment for carers, particularly young carers
- care home placement in other parts of the UK
- expansion of joint financing arrangements for NHS and local authorities.

The Data Protection Act 1998

UK Government 1998 Data Protection Act 1998. The Stationery Office, London. Online. Available: www.opsi.gov.uk/ACTS/acts1998/19980029.htm[†]

- This Act gives applicants the right to:
  - access personal data (about themselves only)
  - know why personal data is held
  - know who else has access to personal data.
- The applicant can obtain a copy of such information and learn its source.
- A fee may be payable.
- There are exemptions which include:
  - no fee has been paid
  - the applicant has not supplied reasonable proof of identification
  - anonymised data or information used entirely for research without any consequences for the data subject
  - where the disclosure of data would lead to the identification of another member of the public – they would also need to consent to disclosure.
- Exemptions do not include:
  - where information is withheld because the professional who contributed or compiled the data may be identified
  - situations where serious harm to a person's mental or physical health would result
  - a request made on behalf of the data subject (e.g. a parent and child) who believes that the information will not be disclosed to the applicant.

The Disability Discrimination Act 1995

UK Government 1995 Disability Discrimination Act 1995. The Stationery Office, London. Online. Available: www.opsi.gov.uk/acts/acts1995/1995050.htm

- The DDA 1995 aims to end the discrimination that many disabled people encounter.
- It gives disabled people rights in the areas of:
  - employment

- education
- access to goods, facilities and services
- buying or renting land or property
- access to transport.

The Disability Discrimination Act 2005

UK Government 2005 Disability Discrimination Act 2005. The Stationery Office, London. Online. Available: www.opsi. gov.uk/ACTS/acts2005/20050013.htm[†]

This Act amends or extends the existing provisions in the DDA 1995, including:

- making it unlawful for operators of transport vehicles to discriminate against disabled people
- making it easier for disabled people to rent property and for tenants to make disability-related adaptations
- making sure that private clubs with 23 or more members cannot keep disabled people out, just because they have a disability
- extending protection to cover people who have HIV, cancer and multiple sclerosis from the moment they are diagnosed
- ensuring that discrimination law covers all the activities of the public sector
- requiring public bodies to promote equality of opportunity for disabled people.

Rights of equal access to health and social care

- The DDA gives disabled people important rights of access to health services and social services. These include doctors' surgeries, dental surgeries, hospitals and mobile screening units.
- A GP should not refuse to let a patient register, or continue with treatment, because of a disability.
- Information about health and social care services should be provided in a format that is accessible – for example, large print or Braille.

Definition

Disabled person – someone who has a physical or mental impairment that has a substantial and long-term adverse effect on their ability to carry out normal day-to-day activities, where

- substantial means neither minor nor trivial
- long term means that the effect of the impairment has lasted or is likely to last for at least 12 months (there are special rules covering recurring or fluctuating conditions)

- normal day-to-day activities include everyday things such as eating, washing and going shopping
- a normal day-to-day activity must affect one of the 'capacities' listed in the Act which include mobility, manual dexterity, speech, hearing, seeing and memory.

Additional points

- Specific exclusions exist and include hay fever and a tendency to set fires.
- The DDA 2005 amended the definition of disability to remove the requirement that a mental illness should be 'clinically well-recognised'.
- People with HIV, cancer and multiple sclerosis will be covered from the point of diagnosis, rather than from the point when the condition has some adverse effect on their ability to carry out normal day-to-day activities.

Weblink Website of the UK government – www.direct. gov.uk.

See also the 'Policy and legislation' section in Chapter 9 (Ethical issues), page 128.

Fairness for all

UK government 2004 Fairness for all: a new Commission for Equality and Human Rights. White Paper (Cm 6185). The Stationery Office, London. Online. Available: www. womenandequalityunit.gov.uk/equality/project/cehr_ white_paper.pdf

This paper signalled the government's intention to create a single public body called the Commission for Equality and Human Rights. This was intended to replace the Commission for Racial Equality, the Disability Rights Commission and the Equal Opportunities Commission.

The Commission would:

- have additional powers to enforce the law in new areas of legislation concerning sexual orientation, religion and age
- represent a single point of contact to tackle discrimination in multiple areas
- have a role in the promotion and enforcement of antidiscrimination regulations
- have an additional role in promoting human rights in general.

The Freedom of Information Act 2000

UK Government 2000 The Freedom of Information Act 2000. The Stationery Office, London. Online. Available: www.opsi.gov.uk/ACTS/acts2000/20000036.htm

---

[†] Crown copyright. Reproduced with permission.

- This Act enables individuals to gain access to information held by public authorities – for example, government departments, NHS trusts, schools and the police. A fee may be payable to gain access.
- An applicant's request for access to information about themselves would more appropriately be made using the terms of the Data Protection Act (1998).
- Every public authority must publish information routinely using a publication scheme.
- In addition, anyone has a right to request information held by a public authority. A response must be made within 20 days.
- The Information Commissioner is an independent regulator with a responsibility to enforce compliance with the Act.

  Exemptions to the Act can include:
- if the information was supplied in confidence by a third party
- sensitive information relating to defence, the economy or law enforcement
- if the information would significantly endanger the mental or physical health of the applicant or any other individual.

The public authority must also decide whether disclosure is in the public interest. It may need to take this into account to override an application or even to outweigh an exemption.

It is the responsibility of the public authority to demonstrate the applicability of these exemptions.

Weblinks Information Commissioner's Office – www.ico. gov.uk/eventual.aspx

Freedom of Information (Scotland) Act 2002 – www.opsi. gov.uk/legislation/scotland/acts2002/20020013.htm:

- Scottish Executive
- Very similar to rest of UK
- Scottish Information Commissioner
- General practitioners specified as public authorities
- Similar exemptions to UK Act.

The Human Rights Act (1998)

UK Government 1998 The Human Rights Act (1998). The Stationery Office, London. Online. Available: www.opsi.gov. uk/acts/acts1998/19980042.htm

The Human Rights Act incorporates most of the European Convention on Human Rights into UK law. Britain signed the convention in 1951. Prior to the introduction of this Act, British citizens had to go to the European Court of Human Rights. Since it was introduced British residents can apply to domestic courts. It is still possible to appeal to Strasbourg if dissatisfied.

The Act applies to public authorities or any organisation carrying out a public function. Courts and Parliament are required to operate within the articles of the Convention. Private citizens can challenge public authorities within a specified time limit if they believe their rights have been infringed upon. Senior judges can also declare laws to be incompatible with the Convention. Medication without consent is permitted in principle, but patients are now better able to challenge what they perceive to be unfair treatment or improper procedure.

Relevant articles include the following:

Article 2: Right to life

- Everyone's right to life is protected by law except in defence against unlawful violence, quelling a riot or arresting a suspect.
- Public authorities must not ignore life-threatening situations (e.g. a suicidal patient).

Article 3: Protection against torture (or degrading treatment or punishment)

- This can include the mistreatment of patients with dementia in elderly care wards (e.g. by tying the patient to a chair).

Article 5: Deprivation of liberty

- There are certain circumstances where a person's liberty can be withdrawn, including 'the lawful detention of persons of unsound mind'.
- The mental disorder must be objectively and expertly diagnosed and judged to be extreme enough to warrant detention.
- There must be regular review.
- Detention must be terminated when it is no longer warranted.
- Tribunal rulings can be challenged if hearings are not arranged timeously.

Article 6: Private and family life

- This deals with protection from interference with correspondence, homes and family.
- Courts have to balance the rights of the individual with the interests and safety of society.
- Issues relevant to this article might include the visiting rights of families and the duties of a service to provide care to maintain a patient in their home environment.

Article 9: Freedom of thought, conscience and religion

- The rights of the individual and the rights of society must be considered.
- Areas of challenge may include dietary requirements, mixed sex wards and facilities for religious observances.

Article 10: Freedom of expression

- Courts must consider '...such...restrictions or penalties as are prescribed by law and are necessary in a democratic society'.

Article 14: Non-discrimination

- This does not deal with discrimination generally, but unequal application of the other rights mentioned in the Convention on grounds of race, colour, sex, language and religion.

    Article 13 was not adopted into UK law by the Act. This would have stipulated that individuals receive an 'effective remedy before a national authority'. Therefore, when UK courts fail to give a satisfactory 'remedy' the individual should appeal to Europe.

See also the 'Policy and legislation' section in Chapter 9 (Ethical issues), page 128.

The Journey to Recovery

> Department of Health 2001 The journey to recovery. The Government's vision for mental health care. DH, London[†]

Mental health, alongside coronary heart disease and cancer, is a top health priority. The main mental health policies are Modernising Mental Health Services, The National Service Frameworks for Mental Health and the chapter on mental health in the NHS Plan.

Modern mental health services

Help at the onset of illness
- Some serious mental health difficulties, such as schizophrenia, usually first occur during the teenage years or the early twenties. Often young people will be unwell for 6 months or more before they get any help.
- To remedy this unacceptable situation, early intervention teams will be able to provide the intensive support and help that every young person who develops a first episode of psychosis needs.
- These teams operate in ways that young people can relate to, providing help and advice on managing symptoms, and will base their care on the belief that engagement, rather than compulsion, is the key to success.

Help in a crisis

- At the moment, the only option for most people needing urgent mental health care is admission to hospital. Often this results in too long a period away from home, work and social networks, and can mean that all of these are damaged or lost.
- In some areas, special crisis resolution teams make an urgent visit to anyone who is thought to need to go into

hospital. Often, the crisis can then be resolved, and by providing intensive treatment at home, a great many hospital admissions can be avoided.
- This type of service is one that many people prefer.

Help for frequent users

- A small number of people use a lot of mental health services. They are frequently admitted to hospital, often compulsorily, but sometimes lose touch with services soon after discharge. Often they suffer from a dual diagnosis of substance misuse and serious mental illness. A small proportion also have a history of offending.
- For this group, assertive outreach teams providing intensive support at home can keep in touch with them, reduce the amount of time they spend in hospital, and help them enjoy a better quality of life.

Community teams

- Community mental health teams (CMHTs) will continue to have an important role to play in supporting service users and families in community settings. They should provide the core around which modern mental health services are developed. Their responsibilities may change over time but, working with primary care, they will be the main pathway for referrals to the more specialist teams.
- CMHTs, in some places known as primary care liaison teams, will also continue to care for the majority of people with moderate to severe mental illness in the community.

Better help in hospital

- Hospitals will also continue to play an important part in mental health care. An effective support system must get the balance right, between better community-based care and high quality, therapeutic inpatient care in good accommodation.
- The NHS has been set three national objectives, which are:
    - to ensure good standards of dignity and privacy for hospital patients
    - to achieve the Patient's Charter standards for segregated washing and toilet facilities
    - safe hospital facilities for patients who are mentally unwell.

Developments

- A campaign called 'Mind Out for Mental Health' to challenge discrimination by raising awareness of mental health, starting with employers, the media and young people.
- The NHS should set an example and health and social services should promote the employment of people with mental health problems in their services.

- Local services must agree plans for health promotion, based on local needs and including schools, the workplace and prisons. The plans must also include action at a local level to reduce discrimination.
- New guidelines for GPs to ensure that all the patients they see with a mental health problem have their psychological needs assessed.
- By 2004 people in all age groups, including children, will have easier access to help if they experience a mental health problem.
- By March 2002, the written care plan for those people on the enhanced CPA must show plans to secure:
  - suitable employment or other occupational activity
  - adequate housing
  - appropriate entitlement to welfare benefits.
- By March 2004 this requirement will apply to everyone on CPA.
- Every health authority in the country must now provide women-only community-based day services, as well as providing women-only accommodation in hospital facilities.
- By March 2002 all patients with a history of severe mental illness or deliberate self-harm must be followed up, by personal contact with a mental health professional, within 7 days of discharge from hospital.
- By March 2002 psychiatric inpatient units must review their physical environment and reduce access to means of suicide.

The Mental Capacity Act 2005

UK Government 2005 The Mental Capacity Act 2005. The Stationery Office, London. Online. Available: www.opsi.gov. uk/acts/acts2005/20050009.htm

This statute to protect and empower vulnerable adults who are unable to make or communicate decisions applies in England and Wales. The government's 1997 green paper Who Decides? sought consultation on earlier recommendations from the Law Commission about reforming the law on capacity for mentally impaired adults.

Following the Bournewood Case in 1998, the House of Lords ruled that people who lack capacity may be admitted to hospital without using the Mental Health Act, if they do not object. The implications of this highlighted the need for safeguards for adults with incapacity.

In 1999 the Lord Chancellor's office published the White Paper Making Decisions containing the government's proposals. The delay in producing a Bill led some to criticise the Lord Chancellor's office. Ten years had elapsed since the Law Commission's initial proposals when the Bill passed into law in 2005.

The Act makes use of five key principles:
- Every adult is presumed to have capacity unless otherwise demonstrated.

- People must be given sufficient assistance to make their own decisions before it can be stated that they are incapable of doing so.
- People are allowed to make unwise decisions.
- Anything done on the behalf of a person without capacity must be in their best interests.
- Anything done for such people must be the least restrictive option available.

The Act deals with assessment of capacity, pointing out that it is decision-specific and time-specific. The person's views, if expressed, must be considered. Carers and family should also be consulted. Restraint is only permitted if proportionate and where it is reasonably believed to be necessary to prevent harm to the person.

The Act describes lasting powers of attorney, which can be conferred by the person before losing capacity. The person can therefore arrange for the attorney to make health and welfare decisions for them in the future as well as financial ones. This replaces the enduring power of attorney under previous arrangements, which only involved financial decisions. The Act establishes a system of court-appointed deputies to replace the current arrangements to do with receivership and the Court of Protection. Deputies can be empowered to take health, welfare and financial decisions on the person's behalf. A new Court of Protection was created to have jurisdiction over capacity matters. A new Public Guardian was appointed to supervise all lasting powers of attorney and court deputies, and to deal with any complaints arising from their operation.

Further provisions designed to protect people who lack capacity include the following:
- Independent mental capacity advocate (IMCA): these can be appointed to represent the views or interests of the person and can challenge the decision-maker on the person's behalf.
- Advance decisions to refuse treatment have safeguards regarding the area of life-sustaining treatment.
- New criminal offence of neglect of a person with incapacity.
- Safeguards to protect people with incapacity from inappropriate research activities.

The Mental Health (Care and Treatment) (Scotland) Act 2003

Scottish Executive 2003 The Mental Health (Care and Treatment) (Scotland) Act 2003. The Stationery Office, London. Online. Available: www.opsi.gov.uk/legislation/scotland/acts2003/20030013.htm

This Act came into effect in October 2005. 'Mental disorder' applies to mental illness, personality disorder and learning disability.

There are 10 guiding principles:

- Non-discrimination: Mentally disordered people retain the same rights as those with different health needs wherever possible.
- Equality: The Act should be applied without preference for or against any specific group – for example, on grounds of race, religion or age.
- Respect for diversity: Care should recognise the patient's ethnic/social background.
- Reciprocity: Obligation of the individual to accept treatment is to be balanced by service's responsibility to provide appropriate, good-quality care which persists after discharge from detention.
- Informal care: This should remain the preferred option when possible.
- Participation: Involvement of service users. Past and present wishes should be considered.
- Respect for carers.
- Least restrictive alternative.
- Benefit: Interventions using the Act should provide a benefit that would not be possible unless the Act was applied.
- Emphasis on child welfare.

There are three main types of detention period:

- Emergency detention: 72-hour period for urgent assessment in hospital. No power to treat provided by Act. Requires any registered doctor to obtain a mental health officer's (MHO) approval unless impracticable. Ought to be reviewed at the earliest opportunity by a doctor with approved medical practitioner status (AMP).
- Short term detention: 28-day period for further assessment and treatment. Requires AMP and MHO approval. Treatment can include drugs, ECT, nursing, psychological treatment and rehabilitation.
- Compulsory treatment order (CTO): Lasts for 6 months initially. Can be extended by another 6 months and then yearly. Can be hospital or community based. Applied for by MHO and requires two medical opinions. Treatment plan usually informs the conditions set by the tribunal when granting the CTO. Stipulations can include that a patient resides at a particular address or receives a certain treatment.

There is provision for nurses holding power and police powers to remove an apparently mentally disordered person from a public place to a place of safety.

Conditions for using the Act are:

- The person has a mental disorder.
- Medical treatment is available to prevent decline or ameliorate the person's symptoms.
- If medical treatment was not provided then there would be a significant risk to the patient or others.
- The mental disorder is significantly impairing the individual's ability to make decisions.
- It is necessary to treat compulsorily.

There are safeguards with regard to ECT, psychosurgery and long-term drug treatment. Carers and service users can request an assessment of the patient's needs. This must be responded to within 14 days. Health boards must also provide age-appropriate care and support services to promote well-being and social development.

The Tribunal consists of a legal member, a doctor with experience in mental health and a lay member. Their role includes consideration of care plans, deciding on CTOs/reviews and listening to patient or advocate challenges. Patients can appoint a named person to support and represent them in proceedings under the Act. As with other mental health service users, those subject to the Act have access to independent advocacy. Tribunals and clinicians must consider advance statements when making treatment decisions.

The Mental Welfare Commission is given more power not only to monitor the operation of the Act in general, but also to enquire into individual cases. Health boards are directed to provide mother and baby units for the care of women with postnatal mental illness when it is clinically appropriate.

The Act also gives courts new options when dealing with mentally disordered offenders. As well as restriction orders and hospital direction, courts may also use Assessment, Treatment, Interim Compulsion and Compulsion Orders.

The Mental Health Bill 2004

Department of Health 2004 Draft Mental Health Bill 2004. Cm 6305-1. DH, London. Online. Available: www.dh.gov. uk/assetRoot/04/08/89/14/04088914.pdf

This Bill was introduced to parliament in September 2004. It applies only to England and Wales. The law required to be modernised to reflect changes in mental health services. The 1983 Act has produced three instances of incompatibility with the European Convention on Human Rights. Consultation on the new Act began in 1998, with a Green Paper *Reform of the Mental Health Act 1983* published in 1999, and a White Paper *Reforming the Mental Health Act* published in 2000. The draft Bill was published in 2002 for consultation.

Key changes made after consultation

- The definition of mental disorder now emphasises the presence of psychological dysfunction rather than merely a causative diagnosis. This means that the effects of the disorder count more than the precise diagnosis.
- The threshold for detention rose from 'health and safety of the patient' to 'for the protection of the patient from suicide, or serious self-harm, or serious neglect by him of health or safety'.
- A requirement for therapeutic benefit from use of formal measures.

- The Tribunal's exclusive power to discharge, grant leave or transfer a patient will be restricted to a small number of significantly high risk patients.
- Compulsion in prison is not to be used as it is not a 'therapeutic environment'.
- Patients over the age of 16 years who have capacity can consent to or refuse ECT. In exceptional emergencies it may still be administered in the face of a patient's refusal.
- Any patient under 16 would only receive ECT if authorised by the courts or the Tribunal.
- The Bill does not now interfere with the common law tradition of parents consenting to treatment on behalf of their children under the age of 16.

Conditions for compulsory treatment

- Presence of a serious mental disorder.
- Treatment necessary to prevent suicide, serious self-neglect or for the protection of others.
- No alternative to the use of the powers in the Bill is available or appropriate.
- Treatment must be available for the individual.

Assessment will include examination by two doctors and an approved mental health professional (often a social worker). There will be consultation with carers. Procedures will necessarily involve written records and time limits. In the next stage the examiners will decide whether or not further assessment and treatment should be provided on a residential basis. The supervising clinician must produce a care plan within 5 days. Treatment can be given without patient consent, but only in a hospital setting.

The Bill would enable some patients to be managed in the community with specified conditions. The requirement for detention is kept under constant review. The initial detention period lasts 28 days. The supervising clinician, in consultation with carers, can then decide whether to apply for a treatment order before the Tribunal. The patient has a right to appeal to the tribunal during the 28-day assessment period.

Treatment orders last for up to 6 months and the Tribunal sets the precise conditions. After a year of continual subjection to treatment orders the tribunal may grant year-long orders.

The Tribunal consists of a legal member, a clinical member and a lay member. Patients and carers have access to specialist independent mental health advocacy services. Provision is made for cross-border transfers (e.g. to Scotland). There are procedures for transfer from prison to hospital or the community for mentally disordered offenders. This would apply to those charged with, or convicted of, minor offences. There are safeguards for minors. There are powers of entry for police to enter property and convey patients to a place of safety. Appeals can be pursued beyond the Tribunal to an Appeals Tribunal and further to the Court of Appeal. The Mental Health Act Commission has been abolished and

responsibilities have been transferred to the Healthcare Commission.

The Royal College of Psychiatrists has expressed serious concerns about the Bill, including:

- the possible extension of compulsory powers to include people with physical illnesses (epilepsy, multiple sclerosis, etc.) and substance misuse problems
- the loose criteria for mental disorder in England when compared with the rest of the UK
- the perceived emphasis on coercive measures which may increase patients' reluctance to seek help
- the possibility of non-consensual treatment of adults who have the capacity to refuse it
- the possibility of detention of personality disordered patients (in particular dissocial personality disorder) even if they have not committed an offence.

In March 2006 the Bill was dropped amid concerns that it was unlikely to pass in its present form. A shorter Bill was therefore prepared with a number of changes. Appropriate treatment should be available for detention to proceed. The definition of mental disorder will be rationalised. The Bill will also be used to amend the 2005 Incapacity Act. This will introduce safeguards for people who lack capacity, but who do not receive the protection of mental health legislation, thus 'closing the Bournewood gap'.

The final details of the Bill were unknown at the time of writing.

Modernising Mental Health Services

Department of Health 1998 Modernising mental health services: safe, sound and supportive. White Paper. DH, London. Online. Available: www.dh.gov.uk/assetRoot/04/04/66/60/04046660.pdf

This Paper proposed local mental health and social services that are:

- safe – to protect patients and the public and provide effective care for those with mental illness at the time they need it
- sound – ensuring that patients and service users have access to the full range of services which they need
- supportive – working with patients and service users, their families and carers, to build healthier communities.

This Paper set 10 guiding principles, i.e. people with mental health problems can expect services that will:

- involve users and their carers in the planning and delivery of care
- deliver high quality treatment and care which is known to be effective and acceptable
- be well suited to those who use them and be non-discriminatory
- be accessible, so that help can be obtained when and where it is needed

- promote their safety and that of their carers, staff and the wider public
- offer choices which promote independence
- be well coordinated between all staff and agencies
- deliver continuity of care for as long as it is needed
- empower and support staff
- be properly accountable to the public, users and carers
- reduce suicides.

The National Service Framework for Mental Health 1999

The Department of Health 1999 The national service framework for mental health: modern standards and service models. DH, London. Online. Available: www.dh.gov.uk/assetRoot/04/01/45/01/04014501.pdf

The NHS Plan (DH 2004) emphasised the role of the NSF in modernising the NHS. The NSF set national standards and set out service models for a defined care group. They contain milestones to measure progress and outline programmes to aid in implementation. They apply to health services in England and Wales.

Since 1998 additional frameworks have been developed and published for older people, diabetes and mental health, among others.

The mental health framework addresses the mental health requirements of adults below the age of 65. It acknowledges that changes may take 5–10 years to implement fully. It makes use of an extra £700 million funding which the government allocated to mental health between 1999 and 2002. It was developed with the input of an External Reference Group. This was chaired by Professor Thornicroft of the Institute of Psychiatry, King's College, London.

The seven standards are as follows:

Mental health promotion, stigma and social exclusion

- All involved organisations in public and private sectors should contribute to population-wide health improvement programmes as well as local individual based strategies.
- Special attention should be paid to vulnerable groups such as:
  - unemployed people
  - ethnic minorities
  - rough-sleepers
  - prisoners
  - other vulnerable populations.
- There should be action to combat discrimination against those with mental health problems.
- Outcome measures will include results of the National Psychiatric Morbidity Survey (NPMS) and rates of suicide.

Primary care and access to services

- 24-hour contact to be available from local services as well as use of NHS Direct.
- Common problems to be managed effectively by primary care with specialist referral for the appropriate minority.
- Use of NICE reviewed protocols for depression, PND, eating disorders, etc.
- Monitoring waiting times for specialist services.
- Liaison, support and education from secondary care.
- Support for families and patients and use of self-help groups.

Effective services for people with severe mental illness

- All service users on CPA should receive care aimed at preventing crises, reducing risk and optimising engagement.
- They should have access to services at all times.
- There should be a written, up-to-date individual care plan given to each service user.
- Appropriate hospital care should be available close to home.
- The type of hospital care provided will depend on the needs of each individual but it should be the least restrictive option.
- Patients should have a copy of their detailed discharge plans with specific advice on further crisis management.
- Training should be provided for staff in risk assessment and management.
- Assertive outreach teams should be developed.
- There is a need to consider the balance between the provision of hospital beds, supported accommodation and home treatment.
- Performance indicators will be:
  - NPMS results
  - rates of suicide
  - frequency of emergency readmissions
  - access to psychology
  - access to rehabilitation services
  - evidence from service users.
- The numbers of prisoners awaiting transfer to hospital and out-of-area inpatient care will also be considered.

Carers

- Carers of a person on CPA should have an annual assessment of their needs as well as a collaborative care plan.
- Outcome measures include:
  - results of NPMS
  - rates of suicide
  - carer satisfaction ratings.

Suicide prevention

- This will be facilitated by delivering on standards detailed above and supporting prison staff in preventing suicides among prisoners.
- Training for staff in risk assessment is to be provided.
- Local systems should be put in place for suicide audit.

See also the 'Policy and legislation' section in Chapter 27 (Service provision), page 406.

The National Service Framework for Mental Health – Five Years On

Department of Health 2004 The National Service Framework for Mental Health – Five Years On. DH, London. Online. Available: www.dh.gov.uk/assetRoot/04/09/91/22/04099122.pdf

- A report detailing the first 5 years of the process of change as set out in the NSF for Mental Health.
- It finds that:
  - suicide rates are at an all-time low
  - many specialist community mental health teams are in operation
  - service users reported increased satisfaction levels
  - there are increased staff numbers
  - atypical antipsychotics are increasingly in use.
- Areas requiring attention are:
  - the care of patients from ethnic minorities without discrimination
  - inpatient wards
  - dual diagnosis (mental illness and substance misuse) services
  - reduction of social exclusion
  - the management of long-term disorders
  - increased availability of psychological therapies
  - new roles for key staff.

See also the 'Policy and legislation' section in Chapter 27 (Service provision), pages 406-407.

National Framework for Service Change in the NHS in Scotland

Scottish Executive Health Department 2005 National framework for service change in the NHS in Scotland. SEHD, Edinburgh. Online. Available: www.show.scot.nhs.uk/sehd/nationalframework/Reports.htm

The Scottish Minister for Health and Community Care asked Professor David Kerr to provide a set of proposals for reshaping the NHS in Scotland over the next 20 years. This followed publication of the Executive's White Paper *Partnership for Care* in 2003.

Following public consultation, seven issues were noted:
- Maintenance of local, high quality services
- Waiting times
- Remote communities
- Empowering clinicians to reform the NHS
- Use of new technology
- Reducing health inequalities
- Value for money.

Final proposals

- All NHS Boards to produce plans to manage more people with long-term conditions at home, or in the community, to reduce the need for hospitalisation.
- Targeted preventative medicine to help reduce inequalities in the future.
- Increased support for patients and their carers to manage their own illness.
- A national IT system to facilitate electronic records and telemedicine.
- Multidisciplinary teams in community casualty departments to provide the bulk of unscheduled care.
- Reduce waiting times and increase patient choice with more day surgery and increased access to diagnostics in the community.
- Specialised, complex care to be provided on fewer sites.
- Networks of rural hospitals.
- Community Health Partnerships to cut through the primary–secondary care barrier and also to work more closely with social services.
- Preventing delayed discharges by reducing emergency admissions.

Challenges to implementation

- An increase in chronic conditions as the Scottish population ages.
- Patients' expectations of local specialised services and distrust of centralisation.
- Ongoing widening of health inequalities.
- Workforce issues such as a reduction in doctors' hours and recruitment/retention problems.

See also the 'Policy and legislation' section in Chapter 27 (Service provision), pages 406-407.

The New NHS

Department of Health 1997 The New NHS: modern, dependable. White Paper. DH, London. Online. Available: www.archive.official-documents.co.uk/document/doh/newnhs/forward.htm

This document was produced within 12 months of the Labour party election win. It outlined the intentions of the government to modernise and improve the NHS.

Three key innovations were:
- NHS Direct: a 24-hour, nurse-led telephone advice line.
- Information technology: an improved NHS information 'superhighway' to facilitate quicker result dissemination, online appointment booking, etc.
- Cancer waiting times: everyone with suspected cancer to be seen within 2 weeks of GP referral.

Other priorities included:
- abolition of the internal market with no return to centralisation
- evidence-based national service frameworks to be introduced
- National Institute for Clinical Excellence to be created to develop guidelines on best practice and cost-effectiveness
- reorganisation of primary care with closer working of GPs and community nurses in primary care groups (PCGs).
- longer-term service agreements between NHS organisations with explicit quality standards
- clinical governance to be given prominence
- a new Commission for Health Improvement (CHI)
- PCGs to take responsibility for their own budget
- management costs to be cut
- incentives to be available to increase efficiency.
- health authorities to be able to withdraw powers from poorly performing PCGs.

See also the 'Policy and legislation' section in Chapter 27 (Service provision), pages 406-407.

The NHS Improvement Plan

Department of Health 2004 The NHS improvement plan: putting people at the heart of public services. White paper. DH, London. Online. Available: www.dh.gov.uk/assetRoot/04/08/45/22/04084522.pdf

This document, applicable in England, lists priorities for the NHS for 2004–2008 and complements *The NHS Plan*.
- Patients are to receive better information and choice to allow them to decide how, where and when they receive treatment.
- Patients will have the choice of at least four healthcare providers subject to certain conditions.
- There is an emphasis on continuing to decrease waiting times.
- More resources are to be devoted to improving the quality of life for people with chronic conditions.

- The rate of suicide is to be reduced by 20% from the 1997 baseline.
- Emphasis to move from hospital to community with greater use of 'community matrons' and GPs with special interests.
- More staff training
- Fewer national targets.
- More locally set priorities.

The NHS Plan

Department of Health 2000 The NHS Plan: a plan for investment, a plan for reform. White Paper. Cm 4818-I. DH, London. Online. Available: www.dh.gov.uk/assetRoot/04/05/57/83/04055783.pdf

This Paper begins with the recognition that the NHS has been insufficiently funded and consequently is increasingly unfit to fulfil its purpose.
- Public consultation showed that people wanted:
  - a larger, innovative and better paid workforce
  - reduced waiting times
  - better hospitals.
- The Plan promised to make use of large funding increases to provide:
  - more than 100 new hospitals by 2010
  - over 3000 renovated health centres
  - clean wards, 'modern matrons' and better food
  - modern IT systems
  - 7500 more consultants
  - 2000 more GPs
  - 20,000 extra nurses
  - 1000 more medical students
  - childcare for NHS staff.
- There is to be involvement of NICE, CHI and a Modernisation Agency to ensure best practice and improve standards. NHS organisations that perform well will obtain more autonomy; failing organisations will face government intervention.
- There is to be reform of doctors' contracts with increasing remuneration and higher productivity. The Plan proposed a ban on private work in the first 7 years after a consultant is registered. Nurses are to have extended roles.
- Patients are to receive copies of correspondence about them. Patient advocates will be available in every hospital.
- Private sector facilities may be used to maintain improvements where necessary.
- Waiting times are to be cut to less than 3 months for outpatients and 6 months for inpatient stays by 2005.
- Cancer, heart disease and mental health services are to be prioritised.

- *The NHS Plan* makes a number of pledges for mental health, including assertive outreach, home treatment and early intervention services for all who need them, more help for people held inappropriately in high secure hospitals or prisons, new services for women and more support for carers.
- By 2004 there will be:
  - 1000 new graduate mental health staff to work in primary care
  - an extra 500 community mental health team workers
  - 50 early intervention teams to provide treatment and support to young people with psychosis and their families
  - 335 crisis resolution teams
  - an increase to 220 assertive outreach teams
  - women-only day services
  - 700 extra staff to work with carers
  - more suitable accommodation for up to 400 people currently in high secure hospitals
  - better services for prisoners with mental illness
  - a care plan and a keyworker for every prisoner leaving prison with serious mental illness.
- Crisis response teams are to be developed for people with mental health problems.
- There is to be free nursing care in nursing homes and zero tolerance for ageism.
- Deprived areas will be targeted to reduce health inequalities.
- Free fruit will be provided in schools for 4–6 year olds.

Our health, our care, our say: a new direction for community services

Department of Health 2006 Our health, our care, our say: a new direction for community services. Cm 6737. DH, London[†]

This Paper aims to bring about improved health and social care. It arose from the Green Paper *Independence, Well-being and Choice.*

It has four main goals:
- Better prevention services and earlier intervention
- More choice and patient empowerment
- Tackle inequalities and improve access to community services
- More support for people with long term needs.
  These goals are to be achieved through:
- Enabling health, independence and well-being:
  - development of an NHS 'life check' with online self-assessment and a pilot
  - new quality outcomes framework measures for health

- Better access to general practice:
  - increased responsibilities for PCTs
  - improved provision of service information
  - review of funding arrangements
  - more responsive hours and services.
- Better access to community services:
  - extended scope of direct payments
  - national bowel screening programme
  - improved choice in maternity services
  - end-of-campus provision for people with learning disabilities
  - end-of-life care networks.
- Shifting resources into prevention.
- Support for people with longer-term needs:
  - improved information services, including helplines for carers
  - short-term home-based respite support for carers
  - personal health and social care plans for those with both social care needs and a long-term condition
  - joint networks and/or teams for management of health and social care needs between PCTs and local authorities.
- More care to take place away from hospital.
- Joined up care – better joining-up of services at the local level.
- Care closer to home.
- Innovative service development informed by local needs.
- Allowing non-NHS providers to compete to provide some services.

Weblink Our health, our care, our say (Executive Summary) – www.dh.gov.uk/assetRoot/04/12/74/69/04127469.pdf

Partnership for Care

Scottish Executive 2003 Partnership for care. Scotland's Health White Paper. Scottish Executive, Edinburgh. Online. Available: www.scotland.gov.uk/Publications/2003/02/16476/18730

This details a major programme of service redesign across Scotland.

It aims to view pathways to care from the perspective of the patients, with services that are more accessible and with less delay.

A wider range of services will be provided in the community, including diagnostic and outpatient services.

The focus is on the development of services within local communities and better working with local authorities. This will require a massive programme of service redesign.

Areas to be tackled are as follows:
1. Health services in the community
   Considerations include:

- support for primary care
- access to services
- developing community health partnerships.

Local Health Care Cooperatives (LHCCs) have been the basis of primary care services and have focused on the development of community health services. LHCCs will evolve into Community Health Partnerships to provide decentralised but integrated health care.

Partnerships will:

- ensure the involvement of patients and healthcare professionals
- work in partnership with local authority services
- have increased responsibility in the use of resources by NHS Boards
- have a key role in local service redesign
- be key in the integration of local health services, both primary and secondary
- have a key role in delivering health improvements in local communities.

2. Partnership with social care
3. Integrated healthcare
   Service redesign including:
   - managed clinical networks
   - regional planning
   - acute services
4. Public involvement
5. Support for service redesign

This Paper proposed the creation of unified NHS Boards in place of NHS Trusts:

- The new Community Health Partnerships (CHPs) will work more closely with social services and be more accountable to the community.
- There will be public involvement through the new Scottish Health Council.
- Guarantees are made for on time treatment for certain procedures.
- Better patient information will be provided.
- There will be a more robust complaints procedure.

The direction of reform and some of the details were clarified in the *National Framework for Service Change in the NHS in Scotland* report published in 2005.

See also the 'Policy and legislation' section in Chapter 14 (Learning disabilities psychiatry), pages 228-232.

Protection of vulnerable adults

Department of Health 2004 Best practice guidance. Protection of vulnerable adults (POVA) scheme in England and Wales for care homes and domiciliary care agencies: a practical guide. DH, London. Online. Available: www. dh.gov.uk/assetRoot/04/09/03/19/04090319.pdf

From July 2004 individuals who have abused, neglected or otherwise harmed vulnerable adults in their care or placed vulnerable adults in their care at risk of harm should be referred to and included on the POVA list.

Employers must make statutory checks against this list and must not offer such individuals employment in care positions.

The POVA scheme will add significantly to current pre-employment checks – including confirming identity, requesting disclosures and obtaining references – that providers of care should carry out before offering individuals employment in care positions.

The scheme will initially apply to registered care homes and registered domiciliary care agencies. It will be extended to adult placement schemes.

The scheme was originally intended to apply to the NHS and independent health sector; however, there is a delay in implementation in the latter.

See also the 'Policy and legislation' section in Chapter 14 (Learning disabilities psychiatry), pages 228-232.

Securing good health for the whole population

HM Treasury 2004 Securing good health for the whole population. The Wanless report. HMSO, Norwich. Online. Available: www.hm-treasury.gov.uk/media/E43/27/ Wanless04_summary.pdf

In 2002 Derek Wanless was asked by the government to undertake a long-term assessment of NHS resource requirements for the next 20 years. This would take into account population health trends. The resulting report – *Securing our Future Health: Taking a Long-term View* – presented three scenarios depending on different assumptions to do with health service productivity and the population's engagement with public health measures. The most optimistic scenario was based on a fully engaged population, resulted in the best health outcomes and was the least expensive.

This report describes the action necessary to achieve the most optimistic scenario. It concluded that:

- individuals are responsible for their own health, as well as that of their children
- individuals require better information and support to make healthy choices
- individuals should balance their right to choose their own lifestyle against any adverse impacts their choices have on others
- socioeconomic and ethnic health inequalities need to be addressed
- the main levers for government to bring about change are taxation, subsidies, service provision, regulation and information
- public health expenditure decisions must be evidence based, with greater use of NICE methodology

- there should be a consultation period to solicit views on the right action to take in the areas of smoking, obesity, nutrition and exercise
- services should target those people in disadvantaged groups to reduce inequalities
- the onus will be on primary care trusts to deliver public health interventions locally and they may need to pool resources
- productivity increases will accrue from the development of the 'expert patient' and greater use of non-medically qualified staff, including community pharmacists
- other productivity gains will be seen from the increased role of genetic medicine and improved IT systems.

This report informed the development of the White Paper *Choosing Health* published later in 2004.

Smoking, Health and Social Care (Scotland) Act 2005

Scottish Executive 2005 Smoking, Health and Social Care (Scotland) Act 2005. The Stationery Office, Edinburgh. Online. Available: www.opsi.gov.uk/legislation/scotland/acts2005/20050013.htm[†]

Diverse provisions

- Smoking prohibition and control, including:
  - a smoking ban in all enclosed public places
  - an offence of permitting others to smoke in no-smoking premises
  - fixed penalties.
  Exceptions include:
  - designated rooms in adult care homes
  - residential (long-term) psychiatric units.
- General dental services, general ophthalmic services, personal dental services, etc.
- Pharmaceutical care services
- Provision of services under NHS contracts
- Discipline
- Payments to certain persons infected with hepatitis C as a result of NHS treatment
- Authorisation of medical treatment – Amendment of Adults with Incapacity (Scotland) Act 2000 – extends the definition of 'the medical practitioner primarily responsible for the medical treatment of an adult' to include a dental practitioner, an ophthalmic optician, a registered nurse and an individual who falls within such description of persons as may be prescribed by the Scottish Ministers.

Joint ventures

- Smoking ban in all enclosed public places except in designated rooms in adult care homes, and residential (long-term) psychiatric units, amongst others.
- Legislation concerning provision of dental and ophthalmic services to the public.
- Compensation for people infected with hepatitis C as a result of NHS treatment.
- Planning of pharmaceutical services.

See also the 'Policy and legislation' sections in Chapter 14 (Learning disabilities psychiatry), page 227.

Social inclusion

The Scottish Office 1999 Social inclusion – opening the door to a better Scotland: Strategy. Scottish Office, Edinburgh. Online. Available: www.scotland.gov.uk/library/documents-w7/sist-00.htm[†]

Describes the government's programme of action to promote social inclusion in Scotland. The report describes the range of issues which make up social exclusion and the current government action to promote social inclusion.

The government aimed to tackle the problem by providing opportunities to participate in society through work or learning, tackling family poverty and health problems.

The principles underlying the government's approach to promoting inclusion are as follows:

- Integration: the connected problems of social exclusion need to be tackled in a coordinated way, driven by the needs of the individual, the family and the community.
- Prevention: there is a need to tackle the long-term causes of exclusion to prevent problems arising, primarily through work with children, young people and families.
- Understanding: action to promote inclusion should be founded on evidence-based principles.
- Inclusiveness: policies and programmes should be developed and implemented in partnership.
- Empowerment: action to promote inclusion should enable and encourage individuals and communities to utilise opportunities and take control of their situations.

Action under the government's programme includes:
- the New Deal for 18–24 year olds
- the New Deal for the long-term unemployed
- employment zones
- 40,000 extra higher education places
- working families tax credit
- increases in child benefit
- minimum income levels for pensioners
- social inclusion partnerships.

Definition

Social exclusion is a shorthand label for what can happen when individuals or areas suffer from a combination of linked problems such as unemployment, poor skills, low incomes, poor housing, high crime environments, bad health and family breakdown.

See also the 'Policy and legislation' sections in Chapter 14 (Learning disabilities psychiatry), page 227.

Supporting people

Office of the Deputy Prime Minister 2003 Supporting people. ODPM, London. Online. Available: www.spkweb.org.uk

• This programme aims to provide housing-related support to different vulnerable members of society, including:
  – people who are homeless or sleeping rough
  – ex-offenders and those at risk of offending
  – people with physical or sensory disability
  – people at risk of domestic violence
  – people with alcohol and drug problems
  – teenage parents
  – elderly people
  – people with HIV and AIDS
  – young people at risk
  – people with learning difficulties
  – travellers and homeless families with support needs.
• Housing-related support aims to develop and sustain an individual's capacity to live independently in their accommodation.
• The support ranges from ensuring that an individual receives their correct benefit entitlement and that they have the skills to maintain their tenancy, to weekly home visits for a short period or a long-term on-site full-time support worker.
• Support is tailored to each individual's specific needs.

Post-traumatic stress disorder

23

Chapter contents

General Topics

War-related psychological stressors and risk of psychological disorders in Australian veterans

Ikin JF, Sim MR, Creamer MC et al 2004 War-related psychological stressors and risk of psychological disorders in Australian veterans of the 1991 Gulf War. British Journal of Psychiatry 185: 116–126

Questions still remain about the long-term health implications of the 1991 Gulf War. Although a number of studies have been performed, the health effects remain unclear and the research into 'Gulf War Syndrome' is ongoing. Several studies have shown that Gulf War veterans self-report higher than expected rates of psychiatric disorders and psychosomatic symptoms.

Method

- Psychological health assessments in a cross-sectional study of an entire cohort of Australian Veterans of the Gulf War were performed.
- Results were compared with a random group of military controls who did not deploy to that conflict.
- Almost 2000 subjects were recruited – the entire cohort of Australian veterans who served from August 1990 until September 1991.

- Postal questionnaires were sent and comprehensive health assessments were carried out by doctors, nurses and psychologists.
- The health assessment measured prevalence of DSM-IV psychological disorders using the Composite International Diagnostic Interview (CIDI).
- The postal questionnaire examined demographic variables.
- Psychological stressor exposure was measured using the military service experience questionnaire.
- Analysis was conducted on males only as there were too few female veterans.

Results

- Gulf War veterans were slightly younger, lower ranked and were less likely to have received tertiary education than controls.
- 44% of the Gulf War veterans reported being involved in at least one other active deployment.
- The two groups varied very little in psychological morbidity prior to Gulf War deployment. 31% of Gulf War veterans, compared with 21% of the comparison group, were likely to develop post-Gulf War psychological problems.
- There was also an increased risk of post Gulf War bipolar disorder, major depression, alcohol dependence or abuse, and drug dependence or abuse.
- There was no increase in somatisation disorder.
- Anxiety disorders were three to five times more likely in the veteran group and included PTSD, OCD, social phobia, panic disorder and agoraphobia.

- On average, Gulf War veterans had twice as many disorders present in the previous 12 months as the comparison group.

Discussion

- Although the study clearly demonstrates an increased risk of the development of several psychological disorders, the majority of Gulf War veterans did not develop any psychological disorder in the period since the Gulf War.
- The excess risk of psychological disorders in Gulf War veterans can be explained only partly as a generalised 'war deployment effect' (although numbers were small).
- The results also show a strong relationship between increasing numbers of psychological stressors experienced during the Gulf War and the resultant psychological disorder.

Hynams KC, Wignall S, Rosewall R 1996 War syndromes and their evaluation: from the US Civil War to the Persian Gulf War. Annals of Internal Medicine 125: 398–405

- Experience of deployment to war can lead to a variety of physical and psychological health problems.

DeFraites RF, Wanat ER, Norwood AE et al 1992 Investigation of a suspected outbreak of an unknown disease among veterans of Desert Shield/Storm, 123rd Army Reserve Command, Fort Benjamin Harrison, Indiana. Walter Reed Army Institute of Research, Washington, DC

- Reported that veterans from the Gulf War experienced various symptoms and illnesses soon after returning from this deployment.

Stimpson NJ, Thomas HV, Weightman AL et al 2003 Psychiatric disorder in veterans of the Persian Gulf War of 1991: systematic review. British Journal of Psychiatry 182: 391–403

- Recently published data from meta-analyses of nine studies investigating PTSD and 11 studies investigating common mental disorders demonstrated increased risks for both measures in Gulf War veterans compared with non-Gulf War veterans.

Treatment – Psychopharmacology

Pharmacotherapy for post-traumatic stress disorder

Stein DJ, Zungu-Dirwayi N, van der Linden GJH, Seedat S 2006 Pharmacotherapy for post-traumatic stress disorder

(PTSD) **(Cochrane Review)**. In: The Cochrane Library, Issue 2. Update Software, Oxford

- 35 trials were suitable for inclusion.
- These were of short duration (under 14 weeks).
- 17 trials found that medication was associated with reductions in the severity of symptoms.
- 13 trials found that medication was more effective than placebo in the treatment of people with PTSD (NNT 4.85).
- SSRIs appeared to be the most effective of the drug classes.
- Treatment with medication was also found to be associated with improvements in core PTSD symptoms, concurrent depression and levels of disability.

Treatment – Psychological Therapies

Eye movement desensitisation and reprocessing: an update

Coetzee RH, Ragel S 2005 Eye movement desensitization and reprocessing: an update. Advances in Psychiatric Treatment 11: 347–354

The process and suggested theories regarding EMDR are discussed in this article and the best evidence from the field of trauma is reviewed. The clinical use of EMDR is justified in patients who have suffered trauma. There is limited evidence for the use of EMDR in other conditions and in children. Many of the studies are single case reports.

The EMDR process consists of:
- Phase 1 – Assessment
- Phase 2 – Preparation: Therapeutic rapport is established, the patient is educated regarding the process and the type of bilateral stimulation is agreed.
- Phase 3 – Assessment of target memory/image: The most distressing image and the associated negative cognitions and the desired positive cognitions are examined.
- Phase 4 – Desensitisation: The target image, linking memories, negative cognitions and associations are held in mind by the patient during the process of bilateral stimulation. Rapid eye movements are produced by the patient following the therapist's finger while sets of approximately 30 movements are made in an agreed direction (horizontal, vertical, diagonal or circular). This process continues until the patient has no emotional or physical response to the image.

- Phase 5 – Installation: The same process is followed while a positive cognition is held in the mind.
- Phase 6 – Body scan: The patient assesses whether any negative or positive sensations are identified and, if so, bilateral stimulation is repeated to desensitise or strengthen, respectively.
- Phase 7 – Closure: Progress is reported on and support and praise offered to the patient. Containment exercises involving anxiety and relaxation techniques are taught, particularly if further sessions are still required.
- Phase 8 – Debriefing.

Van Etten ML, Taylor S 1998 Comparative efficacy of treatments for post-traumatic stress disorder: a meta-analysis. Clinical Psychology and Psychotherapy 5: 126–144

- This analysed the results of 61 treatment outcome trials for PTSD. Psychopharmacology and psychological therapies were compared.
- Pharmacological treatment was associated with a higher dropout rate than the psychological therapies (32% versus 14%).
- EMDR and behaviour therapy were the most effective forms of psychological therapies and SSRIs were the most effective pharmacological agents. These treatments were equally effective.
- The psychological therapies showed some advantage in symptom reduction.
- The SSRIs were more efficacious in treating depression.

Davidson PR, Parker KCH 2001 Eye movement desensitisation and reprocessing (EMDR): a meta-analysis. Journal of Consulting and Clinical Psychology 69: 305–316

- A meta-analysis of 34 studies of EMDR therapy which included only published trials and excluded reports on follow-up outcome to ensure high quality data.
- They found that EMDR was as effective as other exposure techniques.
- Eye movements were not found to be needed.

Maxfield L, Hyer L 2002 The relationship between efficacy and methodology in studies investigating EMDR treatment of PTSD. Journal of Clinical Psychology 58: 23–41

- This meta-analysis reviewed trials that compared EMDR with waiting list controls or standard treatments but not with trauma-focused CBT, the gold standard.
- Only a small number of trials were included.
- The greater the methodological rigour of the study, the greater the effect size in favour of EMDR.

Grant M, Threlfo C 2002 EMDR in the treatment of chronic pain. Journal of Clinical Psychology 58: 1505–1520

- This study found EMDR had beneficial effects on coping with pain, reduction of pain and on pain-related attitudes and beliefs.
- In some cases physiological damage limits the possibility of pain relief.

National Collaborating Centre for Mental Health (NCCMH) 2005 Post-traumatic stress disorder. The management of PTSD in adults and children in primary and secondary care. National Clinical Practice Guideline Number 26. Gaskell and British Psychological Society, London. Online. Available: www.nice.org.uk/pdf/CG026fullguideline.pdf

- This concluded that EMDR is an effective treatment for PTSD, but without the strong evidence base for trauma-focused CBT.
- It is recommended that patients are offered up to 12 sessions.
- Direct comparisons between trauma-focused CBT, exposure CBT and EMDR found that none showed a clear benefit with regard to treatment outcomes, including the speed of onset of benefit.

Psychological debriefing for preventing post-traumatic stress disorder

Rose S, Bisson J, Churchill R, Wessely S 2002 Psychological debriefing for preventing post traumatic stress disorder (PTSD) **(Cochrane Review)**. In: The Cochrane Library, Issue 2. CD000560. Update Software, Oxford

- 15 trials were included.
- Single session individual debriefing was not found to be effective in preventing the development of symptoms of PTSD.
- Single session debriefing did not reduce psychological distress.
- After 12 months one trial reported a significantly higher risk of PTSD in those who received debriefing.
- There was no evidence that the intervention reduced PTSD severity at any time, or that it reduced general psychological morbidity, depression or anxiety.

Psychological treatment of post-traumatic stress disorder

Bisson J, Andrew M 2005 Psychological treatment of post-traumatic stress disorder (PTSD) **(Cochrane Review)**. In: The Cochrane Library, Issue 3. CD003388. Update Software, Oxford

- 29 studies were included.
- Trauma-focused cognitive behavioural therapy/exposure therapy (TFCBT) and stress management (SM) were significantly more effective in reducing clinician-assessed PTSD symptoms than waiting list controls or treatment as usual.
- There was no significant difference between TFCBT and SM.
- TFCBT was significantly better than other therapies (supportive therapy, non-directive counselling, psychodynamic psychotherapy and hypnotherapy).
- Those receiving other therapies did as well as those in the waiting list/usual care control group.
- Group TFCBT was significantly more effective than waiting list/usual care.

Assessment Tools and Rating Scales

Impact of Events Scale (IES)

Horowitz M, Wilner N, Alvarez W 1979 Impact of Events Scale: a measure of subjective stress. Psychosomatic Medicine 41(3): 209–218. Online. Available: www.swin.edu.au/victims/resources/assessment/ptsd/ies.html

- 15-item questionnaire assessing symptoms of intrusion and avoidance.
- Assesses self-reported levels of distress with regard to a specific life event.
- Well validated.
- Revised edition contains seven additional items and is now more widely used.

Guidelines

Post-traumatic stress disorder (PTSD): the management of PTSD in adults and children in primary and secondary care. NICE Clinical Guideline 26*

Screening of individuals involved in a major disaster, programme refugees and asylum seekers

- For individuals at high risk of developing PTSD following a major disaster, consideration should be given (by those responsible for coordination of the disaster plan) to the routine use of a brief screening instrument for PTSD at 1 month after the disaster. [C]

- For programme refugees and asylum seekers at high risk of developing PTSD, consideration should be given (by those responsible for management of the refugee programme) to the routine use of a brief screening instrument for PTSD as part of the initial refugee healthcare assessment. This should be a part of any comprehensive physical and mental health screen. [C]
- Healthcare professionals should not delay or withhold treatment for PTSD because of court proceedings or applications for compensation. [C]
- Healthcare professionals should be aware that many PTSD sufferers are anxious about and can avoid engaging in treatment. Healthcare professionals should also recognise the challenges that this presents and respond appropriately – for example, by following up PTSD sufferers who miss scheduled appointments. [C]
- Healthcare professionals should treat PTSD sufferers with respect, trust and understanding, and keep technical language to a minimum. [GPP]
- Treatment should be delivered by competent individuals who have received appropriate training. These individuals should receive appropriate supervision. [C]

Comorbidities

- When a patient presents with PTSD and depression, healthcare professionals should consider treating the PTSD first as the depression will often improve with successful treatment of the PTSD. [C]
- For PTSD sufferers whose assessment identifies a high risk of suicide or harm to others, healthcare professionals should first concentrate on management of this risk. [C]
- For PTSD sufferers who are so severely depressed that this makes initial psychological treatment of PTSD very difficult (e.g. as evidenced by extreme lack of energy and concentration, inactivity or high suicide risk), healthcare professionals should treat the depression first. [C]
- For PTSD sufferers with drug or alcohol dependence or in whom alcohol or drug use may significantly interfere with effective treatment, healthcare professionals should treat the drug or alcohol problem first. [C]
- When offering trauma-focused psychological interventions to PTSD sufferers with comorbid personality disorder, healthcare professionals should consider extending the duration of treatment. [C]
- People who have lost a close friend or relative due to an unnatural or sudden death should be assessed for PTSD and traumatic grief. In most cases, healthcare professionals should treat the PTSD first without avoiding discussion of the grief. [C]

The treatment of PTSD

Early interventions A number of sufferers with PTSD may recover with no or limited interventions. However, without effective treatment, many people may develop chronic problems over many years. The severity of the initial traumatic response is a reasonable indicator of the need for early intervention, and treatment should not be withheld in such circumstances.

Watchful waiting Where symptoms are mild and have been present for less than 4 weeks after the trauma, watchful waiting, as a way of managing the difficulties presented by individual sufferers, should be considered by healthcare professionals. A follow-up contact should be arranged within 1 month. [C]

Immediate psychological interventions for all For individuals who have experienced a traumatic event, the systematic provision to that individual alone of brief, single-session interventions (often referred to as debriefing) that focus on the traumatic incident should not be routine practice when delivering services. [A]

PTSD where symptoms are present within 3 months of a trauma

- Brief psychological interventions (five sessions) may be effective if treatment starts within the first month after the traumatic event. Beyond the first month, the duration of treatment is similar to that for chronic PTSD.
- Trauma-focused cognitive behavioural therapy should be offered to those with severe post-traumatic symptoms or with severe PTSD in the first month after the traumatic event. These treatments should normally be provided on an individual outpatient basis. [B]
- Trauma-focused cognitive behavioural therapy should be offered to people who present with PTSD within 3 months of a traumatic event. [A]
- The duration of trauma-focused cognitive behavioural therapy should normally be 8–12 sessions; however, if the treatment starts in the first month after the event, fewer sessions (approximately five) may be sufficient. When the trauma is discussed in the treatment session, longer sessions (e.g. 90 minutes) are usually necessary. Treatment should be regular and continuous (usually at least once a week) and should be delivered by the same person. [B]
- Drug treatment may be considered in the acute phase of PTSD for the management of sleep disturbance. In this case, hypnotic medication may be appropriate for short-term use; however, if longer-term drug treatment is required, consideration should also be given to the use of suitable antidepressants at an early stage in order to reduce the later risk of dependence. [C]
- Non-trauma-focused interventions such as relaxation or non-directive therapy, which do not address traumatic memories, should not routinely be offered to people who present with PTSD symptoms within 3 months of a traumatic event. [B]

PTSD where symptoms have been present for more than 3 months after a trauma

- All PTSD sufferers should be offered a course of trauma-focused psychological treatment (TFCBT or EMDR).

These treatments should normally be provided on an individual outpatient basis. [A]

- Trauma-focused psychological treatment should be offered to PTSD sufferers regardless of the time that has elapsed since the trauma. [B]
- The duration of trauma-focused psychological treatment should normally be 8–12 sessions when the PTSD results from a single event. When the trauma is discussed in the treatment session, longer sessions than usual are generally necessary (e.g. 90 minutes). Treatment should be regular and continuous (usually at least once a week) and should be delivered by the same person. [B]
- Healthcare professionals should consider extending the duration of treatment beyond 12 sessions if several problems need to be addressed in the treatment of PTSD sufferers, particularly after multiple traumatic events, traumatic bereavement or where chronic disability resulting from the trauma, significant comorbid disorders or social problems are present. Trauma-focused treatment needs to be integrated into an overall plan of care. [C]
- For some PTSD sufferers, it may initially be very difficult and overwhelming to disclose details of their traumatic event. In these cases, healthcare professionals should consider devoting several sessions to establishing a trusting therapeutic relationship and emotional stabilisation before addressing the traumatic event. [C]
- Non-trauma-focused interventions such as relaxation or non-directive therapy, which do not address traumatic memories, should not routinely be offered to people who present with chronic PTSD. [B]
- For PTSD sufferers who have no or only limited improvement with a specific trauma-focused psychological treatment, healthcare professionals should consider the following options: [C]
  - an alternative form of trauma-focused psychological treatment
  - the augmentation of trauma-focused psychological treatment with a course of pharmacological treatment.

Drug treatment

- Drug treatments for PTSD should not be used as a routine first-line treatment for adults (in general use or by specialist mental health professionals) in preference to a trauma-focused psychological therapy. [A]
- Drug treatments (paroxetine or mirtazapine for general use, and amitriptyline or phenelzine for initiation only by mental health specialists) should be considered for the treatment of PTSD in adults where a sufferer expresses a preference not to engage in a trauma-focused psychological treatment. [B]
- Drug treatments (paroxetine or mirtazapine for general use, and amitriptyline or phenelzine for initiation only by mental health specialists) should be offered to adult PTSD sufferers who cannot start a psychological

therapy because of a serious ongoing threat of further trauma (e.g. where there is ongoing domestic violence). [C]

- Drug treatments (paroxetine or mirtazapine for general use, and amitriptyline or phenelzine for initiation only by mental health specialists) should be considered for adult PTSD sufferers who have gained little or no benefit from a course of trauma-focused psychological treatment. [C]

- Where sleep is a major problem for an adult PTSD sufferer, hypnotic medication may be appropriate for short-term use; however, if longer-term drug treatment is required, consideration should also be given to the use of a suitable antidepressant at an early stage in order to reduce the later risk of dependence. [C]

- Drug treatments (paroxetine or mirtazapine for general use, and amitriptyline or phenelzine for initiation only by mental health specialists) for PTSD should be considered as an adjunct to psychological treatment in adults where there is significant comorbid depression or severe hyperarousal that significantly impacts on a sufferer's ability to benefit from psychological treatment. [C]

- When an adult sufferer with PTSD has not responded to a drug treatment, consideration should be given to increasing the dose within approved limits. If further drug treatment is considered, this should generally be with a different class of antidepressant or involve the use of adjunctive olanzapine. [C]

- When an adult sufferer with PTSD has responded to drug treatment, it should be continued for at least 12 months before gradual withdrawal. [C]

General recommendations regarding drug treatment

- All PTSD sufferers who are prescribed antidepressants should be informed, at the time that treatment is initiated, of potential side effects and discontinuation/withdrawal symptoms (particularly with paroxetine). [C]

Recommendations regarding discontinuation/withdrawal symptoms

- Discontinuation/withdrawal symptoms are usually mild and self-limiting but occasionally can be severe. Prescribers should normally gradually reduce the doses of antidepressants over a 4-week period, although some people may require longer periods. [C]

- If discontinuation/withdrawal symptoms are mild, practitioners should reassure the PTSD sufferer and arrange for monitoring. If symptoms are severe, the practitioner should consider reintroducing the original antidepressant (or another with a longer half-life from the same class) and reduce gradually while monitoring symptoms. [C]

Chronic disease management

- Chronic disease management models should be considered for the management of people with chronic PTSD who have not benefited from a number of courses of evidence-based treatment. [C]

Children

Early intervention

- Trauma-focused cognitive behavioural therapy should be offered to older children with severe post-traumatic symptoms or with severe PTSD in the first month after the traumatic event. [C]

PTSD where symptoms have been present for more than 3 months after a trauma

- Children and young people with PTSD, including those who have been sexually abused, should be offered a course of trauma-focused cognitive behavioural therapy adapted appropriately to suit their age, circumstances and level of development. [B]

- The duration of trauma-focused psychological treatment for children and young people with chronic PTSD should normally be 8–12 sessions when the PTSD results from a single event. When the trauma is discussed in the treatment session, longer sessions than usual are usually necessary (e.g. 90 minutes). Treatment should be regular and continuous (usually at least once a week) and should be delivered by the same person. [C]

- Drug treatments should not be routinely prescribed for children and young people with PTSD. [C]

- Where appropriate, families should be involved in the treatment of PTSD in children and young people. However, treatment programmes for PTSD in children and young people that consist of parental involvement alone are unlikely to be of any benefit for PTSD symptoms. [C]

- When considering treatments for PTSD, parents and, where appropriate, children and young people should be informed that, apart from trauma-focused psychological interventions, there is at present no good evidence for the efficacy of widely used forms of treatment of PTSD such as play therapy, art therapy or family therapy. [C]

A, B and C indicate grades of recommendation; **GPP** indicates a good practice point (see Appendix II for full details). * Reproduced with permission from the National Institute for Health and Clinical Excellence, London.

Primary care

24

General Topics

Providing a primary care service for psychiatric inpatients

Welthagen E, Talbot S, Harrison O et al 2004 Providing a primary care service for psychiatric inpatients. Psychiatric Bulletin 28: 167–170

Aims

A prospective study of the feasibility, acceptability and activity of an innovative weekly primary care service for patients admitted for acute psychiatric care.

Method

- This article describes the first 10 months of a service providing a weekly primary care service to patients admitted to an inner-city mental health unit.
- One doctor provided a weekly 3-hour session for the 67 patients in the three acute adult psychiatric wards at Charing Cross Hospital as well as offering a limited service to the older persons service.
- Referrals were taken from ward staff and the patients themselves.
- After a few months the service exceeded capacity and priority was given to those who were homeless, were not registered with a GP or who had not seen one for more than 6 months, or who had been in hospital for more than 3 months.
- The doctor offering the service also liaised with ward doctors and nurses and offered advice.

- Data were collected for all consultations over a 10-month period, detailing demographic information, complaints and diagnoses, outcomes and treatment.

Results

- 168 appointments were made with a 73.2% attendance rate.
- Half of the patients attending were offered a further follow-up appointment.

Patient characteristics

- 84 patients attended their consultations:
  - 15% were over 65
  - 75% had a physical examination within a week of admission
  - 25% had no examination prior to consultation
  - 80% had U&Es and FBC done, blood tests mainly being requested routinely.
- The main psychiatric diagnosis was severe enduring mental illness, mainly schizophrenia.
- 25 patients had a secondary diagnosis, mainly substance misuse.

Physical complaints

- Patients presented with a wide range of acute and chronic physical complaints.
- One patient was found to have breast cancer after routine review and one was diagnosed with diabetes which had not been found during a 3-month admission.
- One male required an emergency blood transfusion secondary to anaemia.
- Commonly, diabetes and hypertension were poorly controlled.

Interventions

- New medication was prescribed for 66 consultations and existing medication altered.
- 29 patients required referral to other services.
- Almost all the patients received health promotion.

Patients' perspectives

- Three-quarters of patients interviewed felt the psychiatric teams were taking their physical needs seriously.
- Generally patients were satisfied with the additional input.

Phelen M, Stradins L, Morrison S 2001 Physical health of people with severe mental illness. British Medical Journal 322: 443–444

- People with severe mental illness have poor physical health.

Druss BG, Rohrbaugh RM, Levison CM et al 2001 Primary health care service for long stay psychiatric patients. Psychiatric Bulletin 22: 610–612

- An American study.
- Integrating primary health care into a mental health clinic improved the physical health care.

Dean J, Todd G, Morrow H et al 2001 'Mum, I used to be good looking…look at me now.' The physical health needs of adults with mental health problems: the perspective of users, carers and front-line staff. International Journal of Mental Health Promotion 3: 16–24

- Mental health staff in the UK are unclear about the extent of their role in relation to physical health.
- Staff believe service users are disinterested in their physical ailments.

Friedli L, Dardis C 2002 Not all in the mind: mental health service user perspectives on physical health. Journal of mental Health Promotion 1: 36–46

- Service users see their physical health as a priority.
- They lack relevant information and face difficulties in accessing physical health care.

Rigby JC, Oswald AG 1987 An evaluation of the performing and recording of physical examinations by psychiatric trainees. British Journal of Psychiatry 150: 533–535

- Physical examinations performed by trainees are often done badly.

Osborn D, Warner J 1998 Assessing the physical health of psychiatric patients. Psychiatric Bulletin 22: 695–697

- Less than 75% of patients are examined on admission.
- Physical history is rarely taken.

National Institute for Clinical Excellence 2002 Core interventions in the treatment and management of schizophrenia in primary and secondary care. NICE, London

- Stated that primary care professionals are best placed to monitor the physical health of patients with schizophrenia, and should do so frequently.

Beecroft N, Becker T, Griffiths G et al 2001 Physical health of people with severe mental illness: the role of the general practitioner. Journal of Mental Health 10: 53–61

- Found that patients are more satisfied with help received if they are in contact with their general practitioner.

Burns T, Cohen A 1998 Item of service payments for general practitioner care of severely mentally ill patients: does the money matter? British Journal of General Practice 48: 1415–1416

- Found that opportunities for routine health promotion are seldom taken in routine practice.

Fischer N, Roberts J 1998 Primary health care service for long-stay psychiatric patients. Psychiatric Bulletin 22: 610–612

- Highlighted the importance of having primary care doctors in long-stay wards.

See also the National Service Framework for Mental Health in Chapter 22, page 329, and the 'General topics' section in Chapter 30 (Treatment settings), page 429.

Shared care for people with mental illness

Lester H 2005 Shared care for people with mental illness: a GP's perspective. Advances in Psychiatric Treatment 11: 133–141

Shared care is described as a team approach to a patient's care involving primary and secondary care. Good communication is required in the planning of integrated care. Primary care services provide treatment in an accessible setting with low stigma. A general practitioner's desire to be involved in shared care may be affected by the amount of mental health training received.

Shared care models include:
- community mental health teams
- outpatient clinics set in primary care
- mental health workers based within primary care

- the consultation–liaison model
- integrated working.

Brugha TS, Wing JK, Smith BL 1999 Physical health of the long term mentally ill in the community. Is there unmet need? British Journal of Psychiatry 155: 777–781

- 41% of patients with severe mental illness at a psychiatric day centre had ongoing medical health issues.
- A further 44% were found to have unmet health needs.

Singleton N, Bumpstead R, O'Brien M et al 2001 Psychiatric morbidity among adults living in private households, 2000. Office for National Statistics. The Stationery Office, London

- Patients with psychosis are more likely to have physical health problems than the rest of the population (62% versus 42%).

Harris EC, Barraclough B 1998 Excess mortality of mental disorder. British Journal of Psychiatry 173: 11–53

- Calculated standardised mortality rates for all causes of death for people with schizophrenia as 156 in males and 141 in females.

Kendrick T 1996 Cardiovascular and respiratory risk factors and symptoms among general practice patients with long term mental illness. British Journal of Psychiatry 139: 733–739

- Patients with schizophrenia are more likely to have cardiovascular risk factors, such as poor diet and smoking.
- Primary care records are less likely to have these factors recorded in people with schizophrenia.
- People with schizophrenia are also less likely to address such issues as the rest of the population.

Burns T, Cohen A 1998 Item-of-service payments for GP care of severely mentally ill persons. British Journal of General Practice 48: 1415–1416

- People with severe mental illness attend their general practitioners more than four times the rate of the rest of the population.
- In this patient group less information is recorded regarding health promotion.

Brown J, Weich S, Downes-Grainger E et al 1999 Attitudes of inner city GPs to shared care for psychiatric patients in the community. British Journal of General Practice 49: 643–644

- Some general practitioners, particularly those working in inner city practices, can view patients with mental illness as being difficult and work intensive.

Gray R, Parr AM, Plummer S et al 1999 A national survey of practice nurse involvement in mental health interventions. Journal of Advance Nursing 30: 901–906

- This national survey of practice nurse involvement found that approximately half were administering depot antipsychotic medications each month.
- Monitoring of treatment adherence and side effects was performed by approximately one-third of practice nurses.
- The majority of practice nurses (up to 70%) had received no psychiatric training in the preceding 5 years.

Killaspy H, Banerjee S, King M et al 1999 Non-attendance at psychiatric out-patient clinics: communication and implications for primary care. British Journal of General Practice 49: 880–883

- The communication from secondary to primary care regarding patients' non-attendance at follow-up appointments can be problematic.
- There is an association between non-attendance and level of mental illness.

Byng R, Jones R, Leese M et al 2004 Exploratory cluster randomised controlled trial of shared care development for long-term mental illness. British Journal of General Practice 54: 259–266

- A RCT of link working (shared care between general practitioners and CMHTs).
- Link working is associated with lower relapse rates and higher practitioner satisfaction.

Lester H, Jowett S, Wilson S et al 2003 A cluster randomised controlled trial of patient medical records for people with schizophrenia receiving shared care. British Journal of General Practice 53: 197–203

- Patient-held records can improve communication between primary and secondary care.
- Patient-held records may be viewed as stigmatising by patients as well as causing some concern regarding confidentiality.
- They do not have a beneficial effect on patients' symptoms.

Definition

Shared care – the joint participation of general practitioners and hospital consultants in the planned delivery of care for patients with a chronic condition, informed by enhanced information exchange over and above routine discharge and referral letters. (*Source:* Hickman M, Drummond N, Grimshaw J 1994 A taxonomy of shared care for chronic disease. Journal of Public Health Medicine 16: 447–454.)

See also the 'General topics' section in Chapter 30 (Treatment settings), page 429.

Policy and Legislation

Quality and outcomes framework guidance

British Medical Association 2003 Quality and outcomes framework guidance. BMA, London

- Nationally agreed standards for the primary care provision of care across a number of clinical and organisational indicators.
- Fulfilment of the criteria leads to point accumulation and to financial payments.
- Clinical indicators are organised by disease category. The disease categories that are included are ones where:
  - the responsibility for ongoing management rests principally with the general practitioner and the primary care team
  - there is good evidence, and in particular a national guideline, that improved primary care will lead to health benefits
  - the disease area is a priority in a number of the four nations.

Disease categories

- Coronary heart disease
- Stroke and transient ischaemic attacks
- Hypertension
- Hypothyroidism
- Diabetes
- Chronic obstructive pulmonary disease
- Epilepsy
- Thyroid disease
- Cancer
- Asthma
- Mental health.

Organisational indicators

- Records and information about patients
- Information for patients
- Education and training
- Practice management
- Medicines management.

Mental health indicators

Information should be recorded for the following indicators:

Records
- The practice can produce a register of people with severe long-term mental health problems who need and have consented to regular follow-up.

Ongoing management
- The percentage of patients with severe long-term mental health problems where a review is recorded in the last 15 months. This should include the correct prescribed medication, a physical health review and coordinated care arrangements with secondary care.
- The percentage of people with lithium levels recorded in the last 6 months.
- The percentage of lithium patients with serum creatinine and TSH recorded in the last 15 months.
- The percentage of lithium patients with lithium levels in the therapeutic range recorded in the last 6 months.

The small numbers of indicators for mental health reflect the difficulties in collecting information relevant to mental health indicators from the case records. This is noted to 'reflect the complexity of mental health problems, and reflects the complex mix of physical, psychological and social issues that present to general practitioners'.

There are additional indicators for mental health in the organisational indicators. These include significant event audit (e.g. following a death by suicide or a compulsory admission to hospital) and the ongoing care of patients treated with depot medication in the practice.

Treatment – Psychological Therapies

The effectiveness of psychosocial interventions delivered by general practitioners

Huibers MJH, Beurskens AJHM, Bleijenberg G, Schayck CP van 2003 Th e effectiveness of psychosocial interventions delivered by general practitioners **(Cochrane Review)**. In: The Cochrane Library, Issue 2. CD003494. Update Software, Oxford

- Eight studies were included.
- There is good evidence that problem-solving treatment by general practitioners is effective for major depression.
- There is limited evidence regarding:
  - reattribution or cognitive behavioural group therapy for somatisation
  - counselling for smoking cessation
  - behavioural interventions to encourage alcohol reduction.

Effectiveness of teaching general practitioners skills in brief cognitive behaviour therapy

King M, Davidson O, Taylor F, Haines A, Sharp D, Turner R 2002 Effectiveness of teaching general practitioners skills in brief cognitive behaviour therapy to treat patients with depression: randomised controlled trial. British Medical Journal 324: 947–950

Background

Cognitive behaviour therapy is effective when delivered by general practitioners who have received extensive instruction, but most do not have the time or perhaps the inclination to undergo comprehensive training.

Method

In this study, a 4-day training course was offered to GPs. It aimed to increase professional ease and positive attitudes towards managing patients with depression and to enable the acquisition of skills in the application of brief cognitive therapy. GPs completed questionnaires at baseline and 6 months after training. The Depression Attitude Questionnaire and a questionnaire that explores doctors' knowledge of cognitive behaviour therapy and the extent to which they feel confident in applying it in their practice were used.

Consecutive patients aged 18 and over were screened with the hospital anxiety and depression scale. Patients with psychotic disorders, organic brain syndromes, learning disabilities and those who are unable to read English were excluded. Patients completed the Beck Depression Inventory, the State Anxiety Inventory and the Short Form 36 (a brief measure of quality of life). These scales were completed again at 3 and 6 months. Data were also collected on consultation rates, home visits, psychotropic prescribing, referrals to mental health professionals and other health service providers, and certificated absences for sickness.

Results

- After 6 months, the knowledge and attitudes of doctors who had received training was no different from that of those who had no training.
- The training had no discernible impact on the patients' outcomes.
- Some evidence was found of lower scores in intervention doctors, which indicated greater confidence in treating both depression and anxiety.
- Intervention doctors were more likely than control doctors to refer their affected patients and less likely to offer certificates for sickness, but numbers are small.

- These findings run counter to other studies where brief interventions by general practitioners have been regarded as effective in problem drinking and diabetes.

Effectiveness and cost effectiveness of counselling in primary care

Bower P, Rowland N, Mellor Clark J, Heywood P, Godfrey C, Hardy R 2002 Effectiveness and cost effectiveness of counselling in primary care (Cochrane Review). In: The Cochrane Library, Issue 1. CD001025. Update Software, Oxford

- Seven trials were included.
- They showed that clinicians trained in counselling had significantly greater clinical effectiveness in the short term than the 'usual care' group.
- These benefits were not maintained in the long term.
- Patients were more satisfied with counselling.
- Costs were similar over the long term.

Problem-solving treatment in general psychiatric practice

Mynors-Wallis L 2001 Problem-solving treatment in general psychiatric practice. Advances in Psychiatric Treatment 7: 417–425

For general psychiatrists to utilise psychological treatments in their day-to-day work, treatments must be brief, focused and effective. They must be feasible within a busy outpatient clinic.

Problem-solving treatment is a brief psychological intervention that has been shown to be effective in the treatment of major depression and for patients with a broad range of emotional disorders that have not resolved with simple measures. Problem-solving treatment derives from cognitive behavioural principles. It is a brief, structured psychological intervention that focuses on the here and now. It requires active collaboration between patient and therapist. The patient should have an increasingly active role in the planning of treatment and the implementing of activities between treatment sessions. The treatment has been evaluated as an intervention lasting approximately four to six sessions.

Problem-solving treatment encourages the patient to understand the link between their symptoms and their problems. It begins with the definition of the current problems. Patients are taught problem-solving techniques that attempt to resolve problems in a structured way. It is hoped that the experience of problem solving will be a positive one.

Mynors-Wallis LM, Gath DH, Lloyd-Thomas AR et al 1995 Randomised controlled trial comparing problem-solving treatment with amitriptyline and placebo for major depression in primary care. British Medical Journal 310: 441–445

- 91 primary care patients with major depression were randomly allocated to problem-solving treatment, amitriptyline or a placebo treatment involving both drug and psychological placebos.
- All treatments were given in six sessions over 12 weeks.
- At 6 and 12 weeks, problem-solving treatment was as effective in treating depression as amitriptyline, and significantly more effective than the placebo treatment.
- Problem solving was associated with a low dropout rate (only 7% of the sample compared with 19% for the amitriptyline sample) and was rated as helpful or very helpful by 100% of the patients receiving it (compared with 83% of the amitriptyline sample).

Mynors-Wallis LM, Gath DH, Day A, Baker F 2000 Randomised controlled trial of problem-solving treatment, antidepressant medication and combined treatment for major depression in primary care. British Medical Journal 320: 26–30

- A study which compared the effectiveness of problem-solving treatment and antidepressant medication in combination and alone.
- It studied whether problem-solving treatment can be delivered as effectively by suitably trained practice nurses as by general practitioners.

- 151 patients were randomly allocated to receive problem-solving treatment from a GP, problem-solving treatment from a practice nurse, antidepressant medication alone from a GP, or the combination of problem-solving treatment and antidepressant medication from a GP.
- The results from this study at 6, 12 and 52 weeks indicated that there were no significant differences between any of the four treatment groups.

Mynors-Wallis LM, Gath DH 1997 Predictors of treatment outcome for major depression in primary care. Psychological Medicine 27: 731–736

Could not identify specific predictors of which patients might benefit from drug treatment and which might benefit from problem-solving treatment.

Stages of problem-solving treatment

- Stage 1 – Explanation of treatment and its rationale, including
  - recognition of emotional problems
  - recognition of problems making the link between emotional symptoms and problems
- Stage 2 – Clarification and definition of problem
- Stage 3 – Setting achievable goals
- Stage 4 – Generating solutions
- Stage 5 – Choice of preferred solution
- Stage 6 – Implementation of the preferred solution
- Stage 7 – Evaluation.

Psychological therapies

25

Chapter contents

Treatment – Psychological Therapies

Boundary violation and sexual exploitation

> Sarkar SP 2004 Boundary violation and sexual exploitation. Advances in Psychiatric Treatment 10: 312–320

Therapist–patient sexual contact is always unethical and is also inherently harmful. The American Psychiatric Association expels an average of 10 psychiatrists a year for sexual misconduct, a number that has remained stable over the last 10 years. It does not include other cases of misconduct dealt with by temporary suspension, fines, etc. The GMC no longer publishes details of the types of case that its Professional Conduct Committee hears; however, in the past, approximately six cases of sexual misconduct were heard by the GMC each year, with three finding against the doctor. Most reported cases involve male doctors. Doctors most likely to be involved in serious boundary violations are male, older and highly trained/respected. It is also likely that they have repeated such behaviours over time.

It is the therapist's professional identity that is the therapeutic agent for the patient. If the personal identity is revealed, then this can undermine the professional identity. Doctors who abandon their professional identity for their own needs fail to respect the autonomy of their patients. There is a lack of intentionality, understanding and voluntariness, which means that the patient's autonomous authority is so restricted that apparent 'consent' is suspect. While transference remains the cornerstone of any successful therapeutic relationship (particularly in psychoanalysis), it is the management of transference and countertransference that causes most boundary violations. Mishandling transference is arguably the most frequent cause of boundary violations and training in this area may ultimately be the most useful intervention. Supervision, it often has been said, provides the best safeguard against bad practice. Examining the history of offenders in this area often reveals that they worked alone, without a supervisor.

> Gartrell N, Herman J, Olarte S et al 1986 Psychiatrist–patient sexual activity: results of a national survey. I: Prevalence. American Journal of Psychiatry 143: 1126–1131

- A North American study of psychiatrists.
- Found that between 2 and 6% of psychiatrists had a history of sexual involvement with patients.

> Quadrio C 1996 Sexual abuse in therapy: gender issues. Australian and New Zealand Journal of Psychiatry 30: 125–133

- This Australian study of psychiatrists showed a 2–6% history of sexual involvement with patients.

> Royal College of Psychiatrists 2002 Vulnerable patients, vulnerable doctors: good practice in our clinical relationships. Council Report CR101. Royal College of Psychiatrists, London

- Emphasises that it is the meaning of a behaviour to the patient, and not the intentions of the doctor, that determines harm.
- 'Relationships of sexual intimacy between doctor and patient are totally unacceptable.'

Yalom I 1989 Love's executioner and other tales of psychotherapy. Bloomsbury, London, pp 68–86

- Knowing how not to indulge in self-disclosure in the face of seemingly harmless probing is a complex and subtle professional skill, which requires constant attention.

General Medical Council 2001 Good medical practice. GMC, London

- 'You must not use your professional position to establish or pursue a sexual or improper emotional relationship with a patient or someone close to them.'

Simon RI 1995 The natural history of therapist sexual misconduct: identification and prevention. Psychiatric Annals 25: 90–94

- Boundary violations, especially those of a sexual nature, do harm to the patient.
- A major boundary violation does not occur out of the blue as a single event, but rather it is the culmination of many small violations that the therapist allows to take place over time and that progressively erode professional identity.

Boundary violations have harmful consequences for the patient which include:
- emotional turmoil
- shame, fear or rage
- guilt and self-blame
- isolation and emptiness, disengagement from services
- cognitive distortion
- identity confusion
- emotional lability
- sexual dysfunction
- mistrust of authority, paranoia
- depression
- self-harm
- suicide.

Other issues include the loss of trust and damage to self-esteem. There is the resultant loss of the therapist and of therapy. Patients also have the burden of keeping the relationship secret.

Disch E, Avery N 2001 Sex in the consulting room, the examining room, and the sacristy: survivors of sexual abuse by professionals. American Journal of Ortho-psychiatry 71: 204–217

- Only 20% of therapists in one study made a referral to another clinician.
- This failure to provide for ongoing care creates a very real abandonment but also indicates how little therapists who have sex with their patients really care about them as people with psychological needs.

- Sexual relations with physicians are more damaging than with other types of professional, indicating how much trust is lost by this type of behaviour.

Gabbard GO, Peltz ML 2001 Speaking the unspeakable: institutional reactions to boundary violations by training analysts. Journal of the American Psychoanalytic Association 49: 659–673

- Described a particularly malignant variety of abusive experience, in which the violations occurred in the context of the training analyst–candidate dyad.
- This has long-term potential for future harm.
- The term 'poisoning the well' is used.

Garrett T 2002 Inappropriate therapist–patient relationships. In: Goodwin R, Cramer D (eds) Inappropriate relationships. Lawrence Erlbaum, Mahwah, NJ, pp 147–170

- Showed that 85% of a sample of Dutch male gynaecologists and 80–85% of American psychologists reported erotic feelings towards patients.
- Although erotic feelings on both sides are common in caring relationships, only about 10% of therapists act on them.

Definition

Boundary – the distinction between professional and personal identity.

Cognitive analytic therapy

Denman C 2001 Cognitive analytic therapy. Advances in Psychiatric Treatment 7: 243–252

This is a brief focal therapy informed by cognitive therapy, psychodynamic psychotherapy and certain developments in cognitive psychology. Developed by Anthony Ryle, it is based on the procedural sequence model. This attempts to understand aim-directed action. The model proposes that all aim-directed activity is the consequence of aim generation, environmental evaluation, plan formation, action, evaluation of consequences and, if necessary, remedial procedural revision.

Some procedural sequences are faulty and are repeatedly deployed without revision, causing the repetitive difficulties that characterise some psychological disorders. There are three types of unrevised faulty procedure – traps, dilemmas and snags:
- Traps are repetitive cycles of behaviour in which the consequences of the behaviour further increase the initial problem (e.g. the depressed-thinking trap).
- Dilemmas occur where false or limited options are presented, causing the individual to choose an opposing and maladaptive procedure. An example is the placation

trap in which the patient feels increasingly abused and angry until anger has been shown, at which point the patient reverts to the original placatory behaviour of the dilemma.

- Snags occur when the imagined future consequences of an action are so negative that they are capable of halting a procedure before it begins. This means that a hypothesis is never tested.

In some cases there can be undue restriction in the procedural repertoire. The causes of procedural restriction include impoverished environmental opportunities for learning new procedures, deliberate attempts by caregivers to restrict procedural repertoires and difficulty in new emotional learning owing to previously learned faulty procedures.

Reciprocal roles theory was described by Ryle as a more simple explanation of the concepts of countertransference and projective identification. Early learning about the social world is stored in the form of internalised templates of reciprocal roles. These consist of a role for self, a role for others and a paradigm for their relationship. They may be benign and functional or harsh and dysfunctional. Examples include caregiver/care receiver, bully/victim, admiring/admired and abuser/abused. In general, reciprocal roles are commonly shared templates. Therefore, when an individual takes up one role of a reciprocal role pairing, the person with whom they are relating feels pressure to adopt the opposite role. This can occur in the therapy and, if the patient's own reciprocal role repertoire is both unusually harsh and emotionally extreme, the therapist can feel a strong pressure to reciprocate in ego-alien ways.

In borderline personality disorder, CAT is based on abnormalities in the internalised reciprocal role structure. These include abnormalities in the reciprocal role repertoire, in switching smoothly between reciprocal roles and in the capacity for conscious self-reflection.

CAT shares with cognitive therapy a focus on the analysis of the conscious antecedents and consequences of symptoms. A detailed descriptive formulation is produced and shared with the patient. Homework is set with a problem-solving approach to difficulties. Change during therapy and the creation of shared tools for self-reflection are an important collaborative part of the therapy.

Timetable of therapy

Session 1
The therapist concentrates on three key tasks:
- building a therapeutic alliance
- gathering the patient's story
- giving the patient an understanding of the nature, mechanism of action and process of CAT.

The psychotherapy file (a questionnaire that describes common maladaptive procedures) may be given as homework.

Session 2
- Continues the tasks of Session 1.

- Begins to work with the patient on constructing a list of the main problems (known as target problems).
- Homework may include keeping a diary of target problems.

The reformulation letter

This is written by the therapist after three or four sessions. It usually begins with a narrative account of the patient's story and moves on to the current situation, main problems and the repetitive maladaptive procedures that underlie them. Often contains a diagram that lays out the repertoire of reciprocal roles used by the patient, the procedural sequences that they deployed around those roles and the symptomatic consequences of those sequences. Patients are encouraged to adapt the letter so that it becomes the basis for the rest of therapy.

Changing maladaptive procedural sequences

Once a formulation has been established, the task of therapy changes. The aim is for the patient, at first with the help of the therapist and later independently, to become able to recognise the operation of maladaptive procedural sequences or reciprocal roles as they occur in everyday life. This will continue up to 16 or 24 sessions.

Goodbye letter

This is given to the patient at the penultimate session. It briefly outlines the reason the patient came to treatment and recounts the story of the therapy. Patients can write a goodbye letter of their own. A follow-up session is booked for 3 months later.

Sequential diagrammatic reformulation

This is a diagram of reciprocal roles used by each patient.

Ryle A 1998 Transferences and countertransferences: the cognitive analytic therapy perspective. British Journal of Psychotherapy 14: 303–309

- The theory of reciprocal roles and of reciprocal role induction allows CAT to conceptualise the psychoanalytical concepts of transference, countertransference and projective identification in ways that are less mystifying and more practically useful.

Margison F 2000 Cognitive analytic therapy: a case study in treatment development [editorial]. British Journal of Medical Psychology 73: 145–149

- Highlights the lack of randomised controlled trials validating CAT.

Mann J, Goldman R 1982 A case book in time-limited psychotherapy. McGraw-Hill, New York

- CAT conducted by trainees was as effective as Mann's brief psychotherapy.

Definition

Cognitive analytic therapy – a brief (8–25 session) integrative therapy combining elements of CBT and psychodynamic therapies in an active, structured and collaborative approach, based on written and diagrammatic reformulations of the presenting difficulty. (*Source*: Department of Health 2001 Treatment choice in psychological therapies and counselling. DH, London.)

Cognitive behavioural therapy in first-episode and early schizophrenia

Tarrier N, Lewis S, Haddock R et al 2004 Cognitive behavioural therapy in first-episode and early schizophrenia: 18 month follow-up of a randomised controlled trial. British Journal of Psychiatry 184: 231–239

There is growing evidence for the benefits of CBT in symptoms of chronic schizophrenia.

Method and design

- A multicentre, prospective, rater-masked, randomised controlled trial with an 18-month follow-up period.
- The three groups were:
  - treatment as usual (TAU) with CBT
  - TAU with supportive counselling
  - TAU alone.
- Phase 1 lasted 70 days (see below).
- In Phase 2, patients were reassessed with psychiatric interview and examination of records and case notes at 18 months after randomisation.
- The hypothesis was that those who had received CBT would show reductions in:
  - symptoms
  - relapse (psychotic symptoms of greater than 1 week's duration and leading to a change in the patient's management)
  - readmission
  - admission duration.
- It was also hypothesised that there would be increased time to relapse.
- Patients were recruited from three different catchment areas in England once admitted to hospital.
- Medication was assessed with regard to total dose (chlorpromazine equivalents) and compliance.

The therapeutic interventions were carried out independent of assessors:

- CBT was manual based which provided 15–20 hours of treatment within 5 weeks of admission, plus booster sessions at 2 weeks and 1, 2 and 3 months after the initial treatment.
- Supportive counselling was based on previous work by Tarrier et al (1998) and was delivered at the same times as CBT.

Results

- 309 patients were included.
- 225 were interviewed at follow-up.
- Information was available from case notes for 295 patients.
- Hospital admission data were available for 307.
- Medication data were available for 171.
- Treatment with both CBT and supportive counselling significantly improved outcome compared with TAU.
- There was no difference for delusions and auditory hallucinations on the PSYRATS. There was no significant difference between CBT and supportive counselling, although there was a trend towards CBT for hallucinations.
- There was no significant difference in the treatment groups in terms of antipsychotic medication.
- Rates of hospitalisation were:
  - CBT   33%
  - SC   29%
  - TAU   36%.
- Rates of relapse were:
  - CBT   54.6%
  - SC   52.1%
  - TAU   51.1%.
- The median dose and the range in daily medication doses were:
  - CBT   500 mg (0–1250)
  - SC   400 mg (0–1700)
  - TAU   342.9 mg (0–1800).
- Generally compliance was good with no significant differences between groups.
- 19% had poor compliance.
- The results show that psychological treatment is beneficial in terms of symptom profile at follow-up but offers no benefit in terms of relapse or rehospitalisation.

Drury V, Birchwood M, Cochrane R et al 1996 Cognitive therapy and recovery from acute psychosis: a controlled trial. I. Impact on psychotic symptoms. II. Impact on recovery time. British Journal of Psychiatry 169: 602–607

- CBT significantly reduced recovery time by 25–30% in acutely ill patients.
- CBT significantly decreased the proportion of patients with residual symptoms to 5% in the treatment group compared with 56% in the control group.
- Differences were not apparent 5 years later.

Haddock G, Tarrier N, Morrison AP et al 1999 A pilot study evaluating the effectiveness of individual inpatient cognitive-behaviour therapy in psychosis. Social Psychiatry and Psychiatric Epidemiology 34: 254–258

- CBT provided in a period of acute illness resulted in non-significant reductions in rates of relapse and rehospitalisation over 2 years compared with supportive counselling.

Lewis S, Tarrier N, Haddock G et al 2002 Randomised, controlled trial of cognitive-behavioural therapy in early schizophrenia: acute-phase outcomes. British Journal of Psychiatry 181 (Suppl 43): S91–97

- The Study of Cognitive Reality Alignment Therapy in Early Schizophrenia Study – SoCRATES.
- Tested the hypothesis that CBT would lead to reductions in the time to recovery and subsequently protected against the persistence of symptoms and relapse after a first or early acute onset of the disorder.
- It compared TAU with CBT to TAU with supportive counselling, and TAU alone.
- The first phase examined whether CBT significantly reduced the time to recovery compared with the two control groups.
- Significant decreases were seen over the first 7 weeks, with a significant benefit of CBT over TAU at 5 weeks.

Tarrier N, Kinney C, McCarthy E et al 2001 Are some types of psychotic symptoms more responsive to CBT? Behavioural and Cognitive Psychotherapy 29: 45–55

- Found that hallucinations responded poorly to supportive counselling in patients with chronic schizophrenia.

Pitschel-Waltz G, Leucht S, Baumi J et al 2001 The effect of family interventions on relapse and rehospitalisation in schizophrenia: a meta-analysis. Schizophrenia Bulletin 27: 73–92

- Family interventions reduce relapse rates in studies of efficacy and effectiveness.
- The optimal psychosocial management of early schizophrenia would include a combination of CBT and family intervention.

Cognitive-behavioural therapy for refractory psychotic symptoms of schizophrenia resistant to atypical antipsychotic medication

Valmeggia LR, Van der Gaag M, Tarrier N et al 2005 Cognitive-behavioural therapy for refractory psychotic symptoms of schizophrenia resistant to atypical antipsychotic medication. Randomised controlled trial. British Journal of Psychiatry 186: 324–330

No study has examined the effects of cognitive behavioural therapy for inpatients with treatment-resistant psychotic symptoms.

Method

- This study compares CBT, supportive counselling and standard care.
- Patients were receiving long-term inpatient care.
- Patients had illnesses which had not responded to conventional treatments including adequate atypical antipsychotic medication.
- Patients had suffered from residual delusions or auditory hallucinations for at least 3 months and had not had a medication change less than 6 weeks prior to the start of the study.
- Patients had failed to respond to at least two antipsychotics, one of which was an atypical antipsychotic.
- Antipsychotic medication remained unchanged throughout the study period to ensure the changes in symptoms were due to the psychological interventions.
- CBT was delivered from a manual written by the authors.

Results

- Relapse was defined as an increase of more than 10 in the score on the positive symptom subscale of the PANSS, with deterioration lasting longer than 3 days.
- 62 patients were randomly allocated to either CBT or supportive counselling.
- Follow-up was completed by 42 patients.
- Three patients relapsed during the study and were withdrawn.
- CBT was more effective than supportive counselling at the post-treatment assessment in reducing physical characteristics (frequency, loudness, duration and location) and cognitive interpretation of auditory hallucinations.
- No difference was found with regard to emotional characteristics of auditory hallucinations.
- Psychological treatment could induce a change in psychotic symptoms in patients (in hospital) with chronic illness.

Birchwood M, Spencer E 1999 Psychotherapy for schizophrenia: a review. In: May M, Sartorius N (eds) Schizophrenia. Wiley, Chichester, pp 147–241

- Suggested that psychological interventions and rehabilitative efforts can help patients and their relatives cope with the consequences of having schizophrenia.

Pilling S, Bebbington P, Kuipers E et al 2002 Psychological treatments in schizophrenia: I. Meta-analysis of family intervention and cognitive behaviour therapy. Psychological Medicine 32: 763–782

- Increasing number of studies have shown that CBT combined with standard care, including medication, results in significant clinical benefits over standard care alone.

Wahlbeck K, Cheine M, Essali MA 2002 Clozapine versus typical neuroleptic medication for schizophrenia **(Cochrane Review)**. In: The Cochrane Library. Update Software, Oxford

- Clozapine brought about beneficial effects in 32% of patients in terms of producing clinical improvements.

National Institute for Clinical Excellence 2003 Schizophrenia: full national clinical guideline on care interventions in primary and secondary care. NICE, London

- Reported previous RCTs of CBT compared with other psychological therapies showing a NNT of 5.

See also the 'Treatment – Psychological therapies' section in Chapter 26 (Schizophrenia), pages 395-396.

Cognitive therapy for command hallucinations

Trower P, Birchwood M, Meaden A et al 2004 Cognitive therapy for command hallucinations: a randomised controlled trial. British Journal of Psychiatry 184: 312–320

There are few cognitive-based treatment approaches for patients with command hallucination. None has been tested systematically. Cognitive therapy for hallucinations continues to be developed. The authors suggest that command hallucinations are particularly appropriate for this approach.

Method

- A single blind, intention-to-treat randomised controlled trial.
- Cognitive therapy for command hallucination (CTCH) and treatment as usual (TAU) was compared with TAU alone.
- The main hypothesis (and primary outcome) was that by challenging key beliefs about the power of commanding voices, the CTCH group would show a lower level of compliance and appeasement behaviour

with an increase in resistance compared to the control group.
- The secondary outcomes were a lower conviction in power and social rank superiority of voices and the need to comply, and a reduction in depression and distress.
- 38 patients were recruited.
- All patients had command hallucinations on which they had acted, with serious consequences.
- Patients were randomised to CTCH/TAU or TAU.
- They were followed up at 6 and 12 months.

Results

- They found that there were significant reductions in compliance behaviour with the CTCH group.
- Cognitive therapy also appeared to reduce the conviction in power and superiority of the voices and the need to comply.
- There were also differences in the level of distress and depression.
- Differences were maintained at 12-month follow-up.
- No differences in voice loudness, frequency or content were noted.

Shawyer F, MacKinnon A, Ferhall J et al 2003 Command hallucinations and violence: implications for detention and treatment. Psychiatry, Psychology and the Law 10: 97–107

- Command hallucinations are high risk, upsetting and relatively common symptoms of schizophrenia.
- Found a median prevalence of 53% and a compliance rate of 31%.

Byrne S, Trower P, Birchwood M et al 2003 Command hallucinations: cognitive theory, therapy and research. Journal of Cognitive Psychotherapy: An International Quarterly 17: 67–84

- Applied the social rank theory to command hallucinations, describing how it can account for the cognitive content of the specific beliefs of those suffering command hallucinations.

Birchwood M, Meaden A, Trower P et al 2000 The power and omnipotence of voices: subordination and entrapment by voices and significant others. Psychological Medicine 30: 337–344

- Following the principles of social rank theory, the authors developed cognitive therapy for command hallucinations.
- This aims not to reduce the experience of the voices but to reduce the perceived power the voices have to harm the individual or to motivate compliance with them.

See also the 'Treatment – Psychological therapies' section in Chapter 10 (Forensic psychiatry), pages 166-168.

Cognitive therapy for the prevention of psychosis in ultra-high risk patients

Morrison AP, French P, Lewis S 2004 Cognitive therapy for the prevention of psychosis in people at ultra-high risk. Randomised controlled trial. British Journal of Psychiatry 185: 291–297

Early intervention in psychotic disorders has recently generated much interest. A small number of studies have examined the possibility of detecting individuals in the prodromal phase.

Aims

* This study aimed to establish whether psychological intervention could prevent transition into psychosis in the operationally defined high risk group.
* They hypothesised that cognitive therapy would reduce the transition rate significantly in comparison with treatment as usual.
* They also hypothesised that such cognitive therapy would significantly reduce the proportion of people requiring antipsychotic medication, reducing the likelihood of meeting the diagnostic criteria for schizophrenia, and therefore reduce the severity of the presenting prodromal (subclinical) syndrome.

Method

* 60 patients at ultra-high risk of psychosis were recruited (the results from two patients were excluded from further analyses due to current psychotic symptoms).
* 37 patients were assigned to cognitive therapy and 23 to be monitored.
* The PACE criteria for psychosis (based on PANSS) were used.
* Other instruments used included the General Health Questionnaire and the General Assessment of Functioning.

Results

* More than two-thirds of the sample were men.
* The mean age at entry was 22.
* Logistic regression analysis demonstrated that cognitive therapy significantly reduced the likelihood of progressing to psychosis over a period of 12 months.
* Cognitive therapy significantly reduced the likelihood of being prescribed medication and of meeting the DSM-IV criteria for a psychotic disorder.

* There was also a significant reduction in positive symptoms over 12 months compared to TAU.
* The study shows the benefit of a 6-month package of CBT on preventing the emergence of psychotic features over a 12-month period in a help-seeking, high-risk group.
* With only 14% withdrawing, the suggestion is that it is an acceptable intervention in this population.
* Although cognitive therapy was found to reduce the severity of subclinical psychotic experiences over a 12-month period, there was no evidence that the therapy improved the functioning or distress.

Yung A, McGorry PD, McFarlane CA et al 1996 Monitoring and care of young people at incipient risk of psychosis. Schizophrenia Bulletin 22: 283–303

* Pioneered the prodromal approach to prevention in their Personal Assessment and Crisis Evaluation (PACE) clinic.
* Developed operational criteria to identify the four subgroups at ultra-high risk of incipient psychosis.
* 40% of the high risk group developed psychosis within 9 months.

McGorry PD, Yung AR, Phillips LJ et al 2002 Randomised controlled trial of interventions designed to reduce the risk of progression to first episode psychosis in a clinical sample with subthreshold symptoms. Archives of General Psychiatry 59: 921–928

* Showed that specific pharmacotherapy and psychotherapy reduced the risk of early transition to psychosis in young people at ultra-high risk.
* This was in comparison to case management and supportive psychotherapy.
* There was a reduced rate of transition to psychosis at the end of treatment but not at follow-up.

Pantelis C, Velakoulis D, McGorry PD et al 2003 Neuroanatomical abnormalities before and after onset of psychosis: a cross sectional and longitudinal MRI comparison. Lancet 261: 281–288

* Showed structural brain deficits emerging in the high risk participants who went on to develop psychosis.

Bentall RP, Morrison AP 2002 More harm than good: the case against using antipsychotic drugs to prevent severe mental illness. Journal of Mental Health 11: 351 365

* The use of antipsychotics can be stigmatising and can have harmful side effects.
* The ethics of using cognitive behavioural therapy may be less controversial.

Morrison AP, Benthall RP, French P et al 2002 A randomised controlled trial of early detection and cognitive therapy for preventing transitions to psychosis in high risk individuals: study design and interim analysis of transition rate and psychological risk factors. British Journal of Psychiatry 181 (Suppl 43): S78–S84

- Such therapy may be suited to prevention of psychosis.

Drury V, Birchwood M, Cochrane R et al 1996 Cognitive therapy and recovery from acute psychosis: a controlled trial. I. Impact on psychotic symptoms. British Journal of Psychiatry 169: 593–601

- Effects have been demonstrated in acute psychosis.

Senky T, Turkington D, Kingdon D et al 2000 A randomized controlled trial of cognitive-behavioural therapy for persistent symptoms in schizophrenia resistant to medication. Archives of General Psychiatry 57: 165–172

- CBT is useful in patients with chronic, persistent psychotic symptoms

Gumley A, O'Grady M, McNay L et al 2003 Early intervention for relapse in schizophrenia: result of a 12 month randomised controlled trial of cognitive behaviour therapy. Psychological Medicine 33: 419–431

- CBT is helpful in relapse prevention.

See also the 'Treatment – Psychological therapies' section in Chapter 26 (Schizophrenia), pages 395-396.

Dialectical behaviour therapy in the treatment of borderline personality disorder

Blennerhassett RC, O'Raghallaigh JW 2005 Dialectical behaviour therapy in the treatment of borderline personality disorder. British Journal of Psychiatry 186: 270–280

DBT was developed by Marsha Linehan, a clinical psychologist. It addresses the treatment needs of individuals with a diagnosis of personality disorder and a history of parasuicidal behaviour.

Linehan MM, Armstrong HE, Suarez A et al 1991 Naturalistic follow-up of a behavioural treatment for chronically parasuicidal borderline patients. Archives of General Psychiatry 48: 1060–1064

- Linehan's original study demonstrated efficacy for this form of therapy compared with treatment as usual in:

- reducing the frequency of parasuicidal behaviour
- retaining patients in therapy
- reducing inpatient bed days.

Linehan MM, Schmidt H, Dimeff LA et al 1999 Dialectical behaviour therapy for patients with borderline personality disorder and drug dependence. American Journal of Addictions 8: 279–292

- DBT was shown to be effective in reducing drug misuse in those with a diagnosis of BPD.

Koons CR, Robins CJ, Bishop GK et al 2001 Efficacy of dialectical behaviour therapy in women veterans with borderline personality disorder: a randomized controlled trial. Behaviour Therapy 32: 371–390

- The first replication study.
- A small pilot study.
- Provided further support for the efficacy of the model.

The treatment model

Integrates proven techniques from cognitive and behavioural therapies within a philosophical and theoretical framework for understanding borderline pathology.

Its theory and practice borrow from four different orientations:
- biological
- social
- cognitive behavioural
- spiritual.

Both the experiences of the individual and effective therapeutic intervention are central to the theory. In this view, every experience contains simultaneous valid polarities, with the tension between them offering the possibility for change. The fundamental dialectic in this therapy is between validation and acceptance of the patients as they are, within the context of simultaneously helping them to change.

Components are:
- once weekly outpatient individual psychotherapy
- weekly skills training group
- telephone contact with the primary therapist
- weekly consultation session for the therapy team members.

It is a four-stage treatment which involves:
- decreasing life-threatening suicidal behaviours (at least a year)
- decreasing therapy-interfering behaviours (focuses on past trauma)
- decreasing quality-of-life interfering behaviours (works predominantly on self-esteem)
- increasing behavioural skills (develops the capacity for optimum experiencing).

Dialectical behaviour therapy – a longer-term cognitive behavioural treatment devised for personality disorder which teaches patients skills for regulating and accepting emotions and increasing interpersonal effectiveness. (*Source*: Department of Health 2001 Treatment choice in psychological therapies and counselling. DH, London.)

See also the 'Treatment – Psychological therapies' section in Chapter 19 (Personality disorders), pages 294-295.

Emotional and physical health benefits of expressive writing

Baikie KA, Wilhelm K 2005 Emotional and physical health benefits of expressive writing. Advances in Psychiatric Treatment 11: 338–346

Expressive writing as a therapeutic intervention involves patients writing about traumatic or distressing experiences, for 15–20 minutes per day on 3–5 consecutive days. Much of the evidence is drawn from laboratory studies. There are a number of studies which report beneficial effects on physical health and time spent in hospital. Expressive writing may be of benefit in a number of illnesses, with improvements found in:
- lung function in asthma
- disease severity in rheumatoid arthritis
- pain and physical health in cancer
- immune response in HIV infection
- number of admissions for cystic fibrosis
- level of pain in women with chronic pelvic pain
- time to sleep in poor sleepers
- postoperative recovery.

Pennebaker JW, Beall SK 1986 Confronting a traumatic event. Toward an understanding of inhibition and disease. Journal of Abnormal Psychology 95: 274–281

- The first study of expressive writing.
- Students spent 15 minutes per day on 4 consecutive days writing about their most traumatic previous experience.
- This led to a short-term increase in physical arousal.
- Students in the control group wrote about a mundane topic.
- At 4-month follow-up students in the intervention group had objective and subjective benefits in terms of physical health.

Pennebaker JW 1997 Writing about emotional experiences as a therapeutic process. Psychological Science 8: 162–166

- Whilst the experience of writing can cause distress, subjects report the process as being meaningful and valuable.

Greenberg MA, Wortman CB, Stone AA 1996 Emotional expression and physical heath. Revising traumatic memories or fostering self-regulation? Journal of Personality and Social Psychology 71: 588–602

- Improvements in physical health were found in students with a history of trauma following treatment with expressive writing.

Sloan DM, Marx BP 2004 A closer examination of the structured written disclosure procedure. Journal of Consulting and Clinical Psychology 72: 165–175

- Expressive writing in students who had a history of trauma led to beneficial effects on physical health, symptoms of post-traumatic stress disorder and other symptoms of psychological morbidity.

Richards JM, Beal WE, Seagal JD et al 2000 Effects of disclosure of traumatic events on illness behaviour among psychiatric prison inmates. Journal of Abnormal Psychology 109: 156–160

- Found only limited benefits for expressive writing in a population of male psychiatric prison inmates.

Smyth JM, Hockemeyer JR, Anderson C et al 2002 Structured writing about a natural disaster buffers the effect of intrusive thoughts on negative affect and physical symptoms. Australian Journal of Disaster and Traumatic Studies 1. Online. Available: www.massey.ac.nz/~trauma/issues/2002-1/smyth.htm

- Found only limited benefits for expressive writing in survivors of a natural disaster.

Kovac SH, Range LM 2002 Does writing about suicidal thoughts and feelings reduce them? Suicide and Life-Threatening Behaviour 32: 428–440

- Expressive writing was as effective as control group writing in students screened for suicidality.

Range LM, Kovac SH, Marion MS 2000 Does writing about the bereavement lessen grief following sudden, unintentional death? Death Studies 24: 115–134

- Expressive writing was as effective as control group writing in patients who had had a bereavement.

Batten SV, Follette VM, Rasmussen Hall ML et al 2002 Physical and psychological effects of written disclosure among sexual abuse survivors. Behaviour Therapy 33: 107–122

- Expressive writing was found to have detrimental effects for adults who had been abused in childhood.

Gidron Y, Peri T, Connolly JF et al 1996 Written disclosure in posttraumatic stress disorder: is it beneficial for the patient? Journal of Nervous and Mental Disease 184: 505–507

- This study examined the effects of expressive writing in eight Vietnam veterans with PTSD.
- It had detrimental effects.

Weblink Black Dog Institute's general practitioner education programme – www.blackdoginstitute.org.au.

Family intervention for schizophrenia

Pharoah FM, Rathbone J, Mari JJ, Streiner D 2003 Family intervention for schizophrenia **(Cochrane Review)**. In: The Cochrane Library, Issue 3. CD000088. Update Software, Oxford

- Family intervention may lead to reductions in the frequency of relapse (NNT 7; CI 5–16).
- The results are heterogeneous and tending to the null.
- Family intervention is associated with:
  - improved compliance with medication (NNT 7; CI 4–19)
  - improvements in general social function
  - the levels of expressed emotion in the family.
- Family intervention has no effect on dropout rates.
- It was not possible to draw conclusions regarding the impact on suicide rates.

See also the 'Treatment – Psychological therapies' section in Chapter 26 (Schizophrenia), pages 395-396.

Future of cognitive behavioural therapy for psychosis

Birchwood M, Trower P 2006 The future of cognitive behavioural therapy for psychosis: not a quasi-neuroleptic. British Journal of Psychiatry 188: 107–108

There is a growing evidence base regarding psychotherapy for psychosis, with a growing number of trials of CBT for psychosis finding beneficial effects.

The authors suggest a move away from the neuroleptic metaphor, i.e. a treatment that works in one illness and is used for treatment of another. It is suggested that the use of CBT relies too heavily on the assumptions and techniques of CBT for depression.

Targeted interventions that are informed by the growing understanding of the interface between emotion and psychosis should be developed.

The authors feel that the next generation of therapy needs to focus on theory-driven studies of emotional dysfunction and/or behavioural anomaly in psychosis.

Suggested areas of focus for CBT are:
- to reduce distress, depression and problem behaviour associated with persecutory delusions
- to reduce anxiety, depression and interpersonal difficulty in individuals at high risk of developing psychosis
- the relapse prodrome
- to address premorbid depression and social anxiety, including the patient's appraisal of the diagnosis and its stigmatising consequences
- to reduce stress reactivity, increase resilience to life stressors and prevent relapse
- to increase self-esteem and social confidence in people with psychosis.

National Institute for Clinical Excellence 2002 Core interventions in the management of schizophrenia in primary and secondary care. NICE, London

- Recommends CBT for psychosis to:
  - reduce psychotic symptoms
  - increase insight
  - promote medication adherence.

Tarrier N, Beckett R, Harwood S et al 1993 A trial of two cognitive-behavioural methods of treating drug-resistant residual psychotic symptoms in schizophrenic patients. 1. Outcome. British Journal of Psychiatry 162: 524–532

- CBT was initially used to help patients cope better with their psychotic symptoms.

Chadwick PD, Lowe CF 1990 Measurement and modification of delusional beliefs. Journal of Consulting and Clinical Psychology 58: 225–232

- Concluded that it was possible to 'reality test' delusional beliefs.

Turkington D, Kingdon D, Chadwick P 2003 Cognitive-behavioural therapy for schizophrenia: filling the therapeutic vacuum. British Journal of Psychiatry 183: 98–99

- Expressed concerns that CBT for psychosis now refers to a wide range of CBT treatments which vary in length and emphasis.

Birchwood M 2003 Pathways to emotional dysfunction in first episode psychosis. British Journal of Psychiatry 182: 373–375

- There is increasing evidence about the presence of comorbid psychiatric illness in patients with schizophrenia.

- This includes depression, social anxiety and PTSD.
- The process of relapse is complex and may involve cortical processes in affect regulation and common psychological developmental pathways.

Birchwood M, Gilbert P, Gilbert J et al 2004 Interpersonal and role-related schemata influence the relationship with the dominant 'voice' in schizophrenia: a comparison of three models. Psychological Medicine 34: 1571–1580

- The way people make sense of primary psychotic experiences (voices etc.) provides the main causal pathway to distress and depression associated with these experiences.

Iqbal Z, Birchwood M, Chadwick P et al 2000 Cognitive approach to depression and suicidal thinking in psychosis: 2. Testing the validity of a social ranking model. British Journal of Psychiatry 177: 522–528

- How people respond to the diagnosis of schizophrenia is distressing and can lead to the development of post-psychotic depression.
- Affective symptoms may result from the appraisal of the symptoms rather than being 'caused by' the psychotic experience.

Krabbendam L, Janssen I, Bili RV et al 2002 Neuroticism and low self-esteem as risk factors for psychosis. Social Psychiatry and Psychiatric Epidemiology 37: 1–6

- Neuroticism is a risk factor for psychosis.

Owens DGC, Miller P, Lawrie SM et al 2005 Pathogenesis of schizophrenia: a psychopathological perspective. British Journal of Psychiatry 186: 386–393

- Depression and anxiety (particularly social anxiety) are amongst the strongest predictors of relapse.

Trower P, Birchwood M, Maeden A 2004 Cognitive therapy for command hallucinations: randomised controlled trial. British Journal of Psychiatry 18: 312–320

- Command hallucinations are associated with reduced compliance.
- CBT reduced distress without affecting levels of voice activity.

Gumley A, O'Grady M, McNay L et al 2003 Early intervention for relapse in schizophrenia: results of a 12 month randomised controlled trial of cognitive-behavioural therapy. Psychological Medicine 33: 419–431

- There was a reduction in relapse when there was a focus on the earliest affective signs of relapse, and in particular the way in which they were catastrophised by patients.

Implementing the care programme approach in psychotherapeutic settings

Mace C 2004 Implementing the care programme approach in psychotherapeutic settings. Advances in Psychiatric Treatment 10: 124–130

The place for psychotherapeutic interventions within mental health services is ignored or denied in the literature on the implementation of care programming, even when the policy was 'modernised'. The care programme approach has evolved into a system of case management that has not specifically taken the needs of psychotherapeutic settings into account.

Similarities exist between the principles of CPA and the principles of good practice that apply across the psychotherapies, irrespective of the psychotherapist's model.

Good therapeutic practice requires consideration of a number of factors. Before treatment begins the specific needs and areas of vulnerability for each individual should be considered. A careful formulation should be developed and provided by a single therapist. The progress of treatment and the formulation should be regularly reviewed via supervision.

Effective CPA extends beyond the organisation of clinical treatments to the coordination of care to include:

- integration of health and social care
- streamlining of information systems
- responding to carers' needs.

There is the potential for conflict if the integration of health and social care were to become part of the role of the psychotherapist. The need to act as administrator or to be present at multidisciplinary meetings challenges the therapist's attempts to establish and maintain a working relationship that is privileged in its exclusion of others and in the confidences that may be shared.

The streamlining of information systems may require the therapist to follow protocols, such as the use of standardised risk assessments. This is at odds with a psychotherapeutic format where session agendas are not predetermined. If information is shared routinely between disciplines, on a need to know basis, it may well conflict with the therapist's ethical duty to safeguard the very personal disclosures that may be made to them on the patient's behalf and without their active consent.

Psychodynamically trained psychotherapists usually minimise contact with relatives and other carers in order to focus on the inner world of projections and fantasies that their patients present. While systemic therapists expect to work with families, sharp divisions between user and carer are antithetical to attempt to help family members recognise shared responsibilities for joint problems.

A survey of 20 psychotherapy consultants from different services showed that:

- 14 services had implemented CPA for patients receiving psychotherapy
- implementation was not standardised
- 10 services had a written policy for implementation
- 12 services reported having a written care plan for each patient – but two of these services had reported themselves as non-compliant with CPA
- 11 services had designated staff care coordinators, which included all 10 services that had implemented the CPA and were writing care plans
- eight services used a structured risk assessment
- five services used a structured clinical history
- four services made a record of housing and financial circumstances
- only one service, which offered cognitive behavioural therapy, reported that relatives were routinely involved in drawing up care plans
- when asked if care programming had improved the care received by patients, six said that it had and two said they were unsure, leaving a majority reporting no benefit or a net negative impact
- perceived advantages of the approach included observations that decision making was explicit, that risks were reliably recorded, that there was better communication between professionals and that there were clear staff roles
- perceived disadvantages of CPA included time spent on paperwork, possible effects on confidentiality due to centralised records and conflicts with the philosophy of care.

Individual and group-based parenting programmes for improving psychosocial outcomes for teenage parents and their children

Coren E, Barlow J 2001 Individual and group-based parenting programmes for improving psychosocial outcomes for teenage parents and their children **(Cochrane Review)**. In: The Cochrane Library, Issue 3. CD002964. Update Software, Oxford

- Four studies were included.
- Individual and group-based parenting programmes may be effective over a range of outcome measures including mother–infant interaction, language development, parental attitudes, parental knowledge,

maternal mealtime communication, maternal self-confidence and maternal identity.

- The results were limited by the small number of trials and methodological deficiencies.

See also the 'Treatment – Psychological therapies' section in Chapter 5 (Child and adolescent psychiatry), pages 78-79.

Individual psychodynamic psychotherapy and psychoanalysis for schizophrenia and severe mental illness

Malmberg L, Fenton M 2001 Individual psychodynamic psychotherapy and psychoanalysis for schizophrenia and severe mental illness (Cochrane Review). In: The Cochrane Library, Issue 3. CD001360. Update Software, Oxford

- No trials of a psychoanalytic approach were identified.
- Little information was found for psychodynamic approaches.
- There is no evidence of any positive effect of psychodynamic therapy and the possibility of adverse effects did not appear to have been considered.

See also the 'Treatment – Psychological therapies' section in Chapter 26 (Schizophrenia), pages 395-396.

Life skills programmes for chronic mental illnesses

Robertson L, Connaughton J, Nicol M 1998 Life skills programmes for chronic mental illnesses **(Cochrane Review)**. In: The Cochrane Library, Issue 3. CD000381. Update Software, Oxford

- Two randomised controlled trials were included.
- Data were sparse and no clear effects were demonstrated.
- Further investigation is required.

Motivational interviewing

Treasure J 2004 Motivational interviewing. Advances in Psychiatric Treatment 10: 331–337

Motivational interviewing is a form of counselling that encourages patients to explore and address ambivalence they might have about changing their behaviour. It takes a directive and patient-centred approach. It stems from the belief that negotiation of change will be more effective if it is led by the patient's own exploration of their behaviour and the associated benefits and costs. The process aims to generate a collaborative and therapeutic relationship between the patient and the therapist that is not based upon conflict.

The principles of motivational interviewing are:
- to express empathy via reflective listening
- to recognise and explore the discrepancies between a patient's attitudes and their behaviour
- to use empathy rather than conflict to prevent resistance
- to support the patient's belief that change is possible.

This therapy has been shown to be effective for patients whose difficulties are due to addiction problems, bulimia nervosa and diabetes. The results regarding smoking cessation are equivocal. The intervention is increasingly being adapted for use in other disorders such as psychosis, eating disorders and comorbid drug and alcohol misuse.

Miller W 1995 Increasing motivation for change. In: Hester RK, Miller WR (eds) Handbook of alcoholism treatment approaches: effective alternatives. Allyn and Bacon, Boston, MA

- The style of a therapist's interaction with a patient is the critical component in negotiating change in the patient's behaviour.
- Confrontation by the therapist was associated with the occurrence of resistance.
- Resistance occurred less often with a patient-centred approach.

Miller WR, Benefield RG, Tonigan JS 1993 Enhanced motivation for change in problem drinking: a controlled comparison of two therapist styles. Journal of Consulting and Clinical Psychology 61: 455–461

- Patients who had received therapy based on a confrontation approach had poorer outcomes in terms of drinking after 12 months.
- Low levels of resistance were associated with change.

Brown KL, Miller WR 1993 Impact of motivational interviewing on participation and outcome in residential alcoholism treatment. Psychology of Addictive Behaviours 7: 238–245

- Patients who received a short motivational interviewing intervention (the drinker's check-up) prior to inpatient admission were more likely to participate in their treatment programme and were more motivated.

Project MATCH Research Group 1998 Matching alcoholism treatments to patient heterogeneity: Project MATCH three-year drinking outcomes. Alcoholism, Clinical and Experimental Research 22: 1300–1311

- The largest clinical trial of alcohol dependence.
- A manualised four-session motivational interviewing intervention for alcohol was used.

- 1726 patients were randomised to three different interventions.
- Interventions were 12 sessions of 12-step facilitation therapy, four sessions of motivational interviewing intervention or 12 sessions of CBT.
- Treatment was given in both community and inpatient settings.
- The study concluded that the three interventions were of equal benefit in terms of outcomes up to 12 months after treatment.
- The study had aimed to identify if there were any patient characteristics associated with better outcomes in each of the interventions.
- It found that patients who scored higher on state-trait anger did best with motivational interviewing.

Weblinks
Motivational Interviewing – www.motivationalinterviewing.org.
Project MATCH – www.commed.uchc.edu/match.

Multisystemic therapy for social, emotional, and behavioural problems in youth

Littell JH, Popa M, Forsythe B 2005 Multisystemic therapy for social, emotional, and behavioural problems in youth aged 10–17 (**Cochrane Review**). In: The Cochrane Library, Issue 3. CD004797. Update Software, Oxford

- The pooled results from eight studies showed no significant effects on a number of outcome measures.
- Outcomes included likelihood or duration of restrictive out-of-home placements, proportion of youth who were arrested or convicted, numbers of arrests/convictions within 1 year post-intervention, results from drug testing or self-reported drug use at 6-month follow-up.
- For those who completed the programme, there were no significant between-group differences on self-reported delinquency, peer relations, youth behaviour problems, youth psychiatric symptoms or family functioning.
- There was no evidence that the therapy has harmful effects.

Definition

Multisystemic therapy (MST) – an intensive, home-based intervention for families of youths with social, emotional and behavioural problems. Masters-level therapists engage family members in identifying and changing individual, family and environmental factors thought to contribute to problem behaviour. Intervention may include efforts to improve communication, parenting skills, peer relations, school performance and social networks.

See also the 'Treatment – Psychological therapies' section in Chapter 5 (Child and adolescent psychiatry), pages 78-79.

Parent-training programmes for improving maternal psychosocial health

Barlow J, Coren E, Stewart-Brown SSB 2003 Parent-training programmes for improving maternal psychosocial health **(Cochrane Review)**. In: The Cochrane Library, Issue 4. CD002020. Update Software, Oxford

- Of 26 identified studies, 20 provided sufficient data to calculate effect sizes.
- The five outcomes of depression, anxiety/stress, social support and relationship with spouse/marital adjustment had sufficient data to combine in a meta-analysis.
- All of these outcomes, except for social support, showed statistically significant results favouring the intervention group.
- Some of the studies alone showed no effect.
- There is a lack of evidence as to whether these effects are maintained over time.

Stepped care in psychological therapies

Bower P, Gilbody S 2005 Stepped care in psychological therapies: access, effectiveness and efficiency: a narrative literature review. British Journal of Psychiatry 186: 11–17

A number of studies and papers have suggested 'stepped care' as a solution to the problem of poor access to psychological therapy services. This review considers stepped care, its relation to psychological therapies and the current evidence.

Stepped care model are models of healthcare delivery with two specific principles:
- The recommended treatment should be the least restrictive, while still providing significant health gain. Least restrictive may refer to personal cost, inconvenience, intensity of treatment, etc.
- The stepped care model is self correcting: the results of treatment and decisions about further treatment are monitored systematically and 'stepped up' if current treatments are not achieving significant health gains.

The four qualitatively different steps can be seen as:
- self-help
- guided self-help and group therapy
- brief individual therapy
- longer-term individual therapy.

Decisions about stepping up should not be reliant on professional assessment and should involve guidelines, assessment tools and patients. Stepped care models may be far more appropriate for disorders in which adverse consequences would not result from starting patients on too low a step.

Although practical issues are important, current interest in the stepped care model is based on three fundamental assumptions:
- Equivalence assumption: minimal interventions can provide 'significant health gain' equivalent to that of traditional psychological therapies, at least for a proportion of patients.
- Efficiency assumption: using minimal interventions will allow current healthcare resources to be used more efficiently.
- Acceptability assumption: minimal interventions and the stepped care approach are acceptable to patients and professionals.

There are few published studies of a complete stepped care model.

Kanton W, Von Korff M, Lin E et al 1997 Population based care of depression: effective disease management strategies to decrease prevalence. General Hospital Psychiatry 19: 169–178

- Stepped care standardises systems and procedures with the open aim of improving efficacy.

Scott C, Tacchi MJ, Jones R et al 1997 Acute and one year outcome of a randomised controlled trial of brief cognitive therapy for major depressive disorder in primary care. British Journal of Psychiatry 171: 131–134

- Reported that treatments of different intensity are required.

Dowrick C, Dunn G, Ayuso-Mateos J-L et al 2000 Problem solving treatment and group psychoeducation for depression: multicentre randomised controlled trial. British Medical Journal 321: 1–6

- Minimal interventions can be provided in the form of brief therapies or group treatments.
- CBT is the main candidate for stepped care, having the benefit of consistent operationalised steps.

Rogers A, Hassell K, Nicolaas G 1999 Demanding patients? Analysing the use of primary care. Open University Press, Milton Keynes

- Much informal health care is undertaken by patients in the community without the intervention of mental health services.

Wilson G, Vitousek K, Loeb K 2000 Stepped care treatment for eating disorders. Journal of Consulting and Clinical Psychology 68: 564–572

- Qualified this by exemplifying stepped care as being appropriate for bulimia and binge eating but perhaps not anorexia nervosa.

Lovell K, Richards D 2000 Multiple access points and levels of entry (MAPLE): ensuring choice, accessibility and equity for CBT services. Behavioural and Cognitive Psychotherapy 28: 379–391

- Found the evidence for minimal interventions being best restricted to less severe disorders is not definitive.
- There will be cases in which early intensive treatment is actually more clinically and cost-effective.

Very brief dynamic psychotherapy

Aveline M 2001 Very brief dynamic psychotherapy. Advances in Psychiatric Treatment 7: 373–380

Background

The Nottingham model: three-plus-one (BRF) is a randomised controlled trial which looked at the effect of brief intervention and follow-up in comparison with the standard assessment procedure for dynamic psychotherapy. It aimed to assess whether BRF is beneficial in some patients and whether it is possible to predict which patients need longer therapy.

Method

In BRF the patient is seen for four sessions in total. The initial assessment interview is followed by two therapy sessions during the second, third or fourth weeks. There is a final follow-up session at 3 months. The decision about entry into therapy is made collaboratively at the final session. This is a three-plus-one intervention which compares with a single interview in the standard assessment.

Independent assessment of target problems, symptoms, self-esteem, problems in interpersonal relationships and other relevant aspects was made by a research psychologist at 0, 4, 15 and 36 months.

Results

- 267 referrals for specialist psychodynamic psychotherapy were included.
- Complete data were available for 156 subjects at zero and 4 months.
- The three-plus-one intervention provided sufficient therapy for only 6% of subjects.
- Standard assessment was sufficient therapy in 3% of patients.
- More detailed and patient-informed assessment was done in the three-plus-one intervention.
- More subjects (50%) were judged to be unsuitable for specialist psychotherapy after BRF.

- 21% of patients who received the standard assessment were judged to be unsuitable for specialist psychotherapy.
- Patients preferred the three-plus-one intervention, regardless of outcome.
- While the three-plus-one intervention was resource intensive, there was an overall saving of between 8.5 and 5.7 sessions per patient not put on the waiting list for subsequent therapy.

The therapy

- Both therapist and patient are active in BRF.
- The therapist seeks opportunities for the patient to take 'significant action'.
- Significant action is of personal significance.
- If the patient succeeds in this action then there is a 'corrective emotional experience', the knowledge of which can be used in the future.

Key features of BRF

- Focus on present-day, real-life problems
- Formulation
- Frame focus on what is of central importance
- Flexibility: adapt to what is needed
- Some form of corrective emotional experience
- Crises are opportunities for change
- Reinforces the patient's natural capacity for healing and change.

The formulation aims to move the focus from the symptomatic to the psychological. It seeks the central interpersonal issues. These are derived from detailed examination of recent problematic interactions. Central issues are likely to be recurrent. Issues may pose choices for the patient – for example, to explore or ignore, to change or accept.

Shapiro DA, Firth J 1987 Prescriptive vs exploratory psychotherapy: outcomes of the Sheffield Psychotherapy Project. British Journal of Psychiatry 151: 790–799

- A detailed study of brief psychotherapy.
- Prescriptive and explorative psychotherapy were compared in a 16-week cross-over design with businessmen with moderate depression.
- The subjects had work-related stress.
- Both therapies were effective, with a slight advantage in the treatment population for the directive therapy.

Working with grieving adults

Clark A 2004 Working with grieving adults. Advances in Psychiatric Treatment 10: 164–170

In patients who have been bereaved, pharmacological treatment should be prescribed if indicated as for non-bereaved individuals. It is important to remember that certain medication, particularly anxiolytics, can inhibit the natural grief process.

There is a general lack of literature about effective psychological treatments for grief work. Therapists working with grieving adults can act as a secure base to allow adults to feel safe to explore painful feelings.

> Mitchell A, House A 2000 Adjustment to illness, handicap and bereavement. In: Gelder MG, Lopez-Ibor JJ, Andreassen NC (eds) New Oxford textbook of psychiatry. Oxford University Press, Oxford, pp 1139–1147

- 50% of bereaved spouses meet the criteria for a major depressive episode at some point in the first year following their loss.
- This episode usually resolves by 6 months.
- 10% suffer from depression for the entire year.
- The clinical features which suggest a major depressive episode rather than normal grief are:
  - guilt about things other than actions taken or not taken by the survivor at the time of death
  - thoughts of death except in relation to the deceased
  - feelings of worthlessness
  - psychomotor retardation
  - prolonged and marked functional impairment
  - hallucinations except in relation to the deceased.

> Jacobs S, Hansen F, Kasl S et al 1990 Anxiety disorders during acute bereavement: risk and risk factors. Journal of Clinical Psychiatry 51: 269–274

- In a small study of bereaved spouses it was found that 44% developed an anxiety disorder in the first year.
- 9% developed the symptoms of PTSD.

> Raphael B 1977 Preventative intervention with the recently bereaved. Archives of General Psychiatry 34: 450–454

- Preventative interventions in the early bereavement period were effective for widows at high risk of pathological grief.
- Risk factors selected were lack of support from social networks, previous highly ambivalent relationship with the deceased and the presence of at least three concurrent stressful life events.
- On average, the treatment group received four 2-hour sessions of counselling.
- 77% in the treatment group were improved 13 months after their husband's death compared with 41% in the untreated group.

> Marmar C, Horowitz MJ, Weiss DS et al 1988 A controlled trial of brief psychotherapy and mutual-help group treatment of conjugal bereavement. American Journal of Psychiatry 145: 203–209

- A randomised controlled trial of brief psychodynamic psychotherapy versus a mutual self-help group treatment for widows who had sought treatment for unresolved grief reactions between 4 months and 3 years after the death of their husband.
- It was found that women in both groups experienced a reduction in stress-specific and general psychiatric symptoms as well as improvement in social and work functioning.
- The two treatments were equally effective, although there was greater attrition of numbers in the group treatment.

> Symington J, Symington N 1996 The clinical thinking of Wilfred Bion. Routledge, London

- If the professional can contain the pain of grief, then this can help the patient internalise a sense that their pain can be borne and thought about.

> Mawson D, Marks I, Ramm L et al 1981 Guided mourning for morbid grief: a controlled trial. British Journal of Psychiatry 138: 185–193

- Summarises guided mourning as involving an 'intense reliving of avoided painful memories and feelings associated with bereavement'.
- It is an approach which likens unresolved grief to other forms of phobic avoidance, which are treated successfully with a behavioural approach with exposure to the avoided situation.

Guidelines

Treatment choice in psychological therapies and counselling

> Department of Health 2001 Treatment choice in psychological therapies and counselling. Evidence based clinical practice guideline. DH, London. Online. Available: www.nelmh.org/downloads/other_info/treatment_choice_psychological_therapies.pdf[†]

The guidelines address who is likely to benefit from psychological treatment, and which of the main therapies currently available in the NHS is most appropriate for which patients.

[†] Crown copyright. Reproduced with permission.

The guidelines are relevant to a number of presenting problems, including:

- depression, including postnatal depression and suicidal behaviour
- anxiety and related disorders, including OCD and PTSD
- eating disorders
- personality disorders, including repetitive self-harm
- somatic presentations, including chronic pain, chronic fatigue, gastrointestinal and gynaecological problems.

The guidelines do not address the use of psychological therapies in psychotic disorders, substance misuse, children and adolescents, those with sexual dysfunction and paraphilias, organic brain syndromes and acquired brain injury or learning disability.

A number of general and specific recommendations were made from the best available evidence.

Recommendations

Initial assessment

- Psychological therapy should be routinely considered as a treatment option when assessing mental health problems. [B]
- In considering psychological therapies, more severe or complex mental health problems should receive secondary, specialist treatment. [D]

Therapeutic relationship

- Effectiveness of all types of therapy depends on the patient and the therapist forming a good working relationship. [B]

Treatment length

- Therapies of fewer than eight sessions are unlikely to be optimally effective for most moderate to severe mental health problems. [B]
- Often 16 sessions or more are required for symptomatic relief, and longer therapies may be required to achieve lasting change in social and personality functioning. [C]
- Specific phobias and uncomplicated panic disorder (without agoraphobic symptoms) can respond to brief interventions. [B]

Age, sex, social class and ethnic group

- The patient's age, sex, social class or ethnic group are generally not important factors in the choice of therapy and should not determine access to therapies. [C]
- Ethnic and cultural identity should be respected by referral to culturally sensitive therapists. [C]

Patient preference

- Patient preference should inform treatment choice, particularly where the research evidence does not indicate a clear choice of therapy. [D]

Skill level of therapist

- The skill and experience of the therapist should also be taken into account. More complex problems, and those

where patients are poorly motivated, require a more skilful therapist. [D]

Patient characteristics

- Interest in self-exploration and capacity to tolerate frustration may be particularly important for success in interpretative (psychoanalytic and psychodynamic) therapies, compared with supportive therapy. [C]

Adjustment to life events

- Patients who are having difficulty adjusting to life events, illnesses, disabilities or losses (including childbirth and bereavement) may benefit from brief therapies, such as counselling. [B]

Post-traumatic stress

- Where post-traumatic stress disorder (PTSD) is present, psychological therapy is indicated, with best evidence for cognitive behavioural methods. [A]

Depressive disorders

- Depressive disorders may be treated effectively with psychological therapy, with best evidence for cognitive behaviour therapy and interpersonal therapy, and some evidence for a number of other structured therapies, including short-term psychodynamic therapy. [A]

Anxiety disorders

- Anxiety disorders with marked symptomatic anxiety (panic disorder, agoraphobia, social phobia, obsessive–compulsive disorders, simple phobias and generalised anxiety disorders) are likely to benefit from cognitive behaviour therapy. [A]

Eating disorders

- Bulimia nervosa can be treated with psychological therapy, with best evidence for interpersonal therapy and cognitive behaviour therapy. [A]
- Although individual psychological therapy for anorexia nervosa may be of benefit, there is little strong evidence on therapy type. [B]

Personality disorder

- A coexisting diagnosis of personality disorder may make treatment of the presenting mental health problem more difficult and possibly less effective; indicators of personality disorder include forensic history, severe relationship difficulties and recurrent complex problems. [D]
- Structured psychological therapies delivered by skilled practitioners can contribute to the longer-term treatment of personality disorders. [C]

Somatic complaints

- Cognitive behaviour therapy should be considered as a psychological treatment for chronic fatigue and chronic pain. [B]
- Psychological intervention should be considered for other somatic complaints with a psychological component, such as irritable bowel syndrome and gynaecological complaints (premenstrual syndrome, pelvic pain). [C]

Contraindications

- Routine debriefing shortly after a traumatic event is unlikely to help PTSD and is not recommended. [A]
- Generic counselling is not recommended as the main intervention for severe and complex mental health problems or personality disorders. [D]

A, B, C and **D** indicate grades of recommendation (see Appendix II for full details).

See also the 'Guidelines' sections in Chapter 2 (Affective disorders), page 44; Chapter 3 (Anxiety disorders), page 55; Chapter 16 (Obsessive–compulsive disorder), page 245; and Chapter 23 (Post-traumatic stress disorder), page 340.

Guidance on the use of computerised cognitive behavioural therapy for anxiety and depression. NICE Technology Appraisal Guidance 51*

Guidance

Current research suggests that the delivery of cognitive behavioural therapy via a computer interface (CCBT) may be of value in the management of anxiety and depressive disorders. This evidence is, however, an insufficient basis on which to recommend the general introduction of this technology into the NHS.

To establish the contribution and place of CCBT in the management of anxiety and depressive disorders, including its role within 'stepped care' approaches, the NHS should consider supporting an independent programme of research into CCBT, including carefully monitored pilot implementation projects. The research should include investigations into user preferences, suitability, needs and educational/cultural characteristics.

---

* Reproduced with permission from the National Institute for Health and Clinical Excellence, London.

See also the 'Guidelines' section in Chapter 3 (Anxiety disorders), page 55.

Schizophrenia and related disorders

26

Chapter contents

General topics

The Danish National Schizophrenia Project: prospective, comparative longitudinal treatment study of first episode psychosis

Rosenbaum B, Valbak K, Harder SE 2005 The Danish National Schizophrenia Project: prospective, comparative longitudinal treatment study of first episode psychosis. British Journal of Psychiatry 186: 394–399

It has been suggested that the years which follow an initial episode of psychosis may be critical in the imprinting of biopsychosocial changes with subsequent effects on long-term outcome. Psychosocial interventions that aim to minimise the damaging early effects of illness may have a disproportionate positive impact compared to interventions later in the illness course.

Method

- The Danish National Schizophrenia Project investigated the effects of early, rapid and year-long sustained intervention after the first signs of psychosis.
- A prospective, longitudinal, multicentre investigation of 562 consecutive referrals during a 2-year period.
- Patients were allocated to manualised intervention:
  – supportive psychodynamic psychotherapy as a supplement to TAU

  – integrated, assertive, psychosocial and educational treatment
  – treatment as usual.
- The outcome of improvements in symptoms and social function were studied.
- Interventions focused on the:
  – attitudes toward illness
  – realistic social goals
  – emotional reactions in interpersonal relationships
  – intrapsychic and intrapersonal emotions.
- Manualised psycho-educational family treatment focused on problem solving and the development of skills to cope with aspects of the illness.
- Outcome measures were the Positive and Negative Symptom Subscales and the Global Assessment of Functioning.

Results

- There were no significant differences in outcome at the end of 12 months between any of the groups.
- There was a trend towards greater improvement in social functioning in the integrated treatment group compared with the treatment as usual group.
- Significance was reached for some measures when the confounding effect of drugs and alcohol misuse was included.
- It may be assumed that medication accounted for most of the improvement during the first year of treatment.
- The time frame may have been too short, with some patients only receiving 6 months of individual psychodynamic psychotherapy or social skills training.

- Patients who do not use drugs and alcohol are more receptive to psychotherapeutic interventions.

Martindale B, Bateman A, Crowe M et al 2000 Psychosis: psychological approaches and their effectiveness. Gaskell, London

- Previous studies of first episode psychosis have found positive outcomes for various integrated treatments compared with standard treatment.
- Previous studies comparing psychodynamic psychotherapy and standard treatment are few and have diverse results. None of these studies involved first episode psychosis.

Distinguishing characteristics of subjects with good and poor early outcome in the Edinburgh High-Risk Study

Johnstone E, Cosway R, Lawrie SM 2002 Distinguishing characteristics of subjects with good and poor early outcome in the Edinburgh High-Risk Study. British Journal of Psychiatry 181: S26–S29

Studies of people at high risk of schizophrenia because of family history may provide information regarding the pathogenesis of the disorder. It remains unclear whether abnormalities in language, behaviour and motor development are due to early pathological changes or are vulnerability factors.

Method

- The Edinburgh High-Risk Study recruited young adults aged between 16 and 25 years at high risk of schizophrenia.
- High risk of schizophrenia is determined from having two close relatives with schizophrenia.
- 229 people were identified and, 6 years on, information has been gathered from over two-thirds of the group.
- There are two control groups:
  - 34 age- and sex-matched people with no family history
  - 36 age-matched people with first episode schizophrenia.
- Numbers in the control group reflect the expected number of cases of schizophrenia from the high-risk group (30).
- Groups of patients were identified with good and poor outcomes so far.

- The two groups were compared with regard to:
  - genetic liability
  - baseline neuropsychology
  - baseline neuroanatomy
  - changes from baseline.

Results

- 13 male and 11 female perfects (no scoring on any psychopathological item) at a mean age of 21.2 years were identified.
- Eight males and five females had developed schizophrenia.
- The mean age of ascertaining a diagnosis of schizophrenia was 20.3 years.
- There were no significant differences between the groups in terms of:
  - demographics
  - genetic liability
  - neuroanatomy.
- Being in the good outcome group was associated with better baseline performance on neuropsychological testing.
- Being in the poor outcome group was associated with:
  - impaired memory function
  - a tendency to a reduction in temporal lobe size.

Environmental influences in schizophrenia: the known and the unknown

Leask S 2004 Environmental influences in schizophrenia: the known and the unknown. Advances in Psychiatric Treatment 10: 323–330

It is possible to identify factors that are not obviously a consequence of an individual's behaviour, that are present before any signs of illness or prodrome, and that therefore probably can be seen as independent risk factors for a schizophrenic illness.

Studies using ICD-10 have tended to emphasise geographical differences and supported an increased incidence in urban areas compared with rural areas. Studies in the Caribbean have confirmed a greater incidence in developing countries, but suggest more favourable outcomes in terms of the course and outcome of the illness, despite lack of drugs and healthcare provision. This may relate to social cohesion rather than physical resources.

Numerous studies have described an increased rate of substance misuse in patients with schizophrenia. Unrepresentative samples have often been used or there has been no matched control population. An association is probably there, but whether this is a chance finding, a result of patients self-medicating, the illness predisposing to substance misuse, or vice versa, requires clarification.

Associations have been found between maternal influenza, polio and rubella and an increased risk of schizophrenia. There is no evidence to allow us to establish whether these are specific effects of the infection, the pyrexia, the medications or the maternal immune response.

There is twice the rate of schizophrenia with prenatal maternal stress, unwanted pregnancies and depression in late pregnancy. Schizophrenia is also associated with being in utero during a period of famine.

The association between schizophrenia and environmental factors needs to be further investigated.

Bradbury TN, Miller GA 1985 Season of birth in schizophrenia: a review of the evidence, methodology and aetiology. Psychological Bulletin 98: 569–594

- In the northern hemisphere there is reasonably consistent evidence of a 5–8% excess of births in winter and spring of children who subsequently develop schizophrenia.
- Other studies have suggested that this work is an artefact (as the earlier in the year an individual is born the older they will be).
- This study found an association between winter and spring births unconnected to age.

McGrath J, Welham J, Pemberton M 1995 Month of birth, hemisphere of birth and schizophrenia. British Journal of Psychiatry 167: 783–785

- Similar effect for spring in the northern hemisphere.

Jablensky A, Sartorius N, Ernberg G 1992 Schizophrenia: manifestations, incidence and course in different cultures. A World Health Organization 10-country study. Psychological Medicine Monograph Supplement 20: 1–97

- The incidence of schizophrenia (using ICD-9 and PSE) was significantly higher in developing countries.
- The incidence of schizophrenia as defined by first rank ('nuclear') symptoms was constant across the world.

Faris R, Dunham H 1939 Mental disorders in urban areas. University of Chicago Press, Chicago

- There is an increased risk of developing schizophrenia in urban compared with rural areas.

Marcelis M, Takei N, van Os J 1999 Urbanization and risk for schizophrenia: does the effect operate before or around the time of illness onset? Psychological Medicine 29: 1197–1203

- The greatest association was found between urban birth and schizophrenia as opposed to later urban living.

Odergard O 1932 Emigration and insanity: a study of mental disease among a Norwegian born population in Minnesota. Acta Psychiatrica Neurologica Scandinavica Supplementum 4: 1–206

- There are increased rates of schizophrenia in Norwegian immigrants to the USA.

Harrison G, Owens D, Holten A 1994 A prospective study of severe mental disorder in Afro-Caribbean patients. Psychological Medicine 18: 643–657

- Non-white individuals living in Camberwell are reported to be at a higher risk of schizophrenia than the white population.

Geddes JR, Lawrie SM, Verdoux H 1999 Schizophrenia and complications of pregnancy and labour: an individual patient data meta-analysis. Schizophrenia Bulletin 25: 413–423

- Significant associations were found for:
  - premature rupture of membranes
  - premature birth (< 37 weeks)
  - use of resuscitator or incubator.
- There was a trend towards low birth weight (< 2.5 kg).
- Birth record data of pre-eclampsia and maternal recall of forceps delivery were also significantly associated.

First-episode schizophrenia: a review of cognitive deficits and cognitive remediation

Gopal YV, Variend H 2005 First-episode schizophrenia: a review of cognitive deficits and cognitive remediation. Advances in Psychiatric Treatment 11: 38–44

- No studies were identified of the effects of cognitive remediation on first episode schizophrenia.
- It is not possible to generalise the results from studies of patients with enduring schizophrenia.

Saykin AJ, Shtasel DL, Gur RE et al 1994 Neuropsychological deficits in neuroleptic naive patients with first episode schizophrenia. Archives of Psychiatry 51: 124–131

- This study concluded that the cognitive deficits that occur in first episode psychosis differ from the deficits that occur in long-term illness only in terms of degree of severity.
- Identified memory deficits included impairments in verbal memory and learning.
- Memory deficits did not appear to be caused by anticholinergic medication and were independent of impairments in attention and executive function.

- Attention/vigilance and speeded visuomotor processing were also impaired but not to the same level as memory.

Joyce E, Hutton S, Mutsatsa S et al 2002 Executive dysfunction in first-episode schizophrenia and relationship to duration of untreated psychosis: the West London Study. British Journal of Psychiatry 181 (Suppl 43): S38–44

- This West London study argued that the executive impairment occurring in first episode illness is different from that found in patients with enduring schizophrenia.
- They found significant deficits in spatial working memory, short-term spatial memory and long-term episodic memory in comparison with healthy controls.
- These differences were still significant once IQ was taken into account.
- When timed in tasks of executive function, patients with first episode psychosis were quicker at initiating responses but the overall time to complete a task was the same as for patients with chronic schizophrenia.

Bilder RM, Goodman RS, Robinson D et al 2000 Neuropsychology of first-episode schizophrenia: initial characterisation and clinical correlates. American Journal of Psychiatry 157: 549–559

- It is not clear whether the cognitive deficits in schizophrenia are isolated or part of a more global impairment.
- Patients with first episode schizophrenia who had been stabilised on antipsychotic medication had memory impairments when compared with healthy controls.
- Deficits in executive and motor function were not as great as deficits in memory and attention in patients with first episode schizophrenia.

Mohamed S, Paulsen JS, O'Leary D et al 1999 Generalised cognitive deficits in schizophrenia: study of first-episode patients. Archives of General Psychiatry 56: 749–754

- People with (as yet untreated) first episode schizophrenia had impairments in memory function with impaired immediate and delayed recall.
- Certain cognitive tasks were also impaired and this was particularly the case for cognitive tasks that did not include a motor component.
- There were severe impairments in executive function including sequencing and organisational flexibility.
- There was a weak correlation between negative symptoms and impaired performance.

Hoff AL, Riordan H, Donald W et al 1992 Neuro-psychological functioning of first episode schizophreniform patients. American Journal of Psychiatry 149: 898–903

- Impairments in memory found in a group of patients with first episode schizophrenia were still present once remission was achieved.

Pantelis C, Barnes T, Nelson H et al 1999 A comparison of set shifting ability in patients with schizophrenia and frontal lobe damage. Schizophrenia Research 37: 251–270

- Found that people with chronic schizophrenia have normal initial thinking times but that subsequent responses are slower.

Hoff A, Sakuma M, Weineke M et al 1999 Longitudinal neuropsychological follow-up of patients with first-episode schizophrenia. American Journal of Psychiatry 156: 1336–1341

- A longitudinal follow-up study of 42 patients with first episode schizophrenia.
- Improvements in cognitive performance and improvements in positive symptoms are linked.
- There was no link with changes in negative symptoms or commencement of medication.
- Deficits in verbal memory showed smaller improvements in patients with schizophrenia than healthy controls.

Zipursky RB, Lambe EK, Kapur S et al 1998 Cerebral gray matter volume deficits in first episode psychosis. Archives of General Psychiatry 55: 540–546

- Demonstrated that structural brain abnormalities are present at the time of first episode psychosis.
- They showed changes in grey matter volumes in patients with first episode schizophrenia.

Fannon D, Chitnis X, Doku V et al 2000 Features of structural brain abnormality detected in first-episode psychosis. American Journal of Psychiatry 157: 1829–1834

- This study found that patients with first episode psychosis had significant deficits of cortical and temporal grey matter and changes in cerebrospinal fluid.
- The changes did not appear to be linked to the length of illness or the use of medication.

Ho B-C, Alicata D, Moser DJ et al 2003 Untreated initial psychosis: relation to cognitive deficits and brain morphology in first-episode schizophrenia. American Journal of Psychiatry 160: 142–148

- This study found no correlation between neurocognitive function, MRI brain volumes, brain surface anatomy and duration of untreated illness.
- Patients with a longer than median duration of untreated illness showed significantly greater verbal memory impairment and thinner cortical sulcal depth

when compared with patients with a shorter than median duration of untreated illness.

Bilder RM, Lipschutz-Broch L, Reiter G et al 1992 Intellectual deficits in first-episode schizophrenia: evidence for progressive deterioration. Schizophrenia Bulletin 18: 437–448

- Prospective longitudinal study on cognitive dysfunction and deterioration in cognition in patients with first episode schizophrenia.
- This concluded that the intellectual function in people with schizophrenia included developmental and deteriorative deficits.
- This was more marked in male than in female patients.

Flescher S 1990 Cognitive habilitation in schizophrenia: a theoretical review and model of treatment. Neuropsychological Review 1: 223–245

- Cognitive habilitation consists of:
  - assessing the cognitive impairment and the functionally related disabilities
  - engineering treatment experiences designed to remedy impairments
  - cognitive mediation to help the patient integrate the treatment experience.

Wykes T, Brammer M, Mellers J et al 2002 Effects on the brain of a psychological treatment: cognitive remediation therapy. Functional magnetic resonance imaging in schizophrenia. British Journal of Psychiatry 181: 144–152

- This RCT found that patients with schizophrenia who received cognitive remediation therapy of over 2 years' duration had changes in their prefrontal cortical activity.

Belluci DM, Glaberman K, Haslam N 2003 Computer-assisted cognitive rehabilitation reduces negative symptoms in the severely mentally ill. Schizophrenia Research 59: 225–232

- A computer-assisted cognitive rehabilitation programme in patients with enduring schizophrenia and schizoaffective disorder.
- The programme had significant effects on concentration and verbal/conceptual learning and memory.

O'Carroll R 2000 Cognitive impairment in schizophrenia. Advances in Psychiatric Treatment 6: 161–168

- There is evidence to suggest that the cognitive impairment associated with schizophrenia pre-dates the first episode of illness.
- Errorless learning has been researched in patients with schizophrenia.

- Further investigation is required before the possible benefits are generalised to clinical practice.

Brenner H, Roder V, Hodel B et al 1994 Integrated psychological therapy for schizophrenic patients. Hogrefe and Huber, Toronto

- An integrated psychological therapy in the form of a group-based cognitive remediation technique is described, based on a hierarchy of different skills. Executive function, social perception, verbal communication, social skills and problem solving are addressed.

Pilling S, Bebbington P, Kuipers E et al 2002 Psychological treatments in schizophrenia: II. Meta-analyses of randomised controlled trials of social skills training and cognitive remediation. Psychological Medicine 32: 783–791

- This meta-analysis did not find that cognitive remediation had beneficial effects on attention, verbal memory, planning, cognitive flexibility or mental state.

Definition

Cognitive remediation therapy in schizophrenia is an interventional programme for improving cognitive function by focusing on the specific cognitive deficits of the illness such as poor memory and difficulties in planning and decision making. Alternative names include cognitive habilitation and cognitive rehabilitation.

Influence of carer expressed emotion and effect on relapse

Kuipers E, Bebbington P, Dunn G et al 2006 Influence of carer expressed emotion and effect on relapse in non-affective psychosis. British Journal of Psychiatry 188: 173–179

Background

- The association between high expressed emotion in carers and relapse in patients with psychosis is suggested to occur via affective changes.

Method

- Patients and carers were recruited into the Psychological Prevention of Relapse in Psychosis (PRP) trial.
- This was a multicentre RCT of CBT and family interventions in people with psychosis.
- Patients with non-affective psychosis and their carers (contact of over 10 hours per week, including telephone

contact) were recruited into the trial at the time of relapse. Relapse was taken as the recurrence of positive symptoms within the last 3 months with a score of four or above for at least one positive psychotic symptom on the PANSS at first meeting.
- Carer instruments included the Camberwell Family Interview, the Experience of Caregiving Inventory, the Self-Esteem Scale, the General Health Questionnaire and the COPE Inventory.
- The PANSS, Self-Esteem Scale, the Beck Depression Inventory-II and the Beck Anxiety Inventory were used for patients.

Results

- High expressed emotion in carers is associated with significantly higher levels of anxiety and depression in patients.
- High expressed emotion in carers is not, however, associated with higher levels of psychotic symptoms or lower self-esteem in patients.
- Critical comments by carers were predictive of anxiety symptoms in patients, using linear regression.
- Carers who made critical comments were more likely to have low self-esteem and avoidant coping mechanisms themselves.
- There were also associations between low carer self-esteem, carer depression, carer stress and carer burden.
- Low carer self-esteem was linked to low patient self-esteem.

Longitudinal follow-up in acute and transient psychotic disorder

Pillmann F, Marneros A 2005 Longitudinal follow-up in acute and transient psychotic disorders and schizophrenia. British Journal of Psychiatry 187: 286–287

Method

- A prospective study.
- Two groups of disorders were compared: acute and transient psychotic disorders and schizophrenia.
- The initial hypothesis was that acute and transient psychotic disorders can be differentiated from schizophrenia by a lack of deterioration during the long-term course. They also tested the belief that a subgroup can remain well without further treatment.
- Global functioning was assessed with the Global Assessment Scale (GAS).
- Relapse was defined as the occurrence of major affective syndrome or psychotic symptoms leading to treatment and a disruption of daily living activities assessed using Schedules for Clinical Assessment in Neuropsychiatry.

Results

- There was significant decrease in the GAS from first assessment to the third in the group of patients with schizophrenia.
- Function on the GAS did not change for the group of patients with acute and transient psychotic disorders.
- Both groups had frequent relapses.
- There was no difference in the time to first relapse between the groups.
- The findings clearly supported the idea that the group with acute and transient psychosis had a better prognosis.
- There was, however, no difference in the groups with regard to relapse within the study period.
- At the end of the study, 31% of patients with acute and transient psychotic disorder were regarded as being in stable remission without medication.
- None of the patients with schizophrenia could be regarded as being in stable remission without medication.
- A randomised controlled trial is suggested for improved evidence.

Marneros A, Pillmann F 2004 Acute and transient psychoses. Cambridge University Press, Cambridge

- ICD-10 considered acute and transient psychotic disorders to account for 8–9% of all psychotic disorders.
- They have a benign long-term course.

Metabolic syndrome and schizophrenia

Thakore J 2005 Metabolic syndrome and schizophrenia. British Journal of Psychiatry 186: 455–456

- Metabolic syndrome is a cluster of disorders comprising:
  - obesity (central and abdominal)
  - dyslipidaemia
  - glucose intolerance
  - insulin resistance
  - hypertension.
- This cluster is highly predictive of type 2 diabetes mellitus and cardiovascular disease.

Heiskanen T, Niskanen L, Lyytikainen R et al 2003 Metabolic syndrome in patients with schizophrenia. Journal of Clinical Psychiatry 64: 575–579

- The frequency of metabolic syndrome was two to four times higher in a group of people with schizophrenia, treated with both typical and atypical neuroleptics, than in an appropriate reference population.

American Diabetic Association 2004 Consensus Development Conference of Antipsychotic Drugs and Obesity and Diabetes. Diabetes Care 27: 596–601

- Neuroleptics as a class can induce weight gain, which may explain why people with schizophrenia are more at risk of developing certain features of the metabolic syndrome.
- Aetiology appears uncertain – weight gain may be a risk factor.
- In view of the evidence for increased prevalence of metabolic syndrome in schizophrenia, individuals presenting with a first episode should be screened using one of the sets of diagnostic criteria.
- Monitoring should then take place on a regular basis.

Thakore JH, Vlahoos J, Martin A et al 2002 Increased visceral fat distribution in drug-naive and drug-free patients with schizophrenia. International Journal of Obesity Related Metabolic Disorders 26: 137–141

- Patients with schizophrenia – acute and chronic – have increased levels of intra-abdominal fat.

Ryan MCM, Flanagan S, Kinsella U et al 2004 Atypical antipsychotics and visceral fat distribution in first episode, drug-naive patients with schizophrenia. Life Sciences 74: 1999–2008

- Patients with first episode schizophrenia have more than three times the intra-abdominal fat of controls.

Zhang Z-L, Yao Z-J, Liu W et al 2004 Effects of antipsychotics on fat deposition and changes in leptin and insulin levels: unrelated people with schizophrenia. British Journal of Psychiatry 184: 58–62

- Treatment with risperidone or chlorpromazine for 10 weeks significantly increased fat deposition.
- There were no significant changes in fasting glucose levels with antipsychotic medication.
- This study was not felt to be as methodologically robust as other studies which found differing results.

Lieberman J, Phillips M, Gu H et al 2003 Atypical and conventional antipsychotic drugs in treatment-naive first episode schizophrenia: a 52 week randomized trial of clozapine vs. chlorpromazine. Neuropsychopharmacology 28: 99–103

- A prospective study of drug-naive patients with first episode schizophrenia.
- Fasting glucose levels do not significantly change following either 10 weeks of treatment with risperidone or 52 weeks of treatment with either clozapine or chlorpromazine.

Mukherjee S, Schnur DB, Reddy R 1989 Family history of type II diabetes in schizophrenic patients [letter]. Lancet I: 495

- It may be that diabetes is a feature of schizophrenia itself.
- Unaffected first-degree relatives of people with schizophrenia have high rates of type 2 DM (19–30%), indicating a genetic association between the two disorders.

Ryan MCM, Collins P, Thekadore JH 2003 Impaired fasting glucose and elevation of cortisol in drug naive first-episode schizophrenia. American Journal of Psychiatry 160: 284–289

- Glucose dysfunction was documented in the pre-antipsychotic era, with over 15% of first-episode schizophrenics having impaired fasting glucose levels, hyperinsulinaemia and high levels of cortisol.

Ryan MCM, Sharifi N, Condren R et al 2004 Evidence of basal pituitary–adrenal overactivity in first episode drug-naive patients with schizophrenia. Psychoneuroendocrinology 29: 1065–1070

- Showed that there are higher levels of corticotrophin and cortisol in first episode schizophrenia, suggesting an overactive HPA axis.

Thakore JH (ed.) 2001 Physical consequences of depression. Wrightson, Cambridge

- Indirect support for the hypothesis that chronic stress can lead to metabolic changes comes from the observation that melancholic depression and Cushing syndrome are associated with physical illnesses related to hypercortisolaemia.

See also the 'General topics' section in Chapter 21 (Physical health), page 304.

Origins of cognitive dysfunction

Joyce E 2005 Origins of cognitive dysfunction in schizophrenia: clues from age of onset. British Journal of Psychiatry 186: 93–95

- The age at which someone becomes psychotic is a variable trait related to prognosis.

Suvisaari IM, Haukka J, Tanskanen A et al 1998 Age at onset and outcome in schizophrenia are related to the degree of familial loading. British Journal of Psychiatry 173: 494–500

- Earlier onset of psychosis is associated with a more severe course.

- This is irrespective of the duration of illness.

Cardno AG, Holmans PA, Rees ML et al 2001 A genome-wide linkage study of age of onset in schizophrenia. American Journal of Medical Genetics 105: 439–445

- There is a significant genetic contribution to age at onset.
- There may be sensitive phenotypes for the detection of susceptibility genes or genes that modify the presentation of illness.

Kendler KS, Tsuang MTR, Hays P 1987 Age at onset in schizophrenia: a familial perspective. Archives of General Psychiatry 440: 128–129

- The evidence from studies of twins with schizophrenia suggests that illness onset correlates more strongly in monozygotic than in dizygotic twins.

Kendler KS, MacLean CJ 1990 Estimating familial effects on age at onset and liability to schizophrenia. Acta Psychiatrica Scandinavica 98: 156–164

- Younger age at onset is associated with high familial risk of schizophrenia.

Antilla S, Kampman P, Illi A et al 2003 NOTCH4 gene promoter polymorphism associated with the age of onset in schizophrenia. Psychiatric Genetics 13: 61–64

- Have found a highly significant association between the presence of a NOTCH4 gene promoter polymorphism (T25C) and a younger age at onset.
- This study was of male Finnish patients.
- NOTCH4 patients became unwell at a mean of 4.5 years earlier than patients without the allele.

Verdoux HJ, Geddes JR, Takei N et al 1997 Obstetric complications and age at onset in schizophrenia: an international collaborative meta-analysis of individual patient data. American Journal of Psychiatry 154: 1220–1227

- Obstetric complications have been associated with a younger age of onset, indicating that environmental factors are important.

Rosso IM, Cannon TD, Huttunen T et al 2000 Obstetric risk factors for early-onset schizophrenia in a Finnish Birth Cohort. American Journal of Psychiatry 157: 801–807

- Fetal hypoxia was associated with an increased rate of schizophrenia, specifically related to early onset.
- It is suggested that the hypoxia causes neurotoxic damage to the developing temporal lobe and that this brings forward the age of onset because it reduces the 'psychosis threshold' in adolescence.

Tuulio-Henriksson A, Partonen T, Suvisaari J et al 2004 Age onset and cognitive functioning in schizophrenia. British Journal of Psychiatry 185: 215–219

- Found behavioural evidence relating to genetic and environmental influences on age at onset of schizophrenia.
- Age at onset was significantly and specifically associated with performance of the Californian Verbal Learning Test (CVLT).
- Poorer word list learning and delayed recognition memory were both associated with a younger age of onset.
- Impaired memory may be a risk factor for, as opposed to a consequence of, early onset.
- There was no association between CVLT performance and familial loading, implying that genetic vulnerability and memory impairment were operating as independent risk factors for a younger age at onset.
- Memory impairment might be more related to environmental as opposed to genetic triggers.
- Decreased visuospatial working memory was related to increased genetic susceptibility to schizophrenia.
- This suggests that impaired executive processes (and therefore the integrity of the prefrontal cortex) might be more related to the function of susceptibility or modifying genes than to impaired memory processes.
- Found that executive function was not associated with age of onset; however, the tests focused more on memory than assessing executive function directly.
- There is a trend towards executive function being implicated in risk of early onset.
- The word list in the CVLT consists of groups of words belonging to specific categories. This strategic use of semantic clusters to aid encoding and retrieval is considered a prefrontal function. They found that the degree to which the patients used this strategy was inversely related to a younger age at onset.

Addington J, Addington D 1998 Effect of substance misuse in early psychosis. British Journal of Psychiatry 172 (Suppl 33): S134–S136

- Speculated that drug misuse may bring forward the age of onset by this mechanism.

Partial agonism and schizophrenia

Bolonna AA, Kerwin RW 2005 Partial agonism and schizophrenia [editorial]. British Journal of Psychiatry 186: 7–10

- Aripiprazole is a D2 partial agonist that has recently been licensed in the US and Europe.
- This article reviews the neurochemistry of dopamine in schizophrenia and discusses the theoretical importance of partial agonism as a mechanism for the treatment of the illness.

Ariens EJ 1964 Molecular pharmacology. Academic Press, New York

- Most drugs produce an effect somewhere between agonism and antagonism.
- Such drugs are called 'partial agonists' as they produce an effect of lower intrinsic activity than a full agonist.
- Depending on their environment, they exert different properties. In the presence of agonists they act antagonistically by blocking the receptors; in the absence of these, they are agonists.

Carlsson A, Lindquist M 1963 Effect of chlorpromazine or haloperidol on formation of 3-methoxytyramine and normetanephrine in mouse brain. Acta Pharmacologica et Toxicoliga 20: 140–144

- The original dopamine hypothesis.
- Proposed an excess of dopaminergic activity as the fundamental neurochemical abnormality, based partly on the fact that chlorpromazine alleviated symptoms by antagonising D2 receptors.

Pilowsky L, Costa DC, Elli PJ et al 1992 Clozapine single photon emission tomography and the dopamine D2 receptor blockade hypothesis of schizophrenia. Lancet 340: 199–202; Kapur S, Zipursky R, Jones C et al 2000 Relationship between dopamine D2 occupance, clinical response and side effects: a double-blind PET study of first episode schizophrenia. American Journal of Psychiatry 157: 514–520

- These two studies concluded that newer antipsychotics such as clozapine and quetiapine have relatively low affinity for D2 receptors.
- They are still effective.
- This does not fit with the dopamine hypothesis.

Kerwin RW, Osborne S 2000 Antipsychotic drugs. Medicine 28: 23–25

- Atypical antipsychotic medication is superior to conventional antipsychotics in the treatment of negative symptoms.
- Atypicals are less likely to cause extrapyramidal side effects.

Meltzer HY 1999 The role of serotonin in antipsychotic drug action. Neuropsychopharmacology 21: S106–S115

- Suggested that atypical antipsychotic medication targets other neurotransmitter systems to dopamine, namely serotonin.

Kapur S, Mamo D 2003 Half a century of antipsychotics and still a central role for dopamine D(2)receptors. Progress in Neuropsychopharmacology and Biological Psychiatry 27: 1081–1090

- It is apparent that, to date, all effective antipsychotics incorporate D2 antagonism. The current thinking, therefore, is to identify drugs which target the dopaminergic system with greater therapeutic efficacy.

Thierry AM, Stinus L, Blanc G et al 1973 Some evidence for the existence of dopaminergic neurones in the rat cortex. Brain Research 50: 230–234

- Discovered additional cortical dopamine projections through biochemical and behavioural techniques.
- These projections responded in the opposite way to subcortical dopamine systems.

Carter CJ, Pycock CJ 1979 The effects of 5,7-dihydroxytryptamine lesions of extrapyramidal and mesolimbic sites on spontaneous motor behaviour and amphetamine-induced stereotypy. Naunyn-Schmiedeberg's Archives of Pharmacology 308: 51–54

- Loss of frontal cortical dopamine increased motor activity, the opposite effect of stimulation of dopamine receptors in extrapyramidal and mesolimbic regions.
- Proposed that the fundamental neurochemical lesion in schizophrenia involved a deficit in frontal cortical dopamine and an increase in subcortical dopamine function.

Weinberger DR, Berman KF 1996 Prefrontal function in schizophrenia: confounds and controversies. Philosophical Transactions of the Royal Society of London. Series B, Biological Sciences 351: 1495–1503

- Found that there was an association between hypofrontality and schizophrenia.

Andreasen NC, Rezai KM, Alliger R et al 1992 Hypofrontality in neuroleptic-naive patients and in patients with chronic schizophrenia. Assessment with xenon 133 single-photon emission computed tomography and the Tower of London. Archives of General Psychiatry 49: 943–958

- Showed a correlation between hypofrontality and negative symptoms

Abi Dhargam A, Moore H 2003 Prefrontal dopamine transmission at D1 receptors and the pathology of schizophrenia. Neuroscientist 5: 404–416

- Cortical D1 receptor levels are reduced in patients with schizophrenia.

Breier A, Su TP, Saunders R et al 1997 Schizophrenia is associated with elevated amphetamine-induced synaptic dopamine concentrations: evidence for a novel positron emission tomography method. Proceedings of the National Academy of Sciences USA 94: 2569–2574

- Amfetamine induces excess release of dopamine in the striatum (subcortical region) in patients with schizophrenia compared with controls.
- This overactivity was found to cause positive symptoms.
- It is possible that a dopamine partial agonist could act as a stabiliser by increasing dopamine activity in the frontal cortex and diminishing hyperactive dopamine systems in the subcortical regions.

Elsworth JD, Roth RH 1997 Dopamine autoreceptor pharmacology and function. In: Nerve RL (ed.) Dopamine receptors. Humana Press, Totowa, NJ, pp 232–265

- Described a negative feedback control on dopamine release and/or synthesis which reduces postsynaptic activity.
- Increased dopamine release due to reduced activity of dopamine autoreceptors might be one source of hyperactivity in subcortical systems.

Grunder G, Carlsson A, Wong D 2003 Mechanisms of new antipsychotic medications. Archives of General Psychiatry 60: 974–977

- Partial agonists are potential stabilisers of dysregulated dopamine release in schizophrenia.

Kerwin RW 2000 From pharmacological profiles to clinical outcomes. International Journal of Clinical Psychopharmacology 15: S1–S4

- Suggested that dopamine autoreceptor antagonists (sulpride and amisulpride) stabilise dopamine systems in schizophrenia by increasing dopamine release and selectively blocking D2 and D3 receptors in the limbic system.

Jordan S, Koprivica V, Chen R et al 2002 The antipsychotic aripiprazole is a potent, partial agonist at the human $5HT_{1A}$ receptor. European Journal of Pharmacology 27: 1081–1090

- Found that aripiprazole has affinity at 5HT, $5HT_{1A}$ and $5HT_{2C}$ receptors.
- It acts as an antagonist at $5HT_{2A}$.

Marder SR, McQuade RD, Stock E et al 2003 Aripiprazole in the treatment of schizophrenia: safety and tolerability

in the short-term, placebo-controlled trials. Schizophrenia Research 61: 123–136

- Short-term randomised trials indicate that aripiprazole is efficacious for positive and negative symptoms.
- It has a good safety and tolerability record in patients with acute relapse of schizophrenia or schizoaffective disorder.

Patient-held clinical information for people with psychotic illnesses

Henderson C, Laugharne R 1999 Patient-held clinical information for people with psychotic illnesses (**Cochrane Review**). In: The Cochrane Library, Issue 3. CD001711. Update Software, Oxford

- No studies met the inclusion criteria for review.

Predicting schizophrenia

Johnstone E, Ebmeier KP, Miller P et al 2005 Predicting schizophrenia: findings from the Edinburgh High-Risk Study. British Journal of Psychiatry 186: 18–25

This study examines the hypothesis that schizophrenia is a neurodevelopmental condition. It is a prospective study of young people who are at high risk for schizophrenia (postulated risk of 10–15%). This study examines the premorbid variables distinguishing high risk people who will go on to develop schizophrenia from those who will not. It was predicted that, of 200 high risk individuals, 20 would go on to develop schizophrenia within 10 years. The control group consisted of well young people and those in their first episode of schizophrenia who did not have the family risk. The hypothesis was that those who went on to develop schizophrenia would differ from those who did not long before the development of schizophrenia.

Results

- 12 men and eight women from the high risk group developed schizophrenia within 2.5 years.
- The mean age at diagnosis was 22.8 years for both men and women.
- Psychopathological symptoms were evident in many more of those predicted to develop schizophrenia and it is unlikely that all those in the high risk group who experience psychotic symptoms will go on to develop schizophrenia.

- The whole at-risk group varied from the control group with regard to developmental or neuropsychological variables.
- Those who developed schizophrenia differed from those who did not on social anxiety, withdrawal and other schizotypal features.
- At the time of publication most of the men had passed the period of highest risk.

Hafner H, Maurer K, Loffler W et al 1999 Onset and prodromal phase as determinants of the course. In: Gattaz WF, Hafner H (eds) Search for the cause of schizophrenia. Springer, Berlin, pp 35–58

- Reported that the well-established gender differences in age of onset in schizophrenia are much less in familial cases.

Parnas J, Schulsinger F, Schulsinger H et al 1982 Behavioural precursors of schizophrenia spectrum. A prospective study. Archives of General Psychiatry 39: 658–664; Cannon TD, Mednick SA, Parnas J et al 1994 Developmental brain abnormalities in the offspring of schizophrenic mothers. II. Structural brain characteristics of schizophrenia and schizotypal personality disorder. Archives of General Psychiatry 51: 955–962

- These two studies published results from the Copenhagen High-Risk Study.
- The CHRS is similar in design to the EHRS.
- It examined the children of women with psychotic disorder between the ages of 10 and 19.
- They were followed up at mean ages of 25 and 39.
- The number of cases appeared to increase by four (from 13 to 17 cases) between the two reports.
- It was not expected that many more will go on to develop schizophrenia.

Premorbid adjustment in first episode non-affective psychosis

Larsen TK, Friis S, Haahr U et al 2004 Premorbid adjustment in first episode non-affective psychosis: distinct patterns of pre-onset course. British Journal of Psychiatry 185: 108–115

The pathogenesis of schizophrenia remains unclear. An understanding of premorbid functioning may increase understanding of the pathogenesis by identifying subtypes within this heterogeneous group.

Aims

This study aimed to:
- identify academic and social dimensions

- identify clusters of patients with different time patterns for each of the dimensions
- test the validity of the clusters by comparing them on characteristics at the start of treatment.

Method

- This study combines the Premorbid Adjustment Scale data from four samples of patients with non-affective psychosis.
- Data were collected in Norway and Denmark between 1993 and 2001.
- Cluster analysis was employed to identify patterns of premorbid course.
- Other instruments employed were the DSM-IV SCID, the PANSS, the GAF (symptom and function versions) and the Clinical Rating Scale.
- Drug and alcohol use were calculated.
- Duration of untreated psychosis was also calculated.

Results

- There is some indication that, for many patients, premorbid functioning becomes worse as the onset of psychosis approaches; however, this finding is not uniform.
- Social and academic function constituted fairly independent dimensions.
- Patients with a more stable social course:
  - had a shorter duration of untreated psychosis
  - were older
  - had more friends
  - had fewer negative symptoms.
- Patients with a more stable academic course were older on admission.
- During the pre-morbid period the sample had gradually worsening function on all variables.
- More than three-quarters of patients are stable over time in their childhood level of functioning, especially when that level is either poor or intermediate.
- This is consistent with the repeated finding that neurocognitive deficits are present in people with first episode schizophrenia by the time of onset – so-called static encephalopathy.

Discussion

- The results indicate that the heterogeneity of schizophrenia begins prior to the onset of illness itself.
- 40% reported 'good stable' social functioning which contradicts the argument that schizophrenia is purely a neurodevelopmental disorder, where social dysfunction should be an early manifestation.

Weinberger DR, McClure RK 2002 Neurotoxicity, neuroplasticity and magnetic resonance imaging morphometry: what is happening in the schizophrenic brain? Archives of General Psychiatry 59: 553–558

- The presence of social problems, especially those that worsen over time, is a risk factor for late detection of schizophrenia.

Murray RM, Lewis SW 1987 Is schizophrenia a neurodevelopmental disorder? British Medical Journal (Clinical Research Edition) 295: 681–682

- Queried whether there were underlying neurobiological lesions that later have effects on normal development.

McGlashan TH, Hoffman RE 2000 Schizophrenia as a disorder of developmentally reduced synaptic connectivity. Archives of General Psychiatry 57: 637–648

- Discussed the structural brain changes that may indicate a later neurobiological regressive process (e.g. the loss of synaptic connectivity).
- People with schizophrenia have:
  - reduced brain volume
  - reduced grey matter volume
  - increased extracerebral (sulcal) CSF.

Cannon-Spoor HE, Potkin SG, Wyatt RJ 1982 Measurement of premorbid adjustment on chronic schizophrenia. Schizophrenia Bulletin 8: 470–484

- The premorbid adjustment scale (PAS) defines the premorbid phase from birth to 6 months before the onset of illness.
- A widely used premorbid scale for psychosis.

Social fragmentation, deprivation and urbanicity

Allardyce J, Gilmour H, Atkinson J et al 2005 Social fragmentation, deprivation and urbanicity: relation to first admission rates for psychoses. British Journal of Psychiatry 187: 401–406

A number of studies have shown that areas with greater material deprivation have higher rates of psychosis.

Results

- Areas with high levels of social fragmentation have higher first-ever admission rates for psychosis, independent of deprivation and urban/rural status.
- There was no statistically significant interaction between social fragmentation, deprivation and urban/rural index.

- First admission rates are strongly associated with measures of social fragmentation, independent of material deprivation and urban/rural category.

Allardyce J, Morrison G, McCreadie RG et al 2000 Schizophrenia is not disappearing in south-west Scotland. British Journal of Psychiatry 177: 38–41

- Urban areas have higher rates of psychoses compared with rural areas.

Congdon P 1996 Suicide and para-suicide in London: a small area study. Urban Studies 33: 137–158

- Proposed a census-based index measuring social fragmentation.
- This was used to examine the relative impact of such social fragmentation, material deprivation and urbanicity versus rurality on first admission rates to hospital for psychosis in London over a 5-year period.

Violent behaviour in schizophrenia

Vevera J, Hubbard A, Vesely A, Papezova H 2005 Violent behaviour in schizophrenia. Retrospective study of four independent samples from Prague 1949–2000. British Journal of Psychiatry 187: 426–430

Studies have found associations between schizophrenia and violence.

Method

- This study examined whether there has been an increase in violence in Prague between 1949 and 2000.
- They specifically analysed the relationship between violence, substance misuse and gender.
- Participants had a DSM-IV diagnosis of schizophrenia.
- Aggressive behaviour was measured by the Modified Overt Aggression Scale.
- Patients were considered to be violent if they expressed overt and intentional violence against others or a verbal threat with an accompanying weapon.
- Information on substance misuse was elicited from the case notes.
- Logistical regression was used to investigate trends in the prevalence of violence.

Results

- The following postdiagnosis prevalence rates of violence in patients with schizophrenia were found:
  - 34.8% (1949)

- 44.6% (1969)
- 32.9% (1989)
- 44.4% (2000).
- The overall prevalence for violence was 41.8% for men and 32.7% for women.
- There was no significant linear trend after logistical regression.
- An increase in the rates of violence was not found among those with schizophrenia in the Czech Republic between 1949 and 1989.
- A marginally higher prevalence was found in the sample from 2000.
- The overall prevalence for violence in those with schizophrenia was 42% for men and 33% for women.
- Only a weak association was found between gender and violence – this is similar to other recent studies.
- Family members were involved in half of the assaults, with strangers being attacked in 17%.
- The prevalence of substance misuse was between 2 and 7% which is markedly lower than studies done in Western Europe and America.
- Alcohol misuse remained stable after the fall of communism but illicit substance use increased significantly.
- The data showed that those with schizophrenia did not have a higher rate of substance misuse than the general population.
- No association was found between substance misuse and violence.

Walsh E, Moran P, Scott C et al 2004 Predicting violence in schizophrenia: a prospective study. Schizophrenia Research 67: 247–252

- Although people with schizophrenia are not violent, there appears to be a relationship between this disorder and violence.

Linquist P, Allebeck P 1990 Schizophrenia crime. A longitudinal follow-up of 644 schizophrenics in Stockholm. British Journal of Psychiatry 178: 433–440

- Found the risk of violence in schizophrenia was further increased with associated substance misuse.

Steadman HJ, Mulvey EP, Manahan J et al 1998 Violence by people discharged from acute psychiatric inpatient facilities and by others in the same neighbourhoods. Archives of General Psychiatry 55: 393–401

- The MacArthur Study.
- Suggested that substance misuse is responsible for the rise of violence in people with schizophrenia.

Hodgins S 2001 The major mental disorders and crime: stop debating and start treating and preventing. International Journal of Law and Psychiatry 24: 437–446

- The risk of violence by psychiatric patients in both the community and hospital is increasing.
- This contradicts other studies, which have also suggested that violence is rising in society as a whole.

Hogan MF 2003 The President's new Freedom Commission: recommendations to transform mental health care in America. Psychiatric Services 54: 1467–1474

- Fragmentation of care is responsible for the increasing rates of violence in the US.
- Similarities were noted to the cause of the marginally increased rate in the Czech cohort.

See also the 'General topics' section in Chapter 10 (Forensic psychiatry), page 153.

Treatment – Psychopharmacology

Acute akathisia

Anticholinergics for neuroleptic-induced acute akathisia

Lima AR, Weiser KVS, Bacaltchuk J, Barnes TRE 2002 Anticholinergics for neuroleptic-induced acute akathisia **(Cochrane Review)**. In: The Cochrane Library, Issue 3. CD003727. Update Software, Oxford

- No randomised controlled trials could be included.

Benzodiazepines for neuroleptic-induced acute akathisia

Lima AR, Soares-Weiser K, Bacaltchuk J, Barnes TRE 1999 Benzodiazepines for neuroleptic-induced acute akathisia **(Cochrane Review)**. In: The Cochrane Library, Issue 4. CD001950. Update Software, Oxford

- Two RCTs were included ($n = 27$).
- They were short but found that the use of benzodiazepines may reduce the symptoms of antipsychotic-induced acute akathisia.
- No significant difference was found for adverse effects and no one left the studies early.

Depot medication

Depot flupenthixol decanoate for schizophrenia or other similar psychotic disorders

David A, Adams CE, Quiraishi SN 1999 Depot flupenthixol decanoate for schizophrenia or other similar psychotic disorders **(Cochrane Review)**. In: The Cochrane Library, Issue 2. CD001470. Update Software, Oxford

* There were no trials comparing flupenthixol decanoate to placebo.
* When compared with oral penfluridol there were no clear differences.
* There were no differences when compared with other depot preparations for outcomes of death, global impression, relapse or leaving the study early.
* Two small studies found that depot flupenthixol was associated with lower rates of movement disorders (NNT 5). This was not specific to tremor or tardive dyskinesia.
* When high dose and standard dosages of flupenthixol decanoate were compared, there was no significant difference in relapse rates.
* Further comparison with oral preparations would be useful.

Depot haloperidol decanoate for schizophrenia

Quraishi S, David A 1999 Depot haloperidol decanoate for schizophrenia **(Cochrane Review)**. In: The Cochrane Library, Issue 1. CD001361. Update Software, Oxford

* Data were limited.
* Two small studies comparing oral and depot haloperidol found that the depot formulation was associated with reductions in dropout rates and outcomes of no important improvement in mental state.
* A further comparison of oral and depot haloperidol found no differences between the groups in terms of global impression, mental state or side effects.
* Eight studies compared haloperidol decanoate with other depot medications and found no differences on outcomes of death, global impression, mental state, behaviour or side effects.
* There were no clear differences between haloperidol in its depot form and its oral equivalent.

Depot risperidone for schizophrenia

Hosalli P, Davis JM 2003 Depot risperidone for schizophrenia **(Cochrane Review)**. In: The Cochrane Library, Issue 4. CD004161. Update Software, Oxford

* Only two studies were identified.
* One study comparing depot risperidone with placebo had a 56% dropout rate by 3 months.
* Risperidone had no effect on anxiety symptoms but may reduce agitation.
* Risperidone depot reduced 'psychosis' (NNT 9; CI 7–26) but did not clearly affect hallucinations.
* There was a higher dropout from the placebo group (NNT 6; CI 4–12).
* Severe adverse effects were common (13–23%), but significantly more so in the placebo group (NNT 7; CI 7–70).
* Movement disorders were as common in each group, but it appeared that higher doses of depot had greater levels of movement disorder.
* One study compared risperidone in its oral and depot forms ($n = 640$) in patients with stable and relatively mild illness.
* There was no difference between the groups for 'no global improvement' or mental state measures.
* Adverse effects were found in over half of both groups but were poorly reported.
* Compliance rates in this study were good.

Olanzapine IM or velotab for acutely disturbed/agitated people with suspected serious mental illnesses

Belgamwar RB, Fenton M 2005 Olanzapine IM or velotab for acutely disturbed/agitated people with suspected serious mental illnesses **(Cochrane Review)**. In: The Cochrane Library, Issue 2. CD003729. Update Software, Oxford

* Four trials comparing olanzapine IM with IM placebo ($n = 769$) showed that fewer patients given olanzapine IM had 'no important clinical response' by 2 hours (NNT 4; CI 3–5):
  – those receiving olanzapine IM required fewer subsequent injections after the first dose.
* Two trials compared olanzapine IM with haloperidol IM ($n = 482$):
  – at 2 hours there was no difference for the outcome of 'no important clinical response'
  – there was no difference in the rates of patients requiring subsequent injections
  – those receiving olanzapine required less

anticholinergic medication in the first 24 hours (NNT 8; CI 7–11) than those receiving haloperidol haloperidol was associated with increased akathisia (NNT 6; CI 5–15) than olanzapine.

- Two trials compared olanzapine IM with lorazepam IM ($n = 355$):
  - at 2 hours there was no difference for the outcome of 'no important clinical response'
  - fewer patients receiving olanzapine IM required subsequent injections than those receiving lorazepam IM (NNT 10; CI 6–59)
  - there was no difference between the two groups for anticholinergic medication use
  - patients receiving olanzapine had more movement disorders than those using lorazepam.
- There were no data regarding hospital and service use, nor on patient satisfaction, suicide, self-harm or harm to others. The orodispersable velotab preparation was untested.

Risperidone long-acting injection

Paton C, Okacha C 2004 Risperidone long-acting injection: the first 50 patients. Psychiatric Bulletin 28: 12–14

Risperidone long-acting injectable (RLAI) is the first atypical antipsychotic medication available in depot form. The evidence base remains small.

Method

- Prospective data were collected for 50 patients prescribed RLAI.
- Clinical outcomes, including dose, were measured at 3 and 6 months.

Results

- Patients were prescribed RLAI because of :
  - non-compliance (42)
  - refused oral medication (2)
  - failed to respond to conventional antipsychotics (2)
  - patient choice (2)
  - already receiving RLAI (1).
- Mean dosages were:
  - 32 mg per 2 weeks at 3 months
  - 35 mg per 2 weeks at 6 months.
- There was no difference in dosages between responders and non-responders.
- Patients who were rated much or very much improved over 3 months maintained this improvement at 6 months.
- Half those rated as minimally improved at 3 months were much or very much improved at 6 months.
- The attrition rate at 6 months was 42%.

- Patients seemed to require oral medication for longer than the 3-week lead-in period.
- By 6 months all patients were on monotherapy.
- The cost for a 37.5 mg injection is £148.
- Considerable wastage was found as fridges were not available and the drugs were left unrefridgerated, patients refused the injection after the drug was reconstituted or needles leaked and no spare was provided.
- Given that it is commonly presumed that depots improve compliance, the response rate in this study was poor and the attrition rate high.
- One-fifth of patients were changed by the treating clinician either because they had not improved or had deteriorated.
- There are limitations to dose flexibility as the preparation does not allow small dosage changes; dosage frequency is also inflexible.

Conclusions

- 40% had a good/very good outcome at 6 months.
- 18% fared poorly and were switched.
- 24% failed to comply.
- The remainder had minimal clinical gains.

Geddes J, Freemantle N, Harrison P et al 2000 Atypical antipsychotics in the treatment of schizophrenia: systematic overview and meta-regression analysis. British Medical Journal 321: 1371–1376

- Newer antipsychotics are associated with fewer neurological side effects than the older conventional drugs.

Adams CE, Fenton MKP, Quraishi S et al 2001 Systematic meta-review of depot antipsychotic drugs for people with schizophrenia. British Journal of Psychiatry 179: 290–299

- Non-compliance is a major cause of relapse and rehospitalisation in patients with schizophrenia.
- Depot antipsychotics are still widely used in the UK.

Walburn J, Gray R, Gournay K et al 2001 Systematic review of patients and nurse attitudes to depot antipsychotic medication. British Journal of Psychiatry 179: 300–307

- One in four patients receiving conventional depots are dissatisfied with their treatment.

Faloon RH 1984 Developing and maintaining adherence to long term drug-taking regimens. Schizophrenia Bulletin 10: 412–417

- Compliance rates with depot mediation are 80% compared to 60% with oral antipsychotics.

O'Ceallaigh S, Fahy TA 2001 Is there a role for the depot clinic in the modern management of schizophrenia? Psychiatric Bulletin 25: 481–484

- Compliance rates with atypical depots may be higher. See also the NICE guidelines on schizophrenia (p. 399) and the Cochrane Reviews.

Why aren't depot antipsychotics prescribed more often and what can be done about it?

Patel MX, David AS 2005 Why aren't depot antipsychotics prescribed more often and what can be done about it? Advances in Psychiatric Treatment 11: 203–213

- Non-adherence to medication in schizophrenia is a major cause of ongoing morbidity and potentially a preventable one.

Lindstrom E, Bingefors K 2000 Patient compliance with drug therapy in schizophrenia. Economic and clinical issues. Pharmacoeconomics 18: 106–124

- The effectiveness of antipsychotic medication is related to patients' adherence to their medication regimen.

Hughes I, Hill B, Budd R 1997 Compliance with antipsychotic medication: from theory to practice. Journal of Mental Health 6: 473–489

- Described a 'health belief model' whereby health-related behaviours are determined by benefits, costs and susceptibility to relapse, and secondary benefits of treatment with medication, including compliance.

Cramer JA, Rosenheck R 1998 Compliance with medication regimens for mental and physical disorders. Psychiatric Services 9: 196–201

- Found an average rate of adherence to antipsychotic medication of 58% (range 24–90%).

Young JL, Spitz RT, Hillbrand M et al 1999 Medication adherence failure in schizophrenia: a forensic review of rates, reasons, treatments and prospects. Journal of the American Academy of Psychiatry and the Law 27: 426–444

- This review reported a non-adherence rate of 24% (range 0–54%).

Hogan TP, Awad AG, Eastwood R 1983 A self-report scale predictive of drug compliance in schizophrenics: reliability and discriminative validity. Psychological Medicine 13: 177–183

- This study showed that how a patient feels while taking a medication is more important than what they know about it.

Kemp R, Kirov G, Everitt B et al 1998 Randomised controlled trial of compliance therapy: 18 month follow-up. British Journal of Psychiatry 172: 413–419

- Cognitive behavioural techniques are more beneficial in improving adherence to treatment than simple psychoeducation.

Adams CE, Fenton MKP, Quraishi S et al 2001 Systemic meta-review of depot antipsychotic drugs for people with schizophrenia. British Journal of Psychiatry 179: 290–299

- This meta-analysis examined the relative efficacy and adverse effects of the various depot preparations.
- Overall analysis found only a modest beneficial benefit for depot antipsychotic medication in comparison with oral antipsychotic medication.
- Patients who receive depot medication still have a relapse rate of 20–25%. In these cases non-adherence can be excluded as the cause.
- The review did not show that depot antipsychotic medication has more adverse effects than those taking oral preparations.
- The risk of tardive dyskinesia was not found to be greater in people receiving depot antipsychotic medication. This may reflect the relative lack of long-term studies.

Walburn J, Gray R, Gournay K et al 2001 Systematic review of patient and nurse attitudes to depot antipsychotic medication. British Journal of Psychiatry 179: 300–307

- The acceptability of medication taken via the depot administration route is variable for both patients and clinicians.
- 12 studies were considered in this review.
- 10 of these studies found a positive view of depot antipsychotic medication and one study a negative view. The remaining study was neutral.
- Patients showed a bias in preference towards the drug formulation they were currently receiving.

Pereira S, Pinto R 1997 A survey of the attitudes of chronic psychiatric patients living in the community toward their medication. Acta Psychiatrica Scandinavica 95: 464–468

- This survey of a group of outpatients receiving depot antipsychotics (some also received oral augmentation) found that 87% would choose to continue with their current medication regimen.

Wistedt B 1995 How does the psychiatric patient feel about depot treatment, compulsion or help? Nordic Journal of Psychiatry 49 (Suppl 35): 41–46

- This concluded that 60% of patients who had been changed over from oral to depot medication preferred the depot medication.
- Patients reported that they felt better while taking the depot medication.
- Patient preference may reflect the fact that the injections are easier to remember than daily tablets.

Glazer WM, Kane JM 1992 Depot neuroleptic therapy: an underutilized treatment option. Journal of Clinical Psychiatry 53: 426–433

- Some patients find the depot injections painful, leading to fear.
- Other patients consider depot antipsychotic medication as intrusive and degrading.
- Receiving medication in a depot formulation can be stigmatising, particularly if professionals view those requiring depot medication due to non-adherence as non-compliant or bad patients.

Valenstein M, Copelenad LA, Owen R et al 2001 Adherence assessments and the use of depot antipsychotics in patients with schizophrenia. Journal of Clinical Psychiatry 62: 545–551

- This American study found that black and Hispanic patients were more likely to receive depot medication than white patients.
- This may reflect bias against people from ethnic minorities.
- It may reflect preferential treatment for the white population.

Marland GR, Sharkey V 1999 Depot neuroleptics, schizophrenia and the role of the nurse: is practice evidence based? A review of the literature. Journal of Advanced Nursing 30: 1255–1262

- Concluded that both nurses and patients should be included in the planning of treatment and care.
- This encourages patient autonomy and empowerment.
- It is also beneficial for a satisfactory therapeutic relationship between patients and nurses.

Remington GJ, Adams ME 1995 Depot neuroleptic therapy: clinical considerations. Canadian Journal of Psychiatry 40 (Suppl 1): S5–11

- Depot clinics are cheap to run, particularly if the comparative costs of rehospitalisation are taken in to account.

Tavcar R, Dernovsek MZ, Zvan V 2000 Choosing antipsychotic maintenance therapy – a naturalistic study. Pharmacopsychiatry 33: 66–71

- The prescription of depot antipsychotic medications was most likely in patients who had previous experience of depot antipsychotic medication.

Kane JM, Eerdekens M, Lindenmayer J-P et al 2003 Long-acting injectable risperidone: efficacy and safety of the first long-acting atypical antipsychotic. American Journal of Psychiatry 160: 1125–1132

- RLAI appears to be as effective as oral risperidone and with a similar side effect profile.

Patel MX, Nikolaou V, David AS 2003 Eliciting psychiatrists' beliefs about side-effects of typical and atypical antipsychotic drugs. International Journal of Psychiatry in Clinical Practice 7: 117–120

- A survey of psychiatrists.
- Depot medications were thought to be:
  - old-fashioned (40%)
  - stigmatising (48%)
  - responsible for more adverse effects (38%).
- It was believed that depot medication was less acceptable to patients (69%) and their relatives (49%).
- It was also believed that depot medication had beneficial effects on treatment adherence (81%) and relapse prevention (94%).

Patel MX, deZoysa N, Baker D et al 2005 Depot antipsychotic medication and attitudes of community psychiatric nurses. Journal of Psychiatric and Mental Health Nursing 12: 237–244

- A survey of community psychiatric nurses found that they were more likely than psychiatrists to believe that antipsychotic medication given in a depot formulation compromised a patient's autonomy and involved coercion.

Oral treatment

Amisulpride for schizophrenia

Mona Neto JIS, Lima MS, Soares BGO 2002 Amisulpride for schizophrenia (**Cochrane Review**). In: The Cochrane Library, Issue 2. CD001357. Update Software, Oxford

- 19 RCTs were included ($n = 2443$).
- Four trials ($n = 514$) compared amisulpride with placebo for patients with predominantly negative symptoms.
- They suggested that low dose amisulpride:
  - was more acceptable than placebo (NNT 3; CI 3–7)
  - showed improvement in the patient's global state (NNT 3; CI 2–6)

- could be used for the treatment of negative symptoms (WMD = –10.1; CI 16.6 to –3.5).
- Pooled results from 14 trials (*n* = 651) found that when amisulpride was compared with typical antipsychotics it was more effective in improving:
  - global state (NNT 6; CI 4–11)
  - general mental state (WMD = –4.2; CI –6.5 to –1.9)
  - negative symptoms (WMD = –2.8; CI –4.3 to –1.3).
- Amisulpride was as effective as typical antipsychotics in terms of positive symptoms.
- Amisulpride was less likely to cause at least one adverse effect (NNH 9; CI 6–18), one extrapyramidal side effect (NNH 5; CI 4–19) or to require the use of antiparkinsonian medication (NNH 4; CI 3–6).
- There were no differences found with regard to other adverse effects.
- Patients taking amisulpride were less likely to leave the study early (NNT 16; CI 9–69) than those taking conventional drugs. A publication bias may have caused an overestimation.

Antidepressants for people with both schizophrenia and depression

Whitehead C, Moss S, Cardno A, Lewis G 2002 Antidepressants for people with both schizophrenia and depression **(Cochrane Review)**. In: The Cochrane Library, Issue 2. CD002305. Update Software, Oxford

- Eleven small studies of patients treated with a wide range of antidepressants just after the acute phase of psychosis were included.
- Antidepressants were significantly better than placebo in terms of the 'no important clinical response' outcome.
- When a fixed effects model was used, those receiving antidepressants showed improvement on their depression score.
- There was no evidence that the use of antidepressants worsened psychotic symptoms.
- Overall, the evidence was of poor quality and likely to overestimate the treatment effect.
- Publication bias may be an issue.

See also the 'Treatment – Psychological therapies' section in Chapter 2 (Affective disorders), page 37.

Antipsychotic drugs – information and choice

Olofinjana B, Taylor D 2005 Antipsychotic drugs – information and choice: a patient survey. Psychiatric Bulletin 29: 369–371

Aims

This study aimed to evaluate the extent to which patients were provided with information and involved in the choice of antipsychotic prescribed.

Method

- 30 patients were informally interviewed.

Results

- The results varied.
- The majority of patients did not feel involved in discussions about their antipsychotic medication.
- Only a very small number of patients were given the opportunity to choose.
- Documentation in the notes involving discussion of medication was poor and did not seem to reflect the information given by patients.

Discussion

- In the situation where the patient is deemed incapable of engaging in informed discussion, NICE advise that an advocate or carer be appointed to help them make an informed choice.
- It also stresses full documentation in the notes.
- It has been suggested that information about antipsychotic medication is withheld from patients to aid adherence.

National Institute for Clinical Excellence 2002 Guidance on the use of newer (atypical) antipsychotic drugs for the treatment of schizophrenia. NICE, London

- NICE recommend in their guidelines about schizophrenia that patients be involved in the discussion about antipsychotic medication given to them.

National Schizophrenia Fellowship 2000 A question of choice. NSF, London

- The National Schizophrenia Fellowship (now Rethink) carried out a survey of service users and issued the report entitled *A Question of Choice*.
- 38% of users were offered a choice of medication.
- 40% had no written information about side effects.
- Follow-up a year later reported similar findings.

Brown KW, Billcliff N, McCabe E 2001 Informed consent to medication in long-term psychiatric in-patients. Psychiatric Bulletin 25: 132–134

- Looked at the extent to which consent was given by long-term psychiatric inpatients.
- Only one in five knew the purpose of their medication.

Chaplin R, Kent A 1998 Informing patients about tardive dyskinesia. Controlled trial of patient education. British Journal of Psychiatry 172: 78–81

- Found that informing patients of the long-term side effects of antipsychotics, such as tardive dyskinesia, seems to have little impact on adherence.
- The authors end by commenting that there are many reasons to involve patients in choices about treatment but often prescribers are reluctant to take on this recommended practice. The reasons for this are unclear.

Aripiprazole for schizophrenia

El-Sayeh HG, Morganti C 2006 Aripiprazole for schizophrenia (Cochrane Review). In: The Cochrane Library, Issue 2. Update Software, Oxford

- 15 RCTs of 7110 patients were included.
- There was enormous loss to follow-up over a short period of time.
- Data were poorly recorded.
- No usable data were available regarding death, service outcomes, general functioning, behaviour, engagement with services, satisfaction with treatment, economic outcomes or cognitive functioning.
- In comparison with placebo, aripiprazole significantly decreased relapse in the short and medium term (NNT 5; CI 4–8) and improved compliance with the study protocol (NNT 26; CI 16–239).
- One trial ($n = 305$) suggested aripiprazole may decrease prolactin levels below that expected from placebo (NNT 14; CI 11–50).
- In comparison with typical antipsychotics, there were no significant differences in terms of global state, mental state, quality of life or leaving the study early.
- Rates of adverse effects were similar, except for akathisia (NNT 20) and treatment with antiparkinsonian medication (NNT 2).
- Aripiprazole caused more insomnia than perphenazine (NNH 4; CI 3–9).
- Patients receiving aripiprazole required fewer antiparkinsonian drugs than those receiving 10–20 mg of haloperidol/day (NNT 4; CI 3–5).
- In comparison with olanzapine and risperidone, there were no significant differences for aripiprazole for outcomes of global state and leaving the study early.
- Adverse effects rates were largely similar.
- Treatment with aripiprazole was less likely to cause elevations in prolactin (NNT 2).
- In comparison with risperidone alone, aripiprazole was less likely to prolong QTc interval (WMD = −10.0; CI −16.99 to −3.01).

'As required' medication regimens

Whicher E, Morrison M, Douglas-Hall P 2002 'As required' medication regimens for seriously mentally ill people in hospital (Cochrane Review). In: The Cochrane Library, Issue 1. CD003441. Update Software, Oxford

- No randomised trials comparing 'as required' medication regimens to regular regimens of the same drugs were identified.

Benperidol for schizophrenia

Leucht S, Hartung B 2005 Benperidol for schizophrenia (Cochrane Review). In: The Cochrane Library, Issue 2. CD003083. Update Software, Oxford

- There were insufficient data from RCTs to assess the clinical effects of benperidol.
- More trials are justified for this inexpensive, under-researched drug.

Beta-blocker supplementation of standard drug treatment for schizophrenia

Cheine M, Ahonen J, Wahlbeck K 2001 Beta-blocker supplementation of standard drug treatment for schizophrenia (Cochrane Review). In: The Cochrane Library, Issue 3. CD000234. Update Software, Oxford

- The results from the five studies identified were poorly reported.
- There is very limited good evidence to support the use of beta blockers in the treatment of schizophrenia.

Carbamazepine for schizophrenia and schizoaffective psychoses

Leucht S, McGrath J, White P, Kissling W 2002 Carbamazepine for schizophrenia and schizoaffective psychoses (Cochrane Review). In: The Cochrane Library, Issue 3. CD001258. Update Software, Oxford

- 10 studies with a total of 258 participants were included.
- A study of carbamazepine versus placebo as the only treatment for schizophrenia was terminated early due to high relapse rates.

- Another study comparing carbamazepine alone with antipsychotic medication found no differences in terms of mental state.
- Those receiving antipsychotic medication (perphenazine) had higher rates of extrapyramidal side effects.
- Eight studies compared the addition of carbamazepine versus placebo to antipsychotic medication.
- Although numbers were low, those receiving carbamazepine showed greater overall improvement compared with the placebo groups, but no differences for mental state outcomes.
- There were lower rates of movement disorders in the carbamazepine augmentation group than those receiving haloperidol alone.
- There was no evidence regarding the impact of carbamazepine augmentation on aggressive behaviour, negative symptoms, EEG abnormalities or schizoaffective disorder.

See also the 'Treatment – Psychopharmacology' section in Chapter 4 (Bipolar affective disorder), page 61.

Chlorpromazine versus placebo for schizophrenia

Thornley B, Rathbone J, Adams CE, Awad G 2003 Chlorpromazine versus placebo for schizophrenia **(Cochrane Review)**. In: The Cochrane Library, Issue 2. CD000284. Update Software, Oxford

- 50 studies were included.
- Chlorpromazine reduces relapse over 6 months to 2 years (NNT 3; CI 2.5–4) and promotes a global improvement in a person's symptoms and functioning (NNT 7; CI 5–10).
- The placebo response is also considerable.
- There is no statistical significance in dropout rates although fewer left the chlorpromazine trial early.
- There are many adverse effects.
- Chlorpromazine causes sedation (NNH 5; CI 4–6), increases acute movement disorders (NNH 22; CI 15–46) and parkinsonism (NNH 10; CI 8–16).
- Chlorpromazine may cause seizures.
- It also causes lowering of blood pressure and dizziness (NNH 10; CI 8–15) and considerable increase in weight (NNH 3; CI 2–5).

Clozapine for the treatment-resistant schizophrenic

Kane J, Honigfeld G, Singer J et al 1988 Clozapine for the treatment-resistant schizophrenic: a double blind comparison with chlorpromazine. Archives of General Psychiatry 45: 789–796

Method

- 319 patients with treatment-resistant schizophrenia were identified.
- DSM-III diagnostic criteria were used.
- Treatment-resistance criteria were that patients had had treatment with three different neuroleptics (of at least two different classes and at doses equivalent to 1000 mg/day of chlorpromazine) in the preceding 5 years without effect and that there had been no period of good functioning in those preceding 5 years.
- Patients defined as having treatment resistance received a single blind trial of haloperidol for 6 weeks.
- Patients who did not show improvement ($n = 268$) were then randomly allocated to either clozapine or chlorpromazine treatment for 6 weeks.

Results

- 80% of patients completed the treatment period.
- Mean peak daily doses for clozapine and chlorpromazine were approximately 1200 mg and 600 mg, respectively.
- 30% of patients in the clozapine group showed a response compared to 4% of the chlorpromazine group.
- The significant beneficial effects of clozapine were apparent from the end of the first week of treatment.
- Clozapine showed beneficial effects on the Brief Psychiatric Rating Scale and the Clinical Global Impression Scale. The improvements in the scores were at least three times greater in the clozapine-treated group.
- The clozapine-treated group also showed improvements in the Nurses' Observation Scale for Inpatient Evaluation.
- Improvements were shown for both positive and negative symptoms.
- There were high overall completion rates for both groups.
- The rates and the reasons for dropout were comparable between the groups.
- Prophylactic administration of benztropine reduced the possibility of extrapyramidal side effects.
- Dry mouth and hypotension occurred more commonly in the chlorpromazine-treated group.
- Salivation and tachycardia were more prevalent in the clozapine-treated group.
- There were no cases of agranulocytosis in this short study.

Clozapine versus typical neuroleptic medication for schizophrenia

Wahlbeck K, Cheine MV, Essali A 1999 Clozapine versus typical neuroleptic medication for schizophrenia **(Cochrane Review)**. In: The Cochrane Library, Issue 4. CD000059. Update Software, Oxford

- 31 studies, of a total of 2589 participants, were included.
- The majority of patients were male (74%) with an average age of 38 years.
- This review confirms that clozapine is convincingly more effective than typical antipsychotics in reducing symptoms of schizophrenia, producing clinically meaningful improvements (NNT 6) and postponing relapse in the short term (NNT 20; CI 17–38).
- There was no difference between clozapine and typical antipsychotics for outcomes of mortality, ability to work or suitability for discharge at the end of the study.
- Clozapine was more acceptable than low-potency antipsychotics (e.g. chlorpromazine) but there was no difference for high potency antipsychotics (e.g. haloperidol).
- In the long term, clozapine was more acceptable than conventional antipsychotics (NNT 6; CI 3–111).
- Patients receiving clozapine had higher rates of hypersalivation, temperature increase and drowsiness than those receiving conventional antipsychotics. Despite this, clozapine was more acceptable to patients (NNT 12; CI 7–37).
- Patients receiving clozapine had fewer motor side effects and less dry mouth.
- Clozapine was particularly effective in patients with treatment-resistant schizophrenia (NNT 5; CI 4–7), with 32% of these patients showing a clinical improvement.
- Further study of clozapine should focus on global and social functioning in the community and on specific patient groups, such as those with learning disability.

Haloperidol dose for the acute phase of schizophrenia

Waraich PS, Adams CE, Roque M, Hamill KM, Marti J 2002 Haloperidol dose for the acute phase of schizophrenia **(Cochrane Review)**. In: The Cochrane Library, Issue 2. CD001951. Update Software, Oxford

- 16 randomised trials comparing 19 different dose comparisons were included.
- The studies were small and short.

- No data were available regarding relapse rates or quality of life.
- Low doses of haloperidol (3–7.5 mg/day) did not appear to have lower efficacy than higher doses (7.5–15 mg/day and 15–35 mg/day) in terms of clinically important improvement in global state.
- Low doses of haloperidol (3–7.5 mg/day) had a lower rate of development of clinically significant extrapyramidal adverse effects compared with higher doses.
- Data were particularly limited for the lowest doses of haloperidol (1.5–3.0 mg/day).

Haloperidol versus placebo for schizophrenia

Joy CB, Adams CE, Lawrie SM 2001 Haloperidol versus placebo for schizophrenia **(Cochrane Review)**. In: The Cochrane Library, Issue 2. CD003082. Update Software, Oxford

- 20 out of 74 trials were included.
- Patients receiving haloperidol were more likely to improve in the first 6 weeks of treatment than those given placebo (NNT 3; CI 2–5).
- In eight trials this difference favouring haloperidol was found in the 6- to 24-week period (NNT 3; CI 2–5).
- Small negative studies were not found so results may overestimate.
- Over half of the patients beginning the trials did not complete them, although in the 0- to 6-week period, 10 trials found in favour of haloperidol (NNT 8; CI 5–17).
- The data regarding adverse effects were limited but supported the clinical impression that haloperidol is associated with movement disorders.
- Haloperidol is associated with acute dystonias (NNH 5; CI 3–9), akathisia (NNH 6; CI 4–14) and parkinsonism (NNH 3; CI 2–5).
- The use of haloperidol is supported where no other drug is available, but not if an alternative with less likelihood of EPSEs is available.

Lithium for schizophrenia

Leucht S, McGrath J, Kissling W 2003 Lithium for schizophrenia **(Cochrane Review)**. In: The Cochrane Library, Issue 3. CD003834. Update Software, Oxford

- 20 studies were included ($n = 611$).
- Evidence was limited by small numbers, short length of studies and incomplete reporting.

- Three studies of lithium versus placebo as the only treatment for schizophrenia showed no differences in any outcomes.
- When lithium as the only treatment was compared with antipsychotic medication, there was a higher dropout rate in the lithium group.
- 11 studies comparing lithium augmentation of antipsychotic medication with antipsychotic medication alone showed greater improvements in clinical response in the lithium group.
- This significance became borderline when patients with a diagnosis of schizophrenia were included.
- More patients in the lithium group left the study early.
- Lithium augmentation did not show any significant effects on any specific aspect of mental state.
- Further trials are indicated.

Management of clozapine-resistant schizophrenia

Kerwin RW, Bolonna A 2005 Management of clozapine-resistant schizophrenia. Advances in Psychiatric Treatment 11: 101–106

It is observed that all patients with schizophrenia could be considered treatment resistant as it is unusual to have full remission in this disorder.

Kane J, Honigfeld G, Singer J et al 1988 Clozapine for the treatment-resistant schizophrenic. A double-blind comparison with chlorpromazine. Archives of General Psychiatry 45: 789–796

- This trial compared clozapine and chlorpromazine in treatment-refractory schizophrenia.
- Patients were defined as resistant to treatment if in the last 5 years there had been no response to three different neuroleptics from more than one class (1000 mg chlorpromazine equivalent) and no periods of good functioning.
- They found that the incidence of treatment resistance in schizophrenia was 20%.

Meltzer HY 1992 Treatment of the neuroleptic-nonresponsive schizophrenic patient. Schizophrenia Bulletin 18: 515–542

- This study found that patients can have a delayed response to clozapine.
- 30% were found to respond by 6 weeks.
- A further 20% responded in weeks 6–12.
- An additional 10–20% had responded by 6 months.

Shiloh R, Zemishlany Z, Aizenberg D et al 1997 Sulpride augmentation in people with schizophrenia partially responsive to clozapine. A double-blind placebo-controlled study. British Journal of Psychiatry 171: 569–573

- Using the BPRS and the Scale for the Assessment of Positive Symptoms, sulpride augmentation was found to be beneficial in 28 patients who had shown a partial response to clozapine.

Zink M, Knopf U, Henn FA et al 2004 Combination of clozapine and amisulpride in treatment-resistant schizophrenia: case reports and review of the literature. Pharmacopsychiatry 37: 26–31

- This case series found beneficial effects when clozapine and amisulpride were combined.

Munro J, Matthiasson P, Osborne S et al 2004 Amisulpride augmentation of clozapine: an open non-randomized study in patients with schizophrenia partially responsive to clozapine. Acta Psychiatrica Scandinavica 100: 292–298

- A 1-year open trial of amisulpride augmentation of clozapine therapy.
- Over 50% of patients showed a significant improvement.
- No additional side effects were noted.
- Plasma levels of clozapine were not found to change over the trial period.

Dursun SM, Deakin JF 2001 Augmenting antipsychotic treatment with lamotrigine or topiramate in patients with treatment-resistant schizophrenia: a naturalistic case-series outcome study. Journal of Psychopharmacology 15: 297–301

- 26 patients with treatment-resistant schizophrenia received additional treatment with either lamotrigine (17) or topiramate (9).
- Patients were already receiving a variety of antipsychotic medications.
- Patients who received lamotrigine treatment in addition to risperidone, haloperidol, olanzapine or flupenthixol showed a significant improvement.
- This was not the case for patients who received topiramate in addition to clozapine, olanzapine, haloperidol or flupenthixol.

Tiihonen J, Hallikainen T, Ryynanen OP et al 2003 Lamotrigine in treatment-resistant schizophrenia: a randomized placebo-controlled crossover trial. Biological Psychiatry 54: 1241–1248

- Lamotrigine augmentation in this 14-week study led to significant improvement in positive and general psychopathological symptoms.

- There was no effect on negative symptoms.

Conley RR, Tamminga CA, Bartko JJ et al 1998 Olanzapine compared with chlorpromazine in treatment-resistant schizophrenia. American Journal of Psychiatry 155: 914–920

- Olanzapine was found to be no better than chlorpromazine in treatment-resistant schizophrenia.

Conley RR, Tamminga CA, Kelly DL et al 1999 Treatment-resistant schizophrenic patients respond to clozapine after olanzapine non-response. Biological Psychiatry 46: 73–77

- In this study, 44 patients with treatment-resistant schizophrenia received olanzapine; those who did not respond to olanzapine were then treated with clozapine.
- 5% of patients responded to olanzapine.
- A further 41% responded to clozapine.

Lerner V, Libov I, Kohler M et al 2004 Combination of 'atypical' antipsychotic medication in the management of treatment-resistant schizophrenia and schizoaffective disorder. Progress in Neuropsychopharmacology and Biological Psychiatry 28: 89–98

- A review of the augmentation of clozapine with other atypical antipsychotics.
- There was insufficient evidence and while there may be some benefit, further investigation is warranted.

Kane JM 1996 Factors which make patients difficult to treat. British Journal of Psychiatry 169 (Suppl 31): 10–14

Treatment-resistance factors include:
- available medications and other treatments not being useful in alleviating the target symptoms of schizophrenia
- adverse side effects of medication
- non-adherence to current treatment
- the presence of comorbid conditions such as substance misuse
- the failure of maintenance and relapse despite seemingly adequate doses of antipsychotics.

Managing clozapine-induced neutropenia with lithium

Paton C, Esop R 2005 Managing clozapine-induced neutropenia with lithium. Psychiatric Bulletin 29: 186–188

Lithium has been used to increase white blood cell counts in patients treated with chemotherapy, as has carbamazepine.

National Institute for Clinical Excellence 2002 Guidance on use of newer (atypical) antipsychotic drugs for the treatment of schizophrenia. Technology Appraisal Guidance No 43. NICE, London

Estimate that 30% of those with schizophrenia respond poorly to typical and atypical antipsychotic drugs and therefore warrant a trial of clozapine.

Method

- A literature review of lithium and its effects on white blood cells and the use of lithium for clozapine-induced neutropenia.

Abramson N, Melton B 2000 Leukocytosis: basics of clinical assessment. American Family Physician 62: 2053–2057

- White blood cell levels can drop due to:
  - lack of exercise
  - having not smoked a cigarette
  - having blood taken at the wrong time of day.

Munro J, O'Sullivan D, Andrews C et al 1999 Active monitoring of 12,760 clozapine recipients in the UK and Ireland. British Journal of Psychiatry 175: 576–580

- 0.4% of patients have a pre-treatment WBC that was too low to initiate treatment with clozapine.
- 3% of patients treated with clozapine develop neutropenia:
  - within 18 weeks in 50%
  - within 12 months in 75%
- There is an increased risk of neutropenia with being Afro-Caribbean, young and with a low baseline WBC.
- The risk is not dose related
- Agranulocytosis occurs in 0.7%, with 80% of cases developing in the first 18 weeks.
- Risk factors include increasing age and Asian race.

Dettling M, Schaub RT, Mueleer-Oerlinghausen B et al 2001 Further evidence of human leukocyte antigen-encoded susceptibility to clozapine-induced agranulocytosis independent of ancestry. Pharmacogenetics 11: 135–141

- Some people are genetically predisposed to agranulocytosis.
- It is impossible to predict whether a patient with neutropenia will go on to develop agranulocytosis.

Lapierre G, Stewart RB 1980 Lithium carbonate and leukocytosis. American Journal of Hospital Pharmacy 37: 1525–1528

- Lithium acutely increases the neutrophil count and the total WBC.
- Lithium-induced neutrophilia is not dose related.

Carmen J, Okafor K, Ike E 1993 The effects of lithium therapy on leukocytes: a 1 year follow up study. Journal of the National Medical Association 85: 301–303

- Lithium's effects on white cells can happen over longer periods.
- Lithium-induced neutrophilia is not dose related.

Gerson SL, Lieberman JA, Friedenberg WR et al 1991 Polypharmacy in fatal clozapine-associated agranulocytosis. Lancet 338: 262–263

- Fatal agranulocytosis has occurred in patients receiving lithium treatment.

The use of lithium to increase WBC in patients treated with clozapine is off-label prescribing, and therefore the prescriber is at risk of consequences of off-line prescriptions. There is limited evidence.

Meta-analysis of the efficacy of second-generation antipsychotics

Davis J, Chen N, Glick I 2003 A meta-analysis of the efficacy of second-generation antipsychotics. Archives of General Psychiatry 60(6): 553–564

Background

- The apparent effectiveness of second generation antipsychotic medications may reflect the fact that they have been compared with haloperidol at high dose.
- Some research has concluded that there are no differences between first- and second-generation antipsychotics.
- Clinical guidelines and treatment algorithms recommend SGAs as first-line treatment due to differences in adverse effect profiles.

Method

- A meta-analysis of randomised trials of first (FGAs) and second (SGAs) generation antipsychotic medications.
- The analysis aimed to ascertain whether there:
  - were any differences between FGAs and SGAs
  - were any differences between SGAs themselves
  - was a dose–response relationship for FGAs and SGAs
  - was evidence that comparison with an overly high dose of haloperidol affected results.

Results

- The effect sizes of clozapine, amisulpride, risperidone and olanzapine were 0.40, 0.29, 0.25 and 0.21 greater than those of FGAs with p values of 2×10^{-8}, 3×10^{-7}, 2×10^{-12} and 3×10^{-9}, respectively.
- There were no other significant differences between FGAs and the other SGAs.

- There were no differences in efficacy between amisulpride, risperidone and olanzapine.
- There was no evidence that the dose of haloperidol (or the haloperidol equivalent dose) affected the results for the SGAs when examined by drug or by using a two-way analysis of variance.

Newer atypical antipsychotic medication versus clozapine for schizophrenia

Tuunainen A, Wahlbeck K, Gilbody SM 2000 Newer atypical antipsychotic medication versus clozapine for schizophrenia (**Cochrane Review**). In: The Cochrane Library, Issue 2. CD000966. Update Software, Oxford

- Eight studies were included, with only one of over 12 weeks' duration.
- The equal effectiveness and tolerability of newer atypical drugs in comparison with clozapine is not yet demonstrated due to lack of statistical power.
- There were differences in adverse effect profiles, with clozapine causing increased fatigue, hypersalivation, nausea and orthostatic dizziness, and newer atypical drugs (excepting olanzapine) causing more EPSEs.

Olanzapine for schizophrenia

Duggan L, Fenton M, Rathbone J, Dardennes R, El-Dosoky A, Indran S 2005 Olanzapine for schizophrenia (**Cochrane Review**). In: The Cochrane Library, Issue 2. CD001359. Update Software, Oxford

- 55 trials of more than 10,000 people with schizophrenia were included.
- More than 50% of patients from studies comparing olanzapine and placebo dropped out in the first 6 weeks, making data interpretation difficult.
- Compared with placebo, olanzapine was better for the outcome of 'no important clinical response' (NNT 8; CI 5–27).
- There were increased rates of dizziness and dry mouth in the olanzapine group, but this was not statistically significant.
- The olanzapine group gained more weight.
- There was high attrition in both groups (38%) when olanzapine was compared with typical antipsychotic drugs.
- Olanzapine appeared to be as effective as typical antipsychotics in the short term for the outcome of 'no important clinical response' and was associated with fewer EPSEs.

- Data on weight gain were not statistically significant in the short term.
- By 3–12 months, those receiving olanzapine had gained an average of 4 kg.
- Attrition rates were high when olanzapine was compared with other atypical drugs (23% by week 8, 48% by 3–12 months).
- Olanzapine may cause fewer EPSEs but produces statistically significant levels of weight gain (NNH 5; CI 4–7).
- There were few data regarding the first episode of illness.
- In four trials ($n = 457$) of people with treatment-resistant illness there were no clear differences between olanzapine and clozapine.

Pimozide for schizophrenia or related psychoses

Sultana A, McMonagle T 2000 Pimozide for schizophrenia or related psychoses **(Cochrane Review)**. In: The Cochrane Library, Issue 3. CD001949. Update Software, Oxford

- No data were available for people with delusional disorder.
- 34 studies of patients with schizophrenia were included.
- In comparison with typical antipsychotic drugs for the outcomes of change in global functioning, mental state, relapse rates and dropout rates, pimozide had similar efficacy.
- It was not associated with higher mortality.
- Pimozide was more likely to cause a parkinsonian tremor (NNH 6; CI 3–44) and patients were more likely to receive antiparkinsonian medication (NNH 3; CI 2–5) than other drugs.
- It was less likely to cause sedation (NNH 6; CI 4–16).

Quetiapine for schizophrenia

Srisurapanont M, Maneeton B, Maneeton N 2004 Quetiapine for schizophrenia **(Cochrane Review)**. In: The Cochrane Library, Issue 2. CD000967. Update Software, Oxford

- 12 RCTs of 3443 patients were included.
- There were no data on results of service utilisation, economic outcomes, social functioning and quality of life.
- In studies comparing quetiapine with placebo, over half were lost to follow-up (53% quetiapine versus 61% placebo, NNT 11; CI 7–55), making interpretation of results impossible.

- Those receiving quetiapine did not have any more EPSEs, regardless of dose.
- Two deaths were noted in the high dose quetiapine group (> 250 mg/day).
- In short-term comparisons of quetiapine and typical antipsychotics, approximately 36% of both groups failed to complete the studies.
- Global and mental state (including negative symptoms) outcomes were equivocal.
- Fewer patients allocated to quetiapine required medication for EPSEs (NNT 4; CI 4–5).
- Those receiving quetiapine had higher rates of dry mouth (NNH 17; CI 7–65) and sleepiness (NNH 18; CI 8–181).
- When compared with risperidone, 30% of patients left the study early.
- Four deaths were noted in the quetiapine group.
- There were no clear differences in mental state outcomes.
- Significantly fewer patients receiving quetiapine required medication for EPSEs (NNT 11; CI 10–16).
- Those receiving quetiapine had more dizziness (NNH 14; CI 6–82), more sleepiness (NNH 7; CI 4–17) and more dry mouth (NNH 14; CI 6–82) than those receiving risperidone.

Rechallenge with clozapine following leucopenia or neutropenia during previous therapy

Dunk LR, Annan LJ, Andrews CD 2006 Rechallenge with clozapine following leucopenia or neutropenia during previous therapy. British Journal of Psychiatry 188: 255–263

Treatment with clozapine is contraindicated if there has been an episode of blood dyscrasia during clozapine treatment in the past. Some patients have had a second trial of clozapine, generally where the initial episode was mild or thought unrelated to clozapine treatment.

Between 1989 and 2003, 38,106 patients in the UK and Ireland received clozapine. The rates in this group of neutropenia, leucopenia and agranulocytosis were 1.8%, 0.19% and 0.78%, respectively. There were three deaths where clozapine-induced agranulocytosis was attributed as the cause.

This article discusses the various hypotheses regarding clozapine and blood dyscrasia.

Method

- Patients who had had a previous episode of leucopenia or neutropenia during clozapine therapy and who were given a second course of treatment were investigated.
- 53 patients were included from the UK and Ireland.

Results

- 20 patients had a further episode of leucopenia or neutropenia after rechallenge.
- Of these:
  - 85% had a more severe second episode
  - 60% had a longer episode
  - 85% had quicker onset of the second episode.
- Patients rechallenged with clozapine are 22 times more likely to develop an agranulocytosis than patients who have never received clozapine.
- Of the 53 patients who had a rechallenge, 55% continued on clozapine therapy.
- No specific associations were found between people who a second episode and any of the demographic or outcome measures reviewed.

Risperidone versus olanzapine for schizophrenia

Jayaram MB, Hosalli P 2005 Risperidone versus olanzapine for schizophrenia **(Cochrane Review)**. In: The Cochrane Library, Issue 2. CD005237. Update Software, Oxford

- Most of the trials available were funded by the manufacturing pharmaceutical companies.
- There were no short-term differences for the outcome of 'unchanged or no worse'.
- In terms of mental state, most studies showed the two drugs to be equally effective.
- Risperidone and olanzapine frequently cause adverse effects (at least two-thirds of patients experienced an adverse effect).
- One in five patients experienced anticholinergic effects.
- One in five patients experienced insomnia and approximately one in three experienced sleepiness.
- There was no difference in dropout rates.
- Risperidone is associated with movement disorders and sexual dysfunction.
- Olanzapine is associated with considerable rapid onset weight gain.

Risperidone versus other atypical antipsychotic medication for schizophrenia

Gilbody SM, Bagnall AM, Duggan L, Tuunainen A 2000 Risperidone versus other atypical antipsychotic medication for schizophrenia **(Cochrane Review)**. In: The Cochrane Library, Issue 3. CD002306. Update Software, Oxford

- Nine studies were included. Attrition rates were high and the studies were short.
- Five studies comparing risperidone with clozapine in mainly treatment-resistant patients found that there were no differences in acceptability.
- Confidence intervals were wide, making interpretation difficult.
- Three studies comparing risperidone and olanzapine found largely similar numbers of patients responding to treatment.
- Patients receiving olanzapine were less likely to drop out of the study (NNT 8; CI 4–32) and had fewer EPSEs (NNH 8; CI 5–33).
- Doses of risperidone were higher than those recommended in clinical practice.
- One study compared risperidone with amisulpride. There were no clear differences between the two drugs.

Risperidone versus typical antipsychotic medication for schizophrenia

Hunter RH, Joy CB, Kennedy E, Gilbody SM, Song F 2003 Risperidone versus typical antipsychotic medication for schizophrenia **(Cochrane Review)**. In: The Cochrane Library, Issue 2. CD000440. Update Software, Oxford

- Risperidone when compared with haloperidol was more likely to improve outcomes on the PANSS (NNT 8).
- Long-term studies also favoured risperidone, with reduced relapse rates at 1-year follow-up (NNT 7).
- Risperidone was associated with lower rates of dropout in both the short (NNT 6) and long term (NNT 4).
- Risperidone caused fewer movement disorders (including EPSEs) than those receiving older typical antipsychotics (NNT 3).
- Patients receiving risperidone required less antiparkinsonian medication (NNT 4).
- Four studies ($n = 1708$) showed that risperidone use resulted in increased weight gain and rhinitis (NNT 3) compared with typical antipsychotic use.
- There was no difference between risperidone and haloperidol for sexual problems such as erectile dysfunction.
- Independent studies replicating risperidone's favourable effect on relapse are required.

Schizophrenia, neuroleptic medication and mortality

Joukamaa M, Heliovarra M, Knekt P et al 2006 Schizophrenia, neuroleptic medication and mortality. British Journal of Psychiatry 188: 122–127

Method

- A sample of 7217 Finns aged 30 years and over was studied.
- A thorough medical examination was carried out at baseline.
- Schizophrenia was determined from previous medical records and a current diagnosis with the Present State Examination.
- The association between schizophrenia, treatment with neuroleptic medication and mortality was investigated.

Results

- 99 people with schizophrenia were identified.
- 39 of these people died during the 17-year follow-up period.
- There were significant associations between:
  - heavy smoking and schizophrenia in men and women
  - obesity and schizophrenia in men and women
  - being underweight and schizophrenia in men
  - diabetes and other somatic diseases and schizophrenia in women.
- There were inverse associations between:
  - alcohol intake and schizophrenia in men
  - serum HDL cholesterol and schizophrenia in men
  - exercise and schizophrenia in women
  - systolic blood pressure and schizophrenia in men.
- The relative mortality risk for people with schizophrenia compared to the rest of the population was 2.84.
- The figure was 2.25 when adjusted for potential risk factors for premature death. There was no gender-related difference.
- There was a graded relation between the number of neuroleptics used at baseline and mortality.
- Following correction for age, sex, physical illness and the other noted risk factors for premature death, the relative risk was 2.50 per increment of one neuroleptic.
- This excess could not be explained in terms of known risk factors for premature death or physical illness.

Conclusion

- Further study is required as a priority to ascertain whether the excess mortality associated with schizophrenia is due to neuroleptic medication or to the illness itself.

Waddington JL, Youssef HA, Kinsella A 1998 Mortality in schizophrenia. Antipsychotic polypharmacy and absence of adjunctive anticholinergics over the course of a 10-year prospective study. British Journal of Psychiatry 173: 325–329

- A 10-year follow-up study of 88 people with schizophrenia.

- There is an increase in mortality when patients receive more than one neuroleptic medication at a time.

Sulpride for schizophrenia

Soares BGO, Fenton M, Chue P 1999 Sulpride for schizophrenia **(Cochrane Review)**. In: The Cochrane Library, Issue 1. CD001162. Update Software, Oxford

- 18 trials were included but were short and of poor quality.
- Evidence was limited.
- Side effects may occur less often with sulpride.
- There were no clear findings related to negative symptoms.

Thioridazine for schizophrenia

Sultana A, Reilly J, Fenton M 2000 Thioridazine for schizophrenia **(Cochrane Review)**. In: The Cochrane Library, Issue 2. CD001944. Update Software. Oxford

- 11 studies were included ($n = 560$) comparing thioridazine with placebo:
  - small studies under 3 months found no differences between groups
  - at 6 months two small studies favoured thioridazine ($n = 65$)
  - fewer people left the thioridazine group early (NNT 6; CI 4–10; $n = 510$)
  - there was little difference between the groups with regard to adverse effects.
- 26 studies compared thioridazine to typical antipsychotics ($n = 2397$):
  - there were no clear differences between thioridazine and control typical antipsychotics with regard to the outcome 'no better, no worse'
  - there was no difference with regard to dropout rates
  - there were few differences in adverse effects
  - thioridazine does not cause more anticholinergic-type symptoms or sedation than other drugs
  - in the short term, parkinsonism was less common in the thioridazine group
  - one small study ($n = 40$) found no clear differences between thioridazine and clozapine.

Trifluoperazine for schizophrenia

Marques LO, Lima MS, Soares BGO 2004 Trifluoperazine for schizophrenia **(Cochrane Review)**. In: The Cochrane Library, Issue 1. CD003545. Update Software, Oxford

- 13 studies were included ($n = 1162$) comparing trifluoperazine with placebo:
  - small, short-term studies favoured the treatment group (NNT 3; CI 2–4)
  - there were no differences in loss to follow-up between the groups
  - more people in the treatment group used antiparkinsonian drugs to alleviate movement disorders (NNH 4; CI 2–9).
- 49 studies ($n = 2230$) compared trifluoperazine to another older generation antipsychotic:
  - trifluoperazine was more likely to cause extrapyramidal adverse effects overall when compared with chlorpromazine (NNH 6; CI 3–121). There were no significant differences with regard to loss to follow-up or the outcome 'no substantial improvement'.
  - overall, many adverse effects were found, with identical numbers (~60%) reporting at least one adverse effect.

Valproate for schizophrenia

Bassoon A, Leucht S 2003 Valproate for schizophrenia **(Cochrane Review)**. In: The Cochrane Library, Issue 3. CD004028. Update Software, Oxford

- Five studies ($n = 379$) looked at the effectiveness of valproate as an adjunct to antipsychotics.
- Evidence was limited by small numbers, the short length of the studies and incomplete reporting.
- One study showed a quicker onset of action in the valproate augmentation group.
- This group also showed increased sedation.
- There was no significant effect on patients' global state or general mental state following the addition of valproate.
- Effects of valproate augmentation on aggressive behaviour or in those with schizoaffective disorder are not known.

Zuclopenthixol acetate for acute schizophrenia and similar serious mental illness

Gibson RC, Fenton M, Coutinho ESF, Campbell C 2004 Zuclopenthixol acetate for acute schizophrenia and similar serious mental illness **(Cochrane Review)**. In: The Cochrane Library, Issue 3. CD000525. Update Software, Oxford

- This review did not find any suggestion that zuclopenthixol acetate is more or less effective in controlling aggressive acute psychosis, or in preventing adverse effects than IM haloperidol.
- People given zuclopenthixol acetate were just as likely to be given supplementary antipsychotics.
- There was no evidence that zuclopenthixol acetate had a more rapid onset of action.
- There was no evidence on rates of aggression or harm to self or others.
- There appeared to be no difference in reported adverse effects when using zuclopenthixol acetate versus haloperidol and clotiapine.

Tardive dyskinesia

Anticholinergic medication for neuroleptic-induced tardive dyskinesia

Soares KVS, McGrath JJ 1997 Anticholinergic medication for neuroleptic-induced tardive dyskinesia **(Cochrane Review)**. In: The Cochrane Library, Issue 2. CD000204. Update Software, Oxford

- No data could be extracted from the seven RCTs identified.

Benzodiazepines for neuroleptic-induced tardive dyskinesia

Walker P, Soares KVS 2003 Benzodiazepines for neuroleptic-induced tardive dyskinesia **(Cochrane Review)**. In: The Cochrane Library, Issue 2. CD000205. Update Software, Oxford

- Two small studies were included ($n = 32$).
- Benzodiazepines as adjunctive treatment did not result in any clear changes for a series of tardive dyskinesia medium-term outcomes.
- No information was gathered regarding adverse effects.

Calcium channel blockers for neuroleptic-induced tardive dyskinesia

Soare-Weiser K, Rathbone J 2004 Calcium channel blockers for neuroleptic-induced tardive dyskinesia **(Cochrane Review)**. In: The Cochrane Library, Issue 1. CD000206. Update Software, Oxford

- No trials could be included.
- The effects of calcium channel blockers for antipsychotic-induced tardive dyskinesia are unknown.

Cholinergic medication for neuroleptic-induced tardive dyskinesia

Tammenmaa IA, McGrath JJ, Sailas E, Soares-Weiser K 2002 Cholinergic medication for neuroleptic-induced tardive dyskinesia **(Cochrane Review)**. In: The Cochrane Library, Issue 3. CD000207. Update Software, Oxford

- 11 studies comparing older cholinergic drugs with placebo were included.
- Cholinergic drugs neither improved nor worsened symptoms of tardive dyskinesia.
- Studies were too small and too few to determine the clinical effects of older cholinergic drugs on tardive dyskinesia.
- Studies of newer cholinergic agents would be helpful.

Gamma-aminobutyric acid agonists for neuroleptic-induced tardive dyskinesia

Soares KVS, Rathbone J, Deeks JJ 2004 Gamma-aminobutyric acid agonists for neuroleptic-induced tardive dyskinesia **(Cochrane Review)**. In: The Cochrane Library, Issue 4. CD000203. Update Software, Oxford

- Eight trials were included; all were poorly reported.
- There is no good evidence about the effects of baclofen, progabide, sodium valproate or tetrahydroisoxazolopyridinne (THIP).
- Adverse effects are likely to outweigh any benefits.
- Higher numbers of patients receiving GABA medication failed to complete the trials compared to those receiving placebo; however, this was not statistically significant.
- Adverse effects of ataxia and sedation were noted in the treatment groups when compared with placebo, but again this was not statistically significant.

Neuroleptic reduction and/or cessation and neuroleptics as specific treatments for tardive dyskinesia

McGrath JJ, Soares-Weiser KVS 2006 Neuroleptic reduction and/or cessation and neuroleptics as specific treatments for tardive dyskinesia **(Cochrane Review)**. In: The Cochrane Library, Issue 2. Update Software, Oxford

- Five trials out of 107 were included.
- There was limited good evidence regarding the benefits of neuroleptic reduction or specific neuroleptic medication in the treatment of tardive dyskinesia.

Vitamin E for neuroleptic-induced tardive dyskinesia

Soares KVS, McGrath JJ 2001 Vitamin E for neuroleptic-induced tardive dyskinesia **(Cochrane Review)**. In: The Cochrane Library, Issue 4. CD000209. Update Software, Oxford

- 10 studies were included.
- No clear evidence was found for vitamin E against placebo in terms of clinically relevant improvement or any improvement in TD symptoms.
- However, those people who did not receive vitamin E showed greater deterioration of their symptoms.
- There were no differences in terms of adverse effects or of leaving the study early.

Treatment – Psychological Therapies

Cognitive rehabilitation for people with schizophrenia and related conditions

Hayes RL, McGrath JJ 2000 Cognitive rehabilitation for people with schizophrenia and related conditions **(Cochrane Review)**. In: The Cochrane Library, Issue 3. CD000968. Update Software, Oxford

- Two studies compared cognitive rehabilitation to a placebo intervention and one to occupational therapy.
- All interventions were acceptable to patients with low attrition rates.
- No effects were demonstrated on measures of mental state, social behaviour or cognitive functioning.
- Cognitive rehabilitation had a favourable effect on a measure of self-esteem.
- Data were inconclusive.

See also the 'Treatment – Psychological therapies' section in Chapter 25 (Psychological therapies), page 352.

Music therapy for schizophrenia or schizophrenia-like illnesses

Gold C, Heldal TO, Dahle T, Wigram T 2005 Music therapy for schizophrenia or schizophrenia-like illnesses **(Cochrane Review)**. In: The Cochrane Library, Issue 2. CD004025. Update Software, Oxford

- Music therapy in addition to standard care was more effective than treatment with standard care alone on the outcome of global state.
- Music therapy was also associated with some benefits in terms of general mental state, negative symptoms and social function.
- Results were inconsistent across studies and varied with the number of music therapy sessions.
- Further studies should examine the dose–effect relationship and the long-term effects of music therapy.

Definition

Music therapy – a psychotherapeutic method that uses musical interaction as a means of communication and expression. The aim of therapy is to help people with serious mental illness to develop relationships and to address issues they may not be able to using words alone.

Psychoeducation for schizophrenia

Pekkala E, Merinder L 2002 Psychoeducation for schizophrenia **(Cochrane Review)**. In: The Cochrane Library, Issue 2. CD002831. Update Software, Oxford

- All of the 10 studies included used group education involving family members.
- One study, which used brief group intervention, showed significantly improved compliance with medication at 1 year.
- Other studies showed equivocal or skewed data.
- Any kind of psychoeducational intervention significantly decreased relapse or readmission rates at follow-up (9–18 months) compared with standard care.
- Generally, findings were consistent with the possibility that psychoeducation has a positive effect on a person's wellbeing.
- No impact was found regarding insight, medication-related attitudes or on overall satisfaction of patients or relatives due to the small numbers of studies.
- Psychoeducational approaches are thought to be useful but further studies are needed.

Token economy for schizophrenia

McMonagle T, Sultana A 2000 Token economy for schizophrenia **(Cochrane Review)**. In: The Cochrane Library, Issue 3. CD001473. Update Software, Oxford

- Three RCTs were included.
- It was not possible to draw any conclusions on outcomes of effects on target or non-target behaviour.

- One small study showed improvement in negative symptoms at 3 months.
- It is unclear if the results are reproducible, clinically meaningful and are maintained beyond the treatment programme.

Vocational rehabilitation for people with severe mental illness

Crowther R, Marshall M, Bond G, Huxley P 2001 Vocational rehabilitation for people with severe mental illness **(Cochrane Review)**. In: The Cochrane Library, Issue 2. CD003080. Update Software, Oxford

- 18 RCTs were identified.
- For the primary outcome (number of people in competitive employment) it was found that supported employment led to a significant benefit compared with pre-vocational training.
- Those in supported employment earned more and worked more hours.
- There was no evidence that pre-vocational training led to improvements in helping patients to obtain competitive employment over standard community care.

Definition

Vocational rehabilitation services exist to help mentally ill people find work. Traditionally, these services have offered a period of preparation (pre-vocational training) before trying to place clients in competitive (i.e. open) employment. More recently, some services have begun placing clients in competitive employment while providing on-the-job support (supported employment).

Treatment – Others

Are fish oils an effective therapy in mental illness?

Maidment ID 2000 Are fish oils an effective therapy in mental illness? An analysis of the data. Acta Psychiatrica Scandinavica 102: 3–11

A review

Omega-6 and omega-3 are essential fatty acids. Fish oils have proved a very acceptable therapy to patients. A number of studies have linked low levels of omega-3 fatty acids with depression – no causal relationship has been shown.

There are no data suggesting that omega-3 fatty acids are an effective treatment of depressive disorders. There are some data on the effect of fatty acid supplementation on schizophrenic symptoms. The four trials reported have involved relatively small numbers. The evidence relating to fatty acids and schizophrenia is conflicting.

Maes M, Murphy B, Shay J 1998 Depletion of omega-3 fatty acid levels in red blood cell membranes of depressive patients. Biological Psychiatry 43: 315–319

- In major depression there were lower levels of omega-3 fatty acids, and an increase in monounsaturated fatty acids and the omega-6 fatty acid, docosapentaenoic acid, in serum phospholipids.
- The levels of the omega-6 5 fatty acid (arachidonic acid) were decreased.
- The changes in fatty acids persisted despite successful therapy with fluoxetine.
- Dietary intake of fatty acids was not controlled or measured.

Stoll AL, Severus WE, Reeman MP 1999 Omega-3 fatty acids in bipolar disorder – a preliminary double-blind, placebo controlled trial. Archives of General Psychiatry 56: 407–412

- A preliminary study.
- Patients treated with omega-3 fatty acids had significantly longer periods of remission than those who received placebo.
- There were also significant improvements in the secondary outcome measures of the Ham-D, CGI and the GAS.
- There was a significant drop in depressive symptoms in the fatty acid group
- The study failed to show that omega-3 fatty acids treated manic symptoms.

Mellor JE, Laugharne JDE, Peet M 1996 Omega-3 fatty acid supplementation in schizophrenic patients. Human Psychopharmacology 11: 39–46

- There are substantial data suggesting that the metabolism of both omega-3 and omega-6 fatty acids is disturbed in schizophrenia.
- A greater dietary intake of omega-3 fatty acids was associated with fewer positive symptoms of schizophrenia and a lower incidence of TD.
- There was no relationship between RBC omega-3 fatty acid content and the symptoms of schizophrenia.
- High levels of RBC membrane omega-6 fatty acids resulted in more negative symptoms.
- Fish oil supplementation resulted in improvements in the PANSS and AIMS rating scales.
- Improvements in positive and negative symptoms with fish oil supplementation were noted, but only the improvement in negative symptoms was statistically significant.
- Fish oil supplementation resulted in a significant increase in RBC membrane levels of omega-3 fatty acids and a significant decrease in omega-6 fatty acid membrane levels.
- There is a need for double-blind, placebo-controlled trials.

Vaddadi KS, Courtney T, Gillearde CJ 1989 A double blind trial of essential fatty acid supplementation in patients with tardive dyskinesia. Psychiatry Research 27: 313–323

- Correlation is noted between the low levels of fatty acids in RBC membranes and the severity of TD.
- Efamol supplementation did not cause significant improvement in tardive dyskinesia.
- Efamol supplementation did cause significant improvement in the Comprehensive Psychological Rating Scale compared with placebo, where the significance related to the schizophrenia subscale.
- The main improvement was in negative symptoms; however, the CPRS does not readily show differences in negative symptoms.

Glen AIM, Glen EMT, Horrobin DF 1994 A red cell membrane abnormality in a subgroup of schizophrenic patients: evidence for two diseases. Schizophrenia Research 12: 53–61

- Patients with mainly negative symptoms had significantly reduced levels of arachidonic acid and docosapentaenoic acid.

Shah S, Ramchand CN, Peet M 1998 Eicosapentaenoic acid (EPA) as an adjunct to neuroleptic treatment in the treatment of schizophrenia. Presented at the 9th Schizophrenia Workshop, Davos, 7–13 February 1998

- There was a statistically significant reduction in the general and anergia subscales and the thought disorder and activation subscales of the PANSS.
- There was no statistically significant reduction in the composite, paranoid belligerence, depression and supplemental subscales.
- There was no evidence of effectiveness against depressive symptoms in the population with schizophrenia.

Mellor JE, Peet M 1998 Double blind placebo controlled trial of omega-3 fatty acids as an adjunct to the treatment of schizophrenia. Presented at the 9th Schizophrenia Workshop, Davos, 7–13 February 1998

- Those receiving eicosapentaenoic acid had significantly greater improvement in positive symptoms and the total PANSS score compared to those receiving DHA or placebo.

* Neither EPA nor DHA had a significant effect on negative symptoms.

See also the 'Treatment – Others' section in Chapter 12 (General psychiatry), page 194.

Electroconvulsive therapy for schizophrenia

Tharyan P, Adams CE 2005 Electroconvulsive therapy for schizophrenia (**Cochrane Review**). In: The Cochrane Library, Issue 2. CD000076. Update Software, Oxford

* The review suggests that ECT in combination with antipsychotic drugs may be beneficial in the treatment of people with schizophrenia, in particular when rapid improvements or reductions in symptoms are required.
* Combination therapy with ECT and antipsychotic medication may also be of benefit for people with schizophrenia who have a partial response to medication alone.
* Compared to sham ECT, treatment with ECT was associated with:
  - fewer relapses short term
  - a greater likelihood of being discharged from hospital
  - no clear evidence of the effect being maintained longer term.
* When ECT is directly compared with antipsychotic drug treatment, treatment with medication is associated with greater benefit.
* There was limited evidence that ECT in combination with antipsychotic medication led to greater benefit with regard to mental state than treatment with antipsychotic drugs alone.
* One study concluded that there was an increased risk of transient memory impairment after a course of ECT combined with antipsychotic medication than with medication alone.
* Treatment with both continuation ECT (CECT) and antipsychotic medication led to greater benefits in Global Assessment of Functioning than treatment with antipsychotic medication or CECT alone.
* Unilateral and bilateral ECT were found to be as effective as each other with regard to improvements in global function.

Polyunsaturated fatty acid supplementation

Joy CB, Mumby-Croft R, Joy LA 2003 Polyunsaturated fatty acid supplementation for schizophrenia (**Cochrane**

Review). In: The Cochrane Library, Issue 2. CD001257. Update Software, Oxford

* Five short, small studies were included.
* One small study found that treatment with omega-3 EFA (eicosapentaenoic acid) enriched oil alone may have beneficial effects on psychotic symptom properties when compared to placebo.
* No other studies were of sufficient size as to be of value.
* There was some evidence that for those already receiving antipsychotic medication, supplementation with omega-3 EFA brought about a greater improvement in mental state than placebo supplementation, but this was not significant.
* Omega-3 EFA supplementation was associated with improvements in mental state for patients regardless of whether they were receiving antipsychotic medication or not (NNT 3; CI 2–8).
* One small study looked at the effects of omega-6 EFA compared with placebo for tardive dyskinesia but found no clear effects.
* Large well-designed, conducted and reported studies are required.

Assessment Tools and Rating Scales

Abnormal Involuntary Movement Scale (AIMS)

Guy W 1976 Early Clinical Drug Evaluation Unit (ECDEU) assessment manual for psychopharmacology. Revised. DHEW Publication No. ADM 76-338. US Department of Health, Rockville, MD

* Clinician rated scale which assesses the occurrence of dyskinesia in patients receiving neuroleptic treatment.
* Quick to administer.
* Widely and easily used for assessing TD.

Brief Psychiatric Rating Scale (BPRS)

Overall JE, Gorham DR 1962 The brief psychiatric rating scale. Psychological Reports 10: 799–812

* Structured and unstructured interview.
* Combines observation of patient's behaviour and interactions or information from carers.

- Assesses psychopathology in patients with or suspected of having schizophrenia or psychosis.
- Time period covered is 2–3 days prior to evaluation.
- Takes 15–30 minutes to complete.
- Widely used, frequently revised.
- Traditionally covers 16 items:
  - somatic concern
  - anxiety
  - emotional withdrawal
  - conceptual disorganisation
  - guilt
  - tension
  - mannerisms and posturing
  - grandiosity
  - depression
  - hostility
  - suspiciousness
  - hallucinatory behaviour
  - motor retardation
  - uncooperativeness
  - unusual thought content
  - blunted affect.
- Each item scored 1 (not present) to 7.
- Consistent for broad clinical features.
- Limited in measuring change due to non-linearity of the total score distribution.

Extrapyramidal Symptom Rating Scale (ESRS)

Chouinard G, Ross-Chouinard A, Annable L et al 1980 Extrapyramidal Rating Scale. Canadian Journal of Neurological Sciences 7: 233–239

- Physician rated scale.
- Designed to measure extrapyramidal side effects from antipsychotic medication.
- Six questions about subjective experience of extrapyramidal features (slowness, stiffness and tremor).
- Seven rater-assessed items that address parkinsonian features (rigidity and tremor).
- Does not always differentiate between dystonia and dyskinesia.

Positive and Negative Syndrome Scale for Schizophrenia (PANSS)

Kay SR, Opler LA 1987 The Positive and Negative Syndrome Scale (PANSS) for Schizophrenia. Schizophrenia Bulletin 13: 507–518

- A clinician-administered, 30-item semi-structured interview.
- Provides a balanced representation of positive and negative symptoms.
- Consists of:
  - seven items of positive symptoms (hallucinations, delusions, conceptual disorganisation)
  - seven items assessing negative symptoms (blunted affect, passive/apathetic social avoidance)
  - 16 items assessing global psychopathology (depression, anxiety, lack of insight, guilt).
- Items are scored between 1 (not present) and 7 (severe).
- Well validated.

Scale for the Assessment of Negative Symptoms (SANS)

Andreasen NC 1982 Negative symptoms in schizophrenia. Definition and reliability. Archives of General Psychiatry 39(7): 784–788

- Standardised scale for the assessment of negative symptoms of schizophrenia.
- Six point scale covers a range of negative symptoms.

Guidelines

Schizophrenia: core interventions in the treatment and management of schizophrenia in primary and secondary care. NICE Clinical Guideline 1*

Treatment of the acute episode

Service interventions

- Community mental health teams are an acceptable way of organising community care and may have the potential for effectively coordinating and integrating other community-based teams providing services for people with schizophrenia. However, there is insufficient evidence of their advantages to support a recommendation which precludes or inhibits the development of alternative service configurations. [C]
- Crisis resolution and home treatment teams should be used as a means to manage crises for service users and as a means of delivering high-quality acute care. In this context, teams should pay particular attention to risk monitoring as a high-priority routine activity. [B]

- Crisis resolution and home treatment teams should be considered for people with schizophrenia who are in crisis to augment the services provided by early intervention services and assertive outreach teams. [C]
- Crisis resolution and home treatment teams should be considered for people with schizophrenia who may benefit from early discharge from hospital following a period of inpatient care. [C]
- Acute day hospitals should be considered as a clinical and cost-effective option for the provision of acute care, both as an alternative to acute admission to inpatient care and to facilitate early discharge from inpatient care. [A]

Pharmaceutical interventions

- The dosage of conventional antipsychotic medication for an acute episode should be in the range of 300–1000 mg chlorpromazine equivalents per day for a minimum of 6 weeks. Reasons for dosage outside this range should be justified and documented. The minimum effective dose should be used. [C]
- In the treatment of the acute episode for people with schizophrenia, massive loading doses of antipsychotic medication, referred to as 'rapid neuroleptisation', should not be used. [C]
- Antipsychotic drugs, atypical or conventional, should not be prescribed concurrently, except for short periods to cover changeover. [C]
- When prescribed chlorpromazine, individuals should be warned of a potential photosensitive skin response as this is an easily preventable side effect. [B]
- Where a potential to cause weight gain or diabetes has been identified (and/or included in the Summary of Product Characteristics) for the atypical antipsychotic being prescribed, there should be routine monitoring in respect of these potential risks. [B]

Early post-acute phase: psychological treatments

- Cognitive behavioural therapy (CBT) should be available as a treatment option for people with schizophrenia. [A]
- Family interventions should be available to the families of people who are living with or who are in close contact with the service user. [A]
- Counselling and supportive psychotherapy are not recommended as discrete interventions in the routine care of people with schizophrenia where other psychological interventions of proven efficacy are indicated and available. However, service user preferences should be taken into account, especially if other more effective psychological treatments are not locally available. [C]

Promoting recovery

Service interventions

- Assertive outreach teams should be provided for people with serious mental disorders, including people with schizophrenia. [B]
- Assertive outreach teams should be provided for people with serious mental disorders, including people with schizophrenia, who make high use of inpatient services and who have a history of poor engagement with services leading to frequent relapse and/or social breakdown (as manifest by homelessness or seriously inadequate accommodation). [B]
- Assertive outreach teams should be provided for people with schizophrenia who are homeless. [B]
- Crisis resolution and home treatment teams should be considered for people with schizophrenia who are in crisis to augment the services provided by early intervention services and assertive outreach teams. [C]

Psychological interventions

- Cognitive behavioural therapy should be available as a treatment option for people with schizophrenia. [A]
- In particular, cognitive behavioural therapy should be offered to people with schizophrenia who are experiencing persisting psychotic symptoms. [A]
- Cognitive behavioural therapy should be considered as a treatment option to assist in the development of insight. [B]
- Cognitive behavioural therapy may be considered as a treatment option in the management of poor treatment adherence. [C]
- Longer treatments with cognitive behavioural therapy are significantly more effective than shorter ones, which may improve depressive symptoms but are unlikely to improve psychotic symptoms. An adequate course of cognitive behavioural therapy to generate improvements in psychotic symptoms in these circumstances should be of more than 6 months' duration and include more than 10 planned sessions. [B]
- Family interventions should be available to the families of people with schizophrenia who are living with or who are in close contact with the service user. [A]
- In particular, family interventions should be offered to the families of people with schizophrenia who have recently relapsed or who are considered at risk of relapse. [A]
- Also in particular, family interventions should be offered to the families of people with schizophrenia who have persisting symptoms. [A]
- When providing family interventions, the length of the family intervention programme should normally be longer than 6 months' duration and include more than 10 sessions of treatment. [B]

- When providing family interventions, the service user should normally be included in the sessions, as doing so significantly improves the outcome. Sometimes, however, this is not practicable. [**B**]
- When providing family interventions, service users and their carers may prefer single-family interventions rather than multifamily group interventions. [**A**]

Pharmacological interventions

Relapse prevention: oral antipsychotics
- Targeted, intermittent dosage maintenance strategies should not be used routinely in lieu of continuous dosage regimens because of the increased risk of symptoms worsening or relapse. However, these strategies may be considered for service users who refuse maintenance or for whom some other contradiction to maintenance therapy exists, such as side effect sensitivity.
- Antipsychotic drugs, atypical or conventional, should not be prescribed concurrently, except for short periods to cover changeover. [**C**]

Relapse prevention: depot antipsychotics
- Depot preparations should be a treatment option where a service user expresses a preference for such treatment because of its convenience, or as part of a treatment plan in which the avoidance of covert non-adherence with antipsychotic drugs is a clinical priority. [**B**]
- For optimum effectiveness in preventing relapse, depot preparations should be prescribed within the standard recommended dosage and interval range. [**A**]

Treatment-resistant schizophrenia
- If the symptoms of schizophrenia are unresponsive to conventional antipsychotics, the prescribing clinician and service user may wish to consider an atypical antipsychotic in advance of a diagnosis of treatment-resistant schizophrenia and a trial of clozapine. In such cases, olanzapine or risperidone may be worth considering.
- Service users should be informed that while these drugs may possibly be beneficial, the evidence for improvement in this situation is more limited than for clozapine. [**C**]

Combining antipsychotics
- Antipsychotic drugs, atypical or conventional, should not be prescribed concurrently, except for short periods to cover changeover. [**C**]
- However, the addition of a second antipsychotic to clozapine may be considered for people with TRS for whom clozapine alone has proved insufficiently effective. [**C**]

Employment

- Supported employment programmes should be provided for those people with schizophrenia who wish to return to work or gain employment. However, it should not be the only work-related activity offered when individuals are unable to work or are unsuccessful in their attempts to find employment. [**C**]

Rapid tranquillisation

- Health professionals should identify and take steps to minimise the environmental and social factors that might increase the likelihood of violence and aggression during an episode, particularly during episodes of hospitalisation. Factors to be routinely identified, monitored and corrected include: overcrowding, lack of privacy, lack of activities, long waiting times to see staff, poor communication between patients and staff, and weak clinical leadership. [**C**]

Aims of rapid tranquillisation
- Staff who use rapid tranquillisation should be trained in the assessment and management of service users specifically in this context. This should include assessing and managing the risks of drugs (benzodiazepines and antipsychotics), using and maintaining the techniques and equipment needed for cardiopulmonary resuscitation, prescribing within therapeutic limits and using flumazenil (benzodiazepine antagonist). [**C**]

Training for behavioural control/rapid tranquillisation
- Staff need to be trained to anticipate possible violence and to de-escalate the situation at the earliest opportunity. Physical means of restraint or seclusion should be resorted to 'only after the failure of attempts to promote full participation in self-care'. [**C**]
- Training in the use and the dangers of rapid tranquillisation is as essential as training in de-escalation and restraint. Health professionals should be as familiar with the properties of benzodiazepines as they are with those of antipsychotics. [**C**]
- Specifically, health professionals should [**C**]:
  - be able to assess the risks associated with rapid tranquillisation, particularly when the service user is highly aroused and may have been misusing drugs or alcohol, be dehydrated or possibly be physically ill
  - understand the cardiopulmonary effects of the acute administration of these drugs and the need to titrate dosage to effect
  - recognise the importance of nursing, in the recovery position, people who have received these drugs and also monitoring pulse, blood pressure and respiration
  - be familiar with, and trained in, the use of resuscitation equipment (this is essential as an anaesthetist or experienced 'crash team' may not be available)

– undertake annual retraining in resuscitation techniques

– understand the importance of maintaining an unobstructed airway.

Principles of rapid tranquillisation

- The psychiatrist and the multidisciplinary team should, at the earliest opportunity, undertake a full assessment, including consideration of the medical and psychiatric differential diagnoses. [**C**]

- Drugs for rapid tranquillisation, particularly in the context of restraint, should be used with caution because of the following risks [**C**]:
  – loss of consciousness instead of sedation
  – oversedation with loss of alertness
  – possible damage to the therapeutic partnership between service user and clinician
  – specific issues in relation to diagnosis.

- Resuscitation equipment and drugs, including flumazenil, must be available and easily accessible where rapid tranquillisation is used. [**C**]

- Because of the serious risk to life, service users who are heavily sedated or using illicit drugs or alcohol should not be secluded. [**C**]

- If a service user is secluded, the potential consequences of rapid tranquillisation should be taken particularly seriously. [**C**]

- Violent behaviour can be managed without the prescription of unusually high doses or 'drug cocktails'. The minimum effective dose should be used. The *British National Formulary* recommendations for the maximum doses (BNF – section 4.2) should be adhered to unless exceptional circumstances arise. [**C**]

Route of administration

- Oral medication should be offered before parenteral medication. [**C**]

- If parenteral treatment proves necessary, the intramuscular route is preferred over the intravenous one from a safety point of view. Intravenous administration should only be used in exceptional circumstances. [**C**]

- Vital signs must be monitored after parenteral treatment is administered. Blood pressure, pulse, temperature and respiratory rate should be recorded at regular intervals, agreed by the multidisciplinary team, until the service user becomes active again. If the service user appears to be or is asleep, more intensive monitoring is required. [**C**]

Pharmacological agents used in rapid tranquillisation

- The IM preparations recommended for use in rapid tranquillisation are lorazepam, haloperidol and olanzapine. Wherever possible, a single agent is preferred to a combination. [**C**]

- When rapid tranquillisation is urgently needed, a combination of IM haloperidol and IM lorazepam should be considered. [**C**]

- IM diazepam is not recommended for the pharmacological control of behavioural disturbances in people with schizophrenia. [**C**]

- IM chlorpromazine is not recommended for the pharmacological control of behavioural disturbances in people with schizophrenia. [**C**]

- When using IM haloperidol (or any other IM conventional antipsychotic) as a means of behavioural control, an anticholinergic agent should be given to reduce the risk of dystonia and other extrapyramidal side effects. [**C**]

A, **B** and **C** indicate grades of recommendation (see Appendix II for full details). * Reproduced with permission from the National Institute for Health and Clinical Excellence, London.

Full guidance on the use of newer (atypical) antipsychotic drugs for the treatment of schizophrenia. NICE Technology Appraisal Guidance No. 43*

Guidance

The choice of antipsychotic drug should be made jointly by the individual and the clinician responsible for treatment based on an informed discussion of the relative benefits of the drugs and their side effect profiles. The individual's advocate or carer should be consulted where appropriate.

It is recommended that the oral atypical antipsychotic drugs amisulpride, olanzapine, quetiapine, risperidone and zotepine are considered in the choice of first-line treatments for individuals with newly diagnosed schizophrenia.

The oral atypical antipsychotic drugs (amisulpride, olanzapine, quetiapine, risperidone and zotepine) should be considered as treatment options for individuals currently receiving typical antipsychotic drugs who, despite adequate symptom control, are experiencing unacceptable side effects, and for those in relapse who have previously experienced unsatisfactory management or unacceptable side effects with typical antipsychotic drugs. The decision as to what are unacceptable side effects should be taken following discussion between the patient and the clinician responsible for treatment.

It is not recommended that, in routine clinical practice, individuals change to one of the oral atypical antipsychotic drugs if they are currently achieving good control of their condition without unacceptable side effects with typical antipsychotic drugs.

In individuals with evidence of treatment-resistant schizophrenia (TRS), clozapine should be introduced at the earliest opportunity. TRS is suggested by a lack of satisfactory clinical improvement despite the sequential use of the recommended doses for 6–8 weeks of at least two antipsychotics, at least one of which should be an atypical.

A risk assessment should be performed by the clinician responsible for treatment and the multidisciplinary team regarding concordance with medication, and depot preparations should be prescribed when appropriate.

Where more than one atypical antipsychotic drug is considered appropriate, the drug with the lowest purchase cost (taking into account daily required dose and product price per dose) should be prescribed.

When full discussion between the clinician responsible for treatment and the individual concerned is not possible, in particular in the management of an acute schizophrenic episode, the oral atypical drugs should be considered as the treatment options of choice because of the lower potential risk of extrapyramidal symptoms (EPS). In these circumstances, the individual's carer or advocate should be consulted where possible and appropriate. Although there are limitations with advanced directives regarding the choice of treatment for individuals with schizophrenia, it is recommended that they are developed and documented in individuals' care programmes whenever possible.

Antipsychotic therapy should be initiated as part of a comprehensive package of care that addresses the individual's clinical, emotional and social needs. The clinician responsible for treatment and the keyworker should monitor both therapeutic progress and tolerability of the drug on an ongoing basis. Monitoring is particularly important when individuals have just changed from one antipsychotic to another.

Atypical and typical antipsychotic drugs should not be prescribed concurrently except for short periods to cover changeover of medication.

Psychosocial interventions in the management of schizophrenia. SIGN Publication Number 30** see page 404

See also the 'Guidelines' section in Chapter 25 (Psychological therapies), pages 352-356, 358-360.

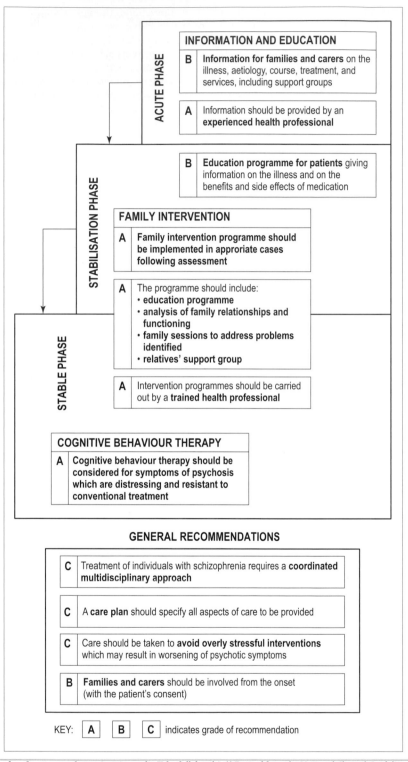

A, B and **C** indicate grades of recommendation (see Appendix II for full details). ** Derived from the National Clinical Guideline recommended for use in Scotland by the Scottish Intercollegiate Guidelines Network (SIGN), Edinburgh. © SIGN, 1998. Reproduced with permission.

Service provison

27

General Topics

General Household Survey

Office for National Statistics. General Household Survey. Social Survey Division. Online. Available: www.statistics.gov.uk/ssd/surveys/general_household_survey.asp

- A multipurpose survey carried out almost continually since 1971.
- Information is collected from people living in private households in Great Britain.
- Data are collected on a range of topics including demographics, household and consumables ownership, employment, education and health.
- The sample size is 13,250 and the format a face-to-face interview.

Results 1971–2002

Households
- The average size of household has decreased from 2.91 to 2.31.
- The number of people living alone has increased from 17 to 31%.
- The number of lone parent households has increased from 5 to 15%.
- The number of people over 65 living alone has remained fairly stable in the last 20 years.

People
- The number of people aged 75 or over rose from 4% in 1971 to 7% 10 years ago, and has remained constant since then.

- The number of children under the age of 16 has decreased from 23 to 20%.

Self-reported illness
- Self-reported chronic illness in adults and children has risen from 21 to 35%.
- Self-reported limiting longstanding illness in adults and children has risen from 15% in 1975 to 21%.
- Changes in self-reported illness may reflect changes in people's expectations about health as much as actual changes in the prevalence of illness.

Integrated care pathways (ICPs)

- These pathways offer the clinician a structured means of developing and implementing local protocols of care founded on evidence-based clinical guidelines.
- Such pathways are helpful to staff as they can enable them to provide a consistent level of care and be aware of the possible complications, outcomes and stages of progress. Evaluation processes can be incorporated.
- Patient versions of the pathways provide improved information and allow patients to be more involved.
- Pathways can be used in staff induction as a tool that provides clear information about service processes.

Definition

An **integrated care pathway** determines locally agreed, multidisciplinary practice based on guidelines and evidence, where available, for a specific client group. It forms all or part of the clinical record, documents care given and facilitates the evaluation of outcomes for continuous quality improvement. (*Source*: Overill S 1998 A practical guide to care pathways. Journal of Integrated Care 2: 93–98.)

Weblinks

Integrated Care Pathway Users Scotland – www.icpus.
  ukprofessionals.com.

National Pathways Association – www.the-npa.org.uk.

NHS National Library for Health: Protocols and Care
  Pathways Specialist Library – www.library.nhs.uk/
  pathways.

Managed clinical networks (MCNs)

This concept arose in a Scottish Health acute services
review in 1998. It was further clarified in *Our National
Health: A Plan for Action, A Plan for Change* with regard to
those suffering with chronic illness.

MCNs aim to improve patient care by enhancing the
coordination of services across organisational boundaries
and disciplines. There is an emphasis on audit, clear
organisational responsibilities and evidence-based processes
leading to measured outcomes. Patients must be involved
alongside clinicians in helping to shape disease-specific, or
problem-specific, service delivery.

These factors should enable all professionals that work
with a particular clinical problem to link up. This will help
to bridge the gap between primary and secondary care.

MCNs exist for learning disabilities psychiatry, diabetes
and coronary heart disease in parts of Scotland. There is a
national MCN for people with cleft lip or palate.

MCNs provide a modern alternative to the now
redundant internal market in the NHS. The Scottish
Executive has repeatedly stated its commitment to working
with clinicians, patients and managers in the development
of more MCNs across Scotland.

Definition

Managed clinical networks – linked groups of health
professionals and organisations from primary, secondary
and tertiary care, working in a coordinated manner,
unconstrained by existing professional and health board
boundaries, to ensure equitable provision of high-quality,
clinically-effective services. (*Source*: The same as you?
Scottish Executive, Edinburgh, 2004.)

The tiered model – a framework for the provision of care

* Tier 0 – Community, public health and strategic
  approaches to care
* Tier 1 – Primary care and directly accessed health
  services
* Tier 2 – Health services accessed via primary care
* Tier 3 – Specialist locality health services
* Tier 4 – Specialist area and regional health services.

See also Promoting health, supporting inclusion (p. 229),
NICE and SIGN guidelines and Addictions (p. 15).

Policy and Legislation

Case management competences

NHS Modernisation Agency and Skills for Health 2005
A case management competences framework for the
care of people with long term conditions. Best Practice
Guidance. NHS Modernisation Agency and Skills for
Health, London. Online. Available: www.dh.gov.uk/
assetRoot/04/11/81/02/04118102.pdf

Over 17 million people in the UK report living with a
chronic condition. While most receive adequate care, there
is evidence that those with more complex needs do not
receive a properly coordinated service. If each component
of a complex condition is dealt with by separate agencies,
then care will fragment, resulting in deficient care and
unnecessary hospital admissions.

'Case management' is the suggested approach to deal
with an individual's problems in a more coordinated
fashion.

This document outlines the competences necessary
for case managers (nurse, social worker or AHP) and
community matrons.

The paper describes a model with three levels:

Level 1

* Applies to approximately 70% of the long-term care
  population.
* Features:
  – supported self-care
  – helping individuals and their carers develop the
    knowledge and skills to manage their own condition.

Level 2

* For high risk patients.
* Features:
  – case manager involved
  – provision of disease-specific, specialist
    multidisciplinary care
  – service delivery in accordance with National Service
    Frameworks.

Level 3

* For high complexity patients.
* Features:
  – identification of very high intensity users of
    unplanned secondary care

- community matron involvement
- case management approach to coordination of health and social care.

The competences are grouped into nine separate domains. These include:

- advanced clinical nursing practice
- managing cognitive impairment and mental well-being
- managing care at the end of life.

These competences can be used as an aid to developing services, compiling job descriptions and providing training. It is hoped the competences will improve health and social care, make them more 'person-centred' and help develop career pathways for staff.

Assessment Tools and Rating Scales

Camberwell Assessment of Need (CAN)

- A measure of assessment of the health and social needs of people with mental health problems.
- Four versions exist for different populations:
  - Adult CAN – for working-age adults
  - CANE – for people over 65 years
  - CANDID – for people with learning disabilities
  - CANFOR – for people with forensic issues.
- Other versions include:
  - CAN-R – research format
  - CANSAS – short appraisal schedule
  - CAN-C – clinical format.
- These instruments measure needs and support over the previous 4 weeks.
- 22 health and social domains are covered:
  - Accommodation
  - Food
  - Looking after the home
  - Self-care
  - Daytime activities
  - Physical health
  - Psychotic symptoms
  - Information
  - Psychological distress
  - Safety to self
  - Safety to others
  - Alcohol
  - Drugs
  - Company
  - Intimate relationships
  - Sexual expression
  - Childcare
  - Basic education
  - Telephone
  - Transport
  - Money
  - Benefits.
- For each domain, one of four responses can be chosen:
  - no need
  - met need
  - unmet need
  - not known
- A need may be met, but only because the adult already receives adequate support.
- When met and unmet needs are identified, then further questioning will investigate how much support the adult receives and needs from formal and informal sources

Weblink Institute of Psychiatry, King's College London – www.iop.kcl.ac.uk.
See also the 'Assessment tools and rating scales' section in Chapter 12 (General psychiatry), page 198.

The Carstairs and Morris index of deprivation

- An index of deprivation calculated from the 1981 Scottish census data.
- It calculated deprivation from four variables of material disadvantage:
  - overcrowding
  - male unemployment
  - social class 4 or 5
  - no car.
- A composite score was created for most postcode areas.
- The index correlates well with a range of health measures.
- McLoone updated the scores for Scotland from the 1991 census information.

See also the 'Assessment tools and rating scales' section in Chapter 12 (General psychiatry), page 198.

Jarman deprivation scores

- A measure of need.
- The scores were calculated from the 1991 census local base statistics.
- They provide a measure of social deprivation.
- Eight variables are used and taken as a proportion of the whole:
  - Unemployment
  - Overcrowding
  - Lone pensioners
  - Single parents
  - Born in the New Commonwealth
  - Children aged under 5
  - Low social class

– 1-year migrants (i.e. people who had a different address 12 months before).

See also the 'Assessment tools and rating scales' section in Chapter 12 (General psychiatry), page 198.

Townsend deprivation Index

- A score of multiple deprivation by area.
- The scores are calculated from the 1991 census.
- Four variables are used:
  - unemployment
  - overcrowding
  - non car ownership
  - non home ownership.

Underprivileged area score (UPA)

- An area-based measure calculated from additional workload or pressure for GPs.
- They were calculated following a survey of UK GPs.
- GPs were asked to weight different variables with regard to their impact on their workload.
- Scores range from −50 to +70.
- Deprived areas are those with a score of 30 or above.

Stigma

28

Chapter contents

Ethical Issues

Independent inquiry into the care and treatment of Daksha Emson

North East London Strategic Health Authority 2003 Independent inquiry into the care and treatment of Daksha Emson. NELSHA, London. Online. Available: www.nelondon.nhs.uk/?ID=3119

In October 2000 Dr Daksha Emson, a psychiatrist with a history of bipolar affective disorder, stabbed her 3-month old daughter and set herself on fire when suffering from a psychotic episode. The baby died at the time of the incident; her mother died 3 weeks later.

Fear of the stigma due to having a psychiatric illness prevented Dr Emson from accessing adequate care. The action plan recommended an antidiscrimination code of practice and appropriate staff training as well as Royal College, GMC and BMA involvement in anti-stigma work.

The Inquiry report also stated that the relationship between treating doctors and doctors undergoing treatment necessitates significant attention. The plan recommended that a protocol should be drawn up for doctor–doctor consultations. It also pointed out the need to improve occupational health services in the NHS.

The postnatal relapse of the illness could and should have been anticipated. Therefore existing guidelines from the Royal College of Psychiatrists on perinatal mental health services should be followed to ensure risks are identified and managed well.

Freya, her daughter, was viewed as an appendage of her mother rather than as an individual. There is a need for a holistic approach to families by mental health services as well as a greater emphasis on child protection issues.

See also the 'General topics' section in Chapter 11 (Gender), page 172.

General Topics

Changing minds at the earliest opportunity

Shah N 2004 Changing minds at the earliest opportunity. Psychiatric Bulletin 28: 213–215

Dr Shah reports on the series of talks about stigma and mental illness that she gave to primary school children aged between 5 and 11 years.

- The youngest children viewed the terms 'mad' and 'crazy' as positive.
- Older children described the September 11 bombers as 'mad'.
- She found that most of the stigma towards people with mental illness occurred in the oldest of the children and in some of the teachers.
- Feedback was received from 50% of the teachers about the sessions.
- There were mixed responses, with 25% of teachers believing the children were better informed.
- She concluded that increasing awareness of mental health and illness in children is unlikely to cause harm, and could be argued to be an important component of primary education.

Wolff G, Pathare S, Craig T et al 1996 Community knowledge of mental illness and reaction to mentally ill people. British Journal of Psychiatry 168: 191–198

- Stigmatising attitudes about mental health are reinforced by lack of knowledge.
- It is suggested that this should be tackled at a young age.
- Stigmatising attitudes can exist from older childhood.

Wilson C, Nairn R, Coverdale J et al 2000 How mental illness is portrayed in children's television: a prospective study. British Journal of Psychiatry 176: 440–443

- Suggested that young people are socialised into stigmatising conceptions of mental illness through children's TV programmes

Weblink The College anti-stigma campaign. Royal College of Psychiatrists 1998 Changing Minds – www.rcpsych. ac.uk/campaigns/changingminds.aspx.

The College Anti-Stigma Campaign 1998–2003

Crisp A, Cowan L, Hart D 2004 The College Anti-Stigma Campaign 1998–2003. Psychiatric Bulletin 28: 133–136

The anti-stigma campaign was conceptualised by the college in 1996, under the presidency of Dr R Kendell. The working party was established in 1997 and decided it would be timely to recognise the differences in public attitudes to the variety of mental illness.

The campaign addressed six disorders:
- anxiety disorders
- depressive disorders
- dementia
- schizophrenia
- eating disorders
- drug and alcohol misuse/addiction.
  Target audiences were:
- doctors
- children and adolescents
- the workplace
- the media
- the general public.

A survey of the British public concerning people with mental illness funded by the Office for National Statistics

The outcomes of the campaign were:
- Mental illness: stigmatisation and discrimination within the medical profession. Royal College of Psychiatrists

Council Report: a collaborative report distributed to undergraduate and postgraduate educational bodies on the UK.
- '1 in 4' cinema film: 2-minute film launched on Mental Health Day 2000 aimed at young adults (15–25) to challenge the preconceptions about mental illness.
- Every Family in the Land. Changing minds – our lives and mental illness: book presenting personal stories of those with mental illness, with commentaries from professionals.
- 'Tube cards' – advertising campaign on the London underground.
- Booklets, statements and the campaign video.
- Changing minds CD-Rom for 13–17 year olds: multimedia CD-Rom for use in schools.
- Reading Lights – four picture books for 4–7 year olds: simple texts encouraging respect and understanding of diversity.
- Articles published in the medical press. The campaign commissioned numerous articles. There are now over 100 referenced in the tool kit.
- A campaign roadshow with international presentation.

See also Department of Health 2001 Mind out for mental health campaign. DH, London.

Iatrogenic stigma of mental illness

Sartorius N 2002 Iatrogenic stigma of mental illness [editorial]. British Medical Journal 324: 1470–1471

The World Psychiatric Association's global programme against the stigma and discrimination associated with schizophrenia began with an investigation into the experiences of patients with schizophrenia and their families. It aimed to identify targets for interventions.

Twenty countries are involved in this long-term programme, with different interventions being adopted in different countries.

Identified targets included accident and emergency departments in Canada, shopkeepers in Italy and the media and the reporting of mental illness in Germany.

Iatrogenic stigma was noted to occur in a number of ways:

Labelling

It is important to establish a diagnosis as the use of a diagnosis allows effective communication between doctors and allied health professionals. However, other disciplines and public sector staff may use diagnostic terms without a full understanding of their meaning and with associated negative attitudes. Diagnostic information should be protected.

Adverse effects of medication

Obvious side effects of medication (e.g. extrapyramidal side effects) may be more stigmatising than the actual illness. The implications of these adverse effects should be considered with other issues, such as cost and treatment guidelines.

Legislation

It is not acceptable to use diagnosis alone when considering whether or not to use specific mental health legislation. Instead, each individual's behaviour and capacity should be taken into consideration, as it is in those who do not have a diagnosis of mental illness.

Mental health staff

Psychiatrists and other staff have in the past secured special terms and conditions including increased annual leave, higher pay and earlier retirement because they have had to work with 'dangerous' patients with mental illness.

Institutions and psychiatric hospitals have rarely ensured that patients have had the opportunity to participate in elections and voting.

These issues have implications as to how people with mental illness are perceived in terms of their capacity and their rights.

Stigma in psychiatry

Gray JA 2002 Stigma in psychiatry. Journal of the Royal Society of Medicine 95: 72–76

* Medical professionals should be aware of their own attitudes, should involve service users in the development of services and stand against discrimination.

Definition

Labelling – the careless use of diagnostic labels.

Stigma: the feelings and experiences of 46 people with mental illness

Dinos S, Stevens S, Serfaty M, Weich S, King M 2004 Stigma: the feelings and experiences of 46 people with mental illness. A qualitative study. British Journal of Psychiatry 184: 176–181

Stigma has been described as a social construct that defines people in terms of distinguishing characteristics or marks and devalues them as a consequence. The majority of the research has focused on the views of the general population about people with mental illness. There has been little subjective investigation of the experiences of people with mental illness.

Goffman E 1963 Stigma: notes on the management of spoiled identity. Penguin, London

According to Goffman's original formulation, the stigma of mental illness can either be:
* discrediting – when it is obvious to others
* discreditable – when it is not obvious to others.

Aims

* A qualitative study.
* Explores the relationship between stigma and diagnosis, and perceptions of illness and treatment, and examines the consequences of stigma on people's lives.

Method

* 46 patients with psychiatric diagnoses were recruited from a variety of settings.
* Their own reports of their diagnoses were considered the most relevant description of their illnesses for the purposes of this study.
* Stigma was not directly talked about in the interviews to avoid leading the subjects.

Results

* Participants talked a great deal about stigma.
* Two distinct subcategories emerged during the discussions:
  – subjective feelings of stigma in the absence of discrimination
  – stigma in the context of overdiscrimination.
* People with psychosis or drug dependence were most likely to report feelings and experiences of stigma and were most affected by them.
* Those with depression and anxiety were more likely to experience patronising attitudes rather than overt stigma.
* Of note is the fact that, of the 46 people interviewed, 39 were able to talk about the positive side to having a mental illness. This mainly covered relief at being given a diagnosis, which was more prominent in those with depression and/or anxiety.
* Concern about disclosure of a mental illness emerged as a major theme, supporting Goffman's views that the need to manage a discreditable identity can be a powerful source of anxiety.

Jacoby A 1994 Felt versus enacted stigma: a concept revisited. Evidence from a study of people with epilepsy in remission. Social Science and Medicine 38: 269–274

- Found that 'feeling stigmatised can occur in the absence of any direct discrimination'.
- Participants' attempts to avoid disclosure resulted in stress, isolation and a sense of shame.

Stigmatisation of people with mental illnesses

Crisp AH, Gelder MG, Rix S 2000 Stigmatisation of people with mental illnesses. British Journal of Psychiatry 177: 4–7

This survey aimed to collect baseline data regarding the views of the UK population on people with mental illness. The results would guide the 'Changing Minds' campaign, begun by the Royal College of Psychiatrists in 1998 to reduce the stigma of mental illness.

Method

- 1737 adults were surveyed about seven common mental disorders: severe depression, panic attacks, schizophrenia, dementia, eating disorders, alcoholism and drug addiction.

Results

- People with schizophrenia, alcoholism and drug dependence were viewed as unpredictable (80%) and dangerous (70%).
- Alcoholism and drug dependence were believed to be self-inflicted.
- Only 7% of respondents thought that people with schizophrenia were responsible for their illness and capable of helping themselves.
- People with mental disorders were viewed as difficult to talk to.
- 63% of the adults surveyed felt that people with severe depression were hard to talk to.
- There appeared to be a reasonable understanding of the role of medication and prognosis of mental disorders.

- Approximately half of the respondents knew someone with a mental illness, but their attitudes did not differ significantly from the rest.

Policy and Legislation

Mental health and social exclusion

Office of the Deputy Prime Minister 2003 Mental health and social exclusion. Social Exclusion Unit Report. ODPM, London. Online. Available: www.socialexclusion.gov.uk/downloaddoc.asp?id=134

- Proposes that health services address the social needs of those excluded from wider society by mental illness, not just their medical needs.
- The 5-year plan includes ambitious anti-stigma and discrimination campaigns. These campaigns for employers, schools and the media aim to challenge beliefs that people with mental illness are dangerous, unstable and unemployable.
- Links between trusts and job centres are to be established or strengthened.
- Benefits agency and job centre staff will be given mental health awareness training.
- The transition to work will be improved by ensuring clear benefits advice is available.
- Psychiatric inpatients are to receive employment advice and support.
- NHS day centres must focus on the reintegration of patients into their communities via job training, employment advice or voluntary work.
- People with mental illness should have the same opportunities as the general public and will no longer be excluded from sitting on a jury or for standing as a school governor.

Suicide and self-harm

29

Chapter contents

General Topics

Management of self-harm in adults

Kapur N 2005 Management of self-harm in adults: which way now? British Journal of Psychiatry 187: 497–499

Published documents emphasised the role of psychosocial assessments, multidisciplinary approaches to working, adequate training and supervision, and the organisation of services for self-harm. The provision of services has, however, remained extremely variable. Two guidelines (below) have since been published. Self-harm has replaced the term deliberate self-harm.

Various treatments have been evaluated for self-harm but few have led to clinically significant reductions in repetition. A number of interventions warrant investigation in large clinical trials. These include problem-solving therapy, interpersonal therapy and emergency card type interventions. Treatments helpful in subgroups of patients include DBT for those who repeatedly self-harm and group therapy for adolescents.

This editorial suggests that service providers' attitudes need to change in order to ensure appropriate management. A reduced preoccupation with risk may improve the general hospital management of self-harm.

Risk prediction regarding future suicidal behaviour following self-harm remains difficult because the outcomes are rare and the assessment tools relatively crude. Prompt follow-up is essential, given that of those who self-harm again within a year, about a quarter do so within the first 3 weeks.

National Collaborating Centre for Mental Health 2004 Self-harm: the short term physical and psychological management and secondary prevention of self-harm in primary and secondary care. Clinical Guideline 16. Gaskell and the British Psychological Society, London

- A comprehensive document that considers the short-term physical and psychological management of self-harm.
- Recommendations cover components of good practice.
- Some recommendation may be difficult to implement – for example, all those who self-harm should be assessed by a mental health specialist.
- Patients at risk of repetition should have intensive therapeutic intervention combined with outreach. This includes 3 months of therapy with telephone contact and home treatment as necessary.
- These recommendations appear unrealistic.
- Little of the evidence was based on verification other than clinical experience.
- The majority of recommendations are good practice points.
- The focus has shifted to 'needs assessment' rather than 'risk assessment.'
- Needs assessment aims to identify psychosocial factors that might explain any act of self-harm leading to a formulation (describing short- and long-term vulnerability factors and precipitating factors) that will direct the management plan.

Royal College of Psychiatrists 2004 Assessment following self-harm in adults. Royal College of Psychiatrists, London

- The required general skills for the care of people who self-harm include assessment and treatment of the patient's physical condition, preliminary psychosocial assessment and basic understanding of medicolegal issues.
- Specialist skills include providing diagnostic formulation, assessing risk and drawing up and implementing a treatment plan.
- The report also provides standards for organising services, clinical procedures and facilities and training, and supervision in a variety of settings.
- The report seems especially relevant to those planning a service.

Sheldon TA, Callum N, Dawson D et al 2004 What's the evidence that NICE guidance has been implemented? Results from a national evaluation using time series analysis, audit of patients' notes and interviews. British Medical Journal 329: 999–1004

- Guidelines are more likely to be adopted when there is:
  - strong professional support
  - no associated increase in costs
  - a system in place to monitor take-up with a background of strong evidence.

James A 2004 Psychiatrists rebuke colleagues over remarks on self-harming patients. Online. Available: www.psychminded.co.uk.news (archive 26 August 2004)

- Noted that there is still a body of professionals who view the actions of those who self-harm as immature and diverting resources away from those with 'serious' illness.

Simpson EL, House AO 2003 User and carer involvement in mental health services: from rhetoric to science. British Journal of Psychiatry 183: 89–91

- The negative attitudes of staff could be addressed if users and carers are involved in professional training, service delivery and service evaluation.

Kapur N, Cooper J, Rodway C et al 2005 Predicting the risk of repetition after self-harm: cohort study. British Medical Journal 330: 394–395

- Care must be taken when focusing attention on those deemed to be 'high risk' as those assessed as 'low risk' actually account for the majority of repeat episodes.
- An alternative is suggested whereby basic intervention is offered to all those who have harmed themselves, and a combination of needs and risk assessment is used to identify individuals who might benefit from more intensive treatment.

OPUS study: suicidal behaviour, suicidal ideation and hopelessness among patients with first-episode psychosis

Nordentoft M, Jeppesen P, Abel M et al 2002 OPUS study: suicidal behaviour, suicidal ideation and hopelessness among patients with first-episode psychosis. One-year follow-up of a randomised controlled trial. British Journal of Psychiatry 181: S98–S106

Method

- A Danish RCT that aimed to compare integrated care with treatment as usual in terms of suicidal behaviour and hopelessness.
- Predictive factors for suicidal behaviour were also sought.
- 341 patients with a first episode of psychosis were included.
- The features of integrated care are assertive community treatment and antipsychotic medication for all patients, psychoeducational family treatment and social skills training as appropriate.

Results

- In the 12-month follow-up period, 11% of all of the patients attempted suicide – there were no significant differences between treatment and control groups.
- Treatment in either group was associated with significant reductions in suicidal ideation and reports of suicide during the past 12 months.
- Levels of suicidal ideation and behaviour remained higher than for the general population.
- Suicidal behaviour was associated with:
  - being female
  - hopelessness
  - hallucinations
  - previous suicide attempt reported at baseline.
- Of these, only hallucinations and a previous suicide attempt reported at baseline remained significant following multivariate analysis.
- There were differences in correlates of suicidal ideation and suicidal attempts.
- Integrated treatment was associated with a reduction in hopelessness.

Psychiatry, the law and death on the roads

Gordon H 2004 Psychiatry, the law and death on the roads. Advances in Psychiatric Treatment 10: 439–445; Gunn J, Taylor PJ 1993 Forensic psychiatry: clinical, legal and ethical issues. Butterworth-Heinemann, Oxford

Reckless driving in the late 1980s became the most common type of homicide, causing more deaths than murder and manslaughter.

Cremona A 1986 Mad drivers: psychiatric illness and driving performance. British Journal of Hospital Medicine 35: 193–195

- Human error is the cause of most road traffic accidents.
- Other factors include road conditions, weather and the condition of the vehicle.
- It is suggested that mania will lead to faster driving.
- Impaired concentration in depression with psychomotor retardation may occur.

Raffle PAB 1985 Medical aspects of fitness to drive: a guide for medical practitioners, 4th edn. Medical Commission on Accident Prevention, London

- Less than 1% of road traffic accidents that result in injury involve medical conditions of drivers.

Silverstone T 1988 The influence of psychiatric disease and its treatment in driving performance. International Clinical Psychopharmacology 3 (Suppl 1): 59–66

- Did not find the association between road traffic accidents and psychotic illness that previous studies found.
- Did not find evidence that mania leads to faster driving.
- Patients with depression may show increased suicidality while driving.

Kolowski SJ, Rossiter J 2000 Driving in Somerset. Psychiatric Bulletin 24: 304–306

- Dementia in drivers is associated with an increased accident rate.

Marottoli RA, Cooney LM, Wagner R et al 1994 Predictors of automobile crashes and moving violations among elderly drivers. Annals of Internal Medicine 121: 842–846

- Borderline cognitive impairment in drivers is associated with an increased accident rate.

McKenna P 1998 Fitness to drive: a neuropsychological perspective. Journal of Mental Health 7: 9–18

- Neurological impairment in drivers is associated with an increased accident rate.

Del Rio MC, Gonzalez-Luque JC, Alvarez FJ 2001 Alcohol related problems and fitness to drive. Alcohol and Alcoholism 36: 256–261

- Alcohol intake is one of the most important factors in road traffic accidents.

Bierness DJ 1993 Do we really drive as we live? The role of personality factors in road crashes. Alcohol, Drugs and Driving 9: 129–143

- The combination of alcohol and personality factors such as hostility and aggression can lead to an increased risk of road traffic accidents.

Carter D 2003 The impact of antisocial lifestyle on health. British Medical Journal 326: 256–261

- Described an 'antisocial lifestyle' marked by violent and non-violent offences, drug misuse, promiscuity and reckless driving.

Rasanen P, Hakko H, Jarvelin MR 1999 Early onset drunk driving, violent criminality and mental disorders. Lancet 354: 1788

- Drink driving at a young age is associated with mental illness and violent crime.

Lapham SC, Smith E, C'de Baca J et al 2001 Prevalence of psychiatric disorders among persons convicted of driving while impaired. Archives of General Psychiatry 58: 943–949

- People with drink-driving offences are more likely to:
  - misuse alcohol and other drugs
  - be alcohol dependent
  - have a depressive disorder
  - have post-traumatic stress disorder.

Turnbridge RL, Keigan M, James FJ 2001 The incidence of drugs and alcohol in road traffic fatalities. TRL Report 495. Transport Research Laboratory, Crowthorne

- Fatal road traffic accidents are increasingly linked to drug misuse, cannabis in particular.
- Drug use was associated with being unemployed, under 40 years of age if male and over 40 years of age if female.
- Female drivers were more likely to be driving under the influence of prescribed drugs.

Barbone F, McMahon AD, Davey PG et al 1998 Association of road traffic accidents with benzodiazepines. Lancet 352: 1331–1336

- Users of anxiolytics and hypnotics are at increased risk of road traffic accidents.

McMurray L 1970 Emotional stress and driving performance. The effects of divorce. Behavioural Research in Highway Safety 1: 100–114

- There is an increased risk of a road traffic accident in people who have had a recent life event such as separation or divorce.

Tillman WA, Hobbs GE 1949 The accident-prone automobile driver. American Journal of Psychiatry 106: 321–331

- Described a high accident group of taxi drivers who showed intolerance of and aggression to authority.
- They were more likely to have factors associated with conduct disorder, psychological maladjustment, irresponsible driving and criminal convictions.

Aberg L, Rimmo PA 1998 Dimensions of aberrant driver behaviour. Ergonomics 41: 39–56

- Men are more likely than women to drive dangerously and aggressively.

Moffat GK 2002 A violent heart: understanding aggressive individuals. Praeger, London

- Young, inexperienced drivers are most often involved in fatal road traffic accidents.

Brown P 1993 Mental illness and motor insurance. Psychiatric Bulletin 17: 620–621

- People with mental illness may be refused motor insurance and may drive without the correct insurance.

Rose G 2000 The criminal histories of serious traffic offenders. Home Office Research Study 206. Home Office, London

- Those convicted of dangerous driving and, in particular, those disqualified from driving have profiles similar to mainstream criminal offenders.

Jenkins J, Sainsbury P 1980 Single-car road deaths – disguised suicides? British Medical Journal 281: 1041

- Estimated fatal road traffic accidents as suicide in 2.7% when single vehicle accidents were examined.

Ohberg A, Penttila A, Lonngvist J 1997 Driver suicides. British Journal of Psychiatry 171: 468–472

- 4% of fatal road traffic accidents attributed to suicide led to the death of someone other than the driver.
- Common factors for these drivers included that they were more likely to be young, male, driving alone, to have a head-on collision with a much larger vehicle, to have had recent life events, to have a psychiatric disorder and to have long-term alcohol misuse.

MacDonald JM 1964 Suicide and homicide by automobile. American Journal of Psychiatry 121: 366–370

- This study of suicide and homicide by motor vehicle in Colorado noted that these methods may allow concealment of the crime.

- Of 40 drivers who crashed their car with suicidal ($n = 30$), homicidal ($n = 3$) or combined intent ($n = 7$), the majority ($n = 34$) had hysterical, passive–aggressive or sociopathic personality. Six drivers had a psychotic illness, four had schizophrenia, one had schizoaffective psychosis and one had a depressive illness.

Psychosocial and pharmacological treatments for deliberate self-harm

Hawton K, Townsend E, Arensman E et al 1999 Psychosocial and pharmacological treatments for deliberate self-harm **(Cochrane Review)**. In: The Cochrane Library, Issue 4. CD001764. Update Software, Oxford

- 23 trials were included which had repetition of self-harm as an outcome variable.
- It was not possible to examine other outcome measures such as compliance with treatment, depression, hopelessness, suicidal ideation/thoughts and change in problems/problem resolution.
- There were insufficient numbers in the trials.
- Promising results were found for:
  - problem-solving therapy
  - provision of a card to allow emergency contact with services
  - depot flupenthixol for recurrent repeaters of self-harm
  - long-term psychological therapy for female patients with borderline personality disorder and recurrent self-harm.
- Larger trials are needed.

See also the 'Treatment – Psychological therapies' section in Chapter 25 (Psychological therapies), page 356.

Relationship between alcohol use disorders and suicidality

McCloud A, Barnaby B, Omu N, Drummond C, Aboud A 2004 Relationship between alcohol use disorders and suicidality in a psychiatric population. In-patient prevalence study. British Journal of Psychiatry 184: 439–445

There are mixed results from studies regarding the treatment of alcohol and substance misuse in acute psychiatry settings. It is suggested that there is potential for a reduction in suicide and self-harm in psychiatric populations if treatment is provided for alcohol and substance misuse.

Aims

- The study investigates the prevalence and spread of alcohol use amongst psychiatric patients and the extent to which it is associated with suicidality.

- Hypotheses tested were:
  - alcohol use disorders would be particularly prevalent amongst psychiatric inpatients
  - there would be a positive association between alcohol use disorders and inpatients with a history of suicidality.

Method

- A randomised trial of brief motivational enhancement techniques for alcohol use disorders.
- Sample was obtained from psychiatric admissions over an 8-month period.
- Demographic information, smoking and substance abuse history were assessed.
- The Alcohol Use Disorders Identification Test (AUDIT) was completed.
- Case notes were reviewed to indicate if alcohol use disorders were recorded.

Results

- Just under half of the patients had an AUDIT score of 8 or more, indicating hazardous or harmful drinking.
- Positive scores on AUDIT were associated with being younger and white.
- There were no differences in gender on AUDIT scores.
- There were no differences on other significant variables: diagnosis, having no fixed abode or living alone and on unemployment or sick/disabled.
- Over one in five patients were indicative of severe alcohol dependence.
- There were no differences in gender for severe alcohol dependence.
- Severe alcohol dependence occurred almost exclusively in white people.
- Patients with severe alcohol dependence were less likely to be diagnosed with major mental disorder than patients with lower scores.

Relationship between alcohol use and suicidality

- 52.5% of admissions were related to suicidal ideation or deliberate self-harm.
- The AUDIT score was strongly associated with suicidality.
- 70% of those with a score above 8, and 86.7% of those scoring 16 or above, were admitted with suicidal ideation or deliberate self-harm.
- Suicidality was positively associated with affective disorders and, in women, illicit drug use in the preceding month.
- Suicidality was negatively correlated with psychosis.
- Significant predictors of suicidality were:
  - AUDIT score of ≥ 8

- not having a diagnosis of severe mental illness
- having an irregular sleep pattern.

Platt S, Robinson A 1991 Parasuicide and suicide: a 20 year survey of admissions to a regional poisoning treatment centre. International Journal of Social Psychiatry 37: 159–172

- Alcohol use is a known risk factor for suicide and parasuicide.

Barnaby B, Drummond C, McCloud A et al 2003 Substance misuse in psychiatric inpatients: comparison of a screening questionnaire survey with case notes. British Medical Journal 327: 783–784

- Psychiatrists may miss opportunities to screen for alcohol problems.
- They can hold negative beliefs regarding those perceived to have alcohol problems.

See also dual diagnosis strategy, pages 8 and 13.

See also the 'General topics' section in Chapter 1 (Addictions psychiatry), pages 2-3.

Repeated self-poisoning

Carter G, Reith D, Whyte I, McPherson M 2005 Repeated self-poisoning: increasing severity of self-harm as a predictor of subsequent suicide. British Journal of Psychiatry 186: 253–257

Prediction of suicide is difficult and this is usually attributed to the low base rate of suicide. In some patients the severity of the suicidal ideation and parasuicidal behaviour may increase over time.

Method

- A nested case-controlled study.
- This study aimed to identify and examine changes in clinical presentation predictive of suicide in repeated episodes of hospital-treated self-poisoning.

Results

- Around 30% of self-poisoners to this service had presented before with previous episodes of self-harm.
- 38% of those who subsequently killed themselves had presented to the service on more than one occasion.
- 31 patients who presented on two or more occasions and subsequently committed suicide were included in the study.
- 93 controls were selected.
- Median time from last admission to death was 305 days (4 to 2636).
- People who completed suicide were more likely to have:

- higher scores on coma scales
- taken larger amounts of medication
- taken increasing amounts of medication
- more severe drug and alcohol misuse.
- There were no significant differences between people who completed suicide and controls with regard to:
  - time to presentation, ITU admission or length of stay
  - change in pattern of poison exposure
  - differences in change of length of stay, psychiatric diagnosis or discharge destination.
- The most promising predictor variable was a change in the number of tablets ingested:
  - an increase in the amount of medication taken on subsequent episodes by 70 or more tablets had a high specificity and the best sensitivity of any individual test
  - if an increase in tablet numbers was combined with increasing drug and alcohol misuse, the sensitivity was 47%
  - in combination with a worsening coma the sensitivity increased to 53%, with a specificity of 87%.

Conclusion

- People who have escalating severity of self-poisoning episodes are at greater risk of competed suicide.
- Such patients may warrant additional short- and long-term engagement with clinical services in order to reduce the risk of subsequent suicide.
- These markers should be used in the evaluation of suicide risk.

Powell J, Geddes J, Hawton K et al 2000 Suicide in psychiatric hospital in-patients: risk factors and their predictive power. British Journal of Psychiatry 176: 266–272

- Although tools for assessing suicide have high sensitivity for suicide they may also have low specificity and limited usefulness in practice.

Whyte IM, Dawson AH, Buckley NA et al 1997 Health care. A model for the management of self-poisoning. Medical Journal of Australia 167: 142–146

- People who died by suicide had been treated more than once for deliberate self-poisoning.

Safety First: National Confidential Inquiry into suicide and homicide by people with mental illness

Department of Health Report 2001 Five-year Report of the National Confidential Inquiry into suicide and homicide by people with mental illness. DH, London

Selected key findings include the following:

Suicide

- One in four (*n* = 1500) people in the UK who committed suicide were in contact with mental health services in the year before death.
- The most common methods of suicide were hanging and overdose.
- Schizophrenia, substance misuse, personality disorder and violence were all more common in younger people who committed suicide.
- Most were unemployed and unmarried.
- Being from an ethnic minority and committing suicide is associated with having a severe mental illness.
- Half of the people who were homeless and had committed suicide were on enhanced CPA – approximately two-thirds were out of contact with services.

Psychiatric inpatients

- 10–16% in each region were accounted for by psychiatric inpatients.
- The most common method was self-hanging.
- One in five inpatient suicides were on increased observation levels.
- One-third to one-half of inpatient suicides were on pass at the time of death.
- Specific danger periods were in the 2 weeks following discharge and before the first follow-up appointment.
- Non-compliance and disengagement from services were common features prior to suicide.

Homicide

- A third of perpetrators had a lifetime history of mental disorder.
- The most common mental disorders were substance dependence and personality disorder.
- 2–5% of perpetrators were diagnosed with schizophrenia.
- 9–18% of perpetrators were in contact with mental health services in the year prior to the offence.
- At the final contact with this group, risk of violence was estimated to be low or non-existent in over three-quarters of cases.
- 50% of perpetrators with schizophrenia were out of contact with services.
- Over 90% of perpetrators with personality disorder had no symptoms of mental illness at the time of the offence.

The report combined its key recommendations with those from the 1999 report to produce a 12-point plan for safer services.

New recommendations from this report included:
- a broad-based suicide prevention strategy involving health and social services
- priority groups for suicide prevention to include high risk inpatients, especially those with suboptimal levels

of support at home, recently discharged patients and those who disengage from enhanced CPA
- removal of ligature points from psychiatric facilities
- patients with severe mental illness or a history of deliberate self-harm to be followed up within a week of leaving hospital.
- major overhaul of CPA systems
- improved risk management training
- special attention to:
  - patients with dual diagnosis
  - patients from ethnic minorities
  - mentally disordered offenders
- anti-stigma campaigns to emphasise the relatively low risk to strangers posed by the mentally ill.

Weblink

Department of Health – www.dh.gov.uk/PublicationsAnd Statistics/Publications/PublicationsPolicyAndGuidance

Self-harm in older people with depression

Dennis M, Wakefield P, Molloy C et al 2005 Self-harm in older people with depression. A comparison of social factors, life events and symptoms. British Journal of Psychiatry 186: 538–539

It is recognised that episodes of self-harm in the elderly frequently involve a high degree of suicidal intent. Elderly people who commit suicide and who self-harm have high rates of depression.

Method

- The objective of this study was to determine if there were any high risk factors that could predict suicide and self-harm in older adults.
- Social factors, life events, hopelessness and other symptoms of depression were compared in a group referred with depression following an episode of self-harm and those with depression but no history of self-harm.
- The following assessment tools were used:
  - Beck Depression Inventory
  - Suicide Intent Scale
  - Geriatric Depression Scale
  - Social Contact Schedule
  - Life Events and Difficulties Scale
  - Life Events and Difficulties Schedule.

Results

- Two-thirds of the people in the self-harm group scored 14 or more in the SIS, indicating significant suicidal intent.
- In 67% it was felt that the person had wished to die at the time of the self-harm episode.

- There was little difference in the groups on GDS scores, although the self-harm group was far more likely to report hopelessness and to disagree with the question 'Do you think it's wonderful to be alive now?'
- On the BDI the self-harm group were more likely to report thoughts of suicide and self-harm and rate themselves as sad but were less likely to cry.
- Those in the self-harm group were more likely to:
  - have poorly integrated social networks
  - be lonely
  - lack support from services
  - be poorly integrated into their community.
- Life events are important in the aetiology of depression but there was no excess of events in the self-harm group compared to the control group. Their role in interaction with social support seemed to be influential for the self-harm group but not alone.

Hepple J, Quinton C 1997 One hundred cases of attempted suicide in the elderly. British Journal of Psychiatry 171: 42–46

- There are high rates of completed suicide, particularly in those with persistent depression.

See also the 'General topics' section in Chapter 17 (Old age psychiatry), page 255.

Suicide by hanging

Bennewith O, Gunnell D, Kapur N et al 2005 Suicide by hanging: multi-centre study based on coroners' records in England. British Journal of Psychiatry 186: 260–261

Hanging is the most common method of suicide in England and Wales, accounting for around 2000 deaths per year.

Method

- A large case series.
- It focused on the possibilities for restricting access to means – one of the objectives of the National Suicide Prevention Strategy for England.

Results

- Studied 162 hangings over a 6-month period, across 24 districts.
- The mean ages were 40.6 years for men and 42.2 years for women.
- 6.8% were psychiatric inpatients and 3.1% were prisoners.
- Only 3.1% of inpatients died on the ward.
- 41% were in contact with psychiatric services at the time of death.
- More than half had a diagnosis of affective disorder and 13.3% had schizophrenia.

- 44.7% had previously self-harmed.
- In two-thirds of cases the person hanged themselves at home.
- 16% of people committed suicide in a public place.
- 42% were found by a family member.
- 7% of people were discovered whilst still alive.
- Rope, belts and electrical cord are the most common ligatures in the home.
- Common ligature points were beams, girders and trees.
- All prison hanging took place in cells.
- Torn sheeting was the ligature in 80% of cases.
- Prison and psychiatric ward suicides accounted for only 6%.
- There are limited opportunities for removal of ligatures (ropes, belts, cables) and ligature points (beams, girders, lofts and trees) in community settings.

National Institute for Clinical Excellence 2003 The National Suicide Prevention Strategy for England: Annual Report on Progress 2003. National Institute for Mental Health in England, Leeds

- Non-collapsible bed curtain rails were legally required to be removed by March 2002.
- Nearly half of the suicides did not involve full suspension.
- 4% (seven cases) had also taken an overdose, suggesting that if the treatment focuses on hanging alone, the episode may still be fatal.

Suicide by prisoners

Shaw J, Baker D, Hunt IM et al 2004 Suicide by prisoners. National clinical survey. British Journal of Psychiatry 184: 263–267

Suicide is linked with mental illness and substance abuse. These risk factors occur at a higher rate in prison populations.

Aims

- The first national study of self-inflicted deaths in custody in which detailed clinical data were collected on individual cases.
- The study investigated the timing and methods of prison suicide and the clinical and social antecedents of suicide by prisoners.

Method

- The Safer Custody Group examined information on all self-inflicted deaths in prisons in England and Wales in 1999 and 2000.
- Information was collected for probable suicides and verdicts of misadventure and accidental death.

- The data collection was based on methods used by the National Confidential Inquiry into Suicide and Homicide in People with Mental Illness.
- Questionnaires were completed by prison staff regarding:
  - demographic details
  - details of the suicide
  - events leading to the suicide
  - clinical history
  - history of contact with NHS mental health services
  - contact with prison healthcare and non-healthcare staff
  - assessment of risk of suicide at last contact
  - respondents' views on prevention.
- If the person had seen a psychiatrist, they were then asked to complete a similar questionnaire.

Results

- There were 172 self-inflicted deaths.
- These were:
  - suicide (58%)
  - open verdict (14%)
  - misadventure (10%)
  - accidental death (10%)
  - verdict unavailable (8%).
- Completed questionnaires were returned in 157 cases.
- The average rate of suicide per 10,000 population per year for 1999 and 2000 was 133, the age standardised rate in the general population being 9.4 per 100,000.
- The rate for women was 184 per 100,000 population per year, and for men 129 per 100,000. The age standardised rates in the general population in 1999–2001 were 4.5 per 100,000 in women and 14.5 per 100,000 in men.
- In young age groups, the male suicide rate exceeded 20 per 100,000 in the same 3-year period.
- 32% (55) of suicides occurred within 7 days of reception.
- 11% of suicides were within 24 hours of reception.
- Early suicides were most common in drug-dependent prisoners.
- The commonest method of suicide was hanging or self-strangulation (92%).
- The other methods were:
  - self-poisoning (3%)
  - cutting/stabbing (2%)
  - burning (1)
  - suffocation (1)
  - unspecified (1).
- The commonest ligatures were made from bedclothes and the most frequently used ligature point was window bars.
- 18% of suicides were under 21 years old.

- 21% were charged with or convicted of a violent offence and 49% were on remand.
- 72% had at least one psychiatric diagnosis:
  - drug dependence (27%)
  - schizophrenia (6%)
  - affective disorder (18%).
- In 57%, symptoms of mental disorder were identified at reception.
- 30% were known to have had previous contact with mental health services and 15% had no contact with healthcare staff after reception.
- 17% of suicides occurred in prison healthcare inpatient settings:
  - 81% of these had been admitted because of mental health problems, most often an act of self-harm or expression of suicidal ideation
  - 60% died within 7 days of admission to inpatient care
  - 42% were under medium or high levels of observation at the time of death
  - a further 42% had previous admission to prison healthcare centres.
- In total, 90% of this sample could be considered at high risk of suicide because of a previous history of contact with NHS mental health services, a lifetime history of mental disorder, current symptoms, current treatment or history of drug misuse, alcohol misuse or self-harm.
- However, most people who committed suicide were thought to be at low or no risk at their final contact with services.
- Only 15% were considered preventable.
- Deaths most likely to be seen as preventable were:
  - deaths of those on 'suicide watch'
  - deaths in healthcare inpatient centres
  - deaths in convicted prisoners
  - deaths in people under 21 years of age.
- Suggestions to reduce the likelihood of suicide were:
  - closer supervision
  - better risk assessment training
  - placement in a cell with another prisoner or 'listener'
  - increased staff numbers
  - better prisoner support and clinical management
  - better communication between staff.
- No mention was made of limiting access to ligature points.

Her Majesty's Chief Inspector of Prisons 1999 Suicide is everyone's concern. A thematic review. Home Office, London; Royal College of Psychiatrists 2002 Suicide in prisons (CR99). Royal College of Psychiatrists, London

- Both reports found an increase in the number of suicides in recent years.

Department of Health 2002 National Suicide Prevention Strategy for England. The Stationery Office, London

- Found that prisoners are predominantly socially disadvantaged young men.
- This is a group for whom the suicide rate has increased in society generally.

Liebling A 1994 Suicide among women prisoners. Howard Journal 33: 1–9

- Reported that the prison environment itself may increase suicide risk.

Home Office Prison Statistics 2002 England and Wales. Research, Development and Statistics Department, London

- The ratio of men to women in prison is 18:1.
- 16% are under 21 years old and 19% are on remand.

See also the 'General topics' section in Chapter 10 (Forensic psychiatry), pages 154-155, 157-160, 162.

Suicide following discharge from in-patient psychiatric care

Crawford MJ 2004 Suicide following discharge from in-patient psychiatric care. Advances in Psychiatric Treatment 10: 434–438

The rate of suicide is particularly high in the first few weeks following discharge from inpatient psychiatric care. Interventions to prevent suicide in this period have not been studied.

World Health Organization 2002 Suicide prevention in Europe: the WHO European monitoring survey on national suicide prevention programmes and strategies. WHO Regional Office for Europe, Copenhagen

- There are more than 4500 deaths per year in England and Wales attributed to suicide.

Hawton K, Arensman E, Townsend E et al 1998 Deliberate self-harm: systematic review of efficacy of psychosocial and pharmacological treatments in preventing repetition. British Medical Journal 317: 441–447

- Patients who present to services with an episode of deliberate self-harm are at higher risk of suicide.

Rutz W, Walinder J, Eberhard G et al 1989 An educational program on depressive disorders for general practitioners on Gotland: background and evaluation. Acta Psychiatrica Scandinavica 79: 19–26

- Patients attending primary care services with depression are at higher risk of suicide.

Foster T, Gillespie K, McClelland R 1997 Mental disorders and suicide in Northern Ireland. British Journal of Psychiatry 170: 447–452

- This concluded that most people who commit suicide have a psychiatric illness at the time of their death.
- One in three people who die by suicide have had recent contact with psychiatric services.
- The period following discharge from hospital is noted as the period of greatest risk.

Appleby L, Shaw J, Amos T et al 1999 Suicide within 12 months of contact with mental health services: National Clinical Survey. British Medical Journal 318: 1235–1239

- A review of 2000 suicides.
- One in four deaths by suicide occurs within the 3-month period following discharge from psychiatric hospital.

Goldacre M, Seagroatt V, Hawton K 1993 Suicide after discharge from psychiatric in-patient care. Lancet 342: 283–286

- Estimated that one in 100 patients discharged from psychiatric care will commit suicide in the following 12 months.

Lewis G, Hawton K, Jones P 1997 Strategies for preventing suicide. British Journal of Psychiatry 171: 351–354

- Deaths following discharge from psychiatric care represent 10% of all suicides in the UK.

Appleby L, Dennehy JA, Thomas CS et al 1999 Aftercare and clinical characteristics of people with mental illness who commit suicide: a case-control study. Lancet 353: 1397–1400

- The rate of suicide is at its highest immediately after discharge from hospital.
- 41% of deaths by suicide occur before the first outpatient follow-up appointment.
- Death by suicide was associated with a past history of self-harm.
- Patients who had expressed ideas of post discharge suicide were more likely to commit suicide.
- Patients whose level of care had been decreased were more likely to commit suicide.

Rossau CD, Mortensen PB 1997 Risk factors for suicide in patients with schizophrenia: nested case-control study. British Journal of Psychiatry 171: 355–359

- This study examined the relationship between hospital admission and suicide in 508 people admitted to hospital with first-episode schizophrenia.

- The rate of suicide was at its highest in the 6 months following admission to hospital. It was higher following the first hospital admission than it was for subsequent hospital admissions.
- The rate of suicide was also higher in patients discharged from the medical and surgical wards.

Goldacre M, Seagroatt V, Hawton K 1993 Suicide after discharge from psychiatric in-patient care. Lancet 342: 283–286

- This study reviewed the 134 deaths by suicide that occurred in 14,240 people discharged from hospital.
- 60% of deaths by suicide following discharge from psychiatric hospital occurred in men.
- One in three patients who died by suicide had a diagnosis of a severe mental illness.

Geddes JR, Juszczak E, O'Brien F et al 1997 Suicide in the 12 months after discharge from psychiatric in-patient care, Scotland 1968–1992. Journal of Epidemiology and Community Health 51: 430–434

- Suicide is more common in people with depression and affective disorders.
- This is also true in the post discharge period.

King EA, Baldwin DS, Sinclair JM et al 2001 The Wessex Recent In-Patient Suicide Study, 1. Case-control study of 234 recently discharged psychiatric patient suicides. British Journal of Psychiatry 178: 531–536

- This study of the clinical records of 234 patients who had committed suicide in the 12 months following discharge from psychiatric hospital found associations with a number of clinical and service-related factors.
- The risk of suicide was increased six-fold if the patient's keyworker was on holiday or due to leave the service.
- This study was retrospective and this may have influenced the association.
- There was an association between suicide and a change in consultant at the time of hospital admission.
- Patients' insight and levels of social support were also implicated.

Schwartz RC 2000 Insight and suicidality in schizophrenia: a replication study. Journal of Nervous and Mental Disorders 188: 235–237

- Suicidal ideation and the degree of suicidal intent are associated with higher levels of insight into illness.

Amador XF, Friedman JH, Kasapis C et al 1996 Suicidal behaviour in schizophrenia and its relationship to awareness of illness. American Journal of Psychiatry 153: 1185–1188

- Patients who have a greater awareness of their symptoms and their social situation are more likely to attempt suicide.

Dickinson D, Green G, Hayes C et al 2002 Social network and social support characteristics amongst individuals discharged from acute psychiatric units. Journal of Psychiatric Mental Health Nursing 9: 183–189

- There were no significant differences between levels of social support in patients admitted to psychiatric hospital and those who were not.

Simons L, Petch A, Caplan R 2002 Don't they call it seamless care? A study of acute psychiatric discharge. Scottish Executive Social Research, Edinburgh

- Patients discharged from psychiatric care may feel anxious about discharge home and the reduced social support.
- This was especially true for those discharged after their first admission.

Crawford MJ 2003 Delivering safer services: can suicide and homicide among people in contact with mental health services be predicted? Expert Review of Neurotherapeutics 3: 575–580

- Risk assessment does not allow accurate prediction of future suicide.

Crawford MJ, DeJonge E, Freeman GK et al 2004 Providing continuity of care for people with severe mental illness: a narrative review. Social Psychiatry and Psychiatric Epidemiology 39: 265–272

- The beneficial effects of discharge interventions, such as discharge preparation groups, are not known.
- Impact on suicide post discharge is also not known.

See also the 'General topics' section in Chapter 30 (Treatment settings), page 429.

Suicide in custody

Fruehwald S, Matschnig T, Koenig F, Bauer P, Frottier P 2004 Suicide in custody. A case-control study. British Journal of Psychiatry 185: 494–498

It has been established in international studies that suicide rates in prisons exceed the rates of suicide in the general population.

Aims

- A case-controlled study investigating risk factors for suicide in custody.

- This study matched those who had completed suicide and those who had survived custody over a 25-year period, across Austria.
- Each suicide in the 29 Austrian correctional institutions over 25 years was matched with two cases.
- Matched cases were controlled for institution, gender, nationality, age, custodial sentence and time of admission.
- Comparisons were made between:
  - psychiatric characteristics
  - previous suicidal behaviour
  - criminal history.
- Indicators of social integration were compared.

Results

- The most important predictors for suicide in custody were:
  - a history of suicidality (threats and attempts)
  - the presence of a psychiatric diagnosis
  - treatment with psychotropic medication
  - a highly violent index offence
  - single cell accommodation.

Discussion

- Suicidal behaviour should be taken as seriously in custodial institutions as in other settings.

Studies exploring the risk factors for suicide in custody are detailed in Table 29.1.

See also the 'General topics' section in Chapter 10 (Forensic psychiatry), pages 154-155, 157-160, 162.

Policy and Legislation

National suicide prevention strategy for England

Department of Health 2002 National suicide prevention strategy for England. DH, London. Online. Available: www.dh.gov.uk/assetRoot/04/01/95/48/04019548.pdf [†]

This strategy aims to support the Saving Lives: Our Healthier Nation target of reducing the death rate from suicide by at least 20% by 2010. It is not a one-off document but an ongoing coordinated set of activities which will evolve over several years.

Background

- Around 5000 people commit suicide in England every year. This includes figures for undetermined injury death verdicts.

Table 29.1 Risk factors for suicide in custody

Risk factor	Study
Long sentences after highly violent crime	DuRand C, Burtka GJ, Federman EJ et al 1995 A quarter century of suicide in a major urban jail: implications for community psychiatry. American Journal of Psychiatry 152: 1077–1080
Overcrowding	Marcus P, Alcabes P 1993 Characteristics of suicides by inmates in an urban jail. Hospital and Community Psychiatry 44: 256–261
Isolation	Frottier P, Fruhwald S, Ritter K et al 2001 Deprivation versus importation: ein Erlarungsmodell fur die Zunahme von Suiziden in Halfanstalten. Fortschritte der Neurologie Psychiatrie 69: 90–96
Psychiatric disorder	Marcus P, Alcabes P 1993 Characteristics of suicides by inmates in an urban jail. Hospital and Community Psychiatry 44: 256–261 Bogue J, Power K 1995 Suicide I: Scottish prisons, 1976–1993. Journal of Forensic Psychiatry 6: 527–540 Joukamaa M 1997 Prison suicide in Finland, 1969–1992. Forensic Science International 89: 167–174
Alcohol and drug misuse	Backett SA 1997 Suicide in Scottish prisons. British Journal of Psychiatry 151: 18–221 Dooley E 1990 Prison suicide in England and Wales. 1972–87. British Journal of Psychiatry 156: 40–45

- In the last two decades suicide rates have fallen in older men and in women, but have risen in younger men.
- The majority of suicides now occur in young adult males.
- Suicide is the most common cause of death in men under 35 years.

Goal 1: To reduce risk in high risk groups

Actions to be taken
- Local mental health services will be supported in implementing 12 points to a safer service; these aim to improve clinical risk management.
- A national collaborative is being established for the monitoring of non-fatal deliberate self-harm.
- A pilot project targeting mental health promotion in young men will be established and evaluated from national roll-out.

Goal 2: To promote mental well-being in the wider population

Actions to be taken
- A cross-government network will be developed to address a range of social issues that impact on people with mental health problems (e.g. unemployment and housing).
- The suicide prevention programme will link closely with the NIMHE substance misuse programme to:

  - improve the clinical management of alcohol and drug misuse among young men who carry out deliberate self-harm
  - make available training in suicide risk assessment for substance misuse services.

Goal 3: To reduce the availability and lethality of suicide methods

Actions to be taken
- NIMHE will identify additional steps that can be taken to promote safer prescribing of antidepressants and analgesics.
- NIMHE will help local services identify their suicide 'hotspots' (e.g. railways, bridges) and take steps to improve safety at these.

Goal 4: To improve the reporting of suicidal behaviour in the media

Actions to be taken
- A media action plan is being developed as part of the mental health promotion campaign, Mind Out for Mental Health, which will include:
  - incorporating guidance on the representation of suicide into workshops held with students at journalism schools and round table discussion sessions with leaders in mental health and senior journalists

- a series of roadshows at which frontline journalists can discuss responsible reporting
- a feature on suicide in media journals – for example, Press Gazette, Media Week, British Journalism Review.

Goal 5: To promote research on suicide and suicide prevention

Actions to be taken

- A national collaborative group will oversee a programme of research to support the strategy, including research on ligatures used in hanging and suicides using firearms.
- Current evidence on suicide prevention will be made available to local services through Niche's website and development centres.

Goal 6: To improve monitoring of progress towards the Saving Lives: Our Healthier Nation target for reducing suicide

Actions to be taken

- A new strategy group of experts and other key stakeholders will be established.
- The new strategy group will regularly monitor suicides by age and gender, by people under mental health care, by different methods and by social class.

See also the 'Policy and legislation' section in Chapter 22 (Policy and legislation), page 322.

Saving lives

Department of Health 1999 Saving lives: our healthier nation. White Paper. The Stationery Office, London. Online. Available: www.archive.official-documents.co.uk/document/cm43/4386/4386.htm

An action plan to tackle poor health, with the aim of addressing the health of everyone. The health of the worst off is a particular priority.

The main causes of mortality are the focus, i.e.:
- cancer
- coronary heart disease and stroke
- accidents
- mental illness.

Targets have been set in these priority areas. By 2010 the targets are to reduce the death rate from:
- cancer in people under 75 years by at least a fifth
- coronary heart disease and stroke in people under 75 years by at least two-fifths
- accidents by at least a fifth and serious injury by at least a tenth
- suicide and undetermined injury by at least a fifth.

It is estimated that 300,000 early deaths will be prevented should these targets be met.

Strategies to meet these targets include:
- more money
- addressing smoking
- new healthy citizens programmes, including:
  - NHS Direct
  - health skills programmes
  - expert patient programmes
- partnership of people, communities and government
- health authorities having increased responsibility for the health of the local population
- primary care to have increased responsibilities for public health.

Mental health

Target: to reduce the death rate from suicide and undetermined death by at least a fifth by 2010, saving up to 4000 lives in total.

Suicide is proposed as a proxy measure for the mental health priority area. It is used as it is reliable, measurable and there were no morbidity measures that could be used in its place. It is suggested that promotion of good mental health will lead to a reduction in the number of suicides.

Mental health problems are noted to include depression, anxiety, schizophrenia, bipolar affective disorder, dementia and antisocial personality disorder. The last is noted to contribute to crime and aggression.

Strategies to improve mental health

- National public education campaigns to promote good mental health.
- Better social support, information and education for people who are unemployed, care for relatives with dementia who are isolated or depressed, etc.

Strategies to reduce suicide

- Reduced access to methods of suicide (e.g. smaller packs of paracetamol).
- NHS Direct as a contact for those in mental distress.
- Good assessment and follow-up of people who attempt suicide.
- Development and use of good practice guidelines for the care of people with suicidal ideation in primary and secondary care.
- Training in detection and management of depression and suicidal risk.
- Improved services for those at increased risk of suicide – for example, people with severe mental illness and people in high-risk professions.
- Mental health promotion in schools, workplaces and prisons.
- Responsible reporting of suicide by the media.

- Continued audit of suicide via the National Confidential Inquiry into Suicide and Homicide.
- Anticipation of measures set out in the National Service Framework for Mental Health.

See also the 'Policy and legislation' section in Chapter 22 (Policy and legislation), page 322.

Assessment Tools and Rating Scales

Suicide Intent Scale (SIS)

> Beck A, Schuyler D & Herman J 1974 Development of suicidal intent scales. In: Beck A, Resnik H, Lettieri DJ (eds) The prediction of suicide. Charles, Bowie, MD, pp 45–56

- 15-item questionnaire designed to assess the severity of suicidal intention associated with an episode of self-harm.
- Each item is scored 0–2, giving a score of 0–30.
- The first eight items are concerned with objective 'circumstances' and the remaining seven items are 'self-report' of the patient's feelings and thoughts at the time of the act.

Guidelines

Self-harm: The short-term physical and psychological management and secondary prevention of self-harm in primary and secondary care. NICE Clinical Guideline 16*

Primary care

The management of self-harm in primary care
- Assess risk of further self-harm (consider depression, hopelessness and suicidal intent). [C]
- Inform other relevant staff and organisations of the outcome of this assessment. [C]

When urgent referral to an emergency department is not necessary
- Base your decision on risk and needs assessment, including [C]:
  - social and psychological aspects of the episode of self-harm
  - mental health and social needs
  - hopelessness
  - suicidal intent.

Emergency departments: self-harm

The treatment and management of self-harm in emergency departments includes the following:
Triage
- Consider using a combined physical and mental health triage scale such as the Australian Mental Health Triage Scale. [C]
- Offer psychosocial assessment at triage to determine [C]:
  - mental capacity
  - willingness to remain for further psychosocial assessment
  - distress levels
  - presence of mental illness.

People waiting for physical treatments
- Provide verbal and written information about the care process in a language the service user understands. [C]

People who wish to leave before assessment and/or treatment
- If a person wishes to leave before a psychosocial assessment, assess for mental capacity/mental illness and record assessment in the notes. [C]
- Pass assessment to the service user's GP and to the relevant mental health services as soon as possible, to enable rapid follow-up. [C]
- If mental capacity is diminished and/or the person has a significant mental illness, refer for urgent mental health assessment and prevent the person from leaving. [C]

Emergency departments: repeated self-harm

Support and advice for people who repeatedly self-harm include the following:
Advice for people who repeatedly self-poison
- Do not offer harm minimisation advice regarding self-poisoning – there are no safe limits. [GPP]
- Consider discussing the risks of self-poisoning with service users (and carers, where appropriate) who are likely to use this method of self-harm again. [GPP]

Advice for people who repeatedly self-injure
- Consider giving advice and instructions on [GPP]:
  - self-management of superficial injuries, including providing tissue adhesive
  - harm minimisation issues and techniques
  - appropriate alternative coping strategies
  - dealing with scar tissue.
- Discuss with a mental health worker which service users should be offered the advice above (voluntary organisations may have suitable materials). [GPP]

Psychosocial assessment: specialist mental health professionals

- Record assessment in the service user's notes. [C]
Assessment of needs
- Offer needs assessment to all people who self-harm. [C]
- Include in the assessment [C]:

- social, psychological and motivational factors specific to the act of self-harm
- current intent
- hopelessness
- mental health and social needs assessment.

Assessment of risk

- Assess all people at risk of self-harm. [C]
- Include in the assessment identification of [C]:
  - the main clinical and demographic features known to be associated with the risk of further self-harm and/or suicide
  - the key psychological characteristic associated with risk (depression, hopelessness or continuing suicidal intent).
- Only use standardised risk assessment scales to identify service users of supposedly low risk who are not then offered services. [C]

Referral, admission and discharge following psychosocial assessment

General considerations

- Base decisions about referral, discharge and admission on comprehensive assessment, including needs and risk. [C]

Referral

- Do not refer only on the basis that the patient has self-harmed. [C]

Admission

- Consider offering an intensive therapeutic intervention combined with outreach to people who have self-harmed and are deemed to be at risk of repetition [C]:
  - intensive intervention should allow greater access to a therapist, home treatment when necessary and telephone contact; outreach should include following up the service user when an appointment has been missed
  - continue therapeutic intervention plus outreach for at least 3 months.
- Consider dialectical behaviour therapy for people with borderline personality disorder [C]:
  - do not, however, ignore other psychological treatments for people with this diagnosis that are outside the scope of this guideline.

Discharge

- Decide to discharge a person without follow-up based on a combined assessment of needs and risk. [C]

Special issues for children and young people

Admission

- All children and young people should normally be admitted into a paediatric ward under the overall care of a paediatrician and assessed fully the following day. [C]
- Alternative placements may be needed, depending on [C]:
  - age
  - circumstances of the child and their family
  - time of presentation
  - child protection issues
  - physical and mental health of the child or young person.
- If the young person is 14 years or older, consider an adolescent paediatric ward. [C]
- Occasionally, an adolescent psychiatric ward may be needed. [C]
- After admission, the paediatric team should obtain consent for mental health assessment from the child or young person's parent, guardian or legally responsible adult. [C]
- During admission, the Child and Adolescent Mental Health services team should:
  - provide consultation for the young person, their family, the paediatric team, social services, and education staff [C]
  - undertake assessment, addressing the needs and risk for the child (similar to adults), the family, the social situation of the family and the young person, and child protection issues. [GPP]
- Assessors should be specifically trained and supervised to work with self-harm in this age group. [C]

Other considerations

- For young people who have self-harmed several times, consider offering developmental group psychotherapy with other young people. This should include at least six sessions but can be extended by mutual agreement. [B]

B and C indicate grades of recommendation; GPP indicates a good practice point (see Appendix II for full details). * Reproduced with permission from the National Institute for Health and Clinical Excellence, London.

See also the 'Guidelines' section in Chapter 2 (Affective disorders), page 45.

Treatment settings

General Topics

Assertive community treatment for people with severe mental disorders

Marshall M, Lockwood A 1998 Assertive community treatment for people with severe mental disorders **(Cochrane Review)**. In: The Cochrane Library, Issue 2. CD001089. Update Software, Oxford

- On comparing ACT with standard community care it was found that those receiving ACT were more likely to remain in contact with services, were less likely to be admitted to hospital and spend less time in hospital.
- There were no differences in mental state or social functioning.
- When compared with hospital-based rehabilitation services, those receiving ACT were no more likely to remain in contact with services, were significantly less likely to be readmitted to hospital and spend less time there.
- Those allocated to ACT were significantly more likely to be living independently, but there were no other significant differences in clinical or social outcome.
- In comparison with case management, people allocated to ACT consistently spent fewer days in hospital.
- Data were insufficient to draw other conclusions.

Definition

Assertive community treatment (ACT) was developed in the early 1970s as a response to the closing down of psychiatric hospitals. ACT is a team-based approach aimed at keeping ill people in contact with services, reducing hospital admissions and improving outcome, especially social functioning and quality of life.

Assertive community treatment in UK practice

Kent A, Burns T 2005 Assertive community treatment in UK practice. Revisiting... Setting up an assertive community treatment team. Advances in Psychiatric Treatment 11: 388–397

This article describes the historical background of assertive community treatment. It also discusses the lack of evidence for this treatment in the general psychiatry population in the UK which is in contrast with research performed in America.

There has been no convincing evidence that this treatment model is better than standard community mental health teams with regard to clinical symptoms, social function or quality of life.

Assertive community treatment requires a dedicated team that addresses and provides for the needs of all patients and that is accessible 24 hours a day. The treatment aims to improve daily living skills, including social and vocational skills. Patients are actively and assertively engaged in treatment and follow-up. Treatment is provided in the community setting. Each patient has an adaptable and individualised care plan. Staff have small case loads (no more than 15 patients) and are involved with patients via a collaborating keyworker system. The team should be able to offer a broad mix of therapies over and above those of a standard community mental health team. These could include psychological therapies, family interventions, motivational interviewing and vocational rehabilitation.

> Stein LI, Test MA 1980 Alternative to mental hospital treatment. III. Social cost. Archives of General Psychiatry 37: 400–405

- An early RCT of training in community living.
- Patients who received training in community living had significantly lower readmission rates than patients who received standard care (6% versus 58%, respectively).
- Patients who received training in community living were more likely to live independently in the community, gain employment and have better social function.
- Training in community living was also beneficial in terms of clinical state, adherence to treatment and quality of life.
- There was no increased carer burden.

> Weisbrod BA, Test MA, Stein LI 1980 Alternative to mental hospital treatment. II. Economic benefit–cost analysis. Archives of General Psychiatry 37: 400–405

- Concluded that training in community living was no more expensive than treatment as usual due to reduced time spent in hospital.
- These gains were lost when funding was withdrawn after the study period.

> Tyrer P, Hassiotis A, Ukoumunne O et al 1999 Intensive case management for psychotic patients with borderline intelligence. Lancet 354: 999–1000

- This study found that assertive community treatment was beneficial in the treatment of adults with learning disability in the UK.

> Burns T, Creed F, Fahy T et al 1999 Intensive versus standard case management for severe psychotic illness: a randomised trial. Lancet 353: 2185–2189

- This randomised controlled trial (the largest UK RCT) compared assertive community treatment and standard care.
- The respective case loads were 12 and 32.
- There were no significant differences between the two treatments.

Assessing the value of assertive outreach

> Weaver T, Tyrer P, Ritchie J 2003 Assessing the value of assertive outreach. Qualitative study of process and outcome generation in the UK700 trial. British Journal of Psychiatry 183: 437–445

The UK700 case management trial assessed whether enhanced outcomes could be achieved under CPA by reducing caseload size. Intensive and standard case management practised individual casework, employed assertive outreach with comparable frequency and performed similarly in the outpatient management of emergencies and inpatient discharge. Intensive case management was advantaged in managing some non-compliance and undertaking casework that prevented psychiatric emergencies.

> Tyrer P 2000 Are small case-loads beautiful in severe mental illness? British Journal of Psychiatry 177: 386–387

- The impact of assertive outreach on outcomes remains unclear.

Definition

Intensive case management ratio 1:10–15.

Standard case management ratio 1:30–35.

Care programme approach (CPA)

Introduced in 1991 to provide a framework for community care for people with a serious mental disorder. It is supposed to ensure that statutory health and social services fulfil their duty to assess and provide appropriate services to the individual.

Assessment should inform the creation of a care plan in collaboration with the patient and/or carers. Appointment of a keyworker (often a CPN or social worker) to be patient's first point of contact then follows. The care plan coordinator arranges regular reviews for the patient and issues invitations to all involved in the care of the patient.

The CPA facilitates a multidisciplinary approach that is able to change over time as the patient's needs evolve. It should prevent the patient being lost to follow-up or 'falling through the cracks' between services. It is flexible enough to incorporate MHA statutory aftercare or forensic supervision measures. It specifically involves patients and carers and enables a swift response to any deterioration in patient health.

In England it is routine practice for anyone with a diagnosis regarded as being a serious mental illness to be included in the CPA. In Scotland it is less often employed and tends to be reserved for those with multiple, complex needs, 'revolving door' admission patterns or risky behaviour.

Various recommendations and pieces of legislation have touched on the role of CPA over the past 15 years:
- In 1996, *Building Bridges* (DH) directed that the CPA should apply to all patients accepted by specialist mental health services.

- Further DH guidance in 1999 specified two distinct levels of CPA: standard and enhanced. The enhanced level was envisaged to be reserved for those requiring input from multiple agencies, including patients in the criminal justice system.
- This guidance demanded that crisis plans should be included in the care plan of those with complex CPAs.
- *The NHS Plan* implementation programme from 1999 directed that all patients on CPA have written care plans. The National Service Framework for Mental Health reinforced this (also in 1999).
- *Safety First* (2001) recommended that all patients with schizophrenia should have enhanced CPA as a matter of routine.

Case management for people with severe mental disorders

Marshall M, Gray A, Lockwood A, Green R 1998 Case management for people with severe mental disorders **(Cochrane Review)**. In: The Cochrane Library, Issue 2. CD000050. Update Software, Oxford

- Case management when compared with standard community care increased the numbers remaining in contact with services – one extra person remains in contact for every 15 people who receive case management.
- It also approximately doubled the numbers admitted to psychiatric hospital.
- One study found a positive result with regard to compliance, but no significant advantages on any psychiatric or social outcome variables – mental state, social functioning or quality of life.
- Insufficient data were available to allow cost comparisons.

Characteristics of teams, staff and patients: associations with outcomes of patients in assertive outreach

Priebe S, White I, Watts J et al 2004 Characteristics of teams, staff and patients: associations with outcomes of patients in assertive outreach. British Journal of Psychiatry 185: 306–311

Assertive outreach teams have been introduced in most parts of England to assist with the management of people with severe mental illness. The Pan-London Assertive Outreach Study (PLOA) investigated the routine practice of such teams in terms of patient factors (demographics and patient characteristics) and service organisation (including staff burnout and satisfaction).

Method

- This study examined baseline features and outcomes at 9-month follow-up.
- It aimed to identify predictors of voluntary and compulsory admissions to hospital from assertive outreach services in the UK.
- 24 teams were identified.
- There were 391 existing patients and 189 new patients.
- Rates of admission to hospital were obtained from 487 patients.
- Variables identified as potential predictors covered a wide range of features of the teams and the patients.
- 11 patient characteristics were considered:
  - age
  - gender
  - ethnicity
  - living status
  - total number of previous hospital admissions (0, 1–3, 4–9, 10+)
  - hospitalisation in the 2 years prior to interview
  - alcohol or drug misuse in the past 2 years
  - whether or not the patient had contact with services other than assertive outreach.
- Staff were interviewed for signs of burnout and work satisfaction.
- The outcomes assessed at 9 months were:
  - whether or not patients had been admitted to hospital
  - whether or not they had been admitted voluntarily within the follow-up period.

Results

- Of nine team characteristics, four were significantly associated with outcome and predicted a higher risk of admission:
  - having more clinical staff
  - having more psychiatrist input
  - working out of hours
  - working at weekends.
- In the multivariate adjusted model, only working weekends remained a significant predictor of higher admission rates.
- When adjusted for other factors, working out of hours actually resulted in lower rates of admission.
- Higher scores of staff on personal accomplishment predicted lower admission rates in both univariate and multivariate analysis. This in turn correlated significantly with low depersonalisation.
- Three patient characteristics remained significant after multivariate analysis:
  - patients with more past admissions = increase risk for admission
  - more admissions in the previous 2 years = increased risk for admission

- − contact with other services = protective against admission.
- Compulsory admissions were more likely if there had been previous compulsory admissions and a history of violence and arrests in the past 2 years.

Gandhi N, Tyrer P, Evans K et al 2001 A randomised controlled trial of community-orientated and hospital-orientated care for discharged psychiatric patients: influence of personality disorder on police contacts. Journal of Personality Disorders 15: 94–102

- Suggested such services can reduce contacts with the police but do not address the overall effectiveness of assertive outreach teams.
- The most important outcome from this study is thought to be that certain characteristics of the team, staff and patients were all found to be predictive of outcome.
- The team characteristic of weekend working was a strong predictor of admission, particularly compulsory admission.
- Other team variables often regarded as relevant in the assertive outreach literature, such as multidisciplinary working, high percentage of contacts in the community and integration of health and social care, do not predict outcome when the influence of other factors is controlled for.
- With regard to staff characteristics, job satisfaction did not have an impact on outcome.
- Staff burnout resulted in a higher incidence of admission to hospital, both voluntary and compulsory.
- Previous patient admissions in the past 2 years and physical violence in the past 2 years, as well as no contact with other services, resulted in an increased rate of admission to hospital.
- Patients identified as most in need of such services continue to have the poorest outcomes.
- Contact with other services provided a powerful protective factor, perhaps reflecting a higher level of engagement, a greater willingness to accept support and better skills to seek and receive it.
- The rate for both voluntary and compulsory admissions is reduced by 50% by this additional contact, indicating the importance of multiagency work.

Community mental health teams for people with severe mental illnesses and disordered personality

Tyrer P, Coid, S, Simmonds, S et al 1998 Community mental health teams (CMHTs) for people with severe mental illnesses and disordered personality **(Cochrane Review)**. In: The Cochrane Library, Issue 4. CD000270. Update Software, Oxford

- Patients treated by CMHTs may have lower rates of death by suicide or in suspicious circumstances.
- CMHT management was associated with lower rates of patient dissatisfaction and lower dropout rates.
- There were no clear differences between CMHT management and non-team standard care with regard to:
  - − admission rates
  - − overall clinical outcomes
  - − length of inpatient stay.

See also the 'General topics' section in Chapter 19 (Personality disorders), page 287.

Compulsory community and involuntary outpatient treatment

Kisely S, Campbell LA, Preston N 2005 Compulsory community and involuntary outpatient treatment for people with severe mental disorders **(Cochrane Review)**. In: The Cochrane Library, Issue 3. CD004408. Update Software, Oxford

- Compared with standard care for people with severe mental illness there was little evidence that compulsory treatment was better in terms of health service use, social functioning, mental state, quality of life or satisfaction with care.
- In terms of numbers needed to treat, it would take 85 outpatient orders to prevent one readmission, 27 to prevent one episode of homelessness and 238 to prevent one arrest.
- Compulsory community treatment may not be an effective alternative to standard care.

Crisis intervention for people with severe mental illnesses

Joy CB, Adams CE, Rice K 2004 Crisis intervention for people with severe mental illnesses **(Cochrane Review)**. In: The Cochrane Library, Issue 4. CD001087. Update Software, Oxford

- No trials investigated purely crisis intervention, rather a form of home care for acutely ill people which included elements of crisis intervention.
- Just under half of the crisis/home care group were unable to avoid hospital admission during the treatment period, but perhaps this may help to avoid repeat admissions.
- Crisis/home care reduces the number of people leaving the study early, reduces family burden and is a more satisfactory form of care for patients and families.
- There were no differences in death or mental state outcomes.
- Further evaluative studies are needed.

Day hospital versus admission for acute psychiatric disorders

Marshall M, Crowther R, Almaraz-Serrano A et al 2003 Day hospital versus admission for acute psychiatric disorders **(Cochrane Review)**. In: The Cochrane Library, Issue 1. CD004026. Update Software, Oxford

- Nine RCTs were identified, with individual patient data available from four trials involving 594 people.
- Caring for people in acute day hospitals can achieve substantial reductions in the number of people needing inpatient care, whilst improving patient outcome.
- Combined data suggested that day hospital treatment was feasible for 23% of those currently admitted to inpatient care.
- Compared with controls, people randomised to day hospital care spent significantly more days in day hospital care and significantly fewer days in inpatient care.
- There was no difference in readmission rates between day hospital patients and controls.
- Four of five trials found that day hospital care was cheaper, with cost reductions ranging from 20.9 to 36.9%.

Day hospital versus outpatient care for psychiatric disorders

Marshall M, Crowther R, Almaraz-Serano AM, Tyrer P 2001 Day hospital versus out-patient care for psychiatric disorders **(Cochrane Review)**. In: The Cochrane Library, Issue 2. CD003240. Update Software, Oxford

- One trial suggested that day treatment programmes were better than continuing outpatient care in terms of improving psychiatric symptoms.
- Day care centres may be more expensive than outpatient care.
- One trial suggested that day hospital care was better at keeping patients engaged when compared with outpatient care.
- In general, there were insufficient data regarding clinical or social outcome variables or on costs.

Definition

Day care centres offer structured support to patients with long-term severe mental disorders (mainly schizophrenia) who would otherwise be treated in the outpatient clinic.

Day treatment programmes offer intense treatment for patients who have failed to respond to outpatient care (usually patients with affective disorders).

Transitional day hospitals offer time-limited care to patients who have just been discharged from inpatient care.

Evaluation of a partial hospitalisation programme

Tacchi MJ, Suresh J, Scott J 2004 Evaluation of a partial hospitalisation programme: good news and bad. Psychiatric Bulletin 28: 244–247

Aims

To evaluate an English partial hospitalisation programme during its first 12 months of function with regard to:
- admission rates
- lengths of inpatient stay
- number of repeat admissions.

Main features of the service

- Deprived area with a population of 150,000.
- Core staff: two occupational therapists, two nurses and sessional medical input from existing resources.
- Referrals were from inpatient units, mental health services and psychiatrists.
- Total case load at any one time was 50 but the attendance varied from between 1 hour every 2 weeks to every day.

Aims of the service

- Alternative to inpatient care.
- Transition from hospital to the community.
- Treatment and rehabilitation for those with severe and enduring mental illness and a history of frequent hospital admission, living in the community.

Method

- Data for each referral were examined as well as the effects on the admission unit.
- Pre-coded proforma data were recorded for each referral over the first year of operation.
- Information included:
  - demographics
  - past psychiatric history
  - source and reason for referral
  - frequency of attendance at the PHP or hospital during the course of treatment under the programme
  - patient views using the Client Satisfaction Questionnaire (CSQ)
  - information from the Patient Information Management System (PIMS) to explore the impact of the PHP on the admission unit.

Results

- There were 271 referrals in the first year of operation.
- Nearly three-quarters were from the community, the remainder coming from the hospital:
  - 63% as an alternative to admission
  - 26% were part of early discharge planning
  - 21% were for additional community support.
- Mean referral rate was 23.2 per month.
- Over the year the request for urgent assessment went from 29 to 55%.
- Characteristics of programme attenders:
  - mean age, 42 years
  - mean age at onset of mental disorder, 26 years
  - 45% lived alone
  - 58% were female
  - less than 25% were employed
  - 12% had no prior contact with mental health services
  - 52% had at least one admission in the year prior to referral, almost a quarter under the Mental Health Act
  - 33% had affective disorders
  - 31% had schizophrenia or other psychoses
  - 17% had other Axis I disorders
  - 13% had dual diagnosis
  - 55 had a primary diagnosis of personality disorder.
- 16% required admission to hospital during the period despite being engaged with the programme.

Impact on the inpatient unit

- There were reductions in:
  - median bed occupancy
  - mean bed occupancy rate per month – by 18%
  - the mean number of admissions per month
  - the median length of stay per patient.

Discussion

- A non-blinded, non-randomised trial.
- No causal relationship between the PHP and reduced admission rates could be identified.
- The service does provide a less restrictive alternative.
- 30 individuals who were referred to the programme eventually required admission to hospital; this suggests that the programme may only result in a delay, not prevention of admission.

Department of Health 1999 The National Service Framework for Mental Health. The Stationery Office, London

- Recommend the development of new treatment settings as an alternative to hospital inpatient stays.

Harrison J, Poynton A, Marshall J et al 1999 Open all hours, extending the role of the psychiatric day hospital. Psychiatric Bulletin 23 400–404

- Extended day hospital facilities and home treatment services were beneficial alternatives to inpatient care.

Creed F, Black D, Anthony P et al 1990 Randomised controlled trial of day patient versus inpatient psychiatric treatment. British Medical Journal 300: 1033–1037

- A RCT of day hospital versus inpatient care.
- 40% of people presenting for admission could be diverted to day care without any detrimental effect on outcomes.

Creed F, Mbaya P, Lancashire S et al 1997 Cost effectiveness of day and in patient psychiatric treatment. British Medical Journal 314: 1382–1385

- Day hospitalisation was cheaper than inpatient care.

Intensive case management for psychotic patients with borderline intelligence

Tyrer P, Hassiotis A, Ukoumunne O et al 1999 Intensive case management for psychotic patients with borderline intelligence. Lancet 354: 999–1000

Method

- The UK700 case management trial.
- Compared intensive case management with standard case management.
- 708 patients were followed over a 2-year period.
- Intensive and standard case management are associated with caseloads of 10–15 and 25–35 per worker, respectively.
- The principal outcome measure was days spent in hospital with psychiatric disorders over 2 years.
- Intellectual function was also assessed and the results of the 104 patients with borderline learning disability were reviewed.

Results

- Intensive case management showed no advantages over standard case management for the primary outcome.
- In patients with borderline learning disability, intensive case management was associated with a reduction (by more than half) in subsequent time spent in hospital.
- Patients with borderline learning disabilities and psychosis had significant reductions in bed use and admissions with intensive case management.

Discussion

- The authors felt that the lack of difference between intensive and standard case management in adults with psychosis reflects the improvements in the delivery of the former.

- This was not the case for adults with borderline learning disabilities and psychosis who are in need of more intensive management.

Length of hospitalisation

Johnstone P, Zolese G 1999 Length of hospitalisation for people with severe mental illness **(Cochrane Review)**. In: The Cochrane Library, Issue 2. CD000384. Update Software, Oxford

- Five RCTs were included to answer the question 'Are short or long stays more effective?'
- Patients admitted for planned short stay had no more readmissions, no more losses to follow-up and were more likely to be discharged on time than people who had long stays or received standard care.
- Short-stay patients were no more likely to leave hospital early.
- Short-stay patients were more likely to be in employment.
- Further study is required to look at mental, social and family outcomes, including user satisfaction, deaths, violence, criminal behaviour and costs.

Nidotherapy

Tyrer P, Bajaj P 2005 Nidotherapy: making the environment do the therapeutic work. Advances in Psychiatric Treatment 11: 232–238

Nidotherapy describes a treatment where the environment is adjusted to suit the needs of an individual with chronic psychiatric illness.

The components of nidotherapy are:
- Collateral collocation: The patient's experience of their environment and how that impacts on their functioning is considered. This is helpful in recognising differences in priorities between patients and staff. A detailed list of resulting action points is then created.
- Formulation of realistic environmental targets: Targets that take into account each individual's environmental function.
- Improvement of social function: This primary outcome is achieved indirectly – via environmental changes such as good financial management, enabling good social relationships, better use of recreational time, etc.
- Personal adaptation and control: Using the target list that has been created in collaboration with the patient as a model for treatment gives the patient control of treatment.
- Wider environmental integration and arbitrage: Can include the use of an arbiter between the patient and the

clinical team. An arbiter can be any person respected by both the patient and the clinical team. They are involved at the time when a list of action points is created and their role is in negotiating the different priorities recognised by the patient and the clinical team.

The process of therapy involves identifying the boundaries of therapy, full environmental analysis, implementation of a common nidopathway, monitoring of progress and the resetting of the nidopathway and completion. It is generally given over 10 sessions. Patients often have chronic illness and may have resisted previous attempts at environmental manipulation. The relative gains may be small. Patients can welcome their own priorities and aims being taken seriously, enabling a more collaborative approach.

Nidotherapy can range from purely structural environmental change (a new boiler) to changes to improve social aspects of a patient's life (joining clubs) to longer term goals such as a move to new accommodation. It can exist alongside other treatments.

The nidotherapist can be from any discipline but occupational therapists and music therapists are described as having been effective in this role.

It can be helpful for the patient to have a nidotherapist that is separate from the clinical team and therefore viewed as neutral.

The process of manualisation of this therapy is underway.

Prompts to encourage outpatient attendance for people with serious mental illness

Reda S, Makhoul S 2001 Prompts to encourage outpatient attendance for people with serious mental illness **(Cochrane Review)**. In: The Cochrane Library, Issue 2. CD002085. Update Software, Oxford

- There is evidence that a single reminder to attend the clinic, near to the appointment time, leads to improvements in rates of outpatient attendance.
- A basic letter sent 24 hours prior to the appointment may be better than a telephone prompt in improving attendance rates and can lead to cost savings.
- Further investigation is required.

Psychosocial treatment programmes for people with both severe mental illness and substance misuse

Jeffery DP, Ley A, McLaren S, Siegfried N 2000 Psychosocial treatment programmes for people with both severe mental illness and substance misuse **(Cochrane Review)**. In: The Cochrane Library, Issue 2. CD001088. Update Software, Oxford

- Six studies were identified, but clinically important outcomes such as relapse of severe mental illness, violence to others, patient or carer satisfaction, social functioning and employment were not reported.
- There is no clear evidence supporting an advantage of any type of substance misuse programme for those with serious mental illness over the value of standard care.

See also the 'Treatment – Psychological therapies' section in Chapter 1 (Addictions psychiatry), page 19.

Specialised care for early psychosis

Garety PA, Craig TKJ, Dunn G et al 2006 Specialised care for early psychosis: symptoms, social functioning and patient satisfaction. A randomised controlled trial. British Journal of Psychiatry 188: 37–45

Background

- There are few RCTs of early intervention and only preliminary data have been reported.
- This trial set out to evaluate the effectiveness of a specialist service for early psychosis (the Lambeth Early Onset service) with regard to user satisfaction and clinical and social outcomes over an 18-month period.
- The service comprised an extended hours service using medication, vocational input and psychological therapy (cognitive behavioural and family interventions).
- The aims of the service were to enable the patient to retain or recover function in the educational or employment setting, resume leisure activities and maintain or establish social supports. A family and carers group and a social activity programme were also available.
- An earlier study has shown that the early onset service was more effective than treatment as usual for rehospitalisation over 18 months and rates of contact with services.

Method

- Patients presenting on the first or second occasion (if on the previous occasion had not engaged with services) were randomised to the early onset team or to treatment as usual.
- Patients with non-affective psychosis and schizoaffective and delusional disorders were included.
- Outcomes included symptoms, adherence to treatment, social function, patient satisfaction and quality of life.

Results

- The early onset service was as effective as treatment as usual in terms of improvements in symptoms.
- The early onset service had significant beneficial effects on outcomes of social and vocational (educational or employment-based) functioning, patient satisfaction, quality of life and adherence to treatment.

Conclusion

- This study is one of the first UK-based RCTs reporting on the effects of early intervention services and would support UK policy in recommending the provision of care via early onset services.

Supported accommodation for people with severe mental illness

Macpherson R, Shepherd G, Edwards T 2004 Supported accommodation for people with severe mental illness: a review. Advances in Psychiatric Treatment 10: 180–188

Supported accommodation may benefit three broad groups of patients:
- the 'old long-stay patients'
- the 'new long-stay patients'
- the community care generation.

The number of old long-stay patients is now small and non-existent in some districts. The healthcare system now includes a large group of patients who have responded to treatment, but have residual symptoms and require ongoing care and support, but do not have access to family or similar help. Historically these patients' care pathways would often have involved lengthy hospital admissions. However, in the current system, some of these patients may never have been psychiatric inpatients.

There is no clear method to determine the number of new long-stay patients or to assess the need for supported accommodation among the broader psychiatric population – the community care generation. An overall evaluation is also difficult due to the selection bias that tends to leave the most disturbed patients in the hospital setting. The literature contains few examples of systematic approaches to allocating special needs accommodation at a local level. Patient choice is a key issue in the selection of the type of supported accommodation, with a preference for independent accommodation that allows for privacy.

In order to carry out a meaningful assessment of a locality, an understudying of the total provision of hospital, hostel and supported accommodation should be attempted: levels of different forms of accommodation vary greatly and adequate levels of one form can to some extent compensate for deficiencies in others. It is important that homeless people are not overlooked.

The key issue is the support of the more challenging patients, who may have comorbid substance misuse and/or forensic problems. There is little evidence regarding staffed care homes of core and cluster accommodation. There is little evidence in the literature of differing effectiveness between the various forms of community provision, which is not surprising in a healthcare system where different units are perceived to cater for different types of patients and levels of challenging behaviour.

Lelliot P, Audini B, Knapp M et al 1996 Supported accommodation and main service providers. The mental health residential care study: classification of facilities and descriptions of residents. British Journal of Psychiatry 169: 139–147

Identified the following types of facilities:
- Long-stay wards: usually in large NHS hospitals
- High- and medium-staffed hostels (24-hour nursed-care units): provided variously – directly through the NHS, via the private and voluntary sectors and via the local authority social services departments
- Low-staffed hostels: mostly the private and voluntary sectors (a very few are run by local authority social services departments)
- Staffed care homes: the private and voluntary sectors, with some local authority social services departments
- Group homes: the voluntary sector and local authority social services departments
- Core and cluster/high dependency housing: mostly charitable organisations and housing associations.

Lamb HR 1998 Deinstitutionalistion at the beginning of the new millennium. Harvard Review of Psychiatry 6: 1–9

- The consequences of the loss in the USA of long-term institutions include an increase in rates of severe mental illness in homeless and prison populations.
- A high proportion of mentally ill people found in the criminal justice system resemble in most aspects those who used to be in long-term institutions.
- Lamb notes high rates of disturbance in the residual psychiatric hospital population, and suggests that present-day inpatients have not been 'institutionalised to passivity' by lengthy inpatient treatment.

Lelliot P, Audini B, Knapp M et al 1996 The mental health residential care study: classification of facilities and descriptions of residents. British Journal of Psychiatry 169: 139–147

- Local provision of services is highly varied and largely determined by historical patterns of development.
- Between 1954 and 1996, 110,000 psychiatric hospital beds were closed, with approximately 13,000 places in hostels and homes opened to replace them.

- Individuals who pose a high risk of violence tend to be excluded from community placement, leaving the most difficult patients in increasingly disturbed acute or long-stay NHS wards.

Strathdee G, Jenkins R 1996 Purchasing mental health care for primary care. In: Thornicroft G, Strathdee G (eds) Commissioning mental health services. HMSO, London

- There is no simple system to assess overall need in a locality and no generally recognised instrument to assess housing need at an individual level.

Shepherd G, Muijen M, Dean R et al 1996 Residential care in hospital and in the community – quality of care and quality of life. British Journal of Psychiatry 168: 448–456

- A detailed analysis of 25 residential units in London confirmed higher levels of psychopathology and dependency in hostel residents and rehabilitation patients in hospital than in residents of group homes.
- Also found that staffing ratios bore no relationship to the levels of dependency.

Fitz D, Evenson RC 1999 Recommending client residence: a comparison of the St Louis Inventory of Community Living Skills and global assessment. Psychiatric Rehabilitation Journal 23: 107–112

- The St Louis Inventory of Community Living Skills was developed to help clinicians in recommending residential settings appropriate for people with mental health problems.
- Community living skills, social skills and problem behaviour were primary characteristics affecting adjustment to residential settings.

Bartlett C, Holloway J, Evans M et al 2001 Alternatives to psychiatric in-patient care: a case by case survey of clinicians' judgements. Journal of Mental Health 10: 535–546

- Of the 730 acute admissions analysed, 35% of patients were found to have been inappropriately placed at some time.
- Many patients may have benefited from alternative, mostly community based, services.
- In 24% of cases divertible to community care it was considered that specialist accommodation supported by nurses or care workers would provide an effective alternative to acute hospital care.

Lelliot P, Wing JA 1994 A national audit of new long-stay psychiatric patients. II: Impact on services. British Journal of Psychiatry 165: 170–178

- A UK audit revealed an average point prevalence of 6.1 new long-stay patients per 100,000 population.

- Many English services had few long-stay psychiatric beds.
- 31% of new long-stay patients were housed on acute wards.
- Half the 47% of these patients who were thought to require a community placement remained on acute wards owing to a lack of available resources.

MILMIS Project Group 1995 Monitoring inner London mental illness services. Psychiatric Bulletin 19: 276–280

- Reported 'true' bed occupancy at 130%.

Murphy E 1992 The effects of NHS reorganisation on forensic psychiatric services. Journal of Forensic Psychiatry 3: 13–30

- Argued that the closure of psychiatric hospital beds has led to an increase in mental health problems dealt with in the prison system.

Brooke D, Taylor L, Gunn J et al 1996 The point prevalence of mental disorder in unconvicted male prisoners in England and Wales. British Medical Journal 313: 1524–1527

- Estimated that 880 men in England and Wales required transfer to hospital for psychiatric treatment.

Reed JL, Lyne M 2000 In-patient care of mentally ill people in prison. Results of a year's programme of semi-structured inspections. British Medical Journal 320: 1031–1034

- Patients wait an average of 11 months for transfer from prison to the hospital setting.

Ministry of Health 1962 The hospital for England and Wales. HMSO, London

- This began the hospital closure programme and promoted the development of acute units in general hospitals.

Department of Health and Social Security 1981 Care in the community. HMSO, London

- The responsibility for managing residential care was passed from regional health authorities to local authorities.

UK Government 1990 The NHS and Community Care Act 1990. The Stationery Office, London

- Enabled and encouraged non-statutory agencies to operate residential facilities.

Department of Health 1998 Partnerships in action – new opportunities for joint working between health and social services. A discussion document. The Stationery Office, London

- Promoted joint health and social services commissioning and 'cross-management' arrangements.

Department of the Environment, Transport and the Regions 2001 Supporting people – policy into practice. DETR, London

- Aims to provide housing-related support services to vulnerable people (including those with mental illnesses), robustly funded and planned using a coordinated multiagency approach.
- The advantage of this should be a greater ability to assess and plan for need at a local level assuming that there is sufficient local funding.
- Due to the pressures on overall provision it was proposed that more 24-hour nursed-care beds should be commissioned.

MacPherson R, Jerrom W 1999 Review of twenty-four hour nursed care. Advances in Psychiatric Treatment 5: 146–153

- 24-hour nursed care is associated with an improvement in social functioning, higher levels of social networks and a reduced level of negative symptoms in schizophrenia, but they do not typically affect positive symptoms.
- Most patients and relatives report a higher satisfaction with these units than hospitals; however, for others, stigma and restrictiveness can make this option less attractive.

Keck J 1990 Responding to consumer housing preferences: the Toledo experience. Psychosocial Rehabilitation Journal 13: 51–58

- This North American study showed that an approach which aimed to provide 'normal housing' together with practical assistance was largely effective and was associated with a dramatic decline in hospitalisation.

Nelson G, Brent Hall G, Walsh Bowen R 1997 A comparative evaluation of supportive apartments, group homes and board and care homes for psychiatric consumers/survivors. Journal of Community Psychiatry 25: 167–188

- A comparative evaluation in the US of residents of supported apartments, group homes, and board and care homes all had positive outcomes in terms of work and education.
- Residents in the group facilities reported that they experienced greater support and lower levels of abuse than those in other settings.
- Those in supported apartments and group homes spent less on rent and made more decisions about various aspects of their life.

Leff J 1997 Care in the community: illusion or reality? Wiley, London

Team for the Assessment of Psychiatric Services (TAPS)

- This study by Leff generated extensive evidence regarding the progress of long-stay hospital patients leaving Friern and Claybury hospital in North London.
- A 'funding dowry' was allocated to each discharged patient, who was carefully followed up and evaluated as they moved from long-term care to community care.
- Twelve months after discharge:
  - 49% of the patients were living in large hostels, residential homes or nursing homes
  - 15% were in community inpatient accommodation
  - 12% were living independently
  - 6% were in staffed group homes
  - 4% were in unstaffed group homes
  - the remainder were in sheltered housing or foster care.
- Compared with matched controls remaining in hospital, the community group had reduced negative symptoms, improved social functioning, increased social networks and greatly increased levels of satisfaction.
- There was no difference in positive symptoms, physical health status or rates of suicide and crime.
- Overall costs were slightly lower for the community group.

Shepherd G 1998 System failure? The problems of reductions in long stay beds in the UK. Epidemiology and Social Psychiatry 7: 127–134

- There is a need for a spectrum of solutions that include home-based intensive support and a range of hospital and community facilities, including properly funded 24-hour nursed care and assertive outreach teams.
- In order to meet the overall need for specialist accommodation in a population, it has been argued that a 'systems perspective' should be taken, the aim of which is to generate a 'well coordinated, clearly targeted and efficient system for delivering appropriate housing'.

Audit Commission 1994 Home alone: the housing aspects of community care. Audit Commission, London

- Budgeting for the needs of patients following psychiatric hospital closure was never really adequate.

Definition

New long-stay patients are patients who, despite modern treatment approaches and the ideology of community care, cannot be discharged from hospital, owing to their level of psychopathology, disability or behavioural disturbance. (*Source*: Mann S, Cree W 1976 New long stay patients: a national survey of 15 mental hospitals in England and Wales 1972/3. Psychological Medicine 6: 603–616.)

Supported housing for people with severe mental disorders

Chilvers R, Macdonald GM, Hayes AA 2002 Supported housing for people with severe mental disorders **(Cochrane Review)**. In: The Cochrane Library, Issue 4. CD000453. Update Software, Oxford

- Supported housing where people with severe mental illness are located within one site or building with assistance from professional workers may have benefits for patients who require a stable, supportive environment.
- Supported housing may foster dependence on professionals and lead to patients being excluded from local communities.
- No studies met the inclusion criteria.

Appendix I
Policy and legislation

Green Papers and White Papers

In Commonwealth countries 'White Paper' refers to a proposed policy issued by the government. In the UK they are also called 'Command Papers'. The White Paper may invite consultation and response, but does signal a clear intention from the government to legislate along the lines of the document.

A Green Paper tends to be issued in order to launch a consultation process and may not lead to legislation.

Parliamentary Acts and Bills

An Act of Parliament is a law enacted by the legislative body. Acts of Parliament often begin as White Papers which, if approved, are adopted in the form of a proposed law called a Bill. The Bill is then debated by parliament and may become law in the form of an Act.

Appendix 1

Policy and legislation

Appendix II
Guidelines

Chapter contents

NICE Guidelines: CLINICAL GUIDELINES

Definition NICE 2006

Clinical guidelines are recommendations on the appropriate treatment and care of people with specific diseases and conditions within the NHS in England and Wales.

Clinical guidelines are based on the best available evidence. Guidelines help healthcare professionals in their work, but they do not replace their knowledge and skills.

NICE Guidelines: Grades of recommendation

Grade	Source
A	At least one randomised controlled trial as part of a body of literature of overall good quality and consistency addressing the specific recommendation (evidence levels Ia and Ib) without explanation
B	Well conducted clinical studies but no randomised controlled trials on the topic of recommendation (evidence levels IIa, IIb, III), or without extrapolation from level I evidence

Grade	Source
C	Expert committee reports or opinions and/or clinical experiences of respected authorities. This grading indicates that directly applicable clinical studies of good quality are absent (evidence level IV), or without extrapolation from higher levels of evidence

NICE 2002: Recommendation drawn from the relevant NICE technology appraisal of that year

N	Evidence from NICE technology appraisal guidance

Good practice point

GPP	Recommended good practice based on the clinical evidence of the Guideline Development Group

NICE Guidelines: Key to evidence

Level	Type of evidence
Ia	Evidence obtained from a single large randomised trial or a meta-analysis of at least three randomised controlled trials
Ib	Evidence obtained from a small number of randomised controlled trials or a

Level	Type of evidence
	meta-analysis of less than three randomised controlled trials
IIa	Evidence obtained from at least one well-designed controlled study without randomisation
IIb	Evidence obtained from at least one other well-designed quasi-experimental study
III	Evidence obtained from well-designed non-experimental descriptive studies, e.g. comparative studies, correlation studies and case studies
IV	Evidence obtained from expert committee reports or opinions and/or clinical experiences of respected authorities

NICE guidelines: Technology Appraisals

Technology appraisals are recommendations on the use of new and existing medicines and treatment within the NHS in England and Wales, such as:

- medicines
- medical devices (e.g. hearing aids or inhalers)
- diagnostic techniques (tests used to identify diseases)
- surgical procedures (e.g. hernia repair)
- health promotion activities (e.g. ways of helping people with diabetes manage their condition).

SIGN Guidelines: Good Practice Points

✓ Recommended best practice based on the clinical experience of the Guideline Development Group

SIGN Guidelines: Grades of Recommendation

Note: The grade of recommendation relates to the strength of the evidence on which the recommendation is based. It does not reflect the clinical importance of the recommendation.

A At least one meta-analysis, systematic review of RCTS, or RCT rated as 1++ and directly applicable to the target population; or
A body of evidence consisting principally of studies rated as 1+, directly applicable to the target population, and demonstrating overall consistency of results

B A body of evidence including studies rated as 2++, directly applicable to the target population, and demonstrating overall consistency of results; or
Extrapolated evidence from studies rated as 1++ or 1+

C A body of evidence including studies rated as 2+, directly applicable to the target population and demonstrating overall consistency of results; or
Extrapolated evidence from studies rated as 2++

D Evidence level 3 or 4; or
Extrapolated evidence from studies rated as 2+

SIGN Guidelines: Key to evidence statements and grades of recommendation

Level	Type of evidence
1++	High quality meta-analyses, systematic reviews of randomised controlled trials (RCTs), or RCTs with a very low risk of bias
1+	Well conducted meta-analyses, systematic reviews of RCTs, or RCTs with a low risk of bias
1	Meta-analyses, systematic reviews of RCTs, or RCTs with a high risk of bias
2++	High quality systematic reviews of case control or cohort studies; or High quality case control or cohort studies with a very low risk of confounding or bias and a high probability that the relationship is causal
2+	Well-conducted case control or cohort studies with a low risk of confounding or bias and a moderate probability that the relationship is causal
2	Case control or cohort studies with a high risk of confounding or bias and a significant risk that the relationship is not causal
3	Non-analytic studies, e.g. case reports, case series
4	Expert opinion

Glossary of acronyms

A&E – Accident and Emergency

ACE – angiotensin-converting enzyme

ACT – assertive community treatment

ADD(H) – attention deficit disorder (hyperactivity)

ADHD – attention deficit hyperactivity disorder

ADL – activities of daily living

AHP – allied health professional

AIMS – Abnormal Involuntary Movement Scale

ALT – alanine aminotransferase

AMP – approved medical practitioner

ANH – artificial nutrition and hydration

ASBO – Antisocial Behaviour Order

ASD – autistic spectrum disorder

ASPD – antisocial personality disorder

AST – aspartate aminotransferase

AUDIT – Alcohol Use Disorders Identification Test

BAD – bipolar affective disorder (*see also* BPAD)

BDD – body dysmorphic disorder

BDI – Beck Depression Inventory

BDNF – brain drive neurotrophic factor

BMA – British Medical Association

BME – black and minority ethnic [communities]

BMI – body mass index

BNF – British National Formulary

BPAD – bipolar affective disorder (*see also* BAD)

BPRS – Brief Psychiatric Rating Scale

BPSD – behavioural and psychiatric symptoms of dementia

CAGE – Cut Down–Annoyed–Guilty–Eye opener [acronym formed from the italicised letters in the questionnaire]

CAMCOG – Cambridge Cognitive Capacity Scale

CAMDEX – Cambridge Examination for Mental Disorders in the Elderly

CAMHS – Child and Adolescent Mental Health Services

CAMI – chemical addiction and mental illness

CAN – Camberwell Assessment of Need

CANSAS – Camberwell Assessment of Need Short Appraisal Schedule

CAT – cognitive analytic therapy

CBT – cognitive behavioural therapy

CBT-BED – cognitive behavioural therapy for binge eating disorder

CBT-BN – cognitive behavioural therapy for bulimia nervosa

CCBT – computer-aided cognitive behavioural therapy

CCST – Certificate of Completion of Specialist Training

CCT – Certificate of Completion of Training

CDR – clinical dementia rating

CEMACH – Confidential Enquiry into Maternal and Child Health

CGI – Clinical Global Impression [scale]

CHD – coronary heart disease

CHI – Commission for Health Improvement

CHP – Community Health Partnerships

CHRS – Copenhagen High-Risk Study

CIDI – Composite International Diagnostic Interview

CMHT – community mental health team

COAMD – co-occurring addictive and mental disorders

COSMIC – Comorbidity of Substance Misuse and Mental Illness Collaborative

CPA – care programme approach

CPD – continuous personal development

CPN – community psychiatric nurse

CPR – cardiopulmonary resuscitation

CPRS – Comprehensive Psychopathological Rating Scale

CSA – child sexual abuse

CSF – cerebrospinal fluid

CSM – Committee on Safety of Medicines

CSQ – Client Satisfaction Questionnaire

CT – computed tomography

CTCH – cognitive therapy for command hallucination

CTO – community treatment order; compulsory treatment order

CVLT – Californian Verbal Learning Test

DAD – disability assessment for dementia

DBT – dialectical behaviour therapy

DC-LD – Diagnostic Criteria for Learning Disability

DDA – Disability Discrimination Act

DHA – docosahexaenoic acid
DLRF – Daily Living and Role Functioning [scale]
DBT – dialectical behaviour therapy
DSM-IV – Diagnostic and Statistical Manual, 4th edition
DSPD – dangerous and severely personality disordered
DVLA – Driver and Vehicle Licensing Agency
ECG – electrocardiogram
ECHR – European Convention on Human Rights
ECT – electroconvulsive therapy
EEG – electroencephalogram
EFA – essential fatty acid
EHRS – Edinburgh High-Risk Study
EMDR – eye movement desensitisation and reprocessing
EPA – eicosapentaenoic acid
EPDS – Edinburgh Postnatal Depression Scale
EPS – extrapyramidal symptoms
EPSE – extrapyramidal side effect
ERP – exposure response prevention
ESRS – Extrapyramidal Symptom Rating Scale
EWTD – European Working Time Directive
FAST – fast alcohol screening test
FBC – full blood count
FGA – first-generation antipsychotic
GABA – gamma-aminobutyric acid
GAD – generalised anxiety disorder
GAF – Global Assessment of Functioning
GAS – Global Assessment Scale
GDG – Guideline Development Group
GDS-LD – Glasgow Depression Scale for people with a learning disability
GGT – gamma-glutamyltransferase
GHQ – General Health Questionnaire
GnRH – gonadotrophin releasing hormone
GPP – good practice point
GSH – guided self-help
HAD – Hospital Anxiety Depression Scale
HAM-A – Hamilton Anxiety Rating Scale
HAM-D – Hamilton Depression Rating Scale (*see also* HRSD)
HCR-20 – Historical, Clinical, Risk-20
HDL – high density lipoprotein
HKD – hyperkinetic disorder
HoNOS – Health of the Nation Outcome Scales
HPA – hypothalamic–pituitary–adrenal [axis]
HRA98 – Human Rights Act 1998
HRSD – Hamilton Rating Scale for Depression (*see also* HAM-D)
IADL – Instrumental Activities of Daily Living [scale]
IBQ – Illness Behaviour Questionnaire

ICD – International Classification of Diseases
ICM – intensive case management
ICP – integrated care pathway
IES – Impact of Events Scale
ILS – immediate life support
IM – intramuscular
IMCA – independent mental capacity advocate
IPT – interpersonal therapy
IV – intravenous
LDL – low density lipoprotein
LEDS – Life Events and Difficulties Schedule
LHCC – Local Health Care Cooperative
MADRS – Montgomery–Asberg Depression Rating Scale
MAOI – monoamine oxidase inhibitor
MAPPA – multi-agency public protection arrangements
MAPPP – multi-agency public protection panel
MBU – mother and baby unit
MCI – mild cognitive impairment
MCMI – Millon Clinical Multiaxial Inventory
MCN – managed clinical network
MCV – mean corpuscular volume
MDI – Major Depression Inventory
MHA – Mental Health Act
MHO – mental health officer
MI – myocardial infarction
MICA – mental illness and chemical abuse
MMPI – Minnesota Multiphasic Personality Inventory
MMSE – Mini-Mental State Examination
MOAS – Modified Overt Aggression Scale
MRI – magnetic resonance imaging
MS – multiple sclerosis
MST – morphine sulphate tablets; multisystemic therapy
MSU – medium secure unit
NCCMH – National Collaborating Centre for Mental Health
NHS – National Health Service
NICE – National Institute for Health and Clinical Excellence
NIMHE – National Institu*te* for Mental Health in England
NINCDS–ADRDA – National Institute of Neurologic, Communicative Disorders and Stroke–AD and Related Disorders Association
NINDS–AIRENS – National Institute of Neurological Disorders and Stroke–Association Internationale pour la Recherche et l'Enseignement en Neurosciences
NMD – neurosurgery for mental disorder
NNH – number needed to harm
NNT – number needed to treat
NPI – neuropsychiatric inventory
NPMS – National Psychiatric Morbidity Survey

NP-SAD – National Programme of Substance Abuse Deaths

NRT – nicotine replacement therapy

NSAID – non-steroidal anti-inflammatory drug

NSF – National Service Framework

NTORS – National Treatment Outcome Research Study

OCD – obsessive–compulsive disorder

OLR – Order for Lifelong Restriction

PACE – personal assessment and crisis evaluation

PANSS – Positive and Negative Syndrome Scale

PAS – Premorbid Adjustment Scale

PAS-ADD – Psychiatric Assessment Schedule for Adults with Developmental Disability

PAT – Paddington alcohol test

PCG – primary care group

PCL-R – Psychopathy Check List-Revised

PEG – percutaneous endoscopic gastrostomy [feeding]

PET – positron emission tomography

PHP – partial hospitalisation programme

PIMS – Patient Information Management System

PLOA – Pan-London Assertive Outreach Study

PMETB – Postgraduate Medical Education and Training Board

PND – postnatal depression

POEM – patient-oriented evidence that matters

POVA – protection of vulnerable adults

PRC – potentially reversible cause

PRS – pervasive refusal syndrome

PSE – Present State Examination

PSMS – Personal Self Maintenance Scale

PSYRATS – Psychotic Symptom Rating Scale

PTSD – post-traumatic stress disorder

PVS – persistent vegetative state

QALY – quality adjusted life year

RAVLT – Rey Auditory Verbal Learning Test

RCA – root cause analysis

RCT – randomised controlled trial

RITA – record of in-training assessment

RLAI – risperidone long-acting injectable

RMO – resident medical officer

RRASOR – rapid risk assessment for sex offender recidivism

RRR – relative risk reduction

RSO – Relationship to Self and Others [scale]

RT – rapid tranquillisation

rTMS – repetitive transcranial magnetic stimulation

SAD – seasonal affective disorder

SAD-Q – Severity of Alcohol Dependence Questionnaire

SAD-S mania scale – Schedule for Affective Disorders and Schizophrenia (subscale Mania)

SANS – Scale for the Assessment of Negative Symptoms

SCID – Structured Clinical Interview for DMS-IV Axis I Disorders

SCM – standard case management

SDQ – Strengths and Difficulties Questionnaire

SGA – second-generation antipsychotic

SHAHRP – School Health and Alcohol Harm Reduction Programme

SIGN – Scottish Intercollegiate Guidelines Network

SIS – Suicide Intent Scale

SM – stress management

SMI – severe mental illness

SMR – standardised mortality ratio

SNRI – serotonin–norepinephrine reuptake inhibitor

SPAQ – Seasonal Pattern Assessment Questionnaire

SPC – Summary of Product Characteristics

SPECT – single photon emission controlled tomography

SSRI – selective serotonin reuptake inhibitor

SUDEP – sudden unexpected death in someone with epilepsy

Syst-Eur – Systolic Hypertension in Europe [study]

T-ACE – Tolerance–Annoyance, Cut down, Eye-opener

TAG – Threshold Assessment Grid

TAPS – Team for the Assessment of Psychiatric Services

TAU – treatment as usual

TCA – tricyclic antidepressant

TD – tardive dyskinesia

TFCBT – trauma-focused cognitive behavioural therapy

THIP – tetrahydroisoxazolopyridinne

TMS – transcranial magnetic stimulation

TRS – treatment-resistant schizophrenia

TSH – thyroid stimulating hormone

TWEAK – Tolerance, Worried, Eye-opener, Amnesia, Cut down (K)

U&Es – urea and electrolytes

UPA – underprivileged area score

VNS – vagus nerve stimulation

VRAG – violence risk appraisal guide

WMD – weighted mean difference

Y-BOCS – Yale–Brown Obsessive Compulsive Scale

YMRS – Young Mania Rating Scale

Index

Page numbers in *italics* refer to tables and boxes.